poultry
diseases

For Elsevier:
Commissioning Editor: Joyce Rodenhuis
Development Editor: Rita Demetriou-Swanwick
Project Manager: Gail Wright
Designer: Charles Gray
Illustration Manager: Merlyn Harvey
Illustrator: Hardlines Studio

poultry
diseases SIXTH EDITION

Edited by

Mark Pattison

Barbon, Carnforth
Cumbria, UK

Paul F. McMullin

Poultry Health Services Ltd, Poultry Health Centre
Thirsk, North Yorkshire, UK

Janet M. Bradbury

Department of Veterinary Pathology, University of Liverpool
Neston, UK

Dennis J. Alexander

VLA Weybridge, Department of Virology
Addlestone, Surrey, UK

Foreword by Professor Frank Jordan

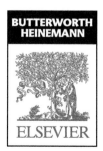

BUTTERWORTH
HEINEMANN

ELSEVIER

Edinburgh | London | New York | Oxford | Philadelphia | St Louis | Sydney | Toronto 2008

SAUNDERS
ELSEVIER

An imprint of Elsevier Limited

First published 1977
Second edition 1982
Third edition   1990
Fourth edition 1996
Fifth edition   2002
Sixth edition   2008

ISBN: 978-0-7020-2862-5

British Library Cataloguing in Publication Data
A catalogue record for this book is available from the British Library

Library of Congress Cataloging in Publication Data
A catalog record for this book is available from the Library of Congress

Notice
Knowledge and best practice in this field are constantly changing. As new research and experience broaden our knowledge, changes in practice, treatment and drug therapy may become necessary or appropriate. Readers are advised to check the most current information provided (i) on procedures featured or (ii) by the manufacturer of each product to be administered, to verify the recommended dose or formula, the method and duration of administration, and contraindications. It is the responsibility of the practitioner, relying on their own experience and knowledge of the patient, to make diagnoses, to determine dosages and the best treatment for each individual patient, and to take all appropriate safety precautions. To the fullest extent of the law, neither the Publisher nor the Authors assume any liability for any injury and/or damage to persons or property arising out or related to any use of the material contained in this book.

The Publisher

Printed and bound in the United Kingdom

Transferred to Digital Print 2010

ELSEVIER your source for books, journals and multimedia in the health sciences
www.elsevierhealth.com

Working together to grow libraries in developing countries

www.elsevier.com | www.bookaid.org | www.sabre.org

ELSEVIER   BOOK AID International   Sabre Foundation

The Publisher's policy is to use **paper manufactured from sustainable forests**

CONTENTS

Contributors   ix
Foreword   xiii
Preface   xv
Dedication   xvii

Section 1 General overview
Edited by Mark Pattison

1 The poultry industry   **2**
Steven Stenhouse

2 How to carry out a field investigation   **14**
Michael J. Alcorn

3 Laboratory investigation to support health programmes and
disease diagnosis   **39**
Chris Morrow

4 Biosecurity in poultry management   **48**
Stephen A. Lister

5 Vaccines and vaccination   **66**
Tibor Cserep

6 Medicines and medication   **82**
Paul F. McMullin

7 Legislation and poultry welfare   **94**
Sue Haslam

Section 2 Bacterial diseases
Edited by Janet M. Bradbury

8 *Enterobacteriaceae*   **110**
Stephen A. Lister, Paul Barrow

9 Infections caused by species of *Pasteurellaceae, Ornithobacterium* and
Riemerella: an introduction   **146**
Magne Bisgaard, A. Miki Bojesen, Jens P. Christensen

10 Fowl cholera   **149**
Jens P. Christensen, A. Miki Bojesen, Magne Bisgaard

11 Infectious coryza and related diseases   **155**
Par J. Blackall, Karl-Heinz Hinz

12 *Gallibacterium* infections and other avian *Pasteurellaceae* 160
A. Miki Bojesen, Jens P. Christensen, Magne Bisgaard

13 *Ornithobacterium rhinotracheale* 164
Paul van Empel

14 *Riemerella* infections 172
Magne Bisgaard, A. Miki Bojesen, Jens P. Christensen

15 Avian bordetellosis (turkey coryza) 176
Karl-Heinz Hinz

16 *Campylobacter* 181
Sarah Evans, Laura Powell

17 Staphylococci, streptococci and enterococci 191
Joan A. Smyth, Perpetua T. McNamee

18 Clostridia 200
Magne Kaldhusdal, Frank T. W. Jordan

19 *Erysipelothrix rhusiopathiae* – erysipelas 215
Frank T. W. Jordan, Magne Bisgaard

20 Avian mycoplasmas 220
Janet M. Bradbury, Chris Morrow

21 Avian chlamydophilosis (chlamydiosis/psittacosis/ornithosis) 235
Zerai Woldehiwet

22 Some other bacterial diseases 243
Frank T. W. Jordan, David J. Hampson

Section 3 Viral diseases
Edited by Dennis J. Alexander

23 *Herpesviridae* 258
Marek's disease virus
Venugopal Nair
Infectious laryngotracheitis
Richard C. Jones
Duck virus enteritis
Richard E. Gough

24 *Retroviridae* 276
Laurence N. Payne

25 *Paramyxoviridae* 294
Paramyxovirinae (Newcastle disease and other paramyxoviruses)
Dennis J. Alexander
Pneumovirinae
Richard C. Jones

26 *Orthomyxoviridae* – avian influenza 317
Dennis J. Alexander

27 *Poxviridae*   **333**
   Michael A. Skinner

28 *Coronaviridae*   **340**
   Jane K. A. Cook

29 *Picornaviridae*   **350**
   Richard E. Gough, M. Stewart McNulty

30 *Birnarviridae*   **359**
   Thierry van den Berg

31 *Adenoviridae*   **367**
   Joan A. Smyth, M. Stewart McNulty

32 *Reoviridae*   **382**
   Reoviruses
      M. Stewart McNulty, Richard C. Jones
   Rotaviruses
      Richard E. Gough, M. Stewart McNulty

33 *Astroviridae*   **392**
   Richard E. Gough, M. Stewart McNulty

34 *Circoviridae*   **398**
   Daniel Todd, M. Stewart McNulty

35 *Parvoviridae*   **405**
   Richard E. Gough

36 *Caliciviridae* and hepeviruses   **410**
   Richard E. Gough

37 Arthropod-borne viruses   **415**
   Ilaria Capua

Section 4 Fungal diseases
Edited by Paul F. McMullin

38 Fungal diseases   **428**
   Thomas Brown, Frank T. W. Jordan with Alisdair M. Wood

Section 5 Parasitic diseases
Edited by Paul F. McMullin

39 Parasitic diseases   **444**
   Alexander J. Trees

Section 6 Diseases of body systems
Edited by Mark Pattison

40 Diseases of the musculoskeletal system   **470**
   Barry H. Thorp

Contents

Section 7 Other diseases, poisons and toxins
Edited by Paul F. McMullin, Mark Pattison

41 Practical epidemiology of poultry disease and multifactorial conditions   **492**
   J.J. (Sjaak) de Wit

42 Nutritional disorders   **510**
   Patrick W. Garland, Steven Pritchard

43 Management as a cause of disease in poultry   **536**
   Chris Morrow

44 Toxicants in poultry   **548**
   Alan Shlosberg

45 Diseases of game birds   **560**
   Tom Pennycott

Appendix 1: Some useful data   **571**
   Frank T. W. Jordan, Paul F. McMullin

Index   **587**

CONTRIBUTORS

Michael J. Alcorn
St David's Poultry Team
Nutwell Estate
Lympstone
Devon, UK

Dennis J. Alexander
Department of Virology
Veterinary Laboratories Agency (Weybridge)
New Haw, Addlestone
Surrey, UK

Paul Barrow
School of Veterinary Medicine & Science
University of Nottingham
Sutton Bonnington
Leicestershire, UK

Magne Bisgaard
Department of Veterinary Pathobiology
Faculty of Life Sciences
University of Copenhagen
Frederiksberg
Denmark

Pat J. Blackall
Department of Primary Industries and
Fisheries
Animal Research Institute
Moorooka
Queensland, Australia

A. Miki Bojesen
Department of Veterinary Pathobiology
Faculty of Life Sciences
University of Copenhagen
Frederiksberg
Denmark

Janet M. Bradbury
Department of Veterinary Pathology
University of Liverpool
Leahurst, Neston
Cheshire, UK

Thomas Brown
Exploratory Drug Safety
Wyeth Research
Andover
Massachussetts, USA

Ilaria Capua
Virology Department
Istituto Zooprofilattico Sperimentale delle
    Venezie
Padova Legnaro
Italy

Jens P. Christensen
Department of Veterinary Pathobiology
Faculty of Life Sciences
University of Copenhagen
Frederiksberg
Denmark

Jane K.A. Cook
Huntingdon
Cambridgeshire, UK

Tibor Cserep
Intervet UK
Walton, Milton Keynes
Buckinghamshire, UK

J.J. (Sjaak) de Wit
GD, Animal Health Service
Deventer
The Netherlands

Sarah Evans
Centre for Epidemiology & Risk Analysis
Veterinary Laboratories Agency (Weybridge)
New Haw, Addlestone
Surrey, UK

Patrick Garland
Alpharma Animal Health
Garden Square
Laarstraat 16

B–2610 Antwerpen
Belgium

Richard E. Gough
Avian Virology
Veterinary Laboratories Agency (Weybridge)
New Haw, Addlestone
Surrey, UK

David J. Hampson
School of Veterinary & Biomedical Sciences
Murdoch University
Murdoch, Perth
Western Australia, Australia

Sue Haslam
Division of Farm Animal Science
School of Veterinary Science
University of Bristol
Langford, Bristol
UK

Karl-Heinz Hinz
Clinic for Poultry
University of Veterinary Medicine
   Hannover
Hannover
Germany

Richard C. Jones
Department of Veterinary Pathology
University of Liverpool
Leahurst, Neston
Cheshire, UK

Frank T.W. Jordan
Department of Veterinary Pathology
University of Liverpool
Leahurst, Neston
Cheshire, UK

Magne Kaldhusdal
National Veterinary Institute
Oslo
Norway

Stephen A. Lister
Crowshall Veterinary Services
Attleborough
Norfolk, UK

Paul F. McMullin
Poultry Health Services
Dalton, Thirsk
North Yorkshire, UK

Perpetua McNamee
Department of Agriculture & Rural
   Development
Omagh, Co. Tyrone
N. Ireland, UK

M. Stewart McNulty
Belfast
N. Ireland, UK

Chris Morrow
At the time of writing:
Aviagen Ltd
Newbridge, Midlothian
Scotland, UK

Currently:
Bioproperties Ltd
Ringwood, Victoria
Australia

Venugopal Nair
Viral Oncogenesis Group
Institute for Animal Health
   Compton
Berkshire, UK

Laurence N. Payne
Sutton Courtenay, Abingdon
Oxfordshire, UK

Tom Pennycott
Scottish Agricultural College Veterinary
   Services
Avian Health Unit
Auchincruive, Ayr
Scotland, UK

Laura F. Powell
Centre for Epidemiology & Risk Analysis
Veterinary Laboratories Agency
   (Weybridge)
New Haw, Addlestone
Surrey, UK

Steven Pritchard
Premier Nutrition
Rugeley
Staffordshire, UK

Alan Shlosberg
Department of Toxicology
Kimron Veterinary Insitute
Bet Dagan
Israel

Michael A. Skinner
Department of Virology
School of Medicine
Wright-Fleming Institute
Imperial College London
London
UK

Joan A. Smyth
Department of Pathobiology & Veterinary
    Science
University of Connecticut
Connecticut, USA

Steven Stenhouse
Aviagen Ltd
Newbridge
Midlothian
Scotland, UK

Barry H. Thorp
Aviagen Ltd
Newbridge, Midlothian
Scotland, UK

Daniel Todd
Agri-Food Biosciences Institute
Stormont
Belfast
N. Ireland, UK

Alexander J. Trees
Liverpool School of Tropical Medicine
University of Liverpool
Liverpool
UK

Thierry van den Berg
Avian Virology & Immunology Unit
Veterinary & Agrochemical Research Centre
    (VAR)
Brussels
Belgium

Paul van Empel
Bio-Manufacturing Support Department
Intervet International BV
Boxmeer
The Netherlands

Zerai Woldehiwet
Department of Veterinary Pathology
University of Liverpool
Leahurst, Neston
Cheshire, UK

Alisdair M. Wood
Veterinary Laboratories Agency (Lasswade)
Pentlands Science Park
Bush Loan, Penicuik
Midlothian
Scotland, UK

FOREWORD

The principal objective of those who have been involved in preparing this edition of *Poultry Diseases* continues to be to provide an up-to-date and concise account of the more common diseases of poultry and of the factors that are important in supporting optimal production.

The first edition was published under the editorship of the late Bob Gordon in 1977 and the regular production of new editions since that time is a reflection of the rapid changes and advances that have taken place in poultry production and in the understanding and control of disease. The use of molecular techniques for rapid diagnosis, for epidemiological tracing and for improved vaccine production is one of the factors that have accelerated the pace of these advances. In addition, greater attention is being given to zoonotic infections, to the advantage of the consumer. The benefits seen by the industry over recent years have been a marked increase in production performance and feed conversion throughout the world and, in many areas, a greater contribution to the quantity and quality of the human food supply. However, there are still challenges to be met. For example, problems have emerged in the control of certain diseases in some countries since the removal of effective drugs.

The editors and contributors to this book are active and renowned in their particular fields and have produced an updated edition that serves a highly useful purpose in providing the latest information on poultry disease and its control.

Frank Jordan

PREFACE

The purpose of *Poultry Diseases* is to provide a standard reference work on health and disease for those involved in the poultry industry.

This book includes information that is relevant to veterinary and agricultural students and their teachers, veterinarians in government and practice, and management staff involved in poultry companies. This is now the sixth edition of the book first edited by the visionary Dr R. F. Gordon in 1977. Its continued success has been a tribute to the zeal, tenacity and scientific standing of Professor Frank Jordan. This is the first edition where he has not been senior editor and the four of us are privileged to continue as his successors.

The poultry industry is very important to the world agricultural economy, and technological innovation has greatly improved the efficiency of poultry production, especially in relation to housing, nutrition, genetics and health management. Hence it was considered necessary to update the content of this book without fundamentally changing its format. For example, the chapter on avian influenza has been expanded and the welfare chapter has been extended to include the European situation. In the bacteriology section, the reclassification of organisms of '*Pasteurella* type' is brought up to date. The importance of biosecurity is now well understood by industry and governments and this is reflected by a complete revamp of the chapter on hygiene.

We would like to acknowledge the helpful suggestions and assistance of numerous colleagues in the production of this new edition.

Carnforth, Thirsk, Liverpool and Addlestone 2007

Mark Pattison
Paul F. McMullin
Janet M. Bradbury
Dennis J. Alexander

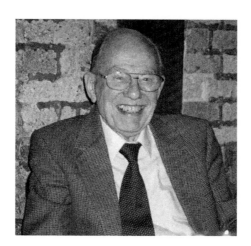

Dedication

This book is dedicated to **Professor Frank Jordan**,
editor of the third edition of *Poultry Diseases*
and co-editor of the second, fourth and fifth editions, and to his late wife,
Bella, who gave him a great deal of help and support.

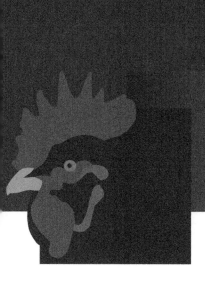

SECTION 1

Mark Pattison

GENERAL OVERVIEW

Chapter **1**   The poultry industry   **2**

Chapter **2**   How to carry out a field investigation   **14**

Chapter **3**   Laboratory investigation to support
health programmes and disease
diagnosis   **39**

Chapter **4**   Biosecurity in poultry management   **48**

Chapter **5**   Vaccines and vaccination   **66**

Chapter **6**   Medicines and medication   **82**

Chapter **7**   Legislation and poultry welfare   **94**

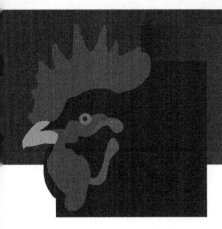

CHAPTER 1

Steven Stenhouse

The poultry industry

WORLD SCENE

In the last few years the poultry industry has faced a number of challenges, including the avian influenza outbreak in Asia that spread west throughout 2005 and early 2006. Despite this and other difficulties, poultry and eggs continue to be a hugely important source of animal protein, with poultry meat production, consumption and trade all increasing steadily since the late 1990s. Although the category of poultry covers many different species, including ducks, geese and ostriches, chicken and turkey are farmed for their meat much more than any other, with chicken alone accounting for over 85% of all poultry meat produced worldwide.

The continuing steady rise in human population, particularly in Asia has helped poultry meat and egg consumption increase consistently over the last few years. The rise in popularity of poultry meat can also be attributed to its versatility, relative low cost in comparison to other meats and the acceptability of poultry meat to all religions.

GLOBAL MEAT TRENDS

Worldwide, pork and poultry meat consumption grew steadily at the end of the 1990s and the beginning of the 21st century while beef and veal consumption remained relatively stable. Beef and veal production rose 5% in the first five years of the 21st century, while pork and poultry production both increased by 10%. In comparison to other meats, global demand for pork has remained steady for over 25 years. In this period of time, around 40% of all meat eaten has been pork and this level of demand is expected to remain for the foreseeable future at least. The biggest change in demand for meat in the last 25 years has been in poultry and beef. In 1980 beef was the second most favoured meat behind pork, almost twice as popular as poultry meat. Since then, the popularity of poultry meat has increased far beyond that of beef, with the result

Table 1.1 Worldwide meat production (million tonnes)

	2000	2001	2002	2003	2004	2005
Beef	50.3	49.6	51.2	50.1	51.3	52.0
Pork	81.8	83.6	86.5	88.9	90.7	92.5
Poultry	55.3	57.1	59.0	59.0	60.7	63.2

Source: United States Department of Agriculture, Foreign Agriculture Service.

Table 1.2 World poultry meat production (million tonnes)

	1994	1995	1996	1997	1998	1999	2000	2001	2002	2003	2004
World	50.9	54.7	56.4	59.8	62.4	65.4	69.2	72.0	74.6	76.4	78.2
Africa	2.2	2.4	2.5	2.7	2.8	2.9	3.1	3.3	3.4	3.4	3.5
North/Central America	15.9	16.7	17.5	18.2	18.6	19.7	20.3	20.9	21.5	21.8	22.4
South America	6.1	6.9	7.0	7.5	8.1	9.0	9.8	10.3	11.0	11.6	12.7
Asia	15.4	17.2	17.7	19.4	20.3	21.2	23.3	24.1	25.1	26.0	25.8
Europe	10.7	10.9	11.1	11.3	11.9	11.8	11.9	12.5	12.7	12.7	12.9
Oceania	0.6	0.6	0.6	0.7	0.7	0.8	0.8	0.8	0.8	0.9	0.9

Source: *Executive Guide to World Poultry Trends* (Watt Publishing).

being that poultry meat is clearly the second favourite choice globally behind pork, with a figure of 30%. The popularity of beef has slipped from 34% in 1980 to 26% in the year 2000 and this fall is expected to continue during this decade and into the 2010s.

The international meat trade continued to grow in the period 2000–05, with beef, pork and poultry meat imports all rising, albeit steadily in the case of beef and pork, with increases of 2% and 3% respectively (Table 1.1). Poultry meat imports rose by 12% in the same time, particularly to the developing African markets. Pork exports grew more quickly than other meats, up over 50% in 5 years, double the rate of both poultry and beef. The main exporters contributing to this were Brazil, China, Canada, the EU and the USA.

POULTRY MEAT PRODUCTION

Global poultry meat production has continued to rise steadily in the last decade. In 1995 the total amount of poultry meat produced was around 55 million tonnes, with the 2005 figure coming in at 45% more, over 80 million tonnes. The continents of North America and Asia account for over 60% of all poultry meat produced around the world. Europe has seen a steady rise year on year, while South America has seen output almost double in the same time. Fewer than 10 years ago, poultry meat production from the developed countries far outweighed that from their developing neighbours. Now however, the situation is reversed, with the developing nations accounting for around 55% of world poultry meat output (Table 1.2).

Chicken meat accounts for more than 86% of all poultry meat produced globally, with every region, Africa, North and Central America, South America, Asia, Europe and Oceania, showing steady growth in production throughout the 1990s and into the new century. In 2004, almost

3

4.7 billion chickens were slaughtered worldwide, 36% in Asia and 25% in North and Central America, the two largest producers of chicken meat. There are three major nations that contribute more than any others to the chicken meat industry, and they are the USA, China and Brazil. Between them, they account for half of total worldwide chicken meat production, amounting to over 33 million tonnes in 2004.

Turkey meat production accounts for just over 6% of global poultry meat production. Output increased steadily throughout the 1990s, reaching a peak of almost 5.5 million tonnes in 2002, before starting to decline. The main regions for turkey meat production are North and Central America and Europe, which account for 90% of the world total. On a country basis, almost half of all turkey meat produced comes from the USA, with France (13%), Germany (7%) and Italy (6%) being the other main contributors.

World duck meat production has increased consistently in the last 10 years, with a rise of around 70% in that time to the 2004 level of 3.25 million tonnes. Asia is the major producer, with over 80% of all duck meat originating from this region. China alone accounts for 60% of world production, with India, Vietnam and Thailand also relatively large contributors. Outside Asia, the largest producer is France, with around 8% of total production.

Goose meat accounts for less than 3% of all poultry meat output. Like other poultry meat, goose meat has seen a steady increase in production levels in recent years, with output in 2004 double that in 1994, at 2.13 million tonnes. China accounts for over 90% of all production, with only Hungary and Egypt producing significant volumes. Other poultry, such as guinea fowl and quail, are also farmed for meat in some countries but the quantities are extremely small.

POULTRY MEAT CONSUMPTION

Between 1992 and 2002, global poultry meat consumption per capita increased at a steady pace, rising 42% to the global average of 11.7 kg. In terms of tonnage, almost 56 million tonnes of broiler meat was consumed in 2005, 40% of which was eaten in China and the USA. Each individual region showed similar growth, with North and Central America up 25%, Europe and Africa both up 30% and Oceania's consumption increased by 36%. Just as in poultry meat production, the largest growth was seen in South America and Asia, with 76% and 73%, respectively. In the early part of the 21st century consumption dipped, mainly because of the outbreaks of avian influenza. Asia particularly suffered, with consumers reacting to the fact that humans could contract avian influenza and the related human deaths that occurred. As avian influenza moves further west towards Europe, consumption in other regions is likely to fall as there is a direct correlation between the proximity of avian influenza and consumption. For instance, consumption in Spain dropped only slightly when avian influenza was reported in Asia but during the outbreak in the Netherlands in 2003, consumption dropped dramatically. It is unlikely, however, that long-term consumption will be badly affected, unlike the huge decrease in beef consumption after the bovine spongiform encephalopathy (BSE) crisis in the 1990s. Evidence of this is backed up by looking at the examples of Thailand and Indonesia, both of which saw substantial drops in consumption following avian influenza outbreaks and related human deaths. Thailand's consumption dropped in 2003 and 2004 but is now on the increase despite higher domestic pricing. This increase in consumption is due to returning consumer confidence in product safety and the continuing competitiveness of poultry prices in comparison to beef and pork. In Indonesia, avian influenza-related human deaths in July 2005 caused consumption to drop 20% in a month but by August 2005 both poultry meat purchases and consumer confidence had began to increase. Consumers very quickly returned to their normal buying and eating habits and the decline was very brief and did not have a negative effect on annual consumption, which in fact increased by 2% from the previous year.

Turkey meat consumption remained fairly constant through the first 5 years of the 21st century, falling slightly from 2.56 million tonnes in 2001 to 2.51 million tonnes in 2005. Between them, the USA and EU consume around 85% of all turkey meat. Outside Europe and the Americas, turkey meat is only eaten in significant amounts in South Africa and Taiwan.

POULTRY MEAT TRADE

World trade in poultry meat has grown very quickly in the last 10 years (Fig. 1.1). In 1995, over 5 million tonnes of poultry meat was imported by all nations combined, rising to more than 9 million tonnes in 2003. This is an increase of more than 70%. Exports increased even more in the same period, going from 5.7 million tonnes to over 10 million, a rise of 75%. Europe is the largest importer of poultry meat (including trade between EU member countries), closely followed by Asia. These two regions account for over 80% of all imports. Europe is also the largest exporter, with 32% of all poultry meat exports worldwide originating from the region, although much of this is among fellow EU members, including the new additions to the EU. The Americas also export vast quantities, with half of all world exports coming from North, Central and South America. Asia also exports in substantial quantities, although trade was affected by the outbreaks of avian influenza in the region, with major exporters such as China and Thailand suffering large setbacks as import bans and tighter restrictions took effect. Exports in Asia are predicted to increase again (for these countries) as they switch to supplying cooked meat, which is not subject to the same regulations as fresh and chilled poultry meat.

The Russian Federation is by far the largest importer of broiler meat, with over 1 million tonnes brought into the country in 2003, which in itself was 200 000 tonnes less than was

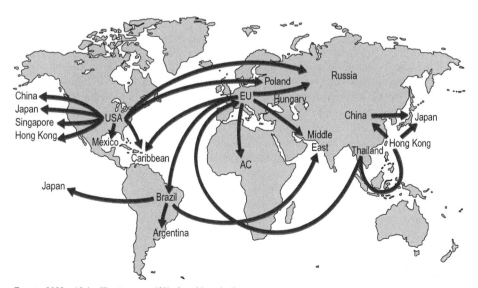

Exports 2003 – 10.1 million tonnes – 13% of world production

Fig. 1.1 Worldwide poultry meat trade.

imported in 2001. The other major importers of chicken meat are China, Japan, Saudi Arabia, Mexico and Hong Kong. Imports into the EU have risen considerably in the last few years as a result of the expansion of the EU. Broiler meat exports are dominated by two nations, Brazil and the USA, which together provide 75% of all exports. The USA has long been the largest exporter, dwarfing every other nation, but since 2000 Brazil has made remarkable improvements to its industry and overtaken its rival to become the largest exporter in 2005. Both nations have strengthened production and exports, responding to high demand within the domestic market and rising international prices. Brazil, however, has a number of advantages over the USA in terms of poultry production, with lower labour and feed costs and the falling value of the local currency. Although the US dollar has devalued recently, Brazil is widely regarded as having the lowest cost broiler production in the world, meaning that it is difficult for any nation to compete on price with Brazil. The other main exporters are the EU, China and Thailand, although the last two nations have suffered setbacks, as discussed earlier in this section.

Mexico is the world's largest importer of turkey meat, with more than 150 000 tonnes brought into the country in 2003. The Russian Federation was previously the largest importer but levels dropped by 30% in 2003. The other main importer of turkey meat is the EU, with much of this being among fellow members. As far as exports go, the USA and the EU lead the way with more than three-quarters of all turkey meat exports originating from these two areas. Brazil has greatly increased exports in recent years, making inroads into the dominant position of the other two areas. It is likely that this growth in Brazilian turkey meat exports will increase so that they will be the major exporting country before long.

Duck meat is mainly imported by Hong Kong, which purchased almost 60 000 tonnes in 2002. The other major importers are Germany and Japan. There is no dominant exporter of duck meat, with China, Hungary, Thailand, Hong Kong and France all exporting relatively substantial amounts.

There are a number of important poultry meat-producing countries and areas that are worthy of a closer look. Over 90% of all poultry meat produced comes from four geographical areas – North and Central America, South America, Asia and the EU – and it is useful to study the major nations in more detail.

USA

The USA is by far the world's largest chicken producer. In 2004 over 15 million tonnes of chicken meat was produced, 6 million tonnes more than China, the second largest producer. While production levels have increased over the last 10 years, the rate of growth has been much slower than that of the other countries in the top five. US production increased 25% between 1994 and 2004, compared with Brazil (108%), China (84%), Mexico (93%) and India (218%). When looking at total consumption within the USA, chicken meat is the most popular meat, followed closely by beef, with pork well behind in third place. Consumption of all meats is predicted to continue to rise in the next 10 years, with chicken meat consumption increasing at a faster rate than either of the alternatives. This is backed up by considering the predicted retail prices of the different meats for the next 10 years. Broiler meat is already 40% cheaper than pork and 60% cheaper than beef per kilogram. With broiler meat prices only expected to rise 5% in the next 10 years there seems to be little doubt which meat will prove to be the most popular in the foreseeable future. Americans eat more meat per capita than any other nation, with almost 123 kg per head consumed in 2005, made up of around 43 kg of beef and veal, 30 kg of beef and 50 kg of poultry.

After being the leading exporter of chicken meat for so long, the USA was overtaken by Brazil in 2005. Export levels had stagnated since the turn of the century and had actually fallen from the record high of 2.5 million tonnes in 2001 to 2.16 million tonnes in 2004. Export levels are expected to increase to keep pace with Brazil in the next few years. The Russian Federation is the largest importer of US chicken meat, with 30% of all US broiler meat ending up there, with Mexico and Canada also large export markets.

Mexico

Mexico is another country that has seen poultry production increase rapidly in the last 10 years, with output levels almost doubling to 2.2 million tonnes. Production is expected to continue to rise steadily in the next decade, and broiler output should top the 3 million tonne mark within this time. The Mexican poultry industry has become more concentrated and modernized in recent years, with more of an emphasis on integration. Domestic producers have struggled to cope with rising demand for chicken in the country and, as a result, import levels have grown to satisfy this increase. Imports have risen by 50% since the year 2000 to 350 000 tonnes, although, as domestic production levels improve, the increasing rate of imports will slow. Mexico is also the leading importer of turkey meat, with more than 150 000 tonnes brought in to the country in 2005, compared with only 14 000 tonnes produced domestically. Consumption of poultry meat has increased quickly in Mexico in recent times, going from 12 kg per person in the early 1990s to 27 kg in 2005. This rise has been driven by the increasing human population, the relative affordability of poultry meat against other meats, improvements in product quality and a sustained marketing campaign highlighting the benefits of poultry meat.

Brazil

Brazil is one of the most important nations in the poultry industry, behind only the USA and China in terms of poultry production (Fig. 1.2). The Brazilian poultry industry has really grown dramatically in the last 10 years, with production more than doubling in this time, from just

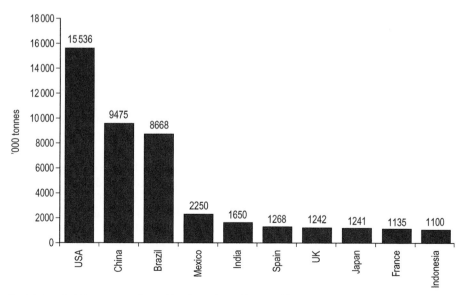

Fig. 1.2 Top 10 chicken meat producers 2004 (*Executive Guide to World Poultry Trends* (Watt Publishing)).

over 4 million tonnes in 1995 to 8.7 million tonnes in 2005. This growth is expected to continue in forthcoming years, albeit at a slower rate, with production predicted to reach 10.6 million tonnes in 2014, comfortably keeping Brazil in third place in the ranking, although still substantially behind the other two nations. Production levels have increased as demand for chicken domestically and internationally has risen. Consumption in Brazil is higher than ever before, with the average person consuming 33 kg per year. Exports have also helped to accelerate the growth of the Brazilian poultry industry, as producers have taken advantage of cheap labour, low feed costs and the falling value of the local currency to provide cheaper chicken meat than elsewhere in the world. Exports from Brazil were less than 900 000 tonnes at the start of the new millennium but within 5 years they had become the leading exporter of chicken meat, overtaking the USA, with more than 2.5 million tonnes. In 1995 domestic consumption accounted for almost 90% of Brazilian production but this figure had dropped to 70% in 2005 as the export market continues to grow, particularly to the lucrative markets in Europe, Saudi Arabia and Japan. Brazil has traditionally had high levels of beef production and consumption, with beef production almost double that of poultry and per capita consumption 20 kg more a decade ago. Poultry production is now level with that of beef and should increase at a greater rate in the near future. Consumption too has almost caught up with beef, with the average Brazilian now eating 33 kg of chicken and 35 kg of beef per year.

Asia

While the USA is the largest single producer of poultry meat, there can be no doubt that Asia produces more poultry meat than any other continent. China, India, Japan and Indonesia are all placed in the top 10 poultry meat producers list. Thailand too has in recent history been an important producer, although production levels have dropped in the last 2 years as the effects of avian influenza and increased barriers to export took effect.

The human population in Asia is expected to grow by more than 350 million in the next 10 years. As the population of North America is predicted to be around 350 million in 10 years' time, it is easy to see why Asia is considered to be a land of opportunity and great potential for many of those involved in the poultry industry, such as breeding companies.

Chicken meat consumption per capita in Asia is very low compared with the other major geographical areas. At present, average consumption per person per year in the region is around 7 kg, as opposed to 19 kg in Europe, 26 kg in South America and 40 kg in North America. The world average is around 12 kg per person. Consumption levels have dipped in the last 2 years in the region due to the avian influenza outbreaks, although levels are beginning to increase again. When the outbreaks first occurred, many people were put off by the few human fatalities from the disease but once it was realised that eating chicken meat didn't cause this, consumer confidence slowly started to return. Consumption is expected to return to and exceed that of the pre-avian-influenza period.

Total meat consumption in Asia is dominated by pork, mainly because of the vast quantities eaten in China. Forty-seven million tonnes of pork meat was consumed in China alone in 2004, dwarfing the 9.5 million tonnes of broiler meat and 7 million tones of beef consumed.

Although Asia is an important region, it is worthwhile looking more closely at some of the major nations within it, as this is where much of the future growth in the poultry meat industry will occur.

China

China is the second largest producer of poultry meat in the world, with output of over 10 million tonnes of chicken meat in 2005, a rise of 80% in 10 years. This rate of growth is expected to slow in the coming years, rising to around 13 million tonnes by 2013. The vast majority of production is used to satisfy demand from the domestic market, where consumption is currently 8 kg per person. While this is a relatively low amount in comparison to other major nations around the world, the huge population of China (1.33 billion, expected to rise to 1.37 billion in 2010) means that even a rise in consumption of 100 g per person would result in production or import levels rising considerably. The processed broiler meat sector in China is expanding quite quickly because of major investment and the increased demand for processed meat and ready meals. This increase in demand has come from those living in the large and medium-sized cities in China, who have seen income levels rise because of a property boom and increases in manufacturing.

As well as being one of the largest producers of chicken meat, China is also one of the largest importers and exporters. Only the Russian Federation and Japan import more, while only four countries (Brazil, USA, the EU and Thailand) export greater quantities. Japan is the largest market for Chinese exports, accounting for over half of all the chicken leaving China. The bulk of China's imports come from the USA, which is the only country able to sell poultry meat products for direct consumption in China's retail sector. The avian influenza outbreaks in Asia have affected exports, with levels down almost 50% since 2002. In order to regain consumer confidence both domestically and internationally, the Chinese poultry industry has implemented a range of new measures and regulations, including the adoption of new disease control methods and safety standards, as well as new drug usage rules.

Thailand

Thailand was one of the major poultry-producing nations through the 20th and into the 21st century but production levels dropped dramatically in 2004 because of the avian influenza outbreaks. In 2003 the country was ranked seventh in the list of chicken meat producers with more than 1.2 million tonnes, yet only a year later they had slipped to 16th, with production slashed by a quarter to less than 900 000 tonnes. Most other nations managed to either increase or maintain production, compounding the slip in rankings. Production of broiler meat in Thailand is export-driven as some 30% of total production has traditionally been sold internationally, especially to the EU and Japan. With many of Thailand's export customers restricting imports, exports fell 60% in 2004 to 215 000 tonnes. In order to avoid some of these restrictions, Thai producers began to export cooked meat, which was not subject to the same barriers as fresh or chilled poultry. Many Thai producers invested in new equipment that allowed them to shift production from fresh to cooked meat. This investment has not proved as successful as anticipated, with demand for cooked meat much lower than predicted. Exports are expected to increase, but it will take a number of years for them to reach pre-avian-influenza levels and it could prove a very difficult few years for many Thai broiler producers. The effects of avian influenza were also seen in domestic consumption levels, with consumption per capita falling from 14 kg in 2002 to 8.4 kg in 2004. Pork has regained its position as the most popular meat in Thailand, although in the next few years demand for chicken meat should return to and indeed overtake previous levels and become the number one choice again.

India

India has in the last decade come from relative obscurity to become the fifth largest poultry producer in the world. Production levels have increased substantially in this time, rising over 200% to 1.65 million tonnes in 2004. All the chicken meat produced in India is for domestic consumption, which has doubled in the last 10 years. Meat consumption is still very low, with only 3 kg of meat per person per year being eaten, 1.5 kg of both chicken meat and beef. There is huge potential for growth in poultry production in India, as the human population has continued to grow quickly and is expected to reach almost 1.2 billion by 2010, a rise of around 10% in 10 years. Like China, if income levels increase, even slightly, then demand will increase and production levels will need to expand to cope. India will be an important country in the poultry industry in the years to come.

Europe

Europe was traditionally the third largest poultry-producing region behind Asia and North America but in the last decade relatively slow growth has seen South America overtake it in overall production. Poultry meat production increased by 15% in Europe in that time whereas the rate of growth in South America was 110%. At the end of the 1990s, poultry meat production in the EU was at record levels, with over 9 million tonnes produced in 1999. Production levels suffered a setback in 2003 with the outbreak of avian influenza in the Netherlands, before climbing back above 9 million tonnes the following year. The rise in poultry meat production was due to an increase in chicken meat production, which reached a record high in 2001 before falling and then picking up again. Turkey meat also reached record production levels in the same year before falling but, unlike chicken, was unable to pick up, finishing 2004 12% down on 2001 figures.

The early part of the 21st century was a period of slow growth for the EU poultry industry. Only Germany and Spain saw any real growth in production, increasing 46% and 35% in total. Of the other major producers, only the UK showed any growth at all, 4%, with France falling 14%, the Netherlands down 8% and Italy down 6%. Outside Germany and Spain, the main growth areas were in eastern Europe, where production levels in Hungary, Poland, Romania, the Russian Federation and Ukraine steadily increased.

At the beginning of 2006, consumer concern over avian influenza lowered poultry meat consumption in the EU. Prior to this, consumption had remained relatively stable in the EU, at 23 kg per capita, 4 kg more than the European average. This was an increase of over 20% in less than 10 years. Pork remains the most consumed meat in the EU, with over 16 million tonnes eaten in 2004, more than double that of beef and almost two and a half times more than chicken.

EGG PRODUCTION

Global egg production has increased consistently in the last 10 years, rising over 40% since 1994, from 41 million tonnes to almost 58 million tonnes in 2004. The number of layers has also increased substantially in this time, up more than 30% to 5435 million birds. Egg production is dominated by Asia, with more than 60% of all production coming from the region – 35 million tonnes in 2004. It is a similar picture in terms of layer numbers, with the region accounting for 60% of world layers, or 3300 million birds.

It is interesting to note a study carried out by Dr Hans-Wilhelm Windhorst, Director of the Institute of Spatial Analysis and Planning at the University of Vechta in Germany. He looked at the 10 leading egg-producing countries between 1974 and 2004 and discovered interesting regional changes (Table 1.3). The change in egg production has been quite dramatic in the last 30 years. The USA produced almost three times as many eggs as China in 1970 yet by 2004 China was responsible for 42% of all global egg production (almost four times the current US figure). The ranking also proves the dominance of Asia, with the five countries in the top 10 producing

Table 1.3	Egg production rankings		
RANKING	**1974**	**1994**	**2004**
1	USA	China	China
2	USSR	USA	USA
3	Japan	Japan	Japan
4	China	Brazil	Russian Federation
5	Germany	India	Mexico
6	UK	Mexico	India
7	France	Germany	Brazil
8	Italy	France	France
9	Spain	Italy	Indonesia
10	Poland	Spain	Turkey

Source: *Poultry International* (Watt Publishing).

50% of the world total. The EU has also seen a huge change in fortunes in the last 30 years. In 1974 five countries were ranked in the top 10, now only France remains. The one positive note for European producers, however, is that, although layer numbers have decreased significantly in the last 10 years, egg production has actually increased slightly, proving how much bird performance has improved during this time.

The potential for the poultry industry in China is huge. With the current population of 1.33 billion people, which is expected to increase by over 40 million by 2010 and improving economic growth, more people will be able to afford to eat better. As a result they will consume more meat and eggs in their diet, increasing the size of the market, not just in China but globally as well.

Although Asian egg production has increased at a remarkable rate in the last decade, most other regions have shown much slower growth, or, in the case of Oceania, no growth at all. Layer numbers have risen in all regions in the same period, with the exception of Europe, with Asia obviously showing the largest increase – up more than 50%. African numbers have increased 30%, North and Central America by 20%, South America by 13% and Oceania by 10%.

EGG CONSUMPTION

Consumer demand for protein is in line with economic development. As income increases, people look to supplement their grain-based diet with protein foods such as eggs. When income increases further, they will then demand processed meat and convenience foods. As a result of this it can be difficult to increase egg consumption in developed countries, which is why the main regions of growth in consumption can be found in Asia, where incomes in the main are nowhere near the levels in regions such as North America, Europe and Oceania.

The global average consumption of eggs per person per year in 2004 was 8.4 kg. Consumption has risen slowly in the last decade, in no small part as a result of the situation in Asia, where consumption levels have increased by almost 50%. This huge rise was balanced by little or no growth in Europe and Africa and declines in South America and Oceania. Consumption in North and Central America stagnated in the early to mid 1990s but has recovered well, showing year-on-year growth since 1997.

EGG TRADE

Europe has traditionally dominated world trade in shell eggs, with Asia in second place. Between them, the two regions account for almost 90% of all shell egg imports and over 90% of all exports. Europe alone is responsible for 63% of all imported shell eggs, with the Netherlands, Belgium, Germany and France accounting for the bulk of these purchases. Asia has seen exports almost treble since 1990 while Europe's exports have fallen slightly in the same period. World shell egg trade showed slight year-on-year growth in the early years of the 21st century, with exports reaching the million tonne mark for the first time in 2003 and imports doing likewise the year after.

THE ROLE OF BREEDING COMPANIES

Through a series of mergers and acquisitions in the 1990s, the number of broiler breeding companies supplying grandparent and parent stock decreased from around 15 to only three or four main companies with the ability to provide stock to international markets. In the main, these companies are moving towards offering a range of products to suit all markets, with particular attention being focused on the high-yield sector.

Breeding companies often supply stock into markets either directly as parent stock or through supplying grandparent stock to a series of distributors. This grandparent stock originates from pure line programmes run by the breeding companies. To ensure consistent progress and development of their pure lines, genetic selection is used. Selection programmes are becoming more and more sophisticated, with new techniques and technology such as X-rays and ultrasound being developed to aid selection in all traits. In the past, selection was made to enhance progress in conventional areas such as live weight, meat yield and egg numbers but with these new methods it is now possible to select for traits such as skeletal strength, disease resistance and heart and lung fitness. The latest selection technique to be developed is in the field of genomics, where it is possible to identify specific genetic markers in chicken DNA that correspond to particular traits.

It is important in any poultry facility that biosecurity is looked upon as vital but in pedigree stock it is critical that the highest possible standards of biosecurity are maintained, to prevent any possible contamination of birds. Breeding companies have a duty to ensure that the high standards of biosecurity demanded by the poultry industry are maintained in order to prevent the possibility of vertically transmitted diseases and pathogens such as *Salmonella* infecting flocks. With avian influenza now being at the forefront of governmental policy and public thought, it is even more important than ever that extensive testing of pedigree and grandparent stock is carried out by the breeding companies and their distributors to meet tighter export controls.

THE ROLE OF THE VETERINARIAN

The veterinary needs of the poultry industry are mostly met by veterinarians who are poultry specialists. Many of the veterinary inputs are key to the successful running of the poultry industry and are tied in with needs that can be legislative or relate to inspection, auditing or accreditation, for example: supply of prescription-only medicines, poultry meat inspection, health certification for export, welfare inspections, compliance with animal by-products orders. Private veterinarians work closely with and within poultry companies to deal with poultry health and welfare, and health planning. Pharmaceutical companies employ poultry veterinarians in support of their products.

There are now far fewer, but larger, poultry companies. This has tended to result in the alignment of some poultry vets with only one or with only a very limited number of poultry companies. Some companies employ their own full-time veterinarian; other companies keep a private veterinary practitioner employed virtually full-time. The geographical spread of many companies means that different veterinarians may be responsible for the health of poultry in different parts of the country. Indeed, some poultry veterinarians spend a lot of time travelling to clients, who may also be in other countries, in which case there is likely to be a senior veterinarian or company employee who coordinates the veterinary inputs and health programmes. Many companies see the veterinarian as having a major role in advising on standards of biosecurity, health status, welfare issues and product quality. These veterinarians are also vital to the investigation of health and production issues and are likely to work closely with production managers, quality control managers and senior management.

Government veterinarians are key to the control of health status in imported and exported poultry stock. They also manage the quarantine process, both from a biosecurity point of view and also by checking that certification is correct. Where an outbreak of a notifiable disease is suspected, such as avian influenza or Newcastle disease, government veterinarians are central to the control and eradication process. All poultry meat goes through an inspection process to ensure that only suitable meat 'fit for human consumption' is supplied to the consumer. This inspection is also the responsibility of specialist state veterinarians.

The investigation of diseases in poultry, unlike most other livestock, is usually based on postmortem examination and often followed up with histopathology, plus other specialist laboratory methods such as bacteriology, virology and serology. Most poultry companies and management systems generate a great deal of routine data. This is likely to include: mortality, production records, condemnations at the processing plant, feed consumption, water consumption, plus routine records of vaccination and the timing of management practices. The analysis of these records is often a key part of health monitoring and any disease investigation. Within the government veterinary organization there are a few veterinary pathologists who have specialized in poultry pathology. These people provide an invaluable referral service enabling the diagnosis of many diseases.

REFERENCES

All the data used in this chapter are available online and are constantly being updated. The sources that were used are:

USDA Foreign Agriculture Service: www.fas.usda.gov

Watt Poultry Executive Guide to World Poultry Trends

Food and Agricultural Policy Research Institute (FAPRI): www.fapri.org

Poultry World – EU Facts and Forecasts 2005

The European Union Online: www.europa.eu.int/

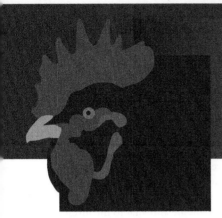

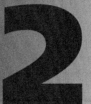

CHAPTER 2

Michael J. Alcorn

How to carry out a field investigation

There is no single 'fits all' protocol for the investigation of disease and production problems in different classes of poultry. The approach taken will depend on the type of flock involved, the nature of the problem and the experience of the person investigating it. In many cases the investigation will stem from the way in which the problem is presented. Often this takes the form of submission of dead or ill birds for laboratory examination. However, in other cases the starting point will be a request to visit the site where the problem is happening, or presentation of information in written or verbal form describing an abnormality.

It is not the intention of this chapter to provide exhaustive lists of differential diagnoses, nor to describe in detail how individual diseases may be diagnosed. Such information is covered by other sections of this book. The intention is to provide broad strategies that may be used to ensure that an investigation has as good a chance as possible of getting to the cause of a problem.

The chapter should be read in conjunction with Chapter 3, which provides an overview of the different laboratory tests available to assist in this process. The diagnosis of poultry problems today is perhaps not the straightforward business involving an infective agent that it was in the early days of the industry. Problems are now often multifactorial in nature, with nutritional, environmental, managemental and genetic undercurrents. Approaches to the use of epidemiological techniques in investigating such problems are described in Chapter 41. Frequently the ill-defined origins of the low-grade but economically important problems may tax or defy the investigator (e.g. a 5% drop in production, shell quality faults, falls in hatchability, leg weakness syndromes or loss of performance). Such problems are frequently more difficult to cope with than classic diseases of an acute or chronic nature involving diagnostic signs, mortality and morbidity.

Basically, there are two categories of problem investigation:

- The relatively straightforward diagnosis of some classical pathological condition. Often this follows a post-mortem or other laboratory test. Here there is often also a specific treatment. Examples of such conditions are coccidiosis, pasteurellosis and red mite infestation

- The 'in-depth' investigation, either to find the underlying cause of an infectious problem or to attempt to define and delineate a more vague, possibly multifactorial condition and determine its origins and remedy.

The development of, and adherence to, standard investigative routines for different problem types will provide the best chance of defining the cause of a problem. Whatever the problem, this type of routine is likely to make use of the following components.

DEFINE THE PROBLEM

Problems generally involve a departure of any measurable parameter from normal. This may refer to anything from mortality numbers to the colour of pigment of a shell. It is therefore essential that the investigator has a clear idea of what the norm is expected to be for the particular type of flock or process being dealt with. In a few cases the problem may simply be an unrealistic expectation of what normal should be.

There is considerable variation in the expected performance for different types of poultry in different management situations. To some extent there can be no substitute for experience in determining the subtleties of this. However, there is much published information that is of value, in particular with regard to the established commercial hybrids that compose the majority of industrial production. Here the breeding companies that produce these strains will publish and regularly update targets for the various aspects of production. These companies are generally happy to provide copies of their publications and often have technical staff who have great experience in how their birds will perform under differing management conditions. Examples of such information are given in Figure 2.1, which clearly illustrates the contrast in egg production numbers and persistence for a modern layer bird, broiler breeder and turkey breeder.

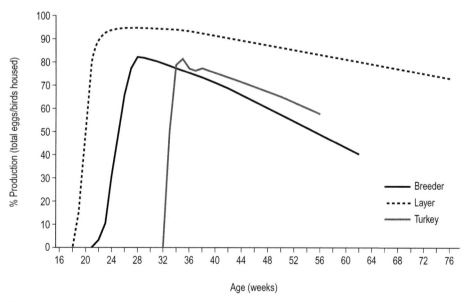

Fig. 2.1 Production figures for different laying flocks.

Similarly, for meat production birds there is generally information relating to expected liveweight gain, feed conversion efficiencies and expected mortality for different ages of bird. However, a rule of thumb is that, for a well-managed flock, first-week mortality should not exceed 1–1.5% and thereafter should never exceed 0.1% on a daily basis. For commercial turkeys, first-week figures may be slightly higher. However, having passed that stage *any* rise in mortality is usually significant.

ESTABLISH THE HISTORY

This is probably the most critical step of the initial investigation into the problem. The clinician should aim to develop a mental or preferably physical checklist for each category of problem. This series of questions should be methodically checked off in every case investigated. In some cases the investigator may be able to fill in answers if familiar with the management practices of the problem farm. However, it is good practice to reinforce ideas by questioning the farmer or fieldsperson involved.

A list of key history points for different types of poultry is given below. While not exhaustive, it should provide a useful basis, which may be modified to suit individual circumstances.

Fattening birds

- Site identification details
- Age (this is a critical piece of information as many problems in fattening birds are strongly age-related)
- Age range on site (critically, is the farm a single or multi-age unit?)
- Number of birds involved and number on the farm (Are all the birds on farm affected or only a subgroup? Often one shed or pen is affected, at least initially)
- Nature of the problem:
  - If mortality is the problem, I collect mortality numbers from the affected group for the previous 5 days and request weekly percentage figures for the period prior to that. Additionally, a subjective impression of the number of sick birds should be sought. A brief description of the signs of illness shown is requested. The last two points are relevant if the flock is showing abnormalities without increased mortality
  - If the complaint reflects a production-related matter such as poor growth or unevenness, a brief indication of the extent and spread of the problem is sought (e.g. How far are they behind target weight? Are all the birds affected?)
- Vaccination/medication history of the flock
- Any previous problems with the flock
- Anything unusual/change in management/what does the farmer think?

Breeding birds

The information sought for fattening stock is relevant. In addition, this category of bird has the capacity to provide problems with egg production and hatchability. The latter may be presented as a hatchery problem. Often the investigator is introduced to the problem by a phrase such as 'failure to attain peak production' or 'a 5% production drop'. In most cases some further enquiry is necessary to fully understand the problem. Often this is best achieved by asking to see a graphical plot of the flock's production or hatchability against the standard normally expected for that breed.

Layer birds

With the exception of hatchability, production-related problems follow a similar pattern to breeders, although the absolute numbers of eggs involved tend to be greater. In laying stock, alterations to the physical appearance of the eggs have a particular significance.

Hatchery

The hatchery provides a testing environment for the investigation of problems. The difference between acceptable performance and disaster can be very subtle. The mechanical systems and procedures involved can be very complex and require specialist knowledge. The key area to define initially is whether a problem involves all or several of the flocks being handled – which suggests a hatchery-based problem. Alternatively, a problem related to a single flock would lead the investigator to suspect a farm-based cause. The issues relating to investigation of a hatchery problem are discussed in more detail later in the chapter.

INVESTIGATION

Collection of a comprehensive history in many cases can lead the investigator to a very narrow spectrum of potential causes. In some cases there may already be a 'prime suspect'. As mentioned earlier, many poultry diseases are strongly age-associated and this often provides a useful narrowing of the list of differential diagnoses.

Where the investigation is laboratory-based, it generally starts with the examination of submitted post-mortem samples.

Often the investigator must examine whatever post-mortem material is submitted. However, it is important to be aware that the sample selection process may have a bearing on the investigator's impression of the flock problem – a wrong impression of a situation may be gained from necropsies carried out on improperly selected specimens, especially if the flock is not seen. Sometimes site managers pick out a few of the 'worst' birds they can find and some of the 'best' birds, neither of which may be typical of the current problem. A few each of dead birds, live ailing birds showing typical clinical signs and sometimes apparently normal birds may be examined in order to obtain a true picture. The owner may badly skew a sample by poor selection (e.g. by removal of birds with conditions s/he recognizes) or by killing sick birds. Culled birds may not be representative of the overall picture.

Where mortality is the problem, fresh, naturally dead material should be examined; if morbidity is the problem, then carefully chosen, live, morbid birds are more representative of what is happening. Usually submission of 8–12 birds represents a good initial balance between the wish to be as comprehensive in examination as possible and the need to limit the time spent per case. It should be borne in mind that additional samples can usually be procured on request.

Killing birds for post-mortem examination

It is important that the investigator is able to kill birds quickly and humanely. The following methods may be employed.

Dislocating the neck

Small or medium-sized birds may be killed in this way but the method is not adequate when the brain is to be examined histologically, as congestion of cerebral vessels ensues. The left hand holds the legs or, alternatively, the base of the wings together over the back, while the right hand grasps the head with the palm against the back of the bird's head, resting in the hollow formed by joining the forefinger and thumb. The head is bent vertically upwards by the thumb under the beak, while at the same time, the head is pulled firmly and steadily forward, stretching the neck, dislocating the skull from the neck and breaking the cord. Stretching must stop as separation is felt (or the head will be pulled off the body); there will be a violent reflex movement of the limbs for a while, during which time the base of the wings should be held or the bird should be placed in a container.

In very young birds the neck may be suitably dislocated by pressure with the thumb against a sharp edge (e.g. of a table), alternatively, by placing the neck between the two shafts of the handle end of a large pair of scissors which are then fully closed.

Large chickens, turkeys and ducks may be similarly dealt with using a Burdizzo forceps.

Injection euthanasia

Pentobarbital solution or some other suitable anaesthetic agent may be injected intravenously, or by the intracardiac, intrathoracic or intraperitoneal routes.

Inhalation euthanasia

Avian species are very susceptible to chloroform, which may conveniently be placed on a thick cottonwool pad at the bottom of a narrow jar; the bird's head is then placed in the mouth of the jar. Care should be taken to allow air to enter the jar (i.e. the bird is anaesthetized and not suffocated) and not to allow the liquid chloroform to fall on to the eye. Death soon follows anaesthesia. This method may be suitable when histological examination of brain tissue is to be carried out.

Post-mortem examination procedures: general

There is no single method for carrying out this procedure and descriptions can be found in various texts. A suggested methodology is described here. However, many equally valid methods exist. What is important is selecting a method that ensures that no system is overlooked. Thereafter follow the same procedure each time. It is preferable to be able to lay out several carcasses for examination at one time. This will allow, for example, an in-depth examination of the initial carcasses to be followed by a more cursory check of subsequent ones where all appear to have a similar condition. Alternatively, it is possible to refer to the initial samples if something becomes apparent later in the procedure and recheck in the light of this. Notes should be made while the birds are still on the table.

Blood sampling procedure

Blood samples are often taken prior to killing and submitted for laboratory examination. Blood is commonly required for serological examination but may also be needed for estimation of cell counts, haemoglobin levels, chemical analysis, microscopic examination or culture.

Blood sampling (for whole blood or plasma) in the fowl may be aided considerably by using heparin solution, whereby a small amount is sucked up into the needle before starting to draw blood. If heparin solution is used, the cells will rapidly settle out and clear plasma is obtained.

When serum samples are required, ready separation of the clot and serum may be ensured by warming the sample after collection. In the field, a polystyrene box with either plastic bags or hot-water bottles will ensure an adequate temperature. Tubes that are turned upside down will cause the clot to adhere to the bung, facilitating aspiration of the serum. If tubes are three-quarters filled and placed on their sides, a larger surface area of sample is available, which increases serum yield.

Intravenous technique

The brachial (wing) vein is usually used. The vein is exposed by plucking a few feathers from the ventral surface of the humeral region. The vein will be seen lying in the depression between the biceps and triceps muscles. Alcohol or saline on the skin facilitates visualization. The needle should be inserted opposite to the direction of blood flow. The wing should be extended and a 19 (metric 1.10) gauge, 19 mm needle used. Passing the needle beneath the wing tendon may facilitate puncture without damage but a haematoma may readily form, obliterating the vein. Excessive suction should not be used or the vein will collapse. A small plug of air (e.g. 0.2 mL) taken into the syringe prior to sampling acts as a pressure buffer, helping to avoid vein collapse. For simple tests, such as for pullorum disease, the brachial vein is punctured with a sharp needle and the blood is collected in a suitable tube.

The jugular vein may also be used. The bird is restrained, beneath the left arm in a right-handed individual, with the head foremost and supported on the raised knee. The neck is held in the left hand with the index finger holding back the mass of neck feathers, some of which may need to be plucked from the vein path. The vein should be stabilized by digital pressure from below. The needle is inserted either with or against the direction of blood flow. The right jugular has a larger diameter than the left and is therefore usually used.

Cardiac puncture may be the method of choice where larger volumes of blood are required. Specimens may be taken when a bird has been killed just prior to post-mortem examination (i.e. when the heart is exposed and is still beating). In live birds the following methods can be used, however to do so without anaesthesia is contrary to welfare principles.

The live bird is placed on its side with the left side facing the operator. A 20/22 (metric 0.9–0.7) gauge needle is used. The site for insertion of the needle is determined by drawing a line at right angles to the keel, at the anterior point of the keel, to the space between the first two ribs. Here the heart may be felt beating and the needle is directed towards the anterior point of the keel.

Alternatively, the bird may be placed upside down, holding the legs in the left hand while stretching the neck over the edge of the table. A 20 (metric 0.9) gauge needle is inserted along the midline between the clavicles at the entrance to the thorax, directed posteriorly and downwards along the line of the keel bone. For older birds, a needle of 17 (metric 1.45) gauge, 5 cm, may be used. For ducks and geese, blood may be taken from the occipital venous sinus.

In day-old or young chicks, blood collection may be made direct from the neck after cutting off or dislocating the head with scissors.

Information on the use of different blood-based tests is given in Chapter 3.

Post-mortem procedure

When specimens have been submitted alive, note is taken of any clinical signs and/or behavioural abnormalities. This is of particular importance when investigating diseases with nervous or locomotor signs.

It is important to examine and weigh the entire carcass before starting dissection. Check for wounds, colour (e.g. jaundice) or pallor and also check for external parasites. This examination is greatly facilitated by immersing each carcass except the head in a dilute solution of disinfectant.

The carcass should now be laid on its back and the angle of the jaw cut through. With the blunt point of scissors inside the oesophagus the cut is continued down the neck, thus exposing the pharynx, oesophageal lining and interior of the crop for examination. The trachea is incised down its length from the larynx and examined. An assessment of the size of the thymus gland can be made at this stage.

Each leg in turn is drawn away from the body and the skin between the leg and the abdomen on each side is incised, the legs are then bent outwards until each femur head is carefully dislocated from its acetabulum. Care is required at this point, especially in young birds, to ensure that abnormalities of the femoral head are not caused by the post-mortem process. The joints of the limbs may then be incised and examined for presence of abnormal amounts or changes to the nature and colour of joint fluid. In addition, the major tendons around the hock joint should be examined for evidence of damage or rupture. The synovial sheaths in this region should also be examined for excess or purulent fluid. In young birds the heads of the long bones may easily be incised with a sharp blade. This will permit checking for abnormalities of bone growth such as dyschondroplasia or regions with abscesses. Multiple sections should be made at these points, as some of the lesions can be quite small. The degree of bend and snap in the long bones should be assessed.

The muscle groups of the thigh should be separated to reveal the sciatic nerve, which can be examined for evidence of change or enlargement.

The skin between the keel and the vent is incised transversely and the cut edge is reflected forwards, exposing the whole ventral aspect of the body and breast muscles. Dehydration will result in this musculature having a 'sticky' feeling and congested appearance. Visceral gout may also be evident. Several diseases such as infectious bursal disease (IBD) also result in surface haemorrhages being evident in this area. However, it should also be noted that haemorrhages may result from agonal changes following cervical dislocation. The muscles of the thigh and sternum, together with other sternal tissues, may be examined. The abdominal wall is incised transversely between the keel and the vent; the breast muscles and rib cage are cut through on each side with scissors or bone forceps forward to the coracoid and clavicle, which are also carefully severed, without cutting the large blood vessels. The sternum may now be removed from the body, exposing the internal organs to full view. The softness or hardness of the ribs should be noted during sectioning and may be examined for evidence of tumours or enlargement of the costochondral junction seen with rickets.

At this stage the exposed organs should be examined in situ. The liver should be checked for enlargement or discoloration. The serosal surfaces and air sacs should be checked for the presence of purulent material. The appearance of the heart and pericardial sac should also be assessed. Any ascitic fluid or effusions into the body cavity will also be evident. At this stage swabs may be taken from exposed organs after searing the surface with a hot knife. Risk of subsequent contamination during handling is thus avoided.

Following examination of the organs in situ, the intestine should be severed at the cloaca and also anterior to the proventriculus, enabling the removal of the whole intestine. This may now be examined along its length, both on its serosal surface and after opening along its lining.

Examination of the organs revealed after removal of the intestinal tract can take place. The ovary and oviduct should be observed, with size, number and condition of follicles being noted in relation to egg production. The kidneys may be examined. The sciatic plexus beneath the kidney should be revealed by removal of kidney tissue by blunt dissection. The bursa of Fabricius should also be checked for inflammation or changes in size. The heart should be incised and the valves examined.

The lungs should be examined and incised to check for consolidation and pneumonia. Again, cultures may be taken if appropriate. The nasal cavities and sinuses may be examined for the presence of exudate by cutting through the upper beak at the appropriate level with sharp scissors.

The brain may be examined and removed for histological examination, if fresh, by removing the head at about the atlanto-occipital area and reflecting the skin forward over the skull and upper mandible. The skull may then be carefully incised in the midline with a sharp, firm scalpel and then likewise transversely. The four quarters of skull bone may be reflected outwards from the middle by grasping with suitable forceps, exposing the entire brain, which may then be removed with small scissors, cutting the nerve attachments carefully. Alternatively, the brain may be fixed in situ following exposure and then removed.

Examination of the spinal cord will require longitudinal section of the vertebral column. This will allow a check to be made for abscesses, tumours or compressive vertebral lesions. A common point at which problems occur is at the T7/T8 junction close to the anterior edge of the kidneys (spondylolisthesis and osteomyelitis, for example). Palpation of the vertebrae from the body cavity can help identify problems here.

During the post-mortem examination tissue samples should be taken for histological and virological examination as required. At this stage it is possible that a tentative diagnosis can be reached and further tests may be undertaken to confirm suspicions or eliminate possibilities. The precise samples taken will depend greatly on the situation, the economic consequences of the disease and often the need to consider the costs of additional tests undertaken. Commonly the following procedures form the next routes of enquiry.

Bacteriology

Often, simple direct plating of swabs on to media such as blood or MacConkey agar, followed by aerobic culture, will suffice for isolating common avian pathogens. More sophisticated technique such as anaerobic culture, specialized media or selective enrichment procedures will be required for certain organisms.

Parasitology

Coccidia

The serosal and mucosal surface of the intestine removed from freshly dead birds should be visually examined throughout its length for evidence of characteristic lesions of the various coccidial species. Wet mount smears of mucosal scrapings from various segments of the intestine may be examined for the presence of oocysts and schizonts. The presence of relatively low numbers of oocysts or of a few intestinal lesions (particularly when associated with certain coccidial types, e.g. *Eimeria acervulina* or *Eimeria maxima*) does not constitute evidence of clinical coccidiosis; rather, it may represent a normal state of affairs, as relatively low numbers of oocysts and some intestinal lesions are commonly found at the 20–40-day stage in broiler birds in the presence of adequate levels of effective anticoccidial drug.

Other protozoa

Wet mounts of preparations should be examined for cryptosporidia, *Histomonas*, *Hexamita* and trichomonads, for example. For flagellates these must be made from a freshly killed bird as motility of the parasites is often lost soon after death of the host.

Worms

In the case of *Capillaria* the mucosal layer of the intestine should be scraped off, emulsified in saline and examined in a strong light on a dark surface or under low-power magnification, or it may be sieved through a fine mesh first to remove debris. The double-poled, lemon-shaped eggs should also be looked for in the faeces or inside female worms. Ascarid worms will be visible in the intestine and *Heterakis* worms in the caeca when the intestine is fully opened.

Histology

Tissue for histology should be taken in thin slices and placed in 10% buffered formal-saline in a ratio of tissue to fixative of 1:15.

Specialized techniques

Where samples are being submitted to another laboratory, for example for virus isolation or polymerase chain reaction (PCR) testing, it is best to seek advice from the laboratory in question as to the best samples to submit and whether any particular transport media or precautions are required. In all cases it must be taken into account that there are regulations covering how pathological samples are packaged. Additional legislation often pertains where the samples must cross a national boundary.

FIELD-BASED TECHNIQUES

Discussion up to this point has been written primarily from the perspective of a laboratory-based examination; however, the majority of the techniques described so far can be used on site as part of a farm-based investigation. A site investigation will be focused by the problems particular to the type of stock involved. Special features of particular relevance to the main types of commercial poultry enterprises will now be considered in more detail.

BROILERS

Numerically, broilers form by far the largest group of poultry farmed commercially. The genetic potential of the modern hybrids for rapid growth, efficient food conversion and production of meat is quite phenomenal. In spite of this, the fact that mortality rates are if anything on the decline is a tribute to the advances made over recent times in the fields of poultry genetics, nutrition and husbandry techniques. However, the characteristics of this type of bird impose a requirement for high standards in all aspects of the bird's care. Often an incidence of disease is secondary to a failing in some aspect of management of the flock. This may be a failure to provide the correct physical environment or nutrition or a deficiency in the vaccination programme of the broiler flock or parents from which the flock derives.

Investigation of a problem involving morbidity or mortality

Most of the methods used to investigate a problem in this type of flock have already been described. The importance of the age at which the problem occurs is especially relevant in this type of stock. The problems of early life such as yolk sac infection are followed by second-week issues such as chick anaemia agent. In the following week, with the waning of maternal antibody, viral diseases such as IBD come to the fore. Finally in the older bird there may be secondary bacterial disease, primarily *Escherichia coli* infection, which represents the end stage of various infectious or environmental insults. Elucidation of the causes of the problem will depend on a combination of pathology and the use of appropriate laboratory tests. These tests are often serological. More recently, PCR tests have proved useful in pathogen detection. Virus and bacteria isolation may also be appropriate. It should be mentioned at this point that the short life of the broiler can cause difficulty with serological tests. Often the bird is killed before antibody titres have a chance to develop. Remaining maternal antibody can confuse results from samples taken earlier in the flock's life. A useful technique is to retain a few birds in isolation after the main flock has been depleted. These can be subsequently tested when titres are more fully developed. Alternatively, suitable (e.g. specific pathogen-free, SPF) sentinel birds can be placed within a flock and later checked for evidence (such as rising serological titres) of exposure to pathogens.

As previously mentioned, deficiencies in the physical environment of the bird can give rise to, or exacerbate, the effects of mild infections. As part of any site-based investigation, time should be dedicated to the assessment of this area. It is important to base opinions on time spent observing the flock (as opposed to reliance on written or computer-generated information). As many senses as possible can be used in this respect. How does the flock behave? Are birds huddling together or clumping near heat sources? Does the flock sound normal? For example are there any coughs or unusual respiratory noises? Alternatively, is the flock unusually quiet? The sense of smell is useful. Are levels of ammonia or dust excessive? Does the litter have an abnormal odour? Examination of farm records is important. Have there been changes to feed or water consumption?

Once again a mental or physical checklist of points will help to ensure that items are not missed.

Investigation of suboptimal performance

In many respects investigation of a problem of excess mortality is the most straightforward problem that can occur with this type of stock. It can be much more difficult to pin down a cause or causes where the problem is that of suboptimal performance, for example in liveweight gain or feed conversion. In many cases the effect may be due to a subtle interaction of several factors. Elucidation of the precise cause may be impossible and the only option left is to make changes that address possible causes of the problem and await a response. There is a great temptation to assume that isolation of a particular virus or discovery of a titre to a particular organism has demonstrated the actual cause. Remember, however, that it is unusual to carry out extensive investigations on flocks that are normal. These flocks may also have yielded similar results to those found during problem periods. It is obviously impossible to demonstrate in every case that a proposed causal agent is beyond doubt the cause; however, a healthy scepticism should be maintained where evidence is incomplete.

In general the depth of investigation should be determined by the severity of economic loss stemming from the problem. It is normal to kill a sample of birds from affected flocks for postmortem examination. Particular attention should be paid to checking for evidence of subclinical coccidiosis problems. Using one of the lesion scoring systems that have been developed can be helpful.

Where concerns exist about the flock's environmental conditions I have found an electronic data logger to be a useful and relatively cheap aid. This may be set to measure environmental conditions such as temperature at preset intervals over long periods. Information gathered in this way can be quite revealing at times, especially in providing detail of what is happening at night when flocks are unsupervised.

It is also useful to carry out a basic analysis of the feed the flock has received. Where samples have been retained from previous feed deliveries, these may provide historical information. It is essential that sampling follows a recognized procedure in case of subsequent dispute. This is described below.

Taking a feed sample

When sampling any kind of feedstuff (e.g. premixes, concentrates, complete feeds) it is essential that samples are taken in a correct manner in order that the sample used is truly representative of the material sampled. Failure to do this renders laboratory analysis or examinations valueless.

Feed samples should not be taken from feed troughs or from under heaters.

The principles of sampling are that from sampled portions (units) of the material, an adequate number of incremental samples are pooled and mixed to form an aggregate sample, from which the final sample is taken. It is a sound practice to hold part of the final sample in storage for reference as needed. Incremental samples may be taken from bulk or bagged material by the use of a sampling spear.

Often the correct procedure is defined in national regulations but in general the method of reducing an aggregate sample is as follows: the material is heaped to form a 'cone', which is then flattened and quartered. Two diagonally opposite quarters are rejected, the remainder is mixed and the quartering and rejection continues as necessary.

Sampling tables indicate the number of incremental samples required for a representative aggregate sample (e.g. if sampling 4–5 tonnes of material, then not less than 10 incremental samples are required).

Investigation of wet litter problems

Problems of this nature are common in broilers. Causes may be managemental, nutritional or other. Poultry managers sometimes confuse 'enteritis' and 'diarrhoea': enteritis is inflammation of the intestine (e.g. as in coccidiosis), diarrhoea is frequent evacuation of watery faeces – often the cause is nutritional.

Poultry faeces

Enteric faeces are normally brown or fawn in colour, with a white urate cap, evacuated 12–16 times in 24 h. Caecal faeces are usually dark brown in colour, semi-liquid, often looking like dark sauce, evacuated only once or twice daily but influenced by the diet. Do not confuse caecal faeces with diarrhoea.

Management

Normal litter should be of uniform consistency (i.e. the surface not markedly different from the subsurface) and it should be friable (i.e. it should crumble when moved about). In a temperate climate, when 'working' correctly and squeezed in the hand, the litter should hold its shape momentarily and then crumble. This 'working' is brought about by bacterial action in the litter.

In contrast, 'wet litter', when squeezed in the hand, retains its shape and exudes moisture.

Water content varies with the age of bird and climate: in a dry, hot climate 5–10% is normal. In older birds 'good' litter is typically 10–30% moisture.

The term 'wet litter' may sometimes be used to mean only surface wetness, stickiness or greasiness, while the litter below may be dry. This is often called 'capped', 'sticky' or 'greasy' litter. The surface may dry out, forming a hard crust on top of the dry 'new' litter beneath (i.e. the litter is not uniform and friable as it should be). Such a litter condition should be avoided by good management or promptly dealt with if it is seen to occur. When areas of litter are wet or sticky, birds will wish to avoid sitting on them; therefore the birds' body heat is not available in that area to get the litter bacteria working and the situation deteriorates. These areas must be promptly turned over by hand or mechanically so that 'new' dry litter from beneath the cap is left on top. Alternatively, fresh litter should be added on top by hand after turning, in order to encourage birds to use the area. Then body heat helps bacterial action and the litter will begin to 'work'. Necessary adjustments should also be made to ventilation, air flow or house temperature to help resolve the situation.

Good broiler house managers will always be on the lookout for early signs of wet litter or patches of wet litter developing and will take prompt action, as described above.

Attention should also be given to drinkers. 'Bell type' drinkers should be set at the correct height for the age of the bird (shoulder level) and with correct (not too deep) water levels in them (not more than 12.5 mm) in order to avoid spillage. Drinker height should be adjusted frequently. Nipple drinkers are less inclined to cause spillage but again the height and pressure require careful adjustment. This type of drinker is not suitable for all types of poultry (e.g. older turkeys).

Control of environment, with the correct balance between house temperature for age, heat input and air flow, is essential in producing good litter.

Note that 1000 mature birds excrete half a tonne of water per day – this must be removed by ventilation. Removal of water by this means is more difficult in cold weather than in warm, because ventilation rates may be reduced to conserve heat. In addition, gas heaters can contribute to higher humidity. Adequate ventilation and heat input must be maintained until the birds are big enough to produce enough body heat to keep the house warm.

Nutrition and wet litter

Water is an important constituent in nutrition. The fowl kidney excretes normal urine in a continual flow that collects in the anterior cloaca as a creamy, thick, mucoid material abundant in urates, which separate out as a semi-solid mass (appearing as a white cap on excreted faeces). A 'flow-back' system along the colon from the cloaca (to as far forward as the caecum) permits water and electrolyte resorption if required (in this so-called 'integrative segment' of bowel), playing an important part in electrolyte balance.

Thus, any factor that increases water consumption will increase the likelihood of wet litter. For example, restriction of feed in replacement breeders tends to cause increased water consumption; thus, water is limited also. Boredom or need for 'gut-fill' causes excessive water consumption, diarrhoea and wet litter. Excessive dietary salt leads to polydipsia, followed by excessive urine flow with no conservation effort in the 'integrative segment'; this in turn will cause loose droppings or diarrhoea.

Drinking water should be of good quality and care must be taken regarding mineral content. Drinkers should be regularly cleaned to avoid microbial build-up.

The mineral level of feed is also very important, especially the mineral cations sodium, potassium and magnesium; sodium and potassium regulate body fluid volume. These three metallic ions may act additively. Thus, excess sodium intake will cause increased water intake and excretion, with increased faecal water (i.e. diarrhoea). A similar effect occurs with excess potassium, of which there are high levels in potato meal, soya and molasses (beet molasses has twice the level of cane molasses). Excess magnesium may be present, for example from dolomitic limestone, which has a high level.

Chloride intake may be limited, in order to reduce water consumption, by partial substitution of sodium bicarbonate for sodium chloride.

Protein in excess, particularly protein of poor digestibility, leads to increased water intake to allow the excretion of higher uric acid levels. Undigested excess protein may be fermented by bacteria in the lower bowel, leading to loose droppings and the condition known as 'hock-burn' in chickens. This has been associated with high levels of soya or other proteins.

Excess levels of undigested or indigestible sugars may lead to osmotic changes, lower bowel fermentation and loose droppings, for example from skimmed milk, high levels of barley or rye (which contain gums (pectins) with water-binding capacity), soya or tapioca.

Ingredients that are variable in composition may in themselves cause trouble at excessive levels (e.g. guar meal, sunflower meal, tapioca).

The sudden introduction of new raw material ingredients should be avoided; such materials should be 'stepped in' gradually in order to allow time for digestion to adapt to the change.

Poor-quality fat, or fat that is poorly digested by poultry, will lead to diarrhoea or a soapy scour and greasy litter. Hence, poor fat digestion may have a significant effect on litter quality: greasy, capped litter may lead to hock burn, breast blisters and subsequent carcass downgrading. Ether extracts from litter (from broiler birds about 6 weeks old) have shown marked differences in birds fed good- and poor-quality fats (e.g. 2.5% and 7.5%, respectively).

Other causes of wet litter

Bacteria, viruses, protozoa and mycotoxins have been implicated. Courses of antibiotics, given via drinking water or feed, may give rise to diarrhoea and, consequently, wet litter by disturbance of the normal, stable gut flora of bacteria.

Consequences of wet or poor litter

These include the following:
- Excess ammonia in the house, because of fermentation of urea (urate in faeces) by urate-splitting bacteria in warm, moist conditions
- Ammonia reduces appetite and damages the respiratory system and consequently predisposes to infection (colibacillosis) and hence to poor performance
- Wet litter predisposes to greater coccidiosis infection and hence to poor performance (coccidial oocysts mature more rapidly in damp conditions)
- Soiling of birds, breast blisters and 'hock burn' in broilers have significant welfare implications as well as resulting in downgrading of carcasses.

EGG-LAYING FLOCKS

Production and egg quality problems form the types of abnormality most specific to this type of poultry. Investigation of problems involving mortality or morbidity follows similar lines to other poultry.

Egg production problems

Broadly speaking, management often plays as great a part in egg production as disease. The care and attention to achieving correct growth rate during the rearing phase sets the tone for subsequent egg production. Hence assessment of condition at transfer to laying accommodation is a very significant aspect of investigation, especially when disease is not suspected. See-saw egg production graphs often indicate a managemental origin; causes are frequently multifactorial and can be very time-consuming to investigate.

In some cases no explanation can be determined for falls in production, especially less serious ones. Transient falls in production of up to 6–8% may occur in layers for quite trivial reasons (e.g. a reduction in feed consumption for 2–3 days), return to normal taking place after several days.

It may be difficult, or impossible, to determine if a 20% egg production loss is due to all birds producing 20% less, half the flock producing 40% less or 20% of birds going out of production. Where there are no clinical signs, it is necessary to find the birds that are not laying, which can be very difficult. However, with birds in cages, each cage without eggs can be marked for three successive mornings, using clothes pegs. Birds can then be selected from any of the cages with three pegs.

If disease is suspected, it is important that any laboratory investigation carried out is relevant, economically justifiable and meaningful. Preoccupation with disease, with a diagnosis based on equivocal findings in one small set of blood samples, may well be misleading and unwise. Alternatively, serological investigation may be an invaluable tool, particularly if it can be done sequentially in time.

As described earlier, many of the problems with this type of flock arise from management inadequacies. Emphasis should be placed on the following areas as part of the investigation.

Rearing management

Information on body weight during rearing should be sought, not only in relation to adherence to target but also with regard to evenness. Checks should be made to ensure that all the birds are of similar age and strain.

Light

The intensity, duration and evenness of light is a key factor. Light should not decrease in intensity or duration during lay. Nor should increases have occurred before the correct stage at the end of rearing. Considerable variation in light intensity can occur from tier to tier in cage houses. In most cases flocks are dependent on artificial light sources controlled by time clocks. Potential for disruption exists because of power failure, or the tampering or breakdown of these units. A gradual reduction in light intensity can result from fused bulbs not being replaced promptly or from a simple build-up of dust on light fittings. Leakage of external light into controlled environment housing can affect the light programme the birds are receiving.

Feeding and nutrition

The correct make up of the feed is vital, as is the physical grist of the ration. As this type of flock is often fed on a simple mash type ration, perhaps made on site, it is possible to see problems arising from incorrect formulation of rations, omission of an ingredient, mineral or vitamin supplement. Problems due to separation of ingredients after mixing can occur. Feed distribution so that all birds in the flock get equal access is also critical. Incorrectly adjusted feeders can result in birds at the end of runs not getting their share. In many cases weighing samples of birds from different areas of the flock, especially if caged, can reveal where this may be occurring. Problems can also occur as a result of the introduction of high-calcium rearing rations too early to rearing birds.

Water

This is an obvious requirement for any flock. Interruption or inadequate supply will result in serious falls in egg production. Such situations can occur because of leaks or pressure fluctuations (e.g. due to use of washing equipment elsewhere on the farm). Birds in cages at the ends of long runs of piping may not be correctly supplied at times of high demand such as during warm weather. Water quality may also occasionally be a problem.

Environment

Birds housed in cages are dependent on the conditions provided for them being correct as they cannot move themselves to a more favourable situation. It is therefore essential, on both production-related and welfare-related grounds, to ensure that temperature, ventilation, humidity and ammonia levels are acceptable to the birds. It is important to ensure that in caged flocks the situation within cages in different parts and levels of the house is monitored rather than simply checking the general house environment. There is also considerable potential for management failure and profound environmental stress in extensive systems.

Pests and vermin

Rats and mice cause nervousness, consume and spoil feed, damage the house, equipment and insulation (causing fires), contaminate eggs and may bite hens on nests. Red mite causes irritation to birds and staff. Production losses will also occur and in heavy infestations death can occur. Insertion of moistened card between crevices in equipment will readily detect this parasite or its faeces. Other mites and lice can be an occasional problem. Flies and moths also cause irritation to birds and staff and can result in moderate production losses (perhaps due to reluctance of staff to spend time in houses).

Human factors

Changes in daily routines, timing, excitement, different staff (at weekends for example) can all have an effect as can sudden noise and disturbance (planes, drills, lorries, dogs, etc.). Recording systems and timing of counts must be similar day to day (so must egg collection times). On occasions problems are the result of faking of records or simple theft of eggs.

Factors affecting egg quality

Table 2.1 summarizes possible causes of poor egg quality.

BROILER BREEDERS

The modern broiler breeder is probably the most challenging of commercial poultry to manage. With this type of bird the aim is to maximize reproductive performance in terms of egg numbers and hatchability in a bird whose genetic background is strongly slanted towards meat production.

Management of this type of stock aims for a controlled but steady increase in weight during rearing. This must be done in an environment that avoids stimulation of sexual maturity until desired. This is achieved through a combination of weight control and restricted day length. When the flock has achieved the desired age and weight profile it is stimulated to come into lay by increasing feed allocation and providing a light stimulus. At this stage the flock is often transferred to laying accommodation and males and females, which have been reared separately until then, are 'mated up'. Thereafter rapid increases are made in feed allocation until the birds

Table 2.1 Egg Quality Problems

ABNORMALITY	POSSIBLE CAUSE
Problem of shell quality	
Soft shell, shell-less	Birds coming into lay; disease e.g. ND/PMV, IB, EDS76, ART; sulphonamides
Misshapen eggs	Genetic causes; disease (ND/PMV, IB); older birds have higher incidence due to inadequate oviduct muscle tone, insufficient protein in thick albumen; birds coming into lay, moving, and also as for ridged waist (see text below)
Ridged waist (equatorial bulge or 'body check')	Uterine damage as egg starting to harden (i.e. in early calcification); activity in early calcification (i.e. in late afternoon); excessive bird density; handling stress (adrenaline (epinephrine) release)
Corrugated eggs	IBV infection; experimental copper deficiency; lathyrism (i.e. beta-aminopropionitrile (BAPN) in legume seeds such as peas (genus *Lathyrus*)) can induce shell abnormalities, increased thin whites and reduced production (toxicity appears similar to copper deficiency)
Flat-sided eggs	Abnormal uterine pressure in early calcification; possibly associated with IB
Thin, porous or soft eggs	Average thickness should be about $330\,\mu m$ in chicken and about $400\,\mu m$ in turkey (measure by micrometer). Genetics; nutrition – calcium or phosphorus lack or imbalance, zinc, manganese or vitamin D_3 lack; separation of feed ingredients, feed intake inadequate; disease (ND/PMV, IB, EDS76, ART); excessive temperature; older birds; disturbance at night; sulphonamides and other antimicrobials
Rough surface	Genetic; disease (ND/PMV, IB); sulphonamides; excessive calcium; young birds coming into lay; older birds (loss of oviduct muscle tone); stress (adrenaline (epinephrine) release)
Mottled eggs	Genetics; humidity extremes; cage marks on freshly laid eggs
Yellow shells	High tetracycline level in feed
Cracked eggs	See above re. shell quality: genetic (not squatting to lay); stocking density; cage design (cage floor, slope, sag, floor lip); collection method, handling; staff; shell thickness or strength or weight per unit area
Loss of colour	Genetic; disease (ND/PMV, IB, EDS76, ART); sulphonamides; nicarbazine, piperazine; high temperature, high production; in free-range birds for unknown reasons (if shut in, colour temporarily restored)
Problems of the egg contents	
Loose air cell	Rough handling; disease e.g. ND/PMV, IB giving rise to poor shell quality and 'watery whites'
'Blood' and 'meat' spots	Genetics; cold environment; marked temperature change; continuous light; older birds; low vitamin K level (especially with sulfaquinoxaline), low vitamin A level; stress at ovulation (30 min after oviposition); following epidemic tremor (for 1 month); mycotoxins; infectious bronchitis
Abnormal yolk colour	Pigment levels in feed (e.g. carotenoids/xanthophylls): oxidative breakdown of natural and/or synthetic carotenoids: gossypol, a toxic phenolic pigment of cotton seed causes mottled red or even olive colour. Malvalic/sterculic acids (cyclopropene fatty acids) from raw or crude cotton seed oil or kapok seed meal cause release of iron from yolk, leading to pink egg contents (and drastic reduction in hatchability, with dead early germs and anaemia), 'pink whites' and putty-like, rubbery, 'golf-ball' yolks. Bacterial contamination can give rise to green or brown discoloration. A similar discoloration arises from unrestricted access to pigmented plants, lush spring grass or other animal feed (e.g. when on free range)

Variable yolk colour	Check that a source of carotenoids is available in feed. Commonly found after disease; oxidative breakdown of natural and/or synthetic carotenoids or bad feed mixing will have similar effects
Decreased yolk colour (with normal carotenoid levels in feed)	Following flock disease, low feed consumption, intestinal parasites, mycotoxins (aflatoxin, ochratoxin, T_2); exposure to coffee bean seed (*Cassia*): oxidative breakdown of natural and/or synthetic carotenoids
Mottled or flecked yolk (a very limited amount of mottling is normal)	Stale eggs; excessive dietary pigment, improper pigment ratios, poor feed mixing – oxidative breakdown of natural and/or synthetic carotenoids; excessive chilling; partial freezing (e.g. free range); high storage temperature (yolks mottled, flaccid and fragile); genetics; nicarbazine, ammonia, gossypol, piperazine, phenothiazine, gallic acid (nut galls) or tannic acid (from bird-resistant sorghums)
Cheesy yolk	Chilling of eggs (free range); raw or crude cotton seed oil, kapok seed meal
Yolk taint (acquired before egg is laid)	Genetics – a fishy taint due to lack of enzyme to convert trimethylamine (TMA) in certain fish meals (and precursor sinapine in certain rape seeds) into the oxide; TMA may also be released by action of enteric bacteria on excess supplementary choline; robenidine, capelin meal (Icelandic herring), certain rapeseed meals; unsaturated fatty acids (fish oils), moulds and certain seed dressings
Yolk and albumen taint (acquired after egg is laid)	Unsuitable detergents; storage near strong odours as the egg cools and respires
Flat yolk	Nicarbazine; poor shell quality; watery white; high storage temperature, excessive storage time; storage blunt end down; weak vitelline membrane
Watery white (Haugh unit score should be 70; <50 is poor)	Genetic; disease (e.g. ND, IB); warm and/or prolonged storage; older birds; ammonia; low protein in ration (also affects egg production and size) (NB. The thin white of a newly laid egg is watery but the thick white is firm)
Pink white	Raw or crude cottonseed oil; kapok seed meal; excessive iron in water or feed; bacterial contamination
Prominent chalazas	Associated with 'watery whites'
Ruptured chalazas	Infectious bronchitis
Prominent vitelline membrane	False impression due to pale, opaque yolk (see 'Decreased yolk colour', above)

ND/PMV, Newcastle disease/*Paramyxovirus*; IB, infectious bronchitis; EDS76, egg drop syndrome 76; ART, avian rhinotracheitis.

approach peak production. Post-peak, feed allocation is reduced gradually to avoid the birds becoming overweight. It is also common to use mechanical systems to feed males and females different amounts of feed and to automatically collect eggs. The vast majority of broiler breeders are housed on deep litter. In addition to the requirements to lay fertile eggs, broiler breeders must have received a suitable vaccination programme not only to ensure their own protection from common diseases but also to pass protection in the form of high levels of maternal antibody to their progeny. As can be discerned, the process briefly described above is a complicated one and great attention to detail is required to ensure success.

The investigation of infectious disease or production problems uses the same methods as described earlier. It is common to have information from routine serological monitoring of parent stock. This is very helpful during investigations. It is a valuable resource to collect and freeze serum samples at intervals during a flock's life, even if they are simply stored without testing. This will allow a retrospective survey of titres to be carried out should it be necessary.

As highlighted above, it is important to ensure that diagnoses are based on sound interpretation of results, not, for example, on a single test result. In addition it is important to remember that it is possible for titres in flocks to rise, especially to diseases against which the flock has been vaccinated, without causing any abnormalities.

Broiler breeders can suffer from most of the conditions afflicting other domestic fowl. In addition, deficits in management can give rise to particular problems. As the birds' feed is restricted through the majority of their lives, it is a key requirement that all birds get an equal chance of receiving their allocation. If this does not occur the stronger birds will thrive at the expense of the weaker. This will result in a large weight range between different birds in the flock. Much of the management effort during rearing should be directed at achieving flock uniformity (e.g. by continual grading of the flock). Measures of the evenness of the flock, such as percentage evenness, or the coefficient of variation (CV) are important. Typically a uniformity of 80% is considered good (i.e. 80% of the flock is within 10% of the target weight). This correlates to a CV of between 7 and 8. Information on this should be available in a well-managed flock and should be sought during any investigation involving this type of stock. A flock with a large weight range indicates either a deficiency in management or alternatively can follow on from various disease insults (such as coccidiosis) to the flock during rearing. The use of attenuated coccidiosis vaccines is commonplace and generally effective. The effects of an uneven flock will extend beyond the rearing phase. Smaller birds will be insufficiently mature to respond when stimulated to lay. Overweight birds are prone to egg peritonitis during early lay. The importance of the rearing phase to the success of later flock production and health is self-evident.

During lay, as described for other laying birds, production drops can occur for various reasons, infectious or otherwise. In general it is usually easier to find the cause of a large drop in production. Often the cause of small drops in production can prove extremely difficult if not impossible to determine. It is also quite normal for there to be no recovery in production following this type of drop, especially with the heavy meat hybrids. With broiler breeders it is especially relevant that veterinary efforts are focused on prevention rather than cure.

TURKEYS

Much of what has been said previously regarding investigation of disease in domestic fowl applies equally to turkeys. With this type of bird there are fewer recognized diseases and consequently a smaller range of tests are available, serological or otherwise. Perhaps because it has been a domesticated species for a shorter time, the turkey is generally a robust animal and will thrive in quite primitive accommodation, particularly after 8 weeks of age.

Breeding birds are generally fed ad libitum throughout their lives and so are spared the efforts required for broiler breeders in this area. During lay production drops can occur as a result of infection with a variety of viruses, such as avian rhinotracheitis (ART), *Paramyxovirus* (PMV3) and turkey haemorrhagic enteritis. Pig strains of influenza virus can produce dramatic losses in production. Falls in production can also follow management failings, in particular inadequate efforts to limit the tendency of the female to become broody, this tendency being exaggerated during very warm weather.

Hatchability is often dependent on the skill of artificial insemination teams and this process should be the first line of investigation if problems occur. Infectious diseases, in particular *Mycoplasma* species, are also of great importance in turkeys.

With regard to fattening stock, ART is of great significance in regions where this disease is present. Secondary infections with *E. coli* and *Ornithobacterium rhinotracheale* are common sequelae to this virus. Other occasional problems include classical infection with bacteria such as *Pasteurella* or *Erysipelas* spp. Viral conditions such as haemorrhagic enteritis occur, as do intoxications, especially with ionophores, to which turkeys are especially sensitive. Various unknown conditions giving rise to the occurrence of wet droppings also exist. These may be investigated as described for broilers but often without a conclusive result.

SPECIAL CONSIDERATIONS FOR FREE-RANGE FLOCKS

There is an increasing trend towards outdoor systems of poultry keeping. While it is perfectly possible to manage such systems successfully, they do present considerable risks and challenges to the manager. In some cases the problems can be heightened by a desire to combine a free-range management system with minimal or no use of drug treatments.

Parasitic disease

This is an obvious risk where the birds have access to an environment that cannot be cleansed and disinfected and where egg, larval stage or intermediate hosts of parasites can persist. In many cases the land to which the poultry have access is limited to that closely surrounding a fixed house. Opportunity to rest or rotate grazing is therefore restricted. All these factors will combine to make parasitic disease of much greater consequence in extensive systems.

Diseases with wildlife hosts

Again it is evident that outdoor systems by their nature will allow contact between the farmed poultry and free-flying birds and other wildlife. It is useful to minimize this contact by maintaining feed and water supplies for the flock indoors. However contact will inevitably occur, with inherent risks of transfer of infection. Avian influenza is a particular candidate for this process. However, other diseases such as *Mycoplasma* infection and Newcastle disease can also be acquired in this way.

Zoonotic infections

A risk of flocks acquiring infections such as *Salmonella* and *Campylobacter* must exist with free-range flocks. The environment to which stock have access is less able to be disinfected between crops and exposure to rodent, wildlife or insect vectors provides a route for infection. However, the epidemiology can be expected to vary with the host, the location and the actual infection.

HATCHERY

Investigation of problems within the hatchery with its complex interdependence between biological and mechanical systems can prove very daunting, especially for the newcomer. Specialists in this field do exist and again poultry breeding companies and hatchery equipment manufacturers can provide useful contacts in this regard. As investigation of hatchery problems can often involve factors outside the disease processes covered in this book, this area will be covered in a little more detail. As elsewhere, a methodical and logical approach can often lead even a relatively inexperienced investigator to a good understanding of where the problem may lie.

Once again a critical part of the process is understanding what is normal. Recent UK surveys show that on average 83% of broiler breeder eggs and 82.5% of turkey eggs produce first-quality

Table 2.2 Hatching failures for broilers and turkeys (%)

	BROILER	TURKEY
Candling waste (infertile and early dead*)	7.0	5.0
Dead in shell	9.0	11.0
Culls	1.0	1.5
Total loss	**17.0**	**17.5**

* The 'expected' infertiles, measured as a percentage of the candling waste, will vary according to the age of the flock (e.g. in chicken about 50% at 30 weeks of age, 70% at 45 weeks and 85% at 55 weeks of age).

Table 2.3 Major causes for hatching failures (%)

	BROILER	TURKEY
True infertility	20	30
Egg storage	25	14
Bacterial or mould contamination ('rots')	12	8
Egg faults or shell damage	10	5
Incubation faults	5	6
Nutritional	10	15
Disease	10	17
Genetic	8	5

chicks or poults. The expected hatchability of a flock changes throughout its laying life, starting at a low level and rapidly rising to a peak level from which there is a gradual decline. It is also typical that heavy meat-strain birds tend to have lower hatchability figures.

Typical figures giving a breakdown of hatchability figures are shown in Table 2.2. It should be noted that hatchability is generally taken to refer to the yield of viable chicks rather than being a measure of all birds that emerge from their shells.

The major causes for eggs failing to hatch are shown in Table 2.3.

Investigation of a hatchery problem

Perhaps more than with any other branch of poultry medicine, this type of investigation is dependent on an initial careful scrutiny of records so that there is a clear understanding of the nature of the problem. It is important to be certain whether the problem is a general one affecting all or a number of flocks supplying the hatchery. It is useful to bear in mind that, as with all biological systems, the same insult may not result in the same degree of loss for all flocks. Thus, for example, an excessive period of egg holding may have serious consequences for very young or very old flocks (where egg size and porosity, respectively, will reduce survivability) but less so for flocks in mid lay. However, it is generally possible to detect a measure of effect on all flocks where a general hatchery problem is at fault. An additional possibility is that problems may be associated with one or more setters or hatchers. Here examination of records over a period of some time may be required before such a trend becomes apparent. In some cases much useful information can be gained if, as sometimes happens, eggs from one source are being hatched at more than one hatchery.

Where a particular supply farm or farms appear to be implicated it is essential to gather as much information as possible. Key points include:

- Breed
- Age of males and females
- Details of disease history and medication on farm
- Details of egg production, with special reference to depression
- Feed and feeding details
- Condition of litter or nest-box litter
- Frequency of egg collection, both on farm and from the farm
- Details of egg washing, dipping or fumigation
- Floor egg numbers as a percentage of totals
- Age of eggs set: oldest and freshest
- Details of storage conditions at farm or hatchery – especially the ability to control temperature and humidity during egg storage.

In some cases clarification of these points may require a visit to the farm itself.

Examination of hatch debris

Having completed an examination of the records the next step is to carry out examination of material from the hatchery. This involves examining retained eggs from hatch debris and examination of the hatch records will allow an estimate of the percentage of the total eggs set that these form. There is a great amount of literature and guidance available to assist with carrying out this procedure. For the novice the amount of detail available can be quite overwhelming; however, illustrated embryo development charts are available for both chickens and turkeys, and are very helpful.

It is often useful at the start of an investigation to use an extremely simple classification of the causes of failure to hatch. I use the following categories:

1. Early mortality – small embryo and egg membrane growth
2. Midterm
3. Late embryonic death
4. Clear eggs
5. Obvious embryonic abnormality (e.g. protrusion of the brain)
6. Positional abnormalities (the normal position for the older embryo is with the head under the right wing with the beak towards the air sac and legs in a 'crouched' position)
7. Obviously contaminated eggs with or without development
8. Cracked eggs.

With this simple categorization in mind, it is possible to examine the contents of at least 50 eggs selected at random from the hatch remnants for a particular flock. By placing the eggs in lines on Keyes trays for each category, a virtual 'bar chart' of the number of eggs falling into each category is quickly built up.

Embryonic mortality is generally highest in two peaks, at about 3–5 days (25%) and again at about 18–21 days (50%). In the chicken, the association of 'normal' embryonic mortality with age of embryo is approximately as follows: 0–4 days, 25%; 4–16 days, 10%; 16–21 days, 65%. In the turkey it is apparent that a higher percentage of midterm (18–24 days) deaths occur.

With the above figures in mind, coupled with the figures provided earlier in the section, it should become readily apparent if the number of eggs in any category is unusually high. This in turn can give a strong indication of where problems may lie. For example:

- **Early death** is frequently due to maladjustment at the critical period of formation of basic organs (e.g. the blood system), which occurs in the first 3–5 days. About 30% of mortality occurs in the first week, the main causes being physical trauma (jarring, often associated with transportation, causing 'loose air cell'), prolonged or poor storage prior to incubation, over-heating or chilling, faulty incubation, improper fumigation, poor hygiene (e.g. shell migration of *E. coli* bacteria) and inadequate turning. Thus, in general, the causes are trauma or stress to the egg, but nutritional factors relevant at this time of vascular development (i.e. 72–96 h) may involve biotin or vitamin E.

- **Midterm death** may be associated with nutritional problems, in which case signs of nutritional inadequacy may be present (e.g. vitamin B_2 deficiency causes clubbed down and oedema). Knowledge of the exact pathology of nutrient deficiencies is quite scanty but it is recognized that phosphorus and zinc may also be of significance in this period. Availability of specific fatty acids such as linoleic acid may also have a significant role in hatchability.

- **Late death** towards full term and at hatching may account for up to about 60% of mortality. Principal causes are incubation faults (temperature, humidity, ventilation), inadequate turning, late transfer, infections such as *Mycoplasma* and prolonged egg storage. Nutritional aspects of significance may involve vitamin B_2, biotin, folic acid, vitamin B_{12} and manganese.

- **Culls** (i.e. second-quality chicks or poults removed after hatching) may occur in up to 1% of chickens, resulting from malformations (old eggs), weak chicks (machine faults, late hatch) or poor chicks (nutrition). In turkeys, incidence may be much higher than in chickens because of unhealed navel (old eggs, high setter temperature, incorrect hatcher humidity) and various defects, including leg abnormalities, undersize, deformity and distended abdomen.

- **Clear eggs**, when examined at hatch, can pose some difficulty in determining which are infertile and which represent very early embryonic death. Where a large number of such eggs are found it is helpful to examine some eggs from the flock during early incubation (4–5 d). At this stage the signs of early development are much easier to distinguish. Where genuine infertility is the issue, factors such as the following should be considered.
  - *Male infertility*: for example due to interference by others during mating because of excess numbers. Inadequate numbers of males can be a cause. However, provided that they are healthy, a remarkably small number of males (e.g. 5–6 per 100 females) can sustain good hatchability. Poorly selected or undernourished males can cause problems (10% below weight leads to loss of fertility, 25% below weight leads to sterility). Males that are too fat can arise from mismanagement of a separate-sex feeding system (i.e. males feeding from female feeders). Infertility can also be due to males who are too old, or unhealthy because of damaged combs and wattles causing difficulty in eating and drinking. Lameness due to, for example, tenosynovitis and sore feet (pododermatitis, etc.) will also interfere with the bird's ability to mate successfully.
  - *Females* can also have a role in fertility, again if they are undernourished or overweight. Fertility will naturally decline during the course of lay. Infectious disease can also have a significant effect.
  - *Husbandry issues*: factors such as stocking density, inadequate feed, water or space allowance can affect fertility, as can lighting patterns in rearing and lay.
  - *Nutrition*: this should be considered in conjunction with both production and hatchability; in general, it has more dramatic effects on hatchability than on fertility.

- *Genetic factors*: these can have an influence both on the innate fertility of particular strains and on physical conformation, which can result in difficult mating.
- *Temperature*: high and very low temperatures depress semen production. High temperature depresses feed intake, requiring higher vitamin and mineral levels.
- *Artificial insemination technique*: this is obviously critical where it is applicable. The interval between inseminations, staff skill and care and how semen is handled during collection, dilution and administration are all key factors.
- *Drugs (especially at incorrect levels) and toxic chemicals*: the following can have deleterious effects – dimetridazole, furazolidone (compounds now banned in many countries), organic mercurials (breakdown products of insecticides), inorganic mercurials, etc. The adverse effect of nicarbazin, even at low levels, on hatchability is well documented.

- **Cracked eggs** normally result from poor handling at any stage from the farm, through transportation to within the hatchery process. Insufficient frequency of egg collection on the farm often gives rise to cracked eggs, especially with automated egg collection systems. Certain disease processes and physical stresses will result in thinner shells; however, visible deterioration of the quality of the shell is usually also evident.
- **Contaminated eggs** most often stem from problems on laying farms. Possible causes include poor floor egg management, poor litter conditions and insufficient frequency of egg collection. It is also possible for exploding eggs ('rots') to contaminate other eggs in the same incubator. A target of less than 0.01% of eggs to be of this type is usual.
- **Anatomical abnormalities** can be genetic in origin or result from poor farm storage, rough handling of eggs or faults in conditions during early incubation.
- **Positional abnormalities** normally arise from inadequate turning of eggs during incubation.

Gaseous environment and hatchability

Although encased in shells the avian embryo has similar respiratory requirements to other living things. Optima for successful hatches are well known – oxygen concentration of 21%, carbon dioxide below 0.5%. Adverse effects of noxious gases on hatchability are documented such as methane (malformations), nitrous oxide (delayed, reduced hatch), carbon monoxide (embryo mortality and brain damage due to hypoxia), automotive exhaust gases (greater effect on mortality than carbon monoxide, with no gross abnormalities).

Control and fine-tuning of the gaseous environment and temperature during incubation is an essential part of the management of any hatchery but is beyond the scope of this chapter.

Nutrition and hatchability

The importance of the nutrition of the dam is indicated by the fact that the egg must contain all the nutrients needed by the embryo.

Development in the egg and for a week or more after hatching is, as far as fat-soluble vitamins and some other factors are concerned, reliant upon supplies from the yolk. Hence, deficiency signs in newly hatched chicks or poults (and often within the next 7–10 d) usually reflect a breeder feed inadequacy rather than a relationship with the starter feed.

It is difficult to affect the relative protein, fat and carbohydrate content of an egg via the diet of the hen but the concentration of vitamins and trace elements in her blood and tissues directly influences that in her eggs. Hence, analysis of egg yolk to determine vitamin and other deficiencies in the breeder may be the preferred and more direct route than blood or tissue sampling of the relevant hens.

Even at acceptable levels of hatchability a proportion of dead-in-shell embryos may exhibit 'nutritional signs', as detailed above, as a result of individual variations in metabolism.

It is of basic importance to realize that hens can produce eggs with dietary levels of vitamins that will not allow the eggs to hatch (except in the case of vitamin A deficiency, in which cessation of production occurs first).

Nutrient deficiencies may give rise to malformed embryos or reduction in hatchability but it may be difficult to identify by examination of the embryo the nutrient deficiency responsible for poor hatchability, since the time of embryonic death will often depend on the degree of deficiency involved. Thus, it has been shown by experiment with pantothenic acid that, while in extreme deficiency hatchability may be totally suppressed, in milder deficiencies a peak of early mortality (1–4 d) occurs but later peaks change according to the amount of pantothenic acid in the diet. Most water-soluble vitamins have a similar effect.

In practice the nutrient deficiencies most likely to give rise to reduced hatchability, unless adequate breeder supplements are used, are vitamin B_2 (riboflavin) and some others of the B group (e.g. biotin), vitamin E, manganese, zinc and phosphorus.

Early death may be related to:
- Biotin
- Vitamin E deficiency (vascular lesions).

Later death (i.e. towards and around midterm) may be related to:
- Riboflavin (anaemia, oedema, micromelia, mesonephros degeneration and clubbed down)
- Phosphorus (no specific abnormalities)
- Zinc inadequacy (faulty trunk, limb, beak, brain and eye development – abnormalities associated with development of the skeletal mesoderm).

Death, during the last few days and at hatching, may be related to deficiencies of the following:
- Vitamin B_2 (clubbed down, curled toe, micromelia, degeneration of the myelin sheath of peripheral nerves, degeneration of embryonic Wolffian bodies)
- Biotin (chondrodystrophy, syndactyly, characteristic skeletal deformities, ataxia and chondrodystrophy in newly hatched chicks)
- Folic acid (chicks may be of normal appearance but die soon after pipping; in severe depletion chondrodystrophy, syndactyly and parrot beak)
- Vitamin B_{12} (malposition, myoatrophy, chondrodystrophy, oedema and haemorrhage)
- Manganese (chondrodystrophy, parrot beak, globular head, cervicothoracic oedema, retarded down feather and body growth, micromelia and ataxia in newly hatched chicks) – bone formation defects are probably associated with abnormal mucopolysaccharide in the organic matrix of bone. Vitamin B_{12} and manganese deficiencies may be associated with extreme reduction in hatchability.

Nutritional deficiencies may be direct (i.e. due to inadequate supply in the feed). This can be as a result of nutrients not being added, badly mixed or badly stored feed. Alternatively, dilution by post-manufacture addition of cereals to formulated rations can be implicated.

Indirect deficiencies can be caused by antagonists such as mycotoxins, inadequate absorption (e.g. parasitism or disease), underconsumption (e.g. overcrowding), or the result of an inappropriate drug inclusion.

While 'nutritional deficiency lesions' are commonly seen in dead-in-shell embryos, incorrect feed manufacture is now seldom incriminated and definitive deficiencies of single nutrients are rare. Instead, a miscellany of lesions suggestive of a number of nutrient shortfalls (see paragraph above) is the commoner finding. It has also been reported that syndromes, which seem to mimic the signs of certain deficiencies, may be evident despite adequate supplies of that nutrient in the feed (e.g. a 'clubbed down' syndrome has been seen in flocks well supplied with vitamin B_2).

Hatchery hygiene survey

This should include appraisal of the following.

- **Hatchery design**: flow of materials and personnel movement. In general, egg reception and storage areas and setters are expected to be the 'cleanest' area of the building. Any areas in which injectable vaccines are prepared need to be especially clean. Chick 'take off' and storage areas are potentially more contaminated. Wash areas for boxes and equipment are deemed 'dirty areas'. Flow of air in the building should reflect this – air should flow from clean to dirty. In a similar way, staff and equipment movement between clean and dirty areas should be controlled.
- **General hygiene**: cleansing and disinfection methods and materials used in all areas within the hatchery should be appropriate and effective. Fumigation is often a key component in this process. Written schedules and checklists are a useful aid to supervision of this process.
- **Bacterial status** of various work areas can be assessed by various methods producing counts of the total number of bacteria, moulds, coliforms and yeasts present on floors, walls, tables, shelves, etc. Airborne contaminant counts can be obtained using special samplers or exposed plates.
- **Personnel**: personal hygiene, clothing policy and hand-washing procedures should be evaluated.
- **Hatcher fluff**: bacteriological examination can provide a useful indicator of the *Salmonella* status of the chicks in that machine.

FURTHER READING

Anon 1998 RossTech98/35. Investigating hatchery practice. Ross Breeders, Newbridge

Boden E (ed) 1993 Poultry practice. Baillière Tindall, London

Chick embryo development chart: obtainable from Jamesway Incubator Company, PO Box 3067, 756 Bishops Street North, Cambridge, Ontario, Canada N3H 4S4

Etches R J 1996 Reproduction in poultry. CAB International, Wallingford, Oxfordshire

Leeson S, Diaz G, Summers J D 1995 Poultry metabolic disorders and mycotoxins. University Books, Guelph, Ontario

MAFF 1972 Avian embryo development. MAFF Technical Bulletin No. 23. HMSO, London

MAFF 1973 Incubation and hatchery practice. MAFF Bulletin 148. HMSO, London

MAFF 1974 Testing of eggs for quality. MAFF Technical Bulletin 28. HMSO, London

MAFF 1982 Egg quality on the farm. MAFF/ADAS Booklet 2382. HMSO, London

MAFF 1982 Environment for laying stock. MAFF/ADAS Booklet 2381. HMSO, London

MAFF 1984 Manual of veterinary investigation laboratory techniques, vols 1 and 2. MAFF/ADAS reference books 389 and 390. HMSO, London

McMullin P F 2004 A pocket guide to poultry health and disease. 5M Publishing, Sheffield

Pattison M (ed) 1993 The health of poultry. Longman, Harlow, Essex

Randall C J 1991 A colour atlas of diseases and disorders of the domestic fowl and turkey, 2nd edn. Wolfe Publishing, London

Saif Y, ed 2003 Diseases of poultry, 11th edn. Iowa State University Press, Ames.

Sainsbury D 1992 Poultry health and management, 3rd edn. Blackwell Scientific, Oxford

Turkey embryo development chart: obtainable from Nicolas Turkey Breeding Farms, 19449 Riverside Drive, PO Box Y, Sonoma, CA, 95476–1209, USA

A range of useful information and links may be accessed at: www.poultry-health.com/

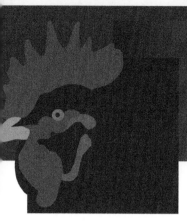

CHAPTER 3

Chris Morrow

Laboratory investigation to support health programmes and disease diagnosis

Laboratory tests are commonly performed by field veterinarians to confirm or exclude diagnoses, to demonstrate freedom from infection (for health programmes or export certification) or to monitor responses to vaccinations. The type of test chosen depends on what is being demonstrated (evidence of the expected infection, toxin or lack or excess of a specific nutrient) and status of the flock being tested. Further, there is little use in testing unless you are going to take action based on the results.

ANTIBODY TESTING

Samples should be taken in tubes suitable for avian blood to clot and then held at room temperature overnight before separation of serum from the clot. Samples should be tested immediately for agglutination tests and then stored for further tests if these are not going to be performed immediately. Routine serological sampling with storage of sera for the life of a flock can provide a useful resource for retrospective analysis and allow comparison between affected and unaffected flocks.

Use of antibody tests to support diagnosis

Demonstration of antibody simply shows that a bird has been in contact with a particular antigen at some time in the past. It does not prove that a clinical syndrome is caused by the organism

Table 3.1 Factors influencing the approach to serological testing of poultry

REASON FOR SEROLOGICAL TEST	NO. OF TEST SAMPLES	ADVANTAGES	LIMITATIONS	FURTHER COMMENT
Diagnosis	10–60	Confirmation of infection supporting diagnosis	Seroconversion must be demonstrated. Timing of sampling is important	Serological variants may give problems in some areas. A back-up test based on a different system (e.g. virus isolation) is useful for confirmation
Health programmes (and export certification)	60	Confirmation of freedom from infection	Tests were often developed to monitor SPF flocks. D-SP* and D-SN† may not be suitable for testing field samples	Testing is usually designed to give 95% confidence that infection of 5% of the animals would be detected
Vaccination response	20–30	Confirmation of vaccine 'take' and prediction of maternal antibody	Wild-strain infection cannot be differentiated from vaccine response. Blocking ELISAs are not intrinsically good at quantifying antibody	Serum antibody is not always correlated with protection. Mean titres and some estimates of variation are needed. Graphical represen-tation of data is useful

*D-SP Diagnostic specificity: the proportion of known infected animals that test positive in the assay. †D-SN Diagnostic sensitivity: the proportion of known uninfected animals that test negative in the assay; ELISA, enzyme-linked immunosorbent assay; SPF, specific pathogen-free.

associated with the particular antigen. For example vaccinated flocks will have antibody from vaccination. Natural infection could also have occurred earlier and not be associated with the clinical syndrome. Paired serum samples (taken at the time of clinical disease and then in con-valescence) provide the most convincing evidence of seroconversion and association of an agent with the clinical signs being seen.

The number of samples needed to be taken will depend on the reason for testing and test characteristics. This is summarized in Table 3.1.

For diagnosis, 10–60 samples per group should be taken. Smaller numbers can be taken from marked birds during paired sampling as demonstration of the seroconversion of individual birds is then possible. More samples are required to show an overall decrease in the number of seronegative birds. The testing of broilers for seroconversion is difficult because of their short life span. Some birds may be grown on to allow clearer seroconversion to be demonstrated or another testing methodology could be used. This is particularly a problem when determining the *Mycoplasma* status.

For confirmation of freedom from infection a maximum of 60 samples per group is needed to give 95% confidence that infection of 5% of the animals would be detected. In this case the observation of one positive result defines the group as infected. In some tests such as *Avian leucosis virus* J-strain (ALV-J) antibody there is an increasing rate of false-positives with age of the flock and therefore the number of positive reactions is usually assessed from 90 samples and interpreted with age and confirmed by virus isolation. This sort of testing can be part of an eradication programme. Day-old chicks and young birds will also have maternal antibody to various agents and this needs to be considered as it may be from vaccination of parent stock rather than wild strain infection.

For vaccination responses 20–30 sera per group are usually tested. The aim is to make the variation of titres observed reflect the variation in response of the birds in the flock rather than the number of samples tested. Repeated testing throughout the life of the flock to monitor vaccination titres is important in some areas for agents such as infectious bursal disease (IBD) and can be used to assess whether revaccination during lay is required.

Serological test interpretation

Serological tests need to be continuously validated (Jacobson 1996) and performance characteristics of the test monitored in the laboratory doing the test. It is not enough that serological test kits are registered – they must be suitable for testing the target population. The usefulness of a diagnostic test will vary according to the infection status of the animals being tested and the cost of testing versus the value of the information. It is usually considered that specificity is more important than sensitivity for surveillance to demonstrate the absence of infection. For diagnosis, sensitivity and repeatability are considered more important than specificity. During eradication programmes, sensitivity is more important early on but, as eradication comes closer, specificity becomes more important. For following vaccination responses repeatability becomes more important than sensitivity. For epidemiological studies sensitivity may be the most important feature of a test.

When serological testing kits are purchased, the manufacturer supplies a criterion for interpreting the test and this may or may not be optimal for the purpose and population being tested. For example, enzyme-linked immunosorbent assay (ELISA) tests for chickens may not be suitable for testing turkey sera because the antichicken-immunoglobulin antibody does not usually react with turkey antibodies.

The diagnostic specificity (D-SP) is the proportion of known infected animals that test positive in a test while the diagnostic sensitivity (D-SN) is the proportion of known uninfected animals that test negative in a test. Combining the D-SN, the D-SP and knowledge of the infection status allows an estimate of the predictive values of a positive (PV^+) or negative (PV^-) result. For example, the PV^+ of one positive reticuloendotheliosis virus ELISA test result in a sample of 60 sera tested may be 0.1: i.e. only once in 10 times will such a result detect an infected flock, the other nine times it will be a false positive. It is not possible to make informed predictions about the infection status of a flock without information on the PV^+ (or PV^-) of that test in the particular population being examined. Inconclusive testing results usually prompt retesting of the flock in 1–2 weeks or the application of alternative tests. In this time false positives may disappear or seroconversion may make the test result more conclusive. During this time the flock may have to be quarantined to prevent the putative infection from being spread to other flocks.

Routine monitoring programmes need to be carefully designed to complement vaccination programmes. For example, *Mycoplasma* serology testing should not be undertaken within 2 weeks of vaccination as this is a well recognized cause of false positives in agglutination and ELISA tests. Enough time must be given between administration of a vaccine and checking the response. In general this period is at least 4 weeks. Where health monitoring testing is regularly performed it is possible to use combined ELISAs to screen sera (for example, a combined *Mycoplasma gallisepticum* and *Mycoplasma synoviae*) and then further test sera that are positive in individual tests. This offers a considerable saving in laboratory resources and time.

Serum banks are useful for retrospective studies and allow one to evaluate whether the infection status of flocks has really changed or whether the test has changed. In the laboratory, calibration of 'working' internal standard sera should be carried out and such sera should be regularly tested. This will allow the identification of changes in the test that may be associated with manufacture or performance of the test. Laboratories should follow good laboratory practice and participate in quality assurance programmes (aiming to maintain precision, repeatability, reproducibility and accuracy).

Yolk testing for antibody is attractive in investigations as the sample is easily obtained from the farm with fewer problems with biosecurity. Immunoglobulin (IgG-like) is the main antibody class in yolk. ELISA tests need to be validated for the use of yolk-derived samples.

OTHER LABORATORY TESTS

Histopathology

Histopathology is a useful tool in the initial investigation of problems. Samples (1 cm³ maximum) should be taken from carefully selected cases usually into buffered formal saline. This test can identify the pathognomonic changes that occur in some diseases such as in fowl pox and infectious laryngotracheitis infection and make definitive diagnosis of many tumour problems (Table 3.2). Also, with other conditions histopathology can be very useful in suggesting possible causes to be investigated. Samples from long-standing cases usually have more definitive gross and histopathological changes and sample selection can influence the success of the investigation. These specimens are usually not the specimen of choice for further microbiological (especially virological) examination. Often it is necessary to plan sampling to optimize the isolation of bacteria and virus after the initial pathological investigation.

The necessity to confirm serological and pathological observations when coming to a diagnosis depends on many factors. These include how common an infection is in the area, the implications of finding the suspected organism and the cost and availability of laboratory support to confirm the presence of the organism. In general if the initial investigation suggests an important agent that has not been or has only rarely been observed in the flock then isolation should be undertaken.

Virus isolation

Isolation of many avian viruses is carried out in fertile eggs. The route of inoculation of the eggs depends on the agent suspected. *Avian influenza virus* (AIV) and *Newcastle disease virus* (NDV) can be grown in the allantoic cavity of fertile eggs and preliminary screening is done by checking for haemagglutination activity. Other agents, including other avian paramyxoviruses and EDS-76 virus, also have haemagglutinating activity so further characterization of putative isolates is necessary. Some viruses can be isolated and identified by primary cell culture, cell culture or tissue culture. Others require direct electron microscopy or a variety of other virological techniques.

Isolation for ubiquitous infections such as *Marek's disease virus* (MDV) is often not attempted. The reasoning is that MDV will be in the birds whether they have tumours or not and current technology to differentiate vaccine strains from field strains is not robust. Finally, further investigation often involves bird experimentation, which takes a long time and is expensive. Practically, MDV isolation is not attempted unless further *in vivo* characterization of the virus is planned.

The isolation of infectious agents is often very useful to provide the materials for epidemiological studies and in some cases to include in autogenous bacterins or new vaccines. One requirement of isolation techniques is that the sample taken must contain the agent. The site of sampling must be where the agent is and the agent must be there at the time of sampling.

Table 3.2 Current preferred methods for investigating some poultry infections

ORGANISM	TO CONFIRM INFECTION STATUS (OR VACCINE RESPONSE)	DISEASE INVESTIGATION	FURTHER TESTING TO PROVIDE MORE INFORMATION	COMMENT
Adenovirus	ELISA, AGID	Histopathology Virus isolation and PCR	Serotyping Sequence comparison	Adenoviruses are part of the normal intestinal flora of young birds
AE	ELISA	Histopathology Paired sera samples to demonstrate seroconversion	Virus isolation or antigen detection	
AIV	HI, AGID	Virus isolation Antigen demonstration and PCR	PCR and sequence analysis, IVPI pathotyping	ELISAs appear to have low specificity (5–10% false positives in field sera)
ALV	GSA (p27) antigen detection* ELISA	Histopathology of tumours	Virus isolation	*Not good for sera (Payne et al. 1993) Genotype of tissue culture must be suitable and defined for VI
APV	ELISA	PCR	Sequence analysis and virus isolation	Blocking ELISAs are not good for quantifying antibody
Avian hepevirus (HSS and BLS)	AGID	PCR	Sequence analysis	
Avibacterium (Haemophilus) paragallinarum	HI test	Culture of early cases	PCR	HI test is serotype specific
Campylobacter carriage or carcass contamination	Microbial culture using selective techniques		MLST	
Escherichia coli	ELISA	PCR	Virus isolation	Blocking ELISAs are not good for quantifying antibody
Escherichia coli	Not applicable	Microbiological culture and serotyping	MLST	*E. coli* is a normal inhabitant of the intestinal tract of birds
EDS-76	HI, ELISA			

Table 3.2 (continued)

ORGANISM	TO CONFIRM INFECTION STATUS (OR VACCINE RESPONSE)	DISEASE INVESTIGATION	FURTHER TESTING TO PROVIDE MORE INFORMATION	COMMENT
Enteric viruses	Negative staining Electron microscopy		Tissue culture	If it can be seen on EM then it probably will not be able to be grown and vice versa
IB	ELISA	PCR and sequencing	HI for serotype specific assays	
IBD	ELISA	Virus isolation and PCR Histopathology		Antibody levels have been used to predict broiler vaccination timing
ILT	SN, ELISA	Histopathology and virus isolation	REA has been of variable utility for epidemiological studies	In some areas field outbreaks are caused by descendants of vaccine strains
Marek's disease	Serology only applicable for testing SPF flocks	Histopathology of tumours and nerves	PCR Real time-PCR	Further investigation requires virus isolation and bird challenge experiments
Mycoplasma gallisepticum	RSA, ELISA	RSA, ELISA, PCR and culture	Sequence analysis for epidemiological studies	False positives associated with recent MS infection and oil-based vaccine administration
Mycoplasma synoviae	RSA, ELISA	RSA, ELISA, PCR and culture	Sequence analysis for epidemiological studies (e.g. vlhA)	False positives associated with oil-based vaccine administration
Mycoplasma iowae	Culture	PCR	No serological test available	
NDV	HI, ELISA	Virus isolation	PCR and sequence analysis, ICPI	Other APMVs can be assayed by homologous HI tests. APMV3 can cause HI cross-reactions with NDV
Pasteurella multocida	ELISA for vaccination responses	Culture	Serotyping	
Pox virus infection	Histology and virus isolation		Bird inoculation studies may be needed. PCR for REV contamination	

Reovirus	ELISA	Virus isolation		Reoviruses are part of the normal intestinal flora of young birds
REV	ELISA		PCR and virus isolation	Many REV-seropositive flocks have no clinical evidence of infection
Rotavirus		EM and PAGE of RNA extracted from faeces		
Salmonella spp.	Microbial enrichment and selective culture (operating at limit of sensitivity)	Microbial culture (including without enrichment)	Serology, PCR and modern antigen-based detection systems	SP and SG are non-motile and might not be detected by selective techniques
Staphylococcus spp.		Bacterial culture	MLST	

AE, avian encephalomyelitis; AGID, agar gel immunodiffusion; AIV, *Avian influenza virus*; ALV, *Avian leukosis virus*; APMV, *Avian paramyxovirus*; APV, *Avian pneumovirus*; BLS, big liver spleen disease; CAV, *Chicken anaemia virus*; EDS, egg drop syndrome; ELISA, enzyme-linked immunosorbent assay; EM, electron microscopy; GSA, group-specific antigen; HI, haemagglutination inhibition; HSS, hepatitis–splenomegaly syndrome; IB, infectious bronchitis; IBD, infectious bursal disease; ICPI, intracerebral pathogenicity index; ILT, infectious laryngotracheitis; IVPI, intravenous pathogenicity index; MDV, *Marek's disease virus*; MLST, multilocus sequence typing; MS, *Mycoplasma synoviae*; NDV, *Newcastle disease virus*; PCR, polymerase chain reaction; REA, restriction endonuclease analysis; REV, *Reticuloendotheliosis virus*; RSA, rapid serum agglutination; SG, *Salmonella gallinarum*; SP, *Salmonella pullorum*; SPF, specific pathogen-free; VI, virus isolation.

Humoral antibody, in contrast, will record the response of the bird with an agent irrespective of which anatomical site in the bird was infected.

Polymerase chain reaction

The use of polymerase chain reaction (PCR) testing to demonstrate the nucleic acid of infectious agents is becoming more common. Sampling is planned to optimize the chance of the organism being found, as for virus isolation or bacterial culture. The sample must be taken from a site where the agent is present. Samples can often be allowed to dry or inactivate and can still be suitable for PCR. Inactivation is typically done by placing the sample on FTA paper (Whatman, http://www.whatman.com/) and then put into a multibarrier bag and stored at room temperature until testing. Another method for tracheal samples is to use cotton swabs and microwave these in an oven for 5 s. Care must be taken using PCR not to cross-contaminate the specimens during sampling or in the laboratory.

Feed

Feed sampling is an art and requires careful planning. Retention feed samples can be useful and in the case of broilers should not be discarded until after the flock is finished. Assaying for manganese is a cheap preliminary method of checking whether premix has been added. Toxicology investigations in the laboratory are usually very specific for the toxin being investigated. Mycotoxins may degrade with storage and this should be considered when interpreting the results of testing. If a feed problem is suspected, changing the feed may give useful diagnostic information and prevent further damage to the birds.

Testing compounded feed for *Salmonella* contamination is insensitive compared with feeding to chickens, but positive results are indicative of gross contamination. Negative results do not mean that the feed is uninfected. Testing raw materials may increase sensitivity and provide evidence for epidemiological studies identifying the source of *Salmonella* infections.

FURTHER CHARACTERIZATION OF AGENTS

The questions under consideration as disease investigations implicate a causal agent are: Where did this infection come from (epidemiological source)? or Why is a disease occurring when a previously successful vaccination or prevention programme is in place? Obviously, there can be problems with vaccine administration: perhaps the challenge is overwhelming or the agent may have changed in some way. For instance, bacteria may have acquired resistance to a previously useful antibiotic. To help differentiate between possible causes, further laboratory work may be performed. In general, epidemiological studies are best undertaken with genome-based analysis. Protection studies are best undertaken using systems that measure the ability of vaccines to provide protection against challenge (so-called protectotype characterization). Other laboratory classification systems may correlate well with these classifications for certain agents and be more readily available, for example, serotyping, subtyping, etc.

MICROBIOLOGICAL TESTING

Bacteriological investigation is an important support for diagnosis and evaluation of the effectiveness of hygiene treatments and biosecurity barriers. The efficacy of cleaning, disinfection and fumigation against all infectious agents can be inferred from total viable counts (TVCs) of bacteria subject to known limitations. New, more rapid methods from food preparation industries are being applied. Commonly these are based on measuring adenosine triphosphate or protein on surfaces as a measure of cleanliness.

MANAGEMENT OF LABORATORY RESULTS

Laboratory information management systems are available for the management of laboratory results as part of flock histories. This allows checking for compliance with planned testing schedules and systematic analysis over time. The following of flock results may allow the identification of changes in test characteristics and help in the selection of vaccines and setting of standards. Monitoring programmes should be designed to fit together with production and vaccination programmes. For example, vaccination of birds for avian encephalomyelitis (AE) at 8 weeks with serological testing at 12 weeks would allow revaccination of nonresponding flocks at 14 weeks and subsequent rechecking well before the onset of lay. Alternatively, all flocks could be vaccinated twice for AE by 12 weeks of age before testing at 16 weeks. The cost of vaccination and testing and the cost of an AE outbreak in lay needs to be analysed when choosing which strategy to adopt.

Knowledge of the test results in affected and unaffected flocks (matched for age, genotype, etc.) is useful, especially when using a new test. This can be aided by the submission of split samples to multiple laboratories (ring tests), submission of split samples to the same laboratory (to test repeatability within one submission and between submissions) and the submission of samples from known uninfected and positively infected flocks. Similar to serological testing laboratories, all laboratories need to quality-control all tests, including PCR testing (especially to identify cross-contamination), histopathology and bacteriological testing (again to identify cross-contamination). For laboratories, participation in ring tests, quality management systems and a healthy scepticism are required.

Laboratories are not infallible and the field veterinarian needs to consider characteristics of the test being used, the precautions against cross-contamination or other laboratory mistake, alternative technologies to confirm the observation, response to therapies and the cost of decisions in coming to a diagnosis.

Finally, syndromes similar to infectious diseases may be the cause of the signs and the reason why no agent can be detected. For example, poor management may cause broiler uniformity problems. Head trauma from male excluder feeding grills may mimic swollen head syndrome. Fine mash diets may cause oral lesions that can be confused with T-2 toxin lesions. Low light intensity during rearing of heavy broiler breeders may mimic reovirus tendon problems. There are many other examples. The reason why a flock may be negative to a diagnostic test could be that it is not infected with that agent. It is up to the field veterinarian to synthesize all the findings (including response to therapies) in coming to a final diagnosis.

REFERENCES

Canon R M, Roe R T 1982 Livestock disease surveys: a field manual for veterinarians. Australian Government Publishing Service, Canberra

Jacobson R H 1996 Principles of validation of diagnostic assays for infectious diseases. In: OIE Manual. OIE, Paris

Payne L N, Gillespie A M, Howes K 1993 Unsuitability of chicken sera for detection of exogenous ALV by the group-specific antigen ELISA. Vet Rec 132: 555–557

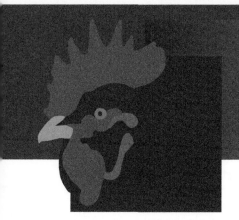
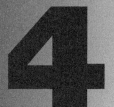

CHAPTER 4

Stephen A. Lister

Biosecurity in poultry management

INTRODUCTION

The impact of disease on poultry production is one of the major limiting factors to successful performance in the poultry industry.

The economics of that production lends itself to larger sites and more dense populations in specific or limited geographical areas. This has many advantages in reducing the costs of live haul, movement of feed and equipment, and flock supervision. However, such densely populated poultry areas present the industry with a daunting challenge in preventing the introduction and persistence of significant disease threats or at least limiting their adverse effects on successful production.

These developments have led to the development of the new 'science' of biosecurity. The term has received various definitions over the last few years but the main philosophy of the approach is to apply this to any procedure or practice that prevents or limits the exposure of a flock to the adverse effects of disease-causing organisms. This may include general on-farm hygiene requirements, vaccination programmes, medication regimes, disease monitoring and the effective use of disinfectants.

In many ways the approach is much more an art than a science, tipping the balance in favour of the birds rather than the bugs.

However, the successful implementation of a biosecurity programme requires considerable technical input. Biosecurity can be directed towards specific targeted organisms or a more generic disease control strategy. While the scope and impact of biosecurity measures may be obvious for large-scale poultry production, its significance for small poultry-keeping situations must not be overlooked; either in their own right or as sources of infection for large commercial flocks.

Table 4.1 Hazard analysis and critical control point (HACCP) principles on the poultry farm

1. Hazard analysis	Conduct a hazard analysis to identify potential hazards that could occur anywhere in the process
2. Critical control points (CCPs)	Identify the CCPs, i.e. those points in the process where potential hazards could occur and then be prevented and/or controlled
3. Critical limits	Establish critical limits or tolerances for each CCP
4. Monitoring	Establish CCP monitoring to ensure each CCP stays within its limits
5. Correction	Establish corrective procedures if monitoring identifies a CCP outside its limit
6. Recording	Establish and maintain an effective recording system
7. Verification	Ongoing audit and review of the HACCP plan, new CCPs, existing limits for existing CCPs and ongoing sampling to ensure compliance

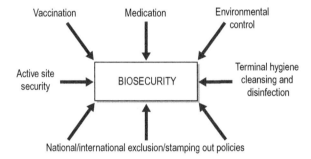

Fig. 4.1 Biosecurity management practices.

Practical biosecurity on the farm requires an accurate assessment of disease challenges and their impact on production. Hazard analysis and critical control point (HACCP) principles are frequently used as a starting point in such assessments (Table 4.1) but practical implementation of targeted interventions is the secret of success, using properly informed risk assessment and risk management.

As a result, an effective biosecurity programme is so much more than just a printed cleansing and disinfection procedure. The concept of biosecurity covers a whole range of procedures and interventions that can, when effectively combined, reduce the impact of disease (Fig. 4.1).

CONCEPTS OF BIOSECURITY

This concept starts at the genetic level. Rapidly growing poultry strains have a relatively naive immune system and much current genetic improvement is aimed at improving intrinsic disease resistance in modern breeds. The focus is on liveability and birds that may be refractory to certain disease challenges. This can be achieved in a variety of ways. Much recent activity has been in developing a more robust immune system to respond generally to a range of disease challenges. Other approaches are aimed at the development of specific resistance markers for specific diseases (e.g. Marek's disease). Future work will attempt to focus more on body systems, such as the respiratory tract to reduce the impact of respiratory pathogens and the gastrointestinal tract to strengthen intestinal integrity.

A second major area relates to environmental control and management. Here, as in many other areas of biosecurity, stockmanship and effective husbandry methods are of paramount importance. This requires the ability of the stockperson to identify health and ill health in flocks under his/her care and respond accordingly. Much of this response requires an assessment of environmental effects, especially in the areas of air quality and litter condition as well as the provision of high-quality feed and clean drinking water. Optimal environmental control reduces insults to the respiratory tract by noxious factors such as ammonia, carbon dioxide, excessive humidity and dust but also helps to excrete unwanted microbiological loads from the house.

Vaccination and medication programmes are very significant contributors to an effective biosecurity programme and are an excellent illustration of the importance of an integrated approach. As an example, efficient vaccines are available for *Salmonella* control but their efficacy is enhanced by an effective strategy of cleansing and disinfection and vermin control to reduce overall challenge pressure and allow the vaccine to work most effectively.

Another significant area is where the vaccination programme is delivered in a coordinated manner designed to prevent generalized infection with agents active in a particular geographical area and contribute to an effective control strategy for a whole region. Examples here are infectious bronchitis, Newcastle disease, Gumboro disease and avian pneumovirus infection. As with many of the other areas, vaccines must be properly applied, in accordance with manufacturers' directions and on the basis of expected challenges, based on accurate diagnostic monitoring.

Medications administered at strategic times can prevent clinical and subclinical effects of secondary disease challenges. This may be with conventional antibiotics or newer developments such as phage treatments. Medications must be used under strict veterinary guidance with clear demonstration of responsible use and should be seen as an adjunct rather than alternative to other biosecurity measures. This requires accurate diagnosis of targeted pathogens, pretreatment testing and appropriate use of products with a narrow spectrum but known efficacy for the target organisms.

The final and major component of any biosecurity programme remains the effective use and application of cleansers, sanitizers and disinfectants and this will be considered in detail later in this chapter. The aim is to use the right product applied in the right way at the right concentration and as part of a complementary programme.

THE NEED FOR BIOSECURITY

The range of disease-causing organisms requiring control vary in their type and impact. At one end of the scale such measures can be the basis for national and international emergency disease control strategies implemented or enforced by national governments. This is clearly important in the control of lethal, highly contagious diseases such as avian influenza and Newcastle disease. However, similar procedures are essential in successful disease control in many other areas, including:

- Control of highly virulent diseases of significant economic impact at a national level (e.g. Gumboro disease, infectious bronchitis, avian pneumovirus infections)
- Reduction of challenge by ubiquitous 'common' organisms known to reduce productivity (e.g. coccidiosis, *Escherichia coli*)
- Reduction or elimination of immunosuppressive diseases that render birds more susceptible to other diseases or environmental effects (e.g. Marek's disease, *Chick anaemia virus* (CAV), Gumboro disease, *Haemorrhagic enteritis virus* (HAV))
- Reduction of contamination of poultry and poultry products with agents of public health significance (e.g. *Salmonella, Campylobacter*).

With this broad requirement for control measures aimed at a range of pathogens there is a need for a focused programme of interventions. This requires a detailed knowledge of the diseases and infectious agents any biosecurity programme is attempting to control. There is a direct relationship between where that infectious agent multiplies in the bird and its mode of transmission from one bird to another, or from one site to another.

- **Respiratory disease organisms** are usually spread via respiratory secretions through aerosols, following sneezing and coughing. Hence, while effective disinfection of all contaminated equipment may be important, the use of strategic vaccination may also be necessary.
- **Enteric diseases** are spread via droppings and litter such that control of faecal spread and effective terminal cleansing and disinfection at depletion are the critical areas.
- **Vertically transmitted infections**, such as mycoplasmas and some *Salmonella* serotypes, require an approach that encompasses the breeder farm, egg hygiene, hatchery hygiene, growing farm procedures, transport and all associated equipment.
- **Highly persistent or resistant infectious agents** (predominantly viral) may require specific measures to control residual site and environmental contamination, and knowledge of disinfectants of known and proven efficacy against the target organisms.

VETERINARY HEALTH AND WELFARE PLANNING

Therefore, although there is no 'one case fits all' strategy for all farms or integrations, a basic approach working as a partnership with a range of technical experts, stockmen and veterinarians can develop an evolving biosecurity programme. This should be formalized as part of the farm veterinary health and welfare plan.

This health plan should be seen as a working document that formalizes agreed actions and procedures. The plan should be a practical document that accurately reflects what is done at the farm level, how it is done, what the aims and targets are and how these will be audited.

In setting baselines and targets for such a programme it is essential to know which disease-causing organisms are present in poultry stock at the breeder and commercial level. A programme should be in place to monitor this, so that the veterinarian and producer can be aware of what challenges are occurring but also to audit the success (or otherwise) of the biosecurity interventions. This is an example of a practical implementation of HACCP principles.

Monitoring and setting baselines

Effective disease monitoring may be achieved by:

1. Regular monitoring of all performance data on farm, including:
   a. Mortality
   b. Culling rate
   c. Daily liveweight gain
   d. Evenness
   e. Food conversion ratio (FCR)
   f. European production efficiency factor (EPEF)
   g. Egg production
   h. Egg quality
   i. Fertility
   j. Hatchability

2. Assessment of processing plant data for levels of:
   a. Carcass damage
   b. Reject rates and criteria
   c. Downgrading
3. Sampling and screening for disease-causing agents:
   a. Serology
      i. Monitor response to vaccination programme
      ii. During a disease outbreak
      iii. Terminal bloods to check exposure to disease agents
      iv. Regular monitoring to confirm freedom from specific organisms
   b. Post-mortem examinations:
      i. During a disease outbreak
      ii. Specific targeted lesion scoring (e.g. for subclinical coccidial challenge monitoring)
      iii. To assess skeletal development
      iv. To screen for subclinical indications of disease, e.g. intestinal damage, presence of parasites, air sac damage
   c. Other samples
      i. Polymerase chain reaction (PCR) swabs for viral/bacterial antigen detection
      ii. Faeces for worm egg count, coccidial challenge, *Salmonella* spp., *Campylobacter* spp.
      iii. Water – water quality testing
      iv. Tissues for virus isolation, residues of extraneous agents, carcass quality
   d. Wild birds and vermin
      i. Screening of reservoirs for disease threats, e.g. avian influenza, *Mycoplasma* spp., *Salmonella* spp.
4. Communication
   a. Awareness of disease challenges in rearing stock
   b. Early warning of disease challenges in other farms in an area
   c. National and international communication on disease threats.

Once baselines are set for disease challenges and trends over time, together with good intelligence as to what major disease risks may be introduced into a particular area, then the veterinary health plan can start to lay down guidance as to what is needed as an effective biosecurity programme. This must be laid down in a logical manner, with aims and objectives produced that are on the one hand effective, but are also able to be achieved under practical conditions.

COMPONENTS OF A BIOSECURITY PROGRAMME

The components of a biosecurity programme can be split into three broad areas. These are:

- **Procedural biosecurity** – this is where the concepts are outlined into an overall strategy of what is trying to be achieved. This may be a multilayered programme such that there is an overarching general disease control programme, to which may be added specific HACCP-type programmes for specific diseases or problems. A good example of one of these specific aspects might be a *Campylobacter* reduction programme. The procedural concepts should outline the strategy and the decision-making procedure and, importantly, identify who within the organization has responsibility for the procedures, their implementation and their audit.
- **Physical biosecurity** – this is the main foundation for the programme. It should consider the structural requirements, farm layouts, specification for all equipment and facilities on farm (e.g. barrier hygiene, showers, provision of wheel and equipment sprays, footdips, structural house design and layout, etc.).

- **Operational biosecurity** – this is where all the procedures are put into practice. The procedural programme should clearly identify personnel responsible for all areas of the operational programme, including production of appropriate paperwork and work recording systems such that it is possible to audit whether what is laid down is actually taking place in practice. Again, there is the requirement for this audit to feed back constantly into the procedural biosecurity strategy.

Procedural biosecurity

Although procedural biosecurity should be based on practical common sense procedures, the use of HACCP principles offers the ability to review all risks and critical control points at the farm and company level and acts as a framework on which to build effective control strategies. Such a system can be developed for small or large sites, or companies operating multiple sites. The complexity of any HACCP system will reflect the risks identified. For disease control, critical control points (CCPs) are the areas or weak points where pathogens may enter the system. Once identified, then procedures can be put in place to reduce or eliminate the hazard posed by these weak points. Hazard analysis is the starting point and can be aimed at general pathogen reduction or at specific threats such as avian influenza, Gumboro disease or *Campylobacter*. The CCPs can then be listed. Examples of the most significant examples for most pathogens are as follows:

- Personnel
- Other poultry
- Vehicles
- Equipment
- Feed
- Litter
- Water
- Vermin
- Insects/beetles
- Wild birds
- Residual site contamination.

Once these have been identified the next stage is to set limits to which the hazard must be reduced. For examples such as avian influenza the target might be total elimination or avoidance, whereas for organisms such as *Campylobacter* targets might be set for reduction in incidence over certain time frames. In assessing whether targets for critical limits have been met there must be effective monitoring of incidence of the organisms under scrutiny over time. On the basis of this monitoring the causes of any noncompliance or failure to achieve targets should be identified and corrective actions put in place. Records must be kept of this HACCP programme with ongoing verification and feedback of success or failure, such that targeted progress can be made. The further aspect of physical biosecurity is aimed at reducing the existence or impact of CCPs, while operational biosecurity procedures should outline the practical and operational steps taken to address known CCPs.

Physical biosecurity

1. Location. Although this may be on a wish list that is not actually achievable, the aim should be to locate farms as well dispersed as possible. A minimum acceptable distance between poultry farms should be 500 m, and preferably 1 km. Consideration should also be given to prevailing wind direction when planning units in relatively close proximity, in

order to minimize the risk of airborne infection. When siting breeder or grandparent farms, this distance should be extended to 8–10 km wherever possible. This should be adequate to limit likely movement of viral diseases spread by aerosol or dust vectors. Increasingly, poultry are sited in densely populated poultry areas, either for historical or logistical reasons. Some degree of compromise is always necessary and this indicates why in some geographical locations there may be added dependence on other aspects of the biosecurity programme. These considerations should extend to the likelihood of poultry litter being spread on agricultural land in the area. It may not always be possible to have control over types of stock or biosecurity measures of third-party producers in a region. As a result, it has to be accepted that airborne respiratory viral challenges will be a feature of the disease load in many areas. In some countries there has been government consideration and restriction of stocking of poultry farms in a particular region in an attempt to break the cycle of infection with highly contagious diseases such as avian influenza.

2. Avoid building sites near waterways, ponds or lakes used by migratory water fowl. This has relevance for a number of diseases but most notably for avian influenza and Newcastle disease, where migrating waterfowl or seabirds may act as potent vectors to introduce disease into a novel area, while themselves showing no clinical signs or illness. If there is local surface water, this should not be used as the source of drinking water for commercial poultry, again because of likely contamination from wild birds with viral pathogens.

3. Avoid putting birds on range, as they will be susceptible to contamination from wild birds and will attract vermin. There is a balance here, with increased interest in the perceived welfare advantages of more extensive production systems, against the risks posed to such flocks, either on their own account or as a focus and source of infection for housed flocks in a given geographical area. Again, flocks which must be kept under such systems require more rigorous actions in other areas of the biosecurity programme to compensate.

4. Locate houses away from major roads that handle high volumes of poultry vehicles (feed lorries, live haul vehicles, etc.).

5. There should be effective waste disposal and removal of used litter as far away from the site as possible. Factories able to burn poultry litter as a source of energy are a valuable method of reducing the infectious agent load in a particular geographical area.

6. The areas around and between houses should be constructed of materials and surfaces that can be cleansed and disinfected to reduce the transmission of all organic material on vehicle, tyres, boots, etc., from the area outside the house into the house. Areas around houses should be kept clear of vegetation to avoid harbouring vermin. Kerbed aprons will help prevent washing of contaminated debris on to surrounding land.

7. Locate poultry sites in well-drained areas to avoid standing water.

8. Use potable drinking water with a low total viable count.

9. House design and site layout should help with the implementation of the biosecurity requirements. There should be a secure perimeter fence such that there is a controlled entry point for all visitors. An amenity block should contain protective clothing and boots as a minimum, but include shower facilities wherever possible for all visitors who must enter the site.

10. Plan the layout of the site to enable feed to be blown into silos/bins on site from outside the perimeter fence, ensuring that feed vehicles can be excluded from the site.

11. Where vehicles must enter a site, consider provision of wheel immersion baths and pressure washing facilities.

Operational biosecurity

The use of HACCP principles should identify all inputs into a site and enable a structured operational procedure to be put in place to ensure that all such inputs are controlled and their impact minimized. These critical control points should be identified by the procedural biosecurity programme. The following are some of the major critical control points to consider in any biosecurity programme.

People

This includes employees, servicemen, lorry drivers, vaccination crews, vets, etc.

1. Staff movements should be as limited as possible. This should be a general consideration but must be strictly adhered to when the disease situation on a particular site or area has deteriorated.
2. Exclude all unauthorized persons. Casual visitors should not be given access to sites. All visitors must make themselves known to site personnel and give details of previous visits. If there are any concerns about the health status of any visitor or previous sites visited they should be excluded from the site. All visitors must be expected to follow the site biosecurity procedures.
3. All visitors must complete an on-site visitors book to allow tracing in the event of a disease outbreak. Wherever possible, visitors should not have visited other poultry sites in the preceding 48–72 h. This is especially necessary at the commercial breeder level and above. Where such downtime is not possible the number of sites visited in a day must be limited and the visits must move from younger to older birds visited through the day.
4. Control site traffic to a minimum. Where possible, all vehicles should be excluded from the site and all visitors should enter on foot through the perimeter fencing, preferably after showering.
5. For vehicles requiring access to the site (e.g. for delivering shavings, chicks, equipment, feed and live bird haulage) there should be facilities for spray disinfection of vehicle wheels and wheel arches situated at the entrance. Without exception, all such visitors should observe standard operating procedures on vehicle cleansing and the use of protective clothing.
6. Any equipment brought on site for use by contractors (e.g. tools, ladders, vermin bait, bait boxes, etc.) should not be contaminated with dust or organic material from sites visited previously. Where possible, dedicated site equipment for use by such personnel should be stored on each farm. Where this is not possible effective cleansing and disinfection should take place before use. All contractors should keep the inside of their vehicles clean and disinfected to reduce contamination or spread on any equipment.
7. All visitors to sites should be provided with adequate protective clothing as clean or disposable boiler suits, footwear and headgear. All visitors should wash their hands prior to visiting birds and use effective hand sanitizers or handwashing facilities between houses on site.
8. When moving between houses on a site care should be taken to avoid contaminating protective clothing or boots from the environment around houses, e.g. avoid walking through standing water or areas with heavy faecal or soil contamination. Use footdips and clean boots with a brush between visits to separate houses.
9. For breeding farms, at least, a shower in, shower out facility must be provided and be used by all visitors.

Poultry

1. Incoming poultry to all sites should be from high-health-status sources.
2. In this regard, the company should have a well-defined health monitoring and audit procedure for breeder supply flocks. This should extend to hatchery hygiene procedures with regular microbiological monitoring.
3. Where possible, multiage sites should be avoided, as this does not allow a natural break in pathogen build-up on site. Where this is not possible, staff on the farm should be dedicated to particular flocks or buildings. For high-value stock a period of quarantine away from other stock on site is advisable, with close clinical monitoring of birds during the quarantine period.
4. Disposal of on farm deaths/culls. On-site incineration prevents the need for removing potentially infected carcasses from the premises or bringing infection on to a site via personnel collecting carcasses from a number of sites. Where this is not possible, any collection system should observe all site biosecurity procedures.

Vehicles

A variety of vehicles visit poultry farms on a regular basis to deliver feed, shavings, staff, contractors, maintenance crews, catching and vaccination teams and equipment, and for carcass collection where necessary.

Wherever possible vehicles should be excluded from the site. Where they must enter the site they should be visibly clean. For vehicles such as feed lorries or for carcass collection, visits should be programmed to avoid moving from lower-health-status to high-health-status sites on the same day. It is desirable to have vehicles dedicated to breeder sites that do not visit commercial flocks. Where there is a known disease risk in an area or site, vehicles visiting such sites should then return to their depot or a third-party cleansing and disinfection facility prior to visiting any other site. Known contaminated sites (e.g. those with *Mycoplasma*) should be visited as a last delivery in the day and vehicles should then return to their depot for immediate cleansing and disinfection and be stood down overnight.

On arrival at the site drivers must make themselves known to site personnel. All drivers will be expected to follow the site's full biosecurity procedures. There should be no exceptions to this rule. Where possible, drivers should change into site protective clothing prior to entering the site.

The vehicle should be disinfected in line with facilities available on site, from disinfectant wheel sprays through to full wheel dips or total vehicle body spray washers.

Equipment

An assortment of equipment may need to move between sites, including egg flats, trolleys and transport crates and modules. Egg flats have been associated with the movement of red mite, *Salmonella* and even infectious laryngotracheitis between egg-laying sites. It is therefore advisable to use disposable 'once-only' trays that can be discarded after one use. Where this is not possible, reusable trays that can be effectively cleaned and disinfected, preferably colour-coded and dedicated to specific sites, may be used, but such cleaning requires very close supervision. Egg trolleys have been cited as vectors of *Salmonella* spp., and live bird transport equipment (and catchers) has been linked to the introduction of *Campylobacter* and *Salmonella* spp. to sites. Transport crates can be very difficult to clean and disinfect because of their design and heavy faecal contamination. In-line systems are usually present at the processing plant but require large amounts of water for full immersion. Systems that recycle wash water and have poor audit of dilution rates and proportioning of disinfectant can in fact increase the bacterial load on 'cleaned' crates and modules. Effective degreasers and the use of contraflow water systems without recycling followed by correct application of a suitable sanitizer are essential.

Feed

As previously discussed, feed lorries can be physical vectors for a number of pathogens. In addition, feed itself can become contaminated with a number of pathogens, predominantly bacterial (e.g. *Salmonella* spp., *E. coli*, *Clostridium* spp.) and fungal (*Aspergillus* spp. and mycotoxins). Contamination can take place via raw materials, during the production process, during storage or in transport vehicles. Feed mills should operate their own established HACCP system at all stages of production, coupled with microbiological monitoring of all raw materials and finished product. High-risk raw materials from known risk sources should be avoided. Heat treatment, extrusion procedures or the addition of organic acids or other acidifiers and mould inhibitors may be useful in reducing feed contamination.

Litter

There is considerable variation in the availability and use of different litter materials for poultry bedding. The best substrate is fresh, dry, white wood shavings. Historically, straw has been a popular material but through contamination during growing, at harvest and in storage microbiological build-up can occur. The most significant is probably fungal contamination with *Aspergillus fumigatus*. This can be dangerous through inhalation of fungal spores and young turkey poults and ducklings are probably the most sensitive species. This can lead to early 'brooder pneumonia' or later debilitating air sacculitis. Only high-quality straw should be used for these species, preferably dust-extracted, and should be avoided in brooding areas. Correct drying and storage after harvest is essential. Straw may also be used for breeder nest box material, where poor-quality material can lead to *Aspergillus* spp. contamination of eggs laid. This can lead to dissemination to the hatchery, leading to rots and bangers, reduced hatchability and brooder pneumonia in chicks exposed to spores on hatcher trays. Spraying of nest box material or eggs immediately after collection with suitable disinfectants can reduce the effects of contamination.

Used litter can be contaminated with a wide variety of pathogens – viral, bacterial and protozoal. As a result, effective disposal methods are recommended. In many agricultural situations used litter is spread on arable land and this can be a potential vector for spread of contagion. This is a special risk for Gumboro disease virus in densely populated broiler growing areas, and has also been implicated in spread of other more sensitive viruses, such as infectious bronchitis virus and avian pneumovirus. Where there are significant problems with a particular disease in a specific area it may be advisable to spray the litter from known infected premises with a virucidal disinfectant prior to removal from the house. Storage of turned litter under cover for up to 6 weeks will help to reduce microbiological load. Where possible, litter should be removed to specialist litter-burning sites for energy production. This reduces the environmental impact and nitrogen loading on agricultural land but also greatly reduces infection pressure in poultry growing areas.

Water

Water systems on poultry farms frequently harbour significant bacterial contamination. Bacteria in feed particles, dust, litter, faeces and nasal or mouth discharges can easily contaminate open drinkers such as bell drinkers. This can act as an efficient focus for infecting other birds. The other aspect that influences the quality of drinking water is the phenomenon of biofilms. It is easiest to understand a biofilm simply as a sludge in which bacteria can hide. They are, in fact, more complex structures involving a honeycomb of cracks and crevices in which bacteria thrive, with water percolating through supplying a source of oxygen and nutrients. The biofilm provides a haven for water-borne pathogens, protected from extremes of water chemistry, temperature and many disinfectants. Controlling the risk of water-borne infections must therefore be aimed at choosing a disinfectant that has proven efficacy against these organisms and is capable of penetrating or removing the protective biofilm. Historically, chlorine-based products have been advocated for water sanitization. However, laboratory and practical work on farm suggests that biofilms result in a more than 3000-fold increase in resistance of certain bacteria to chlorine.

Part of the solution has been to move to closed water systems. The introduction of nipple systems has been shown to have considerable health benefits and it is likely that this is associated with reducing bacterial load. A closely fitting lid to the header tank is also advantageous. The lid helps to exclude:

- Dust, which may carry microorganisms
- Light, which would encourage mould and algal growth
- Birds and rodents, which may carry many microorganisms.

However, even with such systems, water at the bird level may still have a high total bug count. This may relate to primary contamination of the water source or residual contamination in the water system due to ineffective sanitization at flock depletion. The use of sanitizers and disinfectants capable of removing biofilms and then achieving good bacterial kill is essential.

Vermin

Rats and mice are attracted to poultry housing by warmth and shelter and the availability of food sources. They can harbour a number of microorganisms, the most significant of which is probably *Salmonella* spp. These pests can infest the fabric of poultry buildings, causing damage to insulation and electrical installations.

Rats and mice are known to be carriers of significant *Salmonella* serovars such as Enteritidis and Typhimurium. The infective dose for these pests is low and affected vermin can act as latent carriers, only intermittently excreting *Salmonella* in their droppings without being affected themselves. If such vermin are pregnant they can pass infection to their unborn offspring. There is also evidence that virulence for poultry is enhanced by passage through infected vermin.

House design should be such as to prevent access for vermin and areas around poultry houses should be kept clear of vegetation and disused equipment, which can provide shelter for vermin approaching houses. Clearing up all feed spillages is essential, as is the storage of all feed in vermin-proof bins to discourage vermin from visiting sites.

Maintain an effective, audited rodent and wild bird control programme, using proven baits, properly and safely distributed inside and outside houses. This should be supplemented by monitoring for vermin activity such as damage done to buildings, the presence of vermin droppings and the take-up of bait. Increase vermin control strategies and baiting prior to site depletion, when vermin may leave a site temporarily if feed and heat are removed, thus evading the site's terminal cleansing and disinfection programme.

Insects and beetles

Red mite infestations can themselves be associated with anaemia, reduced production and even mortality. Darkling (alphitobious) beetles are cited as vectors of virus diseases such as Gumboro disease and Marek's disease and bacterial infections including *Salmonella* and *Campylobacter*. Flies have been implicated as seasonal vectors of *Campylobacter* spp. Control here is directed at preventing entry into poultry houses, effective use of residual parasiticides and insecticides and basic house design to reduce entry and persistence.

Wild birds

The most significant risk from wild birds to commercial poultry is the highly virulent strains of avian influenza and Newcastle disease. Wild birds, especially migratory waterfowl, are a specific problem by virtue of the fact that they can act as symptomless carriers that, during their migratory season, can travel large distances and circumvent national and international borders.

In addition to these viral diseases, wild birds have also been implicated in the introduction and spread of *Mycoplasma*, *Salmonella* and *Campylobacter* infections, yersiniosis and avian tuberculosis.

All poultry units should be birdproofed using wire mesh over any vents or open sidewalls. All doors should be kept closed. All feed spillages should be cleared up immediately they occur. Poultry houses should not be sited near open water known to attract wild birds and if these are already present close to a unit they should be netted to keep wild birds from alighting. Bird scarers may be appropriate in some situations.

Site decontamination

1. Effective cleaning and disinfection reduce the number of pathogens and the weight of disease challenge and hence greatly enhance biosecurity programmes.
2. Effective cleaning and disinfection can only be achieved with sufficient turnaround/down time to allow removal of all litter and the required contact times for the disinfection products used prior to restocking.
3. Cleaning and disinfection should include the houses, surrounding concrete apron and equipment. Kerbing will prevent wash-off of contaminated material on to surrounding land as well as containing foul water.
4. Maintain a closed water system with lids on all header tanks. There should be effective cleaning and disinfection of the water system at turnaround to remove the greasy biofilm from the inside of the system that will harbour and protect pathogens.
5. Effective cleaning and disinfection of the total feed system should include bins and delivery systems. Feed delivered to the site must be of high health status with vermin protection. Specification for feed supplies should be to exclude all vermin to protect finished feed and stored raw materials, especially cereals. Raw materials and finished feed should be sampled regularly for *Salmonella* spp. Any 'high-risk' raw materials or sources identified by such monitoring should cease to be used.
6. Use only disinfectants with proven broad-spectrum efficacy against all viral and bacterial pathogens. These products should be used at the manufacturer's stated dilutions.

Operational biosecurity can therefore be seen to span two distinct but overlapping areas of operation. The first is the ongoing site security with procedures aimed at countering the effects of the hazard posed by the CCPs identified. This can involve vaccination programmes, medication strategies, environmental control and management/husbandry activities. These are represented by the critical control points listed at A–I above. The second aspect relates to site decontamination or so-called terminal cleansing and disinfection. The latter is a major contribution to breaking the cycle of infection and is worthy of more detailed description.

DISINFECTION PROCEDURES

Disinfectants and disinfection procedures have been widely used for many years in the poultry industry. Natural disinfection agents such as sunlight, heat or just simply resting a premises are no longer considered to be of much practical use. Increasing evidence of the prolonged survival time of a number of significant avian pathogens outside the bird, coupled with ever-increasing economic pressure for quicker restocking of units, has led to an increasing dependence on chemical disinfectants.

Selection of a disinfectant

For many years a range of basic chemicals have been used as disinfectants within the industry, often achieving only limited results. This is due in the main to the limited spectrum of activity of these chemicals in the field situation. However, contributory factors to the generally poor results achieved with disinfection in the past were the areas of application and methods employed. These were often limited by the toxic or corrosive nature of some of the chemicals. In addition, many of these chemicals could be considered by present-day standards to be harmful to the environment. More recently there has been growing concern for the safety of operators applying aldehydes (formaldehyde and glutaraldehyde) as disinfectants, still the most widely used of the basic chemicals. Information on the potential danger of using this group of chemicals is increasing.

Modern broad-spectrum disinfectants with independently proven activity are now available to enable producers to protect their stock against infections while satisfying increasingly stringent user safety requirements.

Selection of an effective and economical disinfectant can appear to be a complicated procedure. A number of considerations have to be taken into account, primarily influenced by the proposed area of application. These will include the nature of the surface to be disinfected, the level of residual organic soiling, temperature, water quality, contact time and the required spectrum of activity. It is essential that these factors are considered in the choice and application of a disinfectant.

- **Type of surface**. Many poultry houses are constructed with materials that have a rough or absorbent surface, such as timber and earth or sand floors. In these cases the physical properties of the disinfectant, such as ability to penetrate such surfaces, become significant.
- **Organic soiling**. Whereas residual organic soiling on surfaces will have a negative effect on all chemical disinfectants, some systems are far more resistant to this challenge than others. For example, quaternary ammonium compounds (QACs), iodophors and formaldehyde are more affected by organic soiling than phenolics and glutaraldehydes. Basic cleaning and washing of surfaces before the application of a disinfectant is the single most important aspect of effective hygiene and disinfection. However, some surfaces are easier to clean than others and, where it is considered that a residual level of organic soiling is unavoidable, it is important to consider the degree to which the activity of the selected disinfectant is potentially lowered. This may influence the choice of product, its method of application and the dilution rate for application.
- **Temperature**. The activity of most disinfectants increases with a rise in temperature. This is often referred to as the temperature coefficient, which is a measure of the change in killing time per degree rise in temperature. This can vary significantly with different chemical systems: for example, glutaraldehydes show a marked temperature-dependent activity. In practice it is necessary to consider the temperature when determining the selection of a disinfectant,

as well as the dilution rate of the selected agent for optimal activity at the anticipated temperature. A common mistake in practice is to overlook the fact that it is the temperature of the surface to be treated that is relevant rather than the air temperature of the house. Short periods of heating a house prior to application of a disinfectant may do little to raise the temperature of a concrete floor. Increased contact time and lower dilution rates may be necessary during the winter months.

- **Water quality**. Water hardness can have a significant effect on the activity of some disinfectants and is therefore a factor to be taken into consideration. For example, phenolic compounds are far less affected by hard water than iodophors or QACs.
- **Contact time**. The contact time required for various disinfectants to achieve an acceptable reduction in surface count can also vary considerably. For example, oxidizing systems are generally very fast-acting; aldehydes tend to be much slower. For most disinfectants the main effect on organisms is while the chemical system is in an aqueous phase, i.e. while the surface remains wet.
- **Spectrum of activity**. Poultry can be challenged by a wide spectrum of pathogens, including varied bacterial, viral, fungal and protozoal species. In vitro activity test results against the most common poultry pathogens are available for many disinfectants. In assessing the results of any activity test it is vital to understand the conditions used in the test and its relevance to a field situation. There are a number of official test systems used by different countries to determine disinfectant activity and these can vary significantly, for example in the nature of the organic challenge used, test temperature, contact time, etc. When attempting to compare the activity and efficacy of disinfectants by reference to such results it is vital to ensure that comparisons are being made under similar test conditions. In the UK, the Department of Environment, Food and Rural Affairs (DEFRA) has a disinfectant approval system under which commercially available disinfectants can be submitted for examination for activity against a number of viruses causing notifiable diseases and for a category covering bacterial activity, so-called 'General Orders'. DEFRA publish lists of approved disinfectants on a regular basis.

From the user's point of view, the main features of a disinfectant to be considered can be divided into three main areas as follows.

- **Efficacy and efficiency**:
  - The biocidal spectrum should control all the pathogens (viral, bacterial and fungal) likely to affect the stock in question
  - Proof of efficacy must be confirmed by independent tests
  - There should be proof of efficacy under farm conditions, including organic soiling, hard water and low temperatures
- **Safety**: the product must:
  - Be safe for the operators to use
  - Be safe for the livestock and leave no potentially harmful residues or taints
  - Not corrode the equipment or fittings
  - Not result in environmental residues or damage
- **Cost**: as with any proposed method of disease control, it must be cost-effective and produce benefit to the user in terms of improved production, e.g. reduced mortality, increased live weight gain and food conversion.

Application of disinfectants

Spread of pathogens on static surfaces in poultry houses can transfer disease from one flock to the next. The survival time of many pathogens on inadequately disinfected inanimate surfaces can run into months. Rodent and insect vectors are often responsible for the transfer of both viral and bacterial infection between houses and sites. These key considerations can be dealt with by the process generally known as terminal disinfection. Apart from the selection of an effective disinfectant, the success of any programme depends on careful attention to every detail of the steps set out below. The procedures required are generally well understood but the expected result is often compromised by a failure to pay sufficient attention to detail. This may be due to the pressure created by short turn-around intervals or purely to a failure to appreciate the import-ance of the steps involved.

Terminal disinfection of poultry houses

In all cases the terminal disinfection programme should follow all, or as many as possible, of the following basic procedures.

1. **Dry clean.** This involves the removal of any residual food from the feeder system and silo. Portable equipment for cleaning and sanitizing should be placed outside the house or pen. Provision of concrete aprons outside houses for this purpose should be considered in the design of new, or improvements of existing, buildings. Litter should be thoroughly removed from the house and transported to a safe area away from stocked houses. Surface dust from ceilings, water pipes, etc., should normally be blown down and then all loose debris from the floor should be blown out after removal of the litter. The use of gantries and other equipment is essential to ensure that all high ledges, pipework, etc. are adequately cleaned. Bulk feed bins should be blown down or washed at this stage.

2. **Sanitize the drinking water system.** This is a procedure sometimes neglected or inadequately carried out but essential in order to avoid the transfer of infection from crop to crop via the drinking system. The header tank should be drained and checked to ensure that it is free of debris. The tank should then be filled with the required quantity of water and disinfectant added to achieve the required dilution. This solution should be allowed to fill the drinking system and left to stand for at least 1 h. After this the system should be thoroughly flushed and drained. Once filled with fresh water all tanks should be covered to reduce recontamination.

3. **Pre-clean the house or pen and equipment.** Use a detergent sanitizer to effectively clean surfaces to minimize organic challenge and reduce the bacterial load prior to disinfection. All surfaces should be sprayed with the solution at low pressure, ensuring thorough wetting. This must include coverage of pipe lines, feeders and drinkers. Externally, loading areas must be included. An alternative method of application favoured by some is by the use of a foam lance. Following the detergent application, cleaning should be completed with high-pressure water until all the areas mentioned are visibly clean.

4. **Disinfection of the house or pen and equipment.** This involves the thorough application of the selected broad-spectrum disinfectant to all surfaces and equipment in the house or pen, taking full consideration of the required dilution rate, application rate and contact time. Application can be with any suitable spraying equipment. If a pressure washer is used it should be set to a low pressure and if possible a fan jet should be employed. In recent years a number of larger operations have used equipment designed for orchard spraying, which can be very effective and time-saving. Choose the dilution at which the disinfectant has been independently proven to be effective against disease organisms. Ensure that the dilution rate is established by a test system incorporating an organic challenge. Always select the highest concentration necessary to eliminate the most resistant actual or potential pathogen. Effective disinfection requires surfaces to be thoroughly wet. An application rate

of 250–300 ml/m^2 is the minimum acceptable for any disinfectant. A higher rate is required on rough or very absorbent surfaces. All disinfectants need to remain in contact with the disease organisms for 'a minimum contact time'. In practice at least 30 min contact time is generally required for effective disinfection. Selection of disinfectant products should take account of other sanitizers and chemicals used in the terminal disinfection process. This selection should ensure full compatibility and prevent inadvertent loss of efficacy due to unintended adverse interactions.

5. **Setting up the house.** All equipment removed from the house, after being cleaned and disinfected, is replaced and litter is spread.

6. **Fumigating, misting or fogging.** After setting up the house this is a final biosecurity measure. In many cases the traditional method of formaldehyde fumigation has been replaced by safer chemicals, applied either with thermal fogging machines or as a fine mist or spray. After this final process, ensure that the house is closed and secured immediately these steps are completed to prevent the reintroduction of pathogens.

Effective control of insects, particularly litter beetle, is essential. They are known vectors of disease, e.g. Gumboro, salmonellosis and Marek's disease. When an insect problem has been identified, it is advisable to 'band spray' the house immediately on depopulation ahead of the migration of the bulk of the insects, which commences as soon as the house begins to cool. Application of a residual insecticide to the walls and floor of the house after completion of the disinfection procedures will further assist in the control.

Similarly, well-disinfected houses can be rapidly recontaminated by rats or mice, particularly with *Salmonella* spp. Effective rodent control measures are therefore essential. Baiting of premises at a time when other food supplies are not present is logical. However, it must be borne in mind that the disturbance of litter removal will often cause a resident rodent population to migrate from the houses only to return after the houses are set up. Therefore, especially in the case of breeder and layer housing, an effective rodent 'knock down' prior to site depletion with intensive baiting several weeks before birds are removed can help to remove this residual population.

Supervision and checking of the terminal disinfection procedures is essential. In large integrated operations this responsibility has not always been well defined. The introduction of HACCP and its verification steps allows a structured approach in this area.

HATCHING AND HATCHERY HYGIENE

Breeder house hygiene and hatching egg care

The ultimate success of hatching depends largely on the quality of the egg. Egg hygiene starts at the farm and requires consideration to be given to nest boxes and their management, and to nest box material, as well as egg handling and storage. All need to be carried out to the highest standards. Good breeder flock management is vital to ensure the production of a high percentage of clean hatching eggs. In many areas demand for hatching eggs is such that the undesirable practice of setting floor and other soiled eggs is required. Minimizing the percentage of these must be a basic management aim for any flock. Improved technology has developed a number of very effective automated nesting systems, which ensure a very high standard of egg hygiene, but the high capital cost involved may prohibit many producers from considering this possibility.

Nest boxes must be kept clean and the litter replaced on a regular basis. Where possible the use of hay or straw should be avoided as these can often be the source of *Aspergillus* spores.

When available, soft wood shavings are the material of choice. Frequent egg collection is vital and should be done at least four times a day. Nest boxes should be well maintained and given special attention during the terminal disinfection procedure.

Early sanitation of the hatching egg, as soon as possible after collection, has been shown to significantly improve hatching results and reduce the incidence of hatchery culls, omphalitis and other causes of early chick mortality. The increasing awareness of the health risks associated with aldehydes has led to the investigation of alternatives to formaldehyde fumigation of eggs. In some areas, egg washing has become a popular procedure, particularly in the wake of concerns over *Salmonella* infection. However, this does not always produce the best results if the procedure is not done well. This has led to the consideration of methods of sanitizing clean nest eggs by means of chemical sprays, this presenting less risk than egg dipping.

Hand hygiene is an important consideration throughout the various stages of handling hatching eggs from egg collectors to hatchery staff. The provision of adequate facilities and materials for this is essential.

Cleaning, disinfection and regular fogging of farm egg stores and equipment is essential, particularly where eggs are stored on farms for any period. Equally, a high standard of hygiene is required for egg transport vehicles. These high standards must be maintained during egg handling on arrival at the hatchery and during subsequent storage.

Hatchery management considerations

The hatchery is the focal point receiving eggs and equipment from a number of sites, which may vary in their geography, standards of biosecurity and pathogen load. The hatchery therefore has the greatest potential to magnify these contaminations, being the point source common factor for every broiler farm in a given company.

As with farms, there are a number of basic management practices that can assist significantly in achieving the desired hygiene standards within a hatchery.

- **Location**. Where possible a hatchery should be located at a distance from poultry farms, while giving consideration to the ease of access to breeder farms for egg collection.
- **Layout**. Careful planning of the working areas of the hatchery can greatly assist in allowing hygienic work practices by separating 'clean' and 'dirty' areas.
- **Ventilation**. Proper ventilation, with air flow patterns in one direction designed to minimize the transfer of infection, are essential. Machines must receive adequate clean fresh air and the air from them should be discharged outside the hatchery in such a way as to minimize recycling. Similarly, air inlets should be sited as far away as possible from any waste handling equipment.
- **Waste disposal**. By making proper arrangements for the disposal of hatchery waste, the risk of contamination of nearby poultry units or creating an environmental nuisance can be minimized.
- **Site security**. As with farms, proper security and control of visitors is essential. This should include the proper provision of shower facilities, or at least adequate protective clothing.

Hatchery cleaning and disinfection

The cleaning and disinfection of hatchery premises needs to be a well-planned and disciplined operation. As with the farm situation, a full HAACP programme should be established. Consideration must be given to the provision of suitable cleansing and disinfection equipment and clear instructions laid down for the use of chemicals. The basic criteria mentioned earlier for farms have to be applied. Thorough cleaning, followed by adequate disinfection, giving consideration to dilution and application rates, is vital in all areas for rooms and equipment. Instructions should include details of the frequency with which procedures should be applied, which in many areas will be influenced by the frequency of hatch days. All equipment and chemical proportioning machinery should be regularly calibrated and maintained. Regular bacteriological monitoring of all hatchery areas is essential to comply with HACCP monitoring and verification procedures.

Biosecurity is equally important and where possible the hatchery should be planned to allow workers to be restricted to particular areas of the operation. Finally, the chick delivery vehicles should be given the same considerations as the hatchery building.

Hatchery planning should aim at providing a workable flow pattern, both for staff and eggs and chicks. Basically a division should exist if possible between what can be defined as 'clean' and 'dirty' areas. The flow of eggs, equipment, personnel and ventilation system should be designed to move only from clean to dirty areas, without backtracking. Improved hygiene standards will be achieved if these areas and the staff working within them are separated as much as possible.

Detailed knowledge of the flow pattern of activities within the hatchery enables a HACCP analysis to be undertaken, which allows effective standard operating procedures and a structured targeted cleansing and disinfection programme to be put in place.

CONCLUSIONS

Biosecurity should be seen as one of the most significant areas of successful poultry management. The application of a wide range of procedures and practices aimed at preventing or limiting the exposure of a flock to the adverse effects of disease-causing organisms is the foundation of economic success in poultry production. Biosecurity procedures require detailed planning and should be built into a practical and responsive veterinary health and welfare plan. Proper application and audit of these procedures can be cost-effective in achieving the goal of reducing the impact of diseases of clinical animal health and public health importance.

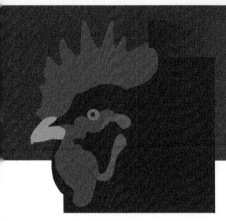

CHAPTER

5

Tibor Cserep

Vaccines and vaccination

Vaccination plays a key role in the modern poultry industry. Without vaccination its productivity would not have progressed so successfully and as rapidly as it has over the last few decades. The reason for this is quite simple. Many infectious diseases are ubiquitous worldwide and airborne pathogens are difficult to control even with very good biosecurity measures. For the poultry industry the main practical method of controlling infectious diseases is vaccination.

The primary reason for vaccinating poultry is to reduce the losses due to morbidity and mortality caused by infectious agents. In addition, layer and breeder birds need protection against diseases causing egg production drops and eggshell deformities.

Vaccination of breeders can also reduce vertical transmission of certain pathogens from breeders to progeny, thus preventing early outbreaks of diseases. Vaccinated breeders can pass maternal antibodies to their progeny to protect them against infections during the first weeks of their life. Increasingly, the aim of vaccination will be to prevent dissemination of zoonoses such as salmonellosis.

Vaccines can contribute greatly to the welfare of domestic and wild animals as well. However, vaccination can never provide 100% protection against infectious diseases. It is only one but a very important part of a complex preventive policy, of which biosecurity and hygiene are equally essential components.

There are now a large number of vaccines available for poultry. Disease control by vaccination is more effective for some diseases than others and programmes and requirements may vary considerably in different parts of the world. The diseases for which vaccines are available are: Newcastle disease (ND), infectious laryngotracheitis (ILT), fowl pox (FP), infectious avian encephalomyelitis (AE; epidemic tremor), Marek's disease (MD), egg drop syndrome (EDS 76), viral arthritis (reovirus), turkey avian rhinotracheitis (TRT/SHS), infectious bronchitis (IB), infectious bursal disease (IBD), chicken infectious anaemia (CIA), infectious coryza (*Haemophilus paragallinarum*), fowl cholera (*Pasteurella multocida*), mycoplasmosis (*Mycoplasma gallisepticum* and *Mycoplasma synoviae*), erysipelas (*Erysipelothrix insidiosa*), salmonellosis (*Salmonella* Enteritidis, *Salmonella* Typhimurium and *Salmonella* Gallinarum), colibacillosis

(*Escherichia coli*), coccidiosis, haemorrhagic enteritis, *Ornithobacterium rhinotracheale* and avian influenza.

TYPES OF VACCINE

At present there are two main types of vaccine available for poultry: live or killed. Vaccines against different diseases are combined in a programme to give protection against a number of viral or bacterial diseases.

Killed vaccines consist of a high dose of inactivated antigens combined with an oil emulsion or aluminium hydroxide adjuvant. They give high and prolonged levels of immunity, especially when used after 'priming' with live vaccine. They must be injected in each individual bird and often antigens of two or more different disease organisms are included in one vaccine (multivalent vaccine).

Live vaccines, on the other hand, usually contain only one antigen and may be administered by spray (aerosol), via drinking water, eye drop or in some cases by injection. The antigen may either be the disease organism, which has been deliberately attenuated, i.e. made less virulent by some suitable means (e.g. H120 strain of infectious bronchitis virus (IBV)) or a naturally occurring mild strain of the organism (e.g. B1 strain of *Newcastle disease virus* (NDV)).

A smaller amount of antigen is required in live vaccines because the organism will multiply rapidly in the target organ(s). This organ is the respiratory tract for viruses such as TRT and IB, or the intestine for AE and the bursa of Fabricius for IBD. Live vaccines may stimulate the production of local or mucosal immunity as well as general (systemic) immunity. Multiplication of the vaccine organism in vaccinated birds is important and excretion may be helpful in producing a good flock immunity by bird to bird transmission. For example, cycling of vaccine virus is advantageous in achieving good flock immunity to IBD, ND and IB. However, cycling is undesirable with TRT or ILT. Lateral spread of vaccine virus can be very undesirable on multiage sites. For example, if AE or IB H52 strain spread into older, unvaccinated groups of birds in lay, the vaccine itself may then cause production problems. Occasionally, birds show a reaction after the administration of live vaccine, for example mild coughing or 'snicking' after NDV vaccination, indicating that the vaccine has 'taken'. Unless concurrent bacterial or mycoplasma challenge is present this mild reaction disappears in a few days time and is not a cause for concern.

Vaccination programmes are designed to prevent or reduce losses caused by disease in vaccinated birds and/or their progeny. In devising a vaccination programme, both immunological and commercial factors must be considered, including the following:
- The general health of the flock and the local pattern of disease – vaccine must not be administered to sick birds
- The genetic type and function of the bird
- The cost–benefit of vaccination against potential loss
- The short- or long-term protection required
- The vaccinations or diseases that occurred in the previous generation and would influence maternal antibody status. Maternal antibody may have a significant effect on the design of a vaccination programme. For example, the level of maternal antibody against IBD virus determines the timing of vaccination with different types of IBD vaccines. For TRT, maternal antibody has no effect on vaccination.

Having decided on the types of vaccine required, the method and frequency of administration must be considered, and how these can be integrated into a vaccination programme.

Vaccination programmes are not universal. They have to be designed individually according to the type of birds, production systems and local disease conditions of an area or of a country.

METHODS OF ADMINISTRATION

Live vaccines are usually supplied in vials in freeze-dried form. They should be kept at 4–8°C and protected from heat and light. Cell-associated MD vaccine is stored and supplied in liquid nitrogen. After thawing, it is a suspension of living cells containing the MD virus ('wet' vaccine).

Most live vaccines are applied by mass application techniques such as drinking water and spray.

Drinking water

Vaccines should be reconstituted in clean, cold water. If the water contains chlorine, skimmed milk powder should be dissolved in it at the rate of 2 g/L or skimmed milk added in the ratio of 2:100. The milk powder or milk should be mixed with the water 20–30 min before adding the vaccine to give time for neutralization of any damaging components in the water such as chlorine or metallic ions. There are also various 'water stabilizer' tablets and powders available that neutralize the chlorine in the drinking water and at the same time change the colour of water to light blue or green.

It is not recommended that vaccine solution is put into metal storage tanks. It is essential to ensure that the whole drinking water system is clean and does not contain any debris such as rust or dirt and that there are no residues of any sanitizer, which may inactivate the vaccine viruses. Plastic header tanks or bins are therefore preferred as they can be thoroughly cleaned.

The vaccine should be used as soon as possible after reconstitution and certainly within 2 h.

The procedure of administration is critical as uptake of one full dose (protective dose) by the individual bird is essential. The most effective uptake of vaccine from nipple drinkers can be achieved as follows:

1. The day before vaccine is due to be administered, the water meter should be read hourly to determine the pattern of drinking, especially in relation to the timing of the feeders. This will give an idea of the best time to vaccinate the birds and also the volume of water required. In the absence of a water meter, the water consumption can be estimated by measuring the water level in the header tanks, or by other methods. (On farms where bell or trough drinkers are used the drinkers should be cleaned but not disinfected.) Water sanitizers should be withdrawn from the drinker system 2 days before vaccine is administered.
2. On the morning of vaccination the main tap to the drinker system should be turned off and the drinker system should be raised and drained. If this is not possible the birds should drink as much water out of the system as possible. It is advisable to remove the filters from the water line where vaccine passes through. Slime and dirt building up on filters can concentrate residue of sanitizers, which can reduce the efficacy of the vaccine. When the drinkers are dry they should be raised, preferably 30–60 min prior to feeder activation. The vaccine should be mixed in the calculated volume of water, which is treated with milk or alternative neutralizing products if mains water is used, plus the volume of residual water within the lines (the drinker lines in a shed may contain as much as 250 L of water). Once the vaccine is mixed, each drinker line should be drained until the milk or dye-stained water is visible at the end of each line (priming of the lines). The vaccine can be made more visible by adding colouring food dye tablets to the mix.
3. When all the lines have been drained and primed, they should be lowered to bird level to coincide with the feeders activating. Preparation of the lines in this way ensures that birds at the far end of the water lines also receive vaccine and not just plain water.
4. Walk along the sides of the shed to stimulate birds to move towards feeders and drinkers.

Table 5.1	Volumes of vaccine-containing water (guide only)
AGE (WEEKS)	**L/1000 BROILERS**
2	14
3	21
4	28

5. Ensure that the main tap of the water system is reopened when vaccinated water is consumed just before the header tank runs dry.

Dosing machines (proportioners) are also used for administering vaccine and are more useful where ad libitum feeding is practised, as the water consumption tends to be constant over time. If timed feeding is practised it is more effective to use the method described above to ensure that the majority of birds receive vaccine timed to coincide with maximum water consumption. Proportioners have their advantages and disadvantages but for certain types of poultry sheds they are the only way in which vaccines or medications can be administered. Unfortunately, the recommended concentration of milk necessary to protect the vaccine virus in the water cannot be achieved using proportioners. To achieve the recommended 2% milk concentration in the drinker lines one has to use pure skimmed milk for stock solution. Alternatively, the recommended amount of neutralizing powder or tablets per litre needs to be mixed into the stock solution.

(Where bell or trough type drinkers are used, the freshly prepared vaccine solution should ideally be poured into clean drinkers within a short period of time, ensuring that each bird in the shed has an opportunity to take the protective dose of vaccine.)

The appropriate volumes of vaccine-containing water to be used for broilers are given in Table 5.1.

Spray

The other method of mass administration of live vaccine involves application by spray or aerosol. An aerosol generally contains mainly particles of less than 5 μm diameter at bird level (approx. 50 μm when they leave the sprayer), which can penetrate deeply into the respiratory tract. This may initiate a severe vaccine reaction with bacteria such as *E. coli*, resulting in septicaemia. Therefore, in certain circumstances a coarser spray with particles greater than 100 μm diameter when they leave the sprayer is generally preferable to an aerosol and is less likely to cause an adverse reaction. Aerosol vaccination is recommended for vaccinating birds in areas where ND is endemic but only after 'priming' with ND vaccine in the form of coarse spray.

It is very difficult to measure droplet size accurately under field conditions but with water-sensitive paper (WSP) a good enough assessment for vaccination purposes can be made. WSP is a rigid paper with a specially coated, yellow surface. This surface is stained a dark blue colour when aqueous droplets come into contact with it.

After application of a spray, the WSP is retrieved from the target area and, once dry, the droplet pattern can be examined. The size of the blue spots reflects the size of spray droplets landing on the target area. Comparison can be made with known standards or the spots can be assessed manually using a pen microscope (Fig. 5.1).

Suitable sprayers for on-farm use are knapsack sprayers or sprayers based on the spinning disc system (Fig. 5.2). There are also specially designed sprayer cabinets for use in hatcheries for the administration of IB, and ND, TRT or coccidiosis vaccines to day-old chicks (Fig. 5.3).

Vaccine should be reconstituted in distilled or deionized water, not tap water, as the latter can contain sanitizer (chlorine), dissolved solids and salts, which concentrate rapidly as spray droplets evaporate and this can be harmful to the vaccine virus. The volume of water is determined by the age of the birds and type of sprayer. For day-old vaccination 200–400 mL of water per 1000 chicks or poults is generally sufficient. If knapsack sprayers are used during rearing or lay 500–1000 mL of water per 1000 birds may be required to achieve uniform vaccine cover. The volume of water for spinning disc sprayers is much less than this and the manufacturer's recommendations should be followed.

Spray vaccine is generally more effective in a controlled environment than in open-sided houses. In closed houses, fans should be turned off with the inlets and outlets closed, the lights should be dimmed and the birds allowed to settle quietly before spraying commences.

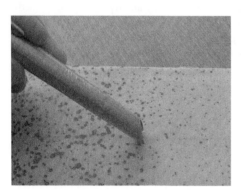

Fig. 5.1 Blue spots on WSP examined by a pen microscope.

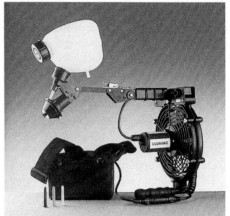

Fig. 5.2 Ulvavac fan sprayer for spray vaccination on the farm. (Courtesy of Micron Sprayers Ltd, UK.)

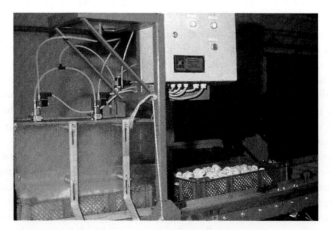

Fig. 5.3 Vaccination of chicks in boxes by overhead spray in the hatchery. (Courtesy of Intervet UK Ltd.)

Eye drop

Of all the methods of administration of live vaccine, the eye drop or intranasal route is probably the most effective, although very time-consuming and labour intensive. Accuracy is important and the vaccine must disappear after a blink (eye drop) or inhalation (intranasal) before the bird is released.

This method is extremely effective for the administration of TRT vaccine, where it is important that each bird receives a full dose of vaccine. It is also used for ILT vaccine and for ND where this is endemic.

Injection

Live vaccines may have to be administered by injection as in the case of MD vaccines (Fig. 5.4), certain *Chicken anaemia virus* (CAV) and reovirus vaccines. The injection route, either intramuscular or subcutaneous, is the only one used for inactivated (killed) vaccines (Fig. 5.5). Automatic syringes are used to a preset dosage. It is important that the equipment is regularly checked to ensure that the dosage is correct and also that the needles are changed regularly (e.g. after each bottle of vaccine or every 500 birds) to minimize the spread of contaminants. A needle sanitizer sleeve containing a biocide-treated sponge can be fitted on to the syringe to ensure aseptic injections up to 500 times. Injection may be subcutaneous in the back of the neck or, more usually, intramuscular into breast or leg. The breast offers a safer target area than the 'drumstick' of the leg where tendons, nerves or blood vessels can be hit above the hock joint, leading to unnecessary suffering and lameness. The tip of the keel bone gives a very good orientation point for breast vaccination. Ideally the needle should be inserted laterally on either side of the breast, approximately 2–3 cm away from the tip of the keel (Fig. 5.6). If the needle is inserted too far from the keel into the flank area or at the tail end of the keel bone, vital organs such as heart or liver can be hit and the bird may die.

In certain countries inactivated vaccines are administered into the muscular part of the tail or subcutaneously into the inguinal flap.

Accuracy is important as incorrect needle placement can result in head swelling, granulomata, liver punctures or lameness, depending on the injection site. The most frequently used needles for inactivated vaccines are 12.5 mm (half inch) long and 1.1 mm (19 gauge) thick.

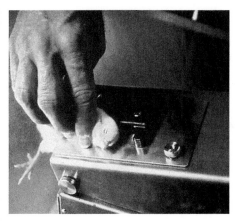

Fig. 5.4 Marek's disease vaccination by subcutaneous injection in the hatchery. (Courtesy of Intervet UK Ltd.)

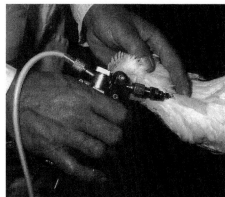

Fig. 5.5 Breeder vaccination by the subcutaneous route. (Courtesy of Intervet UK Ltd.)

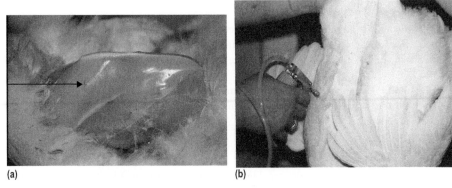

(a)   (b)

Fig. 5.6a,b The ideal area for breast vaccination. (Courtesy of Intervet UK Ltd.)

Wing web

Vaccination via the wing web is the principal method of administration of fowl pox (FP) vaccine. Epidemic tremor vaccine is compatible and sometimes the two products are combined. It is important to use a two-pronged applicator. This provides twice the area inoculated and results in better protection. Care should be taken to avoid the vaccine coming into contact with the bird's eyes or mouth. The application site on the wing web should be examined 5–7 days post-vaccination to ensure a 'take'. This should appear as a slightly raised and swollen area.

In feed

This method has been used for the distribution of live thermostable ND vaccine to widely dispersed small backyard flocks in areas such as India, Ethiopia and south-east Asia. Results have been rather erratic.

In ovo

This system is now being used in a number of countries for the administration of MD and other live vaccines. Fertile chicken eggs are inoculated at 18 days on transfer to the hatchers. It is hoped that this system will ultimately be suitable for administration of a number of live vaccines.

TYPES OF VACCINATION PROGRAMME

Vaccination programmes vary considerably from area to area and country to country, according to the local pattern of disease.

Broilers

Broilers may be killed at any time between 35 and 80 days of age, so vaccine requirements may vary considerably depending on slaughter age.

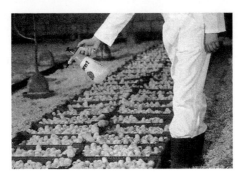

Fig. 5.7 Vaccination of chicks by coarse spray on arrival at the farm. (Courtesy of Intervet UK Ltd.)

The virulent strain of IBD virus is endemic in many countries now and two doses of intermediate strain vaccine are usually required, given at about 17 and 24 days, depending on levels of maternal antibody. Alternatively, one dose of 'intermediate plus' strain vaccine may be given on farms where there is a history of acute IBD with high mortality. This vaccine is given in the drinking water at about 14 days of age but should not be given to birds without maternal antibody. The timing of IBD vaccinations with intermediate plus type vaccine can be more accurately determined using the Kouwenhoven or other formula based on measurement of maternal antibodies by the enzyme-linked immunosorbent assay (ELISA) test. To get meaningful results at least 20 serum samples from 1-day-old chicks from each breeding flock need to be tested. ELISA kit and vaccine manufacturers provide customers with computer software for calculating ideal times for IBD vaccination.

$$\text{Day of vaccination} = \sqrt{\frac{\text{mean ELISA titre (20 sera) - 22.36 + 1}}{2.86}}$$

where $22.36 = \sqrt{350}$ Index units (the threshold at which vaccination is possible); $2.82 =$ half-life of antibody in days; $1 =$ birds placed on farm on first day of life.

IB vaccine is required in most countries to control both variant and classical IB. It is usually administered by coarse spray in the hatchery to day-old chicks or on arrival at the farm while the chicks are still in the boxes (Fig. 5.7) and then a second dose of IB vaccine is given at around 20 days by spray or via drinking water. In most countries the vaccine is of Massachusetts serotype, but local conditions may require the use of other serotypes as well, such as Connecticut, Arkansas, Dutch variants or the UK variant IB 4-91.

NDV challenge is still important in many countries too. The first vaccination can be given as coarse spray in the hatchery. However, if there is a possibility that day-old chicks are infected with *M. gallisepticum* or pathogenic *E. coli*, postvaccinal reaction can occur, particularly if the spray contains fine ($<5.0\,\mu\text{m}$ at bird level) droplets. The second dose of ND vaccine can be given via drinking water or fine spray around 21 days of age. Severe challenge conditions may demand the use of live ND vaccine (spray or eye drop) and a killed oil emulsion ND vaccine (injection) at 1 day old. This combined vaccination usually gives sufficient protection for the short life of broilers. However, in heavy-challenge areas, particularly on multiage farms, a second spray vaccination at 18 days may be necessary.

Table 5.2 | Vaccination programme for broilers (UK)

AGE (DAYS)	VACCINE	ROUTE
1	Infectious bronchitis (H120/Ma5/D274/IBmm/Ark)	Coarse spray
	Newcastle disease (HBI/Clone 30/NDW)	Coarse spray (optional)
	Marek's disease	Injection (optional)
	TRT	Spray (optional)
	Coccidiosis	Spray (optional)
7	TRT	Spray (optional)
10–14 or 14–16	Infectious bronchitis IB 4-91	Water *or* spray (optional)
16	Infectious bursal disease (intermediate plus)	
18	Infectious bursal disease (intermediate)	Water
24	Infectious bursal disease (intermediate)	Water
	Newcastle disease (HBI/Clone 30)	Spray/aerosol (optional)
	Infectious bronchitis (H120/Ma5)	Spray (optional, not necessary if IB 4-91 used at 14–18 days)

MD vaccine is given routinely by injection at 1 day old or in ovo to 18-day-old embryos in countries which reuse litter and therefore have a high residual challenge, or where birds are to be kept to 55 days of age or more.

As a general rule two live vaccines should not be given at the same time but separated ideally by 14 days (minimum 7 days) to avoid the phenomenon of interference.

A vaccination programme for broilers in the UK is given in Table 5.2.

Broiler and layer breeders

All breeders receive MD vaccine at 1 day old. Generally the cell-associated 'wet' vaccine is considered the most effective and it may be either attenuated Marek's disease virus (MDV) or *Turkey herpes virus* (THV) or a combination of both. Rispens (serotype 1) is widely regarded as a very effective vaccine but in some countries SB1 (serotype 2) or various combinations of two or three serotypes may be used. Sometimes a second dose of vaccine is given at around 7–14 days of age and is considered an effective means of preventing disease in areas of high challenge.

Breeding birds are always vaccinated for IB and ND. Live vaccines are administered initially to give protection from disease during the rearing period but also to act as primers for the inactivated vaccine given later. In the UK the first live ND vaccine (B1) is usually given at about 3 weeks and this may be followed by one or more doses of B1, Clone 30, or other strains depending on the local level of challenge. Killed ND vaccine is given around 16–18 weeks of age to provide protection through lay and to give maternal antibody to the progeny. The first dose of IB vaccine (H120 or Ma5) is usually given at 3 weeks of age in the UK. Further doses of H120 or Ma5 vaccine may be used every 6–8 weeks during the laying period if IB infection pressure or challenge is high.

There are a number of live variant strains of IB vaccine available in different countries and these may be used if permitted by the authorities. ND, IB, IBvariant, reovirus, TRT and IBD killed vaccines are used in various combinations and are given at between 16 and 18 weeks,

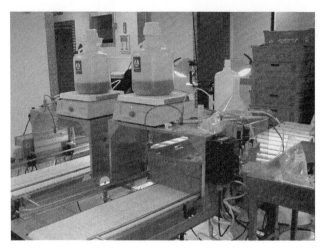

Fig. 5.8 Day-old application of coccidiosis vaccine. (Courtesy of Shering Plough Animal Health.)

normally as one injection. Live and killed TRT vaccines are part of most breeder vaccination programmes and are essential to reduce the impact of challenge by avian pneumovirus, the cause of swollen head syndrome.

IBD vaccine is required in areas of high challenge. Usually an intermediate strain is used at around 3–5 weeks of age. Killed IBD vaccine is given at 16–18 weeks to provide even levels of maternal antibody in the progeny chicks. This helps to plan the timing of IBD vaccination of broilers and layers.

CIA virus live vaccine is now available in many countries and immunization of breeders is very important in preventing the devastating effects of this condition in the progeny. A single dose of live vaccine is given after 6 weeks of age.

Breeders all over the world are given a single dose of live infectious avian encephalomyelitis (IAE) vaccine at around 14 weeks in the drinking water. Again this gives protection to the progeny.

In the UK all broiler breeders have to be vaccinated against *S.* Enteritidis and *S.* Typhimurium. This can be done by two doses of the combined SE + ST inactivated vaccine or by various regimen of live SE and ST vaccines.

Depending on the conditions in the country FP, fowl cholera, ILT, infectious coryza, avian rhinotracheitis, influenza, viral arthritis (reovirus) and EDS vaccines may be required and have to be fitted into the vaccination programme.

Live coccidiosis vaccines are now available worldwide and used successfully in the prevention of coccidiosis. Some of these vaccines are based on precocious strains of *Eimeria* species; others contain more virulent strains. They can be applied in the hatchery by spray at 1 day old, during the first week of life via drinking water or sprayed on feed (Fig. 5.8).

S. Enteritidis and *S.* Typhimurium killed and live vaccines are valuable recent developments and are very effective in reducing transmission of these pathogens from breeders to progeny and further on to humans.

Reovirus vaccine (live and killed) is used in many countries and appears to reduce the incidence of reovirus-associated infections (malabsorption syndrome, viral arthritis and femoral head necrosis) in breeders and their progeny.

Table 5.3 Vaccination programme for broiler breeders (UK)

AGE	VACCINE	ROUTE
1 day	Marek's disease (Rispens + THV)	Intramuscular injection
5 days	Coccidiosis	Drinking water
7–10 days	Marek's disease (THV)	Intramuscular injection (optional)
3 weeks	Newcastle disease (B1/Clone 30)	Spray/drinking water
	Infectious bronchitis (H120/Ma5)	Spray/drinking water
4 weeks	Infectious bursal disease	Drinking water
6–18 weeks	Chicken infectious anaemia (live)	Injection/drinking water (optional)
10 weeks	Newcastle disease (B1/Clone 30)	Spray/drinking water
	Infectious bronchitis (H120/Ma5)	Spray/drinking water
12 weeks	Turkey rhinotracheitis	Spray
	Salmonellosis (SE + ST)	Injection
	Reovirus	Injection (optional)
	Ornithobacterium rhinotracheale	Injection (optional)
14 weeks	Infectious avian encephalomyelitis	Drinking water
18 weeks	Infectious bronchitis (killed)	Intramuscular injection
	Newcastle disease (killed)	Intramuscular injection
	Infectious bursal disease (killed)	Intramuscular injection
	Turkey rhinotracheitis (killed)	Intramuscular injection
	Salmonellosis (SE + ST)	Intramuscular injection
	Reovirus	Intramuscular injection (optional)
	O. rhinotracheale	Intramuscular injection (optional)

The vaccination programme for layer breeders is very similar and may include EDS vaccination at 16–18 weeks of age.
SE, *Salmonella* Enteriditis; ST, *Salmonella* Typhimurium.

Vaccination programmes for breeders in the UK, Asia and South America are given in Tables 5.3, 5.4 and 5.5 respectively.

Commercial layers

The requirements for commercial layers are similar to those for breeders, but there are some differences.

Young egg-laying strains of bird are very susceptible to the virulent forms of IBD infection. Thus up to three doses of intermediate strain vaccine may be given at 14, 21 and 28 days by drinking water. If the level of challenge is very high, a single dose of 'intermediate plus' vaccine has been shown to give protection. Requirements for ND, IB, AE, TRT and MD vaccines are similar to those of breeders. Live respiratory disease vaccines may be sprayed on to birds in cages (Fig. 5.9).

Laying birds are usually kept on multiage sites, so the level of biosecurity is not as good as for breeders. Extra attention should be paid to prevent the spread of certain live vaccines to susceptible birds on the same farm. EDS vaccine may be required and is given by injection at 16 weeks of age as a single dose. EDS immunity is unusual in that it requires only one dose of killed vaccine and no live primer is required. Live ILT vaccine is given by eye drop in areas where ILT is endemic.

Table 5.4 Vaccination programme for broiler breeders (Asia)		
AGE	**VACCINE**	**ROUTE**
1 day	Marek's disease (Rispens)	Intramuscular injection
	Infectious bronchitis (H120/Ma5)	Intraocular/spray
	Newcastle disease (B1/Clone 30)	
35–10 days	Coccidiosis	Drinking water/spray on feed
7 days	Newcastle disease	Intraocular
	Reovirus	Subcutaneous injection
14 days	Infectious bursal disease	Drinking water
3 weeks	Newcastle disease + IB (Ma5 + LaSota/Clone 30)	Intraocular/spray
	Fowl pox	Wing web stab
4 weeks	Avian influenza	Subcutaneous injection
	Infectious bursal disease	Drinking water
6 weeks	Infectious coryza	Intramuscular injection
	Mycoplasma gallisepticum	Intramuscular injection
	Reovirus	Subcutaneous injection
8 weeks	Infectious bronchitis + ND (H120/Ma5 + Clone 30)	Drinking water/spray
	Newcastle disease (LaSota/Clone 30)	Spray
10 weeks	ILT	Intranasal
	Fowl pox + AE	Wing web stab
	Reovirus (live)	Intramuscular injection
12 weeks	Avian influenza	Intramuscular injection
	Fowl pox	Wing web stab
14 weeks	Infectious avian encephalomyelitis	Drinking water
15 weeks	Newcastle disease + IB	Spray/eyedrop
	ND + IB + EDS	Intramuscular injection
	Infectious coryza	Intramuscular injection
16 weeks	Newcastle disease (killed)	Intramuscular injection
18 weeks	*M. gallisepticum*	Intramuscular injection
20 weeks	ND + IB	Eye drop
	ND + IB + IBD + Reovirus	Subcutaneous injection
38 weeks	ND (Clone 30)	Drinking water/eye drop
	Avian influenza	Intramuscular injection

AE, avian encephalomyelitis; EDS, egg drop syndrome; IB, infectious bronchitis; IBD, infectious bursal disease; ILT, infectious laryngotracheitis; ND, Newcastle disease.

Is some countries live or killed *M. gallisepticum* and/or *M. synoviae* vaccines are used, where these diseases have not been eradicated or eradication would be expensive and impractical.

As with breeders, infectious coryza, fowl cholera and pox vaccines are used in endemic areas.

Table 5.5	Vaccination programme for broiler breeders in South America	
AGE	**VACCINE**	**ROUTE**
1 day	Marek's disease (Rispens/HVT + SB1)	Intramuscular injection
	Newcastle disease (killed)	Intramuscular injection (optional)
1–7 days	Infectious bronchitis (H120/Ma5)	Spray/intraocular
	Newcastle disease (La Sota/Clone 30)	Spray/intraocular
7–10 days	Infectious bursal disease	Drinking water/spray/intraocular
7 days	Reovirus (1133)	Subcutaneous injection
18–21 days	Infectious bursal disease	Drinking water/spray/intraocular
25–28 days	Newcastle disease (La Sota/Clone 30)	Drinking water/spray/intraocular
5 weeks	Turkey rhinotracheitis	Spray
8 weeks	Reovirus (1133)	Subcutaneous injection
	Infectious bronchitis (H120/Ma5)	Drinking water/spray/intraocular
	Newcastle disease (La Sota/Clone 30)	Drinking water/spray/intraocular
	Newcastle disease (killed)	Subcutaneous/intramuscular injection (optional)
10 weeks	Turkey rhinotracheitis	Spray
6–14 weeks	Chicken infectious anaemia (P4)	Subcutaneous/intramuscular injection
6–12 weeks	Avian encephalomyelitis/pox	Wing web stab
18 weeks	Newcastle disease (killed)	Subcutaneous/intramuscular injection
	Infectious bronchitis (killed)	
	Reovirus (killed)	
	Infectious bursal disease + variant IBD (killed)	

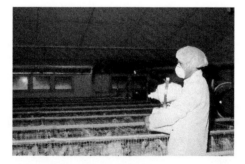

Fig. 5.9 Vaccination of layers in cages by spray. (Courtesy of Intervet UK Ltd.)

Commercial turkeys

In certain European countries, TRT has become endemic and live vaccine is needed as an essential part of the control programme. It can be given by spray or eye drop and is best applied at 1 day old in the hatchery. Sometimes a second dose is given by spray at about 6–10 weeks for birds destined for heavier weights. Fowl cholera vaccine may be required on certain problem farms. Where haemorrhagic enteritis is a problem, in countries such as France, the USA and now in the UK, the impact of the disease can be reduced by a single dose of live vaccine given at 4 weeks of age in drinking water.

ND vaccine may be required in endemic areas.

Turkey breeders

Turkey breeders are normally immunized against ND but this requires more doses of vaccine than for broiler breeders as the turkey seems to be less responsive. Depending on the epidemiological situation at least three doses of live vaccine may be required. The spray method gives a better response than the drinking water route. La Sota or Clone 30 can be used as a primer in turkeys and their 'take' is better than B1. At least two doses of killed vaccine are required. The most difficult problem for immunization is fowl cholera, caused by *P. multocida*. Two doses of killed vaccine are normally given 4 weeks apart during the rearing period, usually between 10 and 24 weeks. In areas of very high challenge it may be necessary to start immunization as early as 8 weeks, with two initial doses of vaccine given 4 weeks apart followed by a third before lay and even a fourth during lay. Two priming doses of live vaccine given orally are used in some countries (e.g. USA) but live cholera vaccines are not licensed in the UK. Pox vaccination is often required for turkeys in hotter climates (e.g. California and Australia). Two doses are given by wing web stab; the timing will depend on when challenge is likely to occur.

Vaccines for rhinotracheitis are now available in the USA, where this condition is caused by *Bordetella avium*, while in Europe TRT, which is a clinically similar disease, is caused by avian pneumovirus. To protect against TRT infection, breeders require live priming vaccine given by spray at 1 day old and about 6 weeks, followed by killed vaccine given at 14 and 22 weeks. The current live TRT vaccines seem to be capable of giving cross-protection against the new 'type C' pneumovirus isolated recently from turkey flocks in the USA.

Paramyxovirus (PMV-3) vaccine is often used to prevent drops in egg production due to this infection.

Table 5.6 gives a vaccination programme for turkey breeders in the UK.

Ducks

For breeders and commercial birds, duck virus hepatitis (DVH) vaccine and duck viral enteritis (DVE) are needed. In some countries they are also vaccinated against fowl cholera (Tables 5.7 and 5.8).

The DVH vaccine referred to here is for DVH type 1. There may be a requirement in some areas for DVH type 2 vaccine.

Game birds

Quail, pheasants and partridges may need ND vaccine in areas of risk. If so, a similar programme to that given for broiler breeders may be followed. Pheasants can carry viruses such as IB and TRT, which are present in chickens or turkeys too. Challenge with these viruses can sometimes result in pheasant mortality as a result of so-called coronavirus-nephritis or respiratory disease similar to swollen head syndrome of chickens. Vaccination of pheasant flocks against these diseases has proved to be successful in certain game units in the UK and might be necessary in the future.

Table 5.6 | Vaccination programme for turkey breeders (UK)

AGE	VACCINE	ROUTE
1 day	Turkey rhinotracheitis (live)	Spray
2 weeks	Newcastle disease (HBI)	Spray
6 weeks	Newcastle disease (Clone 30)	Spray
	Turkey rhinotracheitis (live)	Spray
10 weeks	Newcastle disease (Clone 30)	Spray
	Turkey rhinotracheitis (live)	Spray
	Pasteurellosis and erysipelas* (killed)	Injection
12 weeks	Avian encephalomyelitis (live)	Drinking water
14 weeks	Newcastle disease, TRT, PMV-3 (killed)	Injection
	Pasteurellosis and erysipelas (killed)	Injection
20 weeks	Infectious avian encephalomyelitis	Drinking water
24 weeks	Newcastle disease, TRT, PMV-3 (killed)	Injection
	Pasteurellosis and erysipelas (killed)	Injection

* The combined pasteurella + erysipelas vaccine is no longer available in the UK.

Table 5.7 | Duck breeders

AGE	VACCINE	ROUTE
1–10 days	Duck virus hepatitis (DVH)	Web stab
2–3 weeks	Fowl cholera	Intramuscular injection
6–7 weeks	Fowl cholera	Intramuscular injection
8–9 weeks	Duck viral enteritis	Intramuscular injection
20 weeks	Duck virus hepatitis (DVH)	Intramuscular injection

Table 5.8 | Commercial ducks

DVH IMMUNITY STATUS	AGE	VACCINE	ROUTE
No maternal immunity	1 day	DVH	Web stab
Maternal immunity present	10 days	DVH	Web stab
	2–3 weeks	Fowl cholera	Intramuscular injection

RECOMBINANT VACCINES

Molecular biology has now developed to the extent that techniques are available that make it possible to insert into a vector (either a nonpathogenic virus or bacterium) those genes from a pathogenic organism that are known to be important in conferring protection. Following inoculation into an animal, the vector will replicate and, in so doing, the inserted gene is also replicated and its product is expressed, which can then stimulate an immune response to the insert in addition to the vector. Theoretically, this opens up the possibility of a new generation of vaccines, often called recombinant DNA vaccines, in which the advantage of the safety of killed vaccines is combined with the efficacy of live ones.

The choice of suitable vectors is important. They must be capable of being given by mass application methods and frequently must replicate in the face of maternally derived immunity. Two existing poultry vaccines, herpesvirus of turkeys (HVT) and fowl pox virus (FPV), are suitable for use as vectors and experimental studies have shown that, for example, the F gene of either NDV or TRT virus can be inserted into these vectors and be expressed in the birds following inoculation of the vector and also confer protection against experimental challenge with pathogenic NDV or TRT virus respectively. Thus, the system has potential for commercial use and it is certainly attractive that protection against both the vector (HVT or FPV) and the inserted genes can be achieved in a single vaccination. However, it is still unclear whether these vaccines will have any significant advantages over existing conventional ones in, for example, the type or duration of immunity which they confer. One recombinant DNA vaccine (FPV containing the protective genes of NDV) has recently been licensed for use in poultry in the USA so the performance of such a vaccine can now be assessed under field conditions.

FURTHER READING

Aini I 1990 Control of poultry disease in Asia by vaccination. World's Poult Sci J 46: 125–132

Baxendale W 1996 Current methods of delivery of poultry vaccines. In: Davison T F, Morris T R, Payne L N, eds. Poultry immunology. Carfax, Abingdon, p 375–387

Bosch G 1998 Vaccination in the hatchery. Int Hatchery Pract 12(3)

Box P G 1984 Poultry vaccines – Live or killed? Poult Int May: 58–66

Fletcher O J 1984 Basic considerations in design, implementation of immunisation programmes. Poult Dig 43: 412–415

Grieve D 1992 Evaluation of water, spray vaccinations using a blue dye. Poult Dig November: 28–32

McMillen J K, Cochran M D, Junker D E et al. 1991 The safe and effective use of fowlpox virus as a vector for poultry vaccines. In: Brown F, ed. Recombinant vectors in vaccine development. Dev Biol Stand 82. S Karger, Basel, p 137–145

Sander J E 1994 Basic concepts of broiler, breeder vaccination programmes. Poult Dig March: 10–12

Wigle W J 1990 Proper water vaccination requires certain techniques. Poult Dig March: 30–32

Yadin H 1980 Aerosol vaccination against Newcastle disease: virus inhalation and retention during vaccination. Avian Pathol 9: 163–170

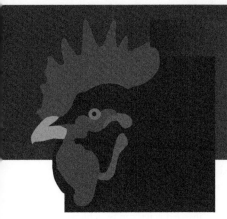

CHAPTER 6

Paul F. McMullin

Medicines and medication

The techniques discussed in the previous two chapters, biosecurity and vaccination, have had a major impact on the occurrence of disease in poultry production. However, disease can still occur. Medication may be intended to target the specific pathogen or an opportunistic bacterial infection secondary to a viral disease. Medication or supply of normal nutrients such as vitamins and electrolytes may also be used to provide symptomatic relief or compensate for the effects of reduced feed intake. The primary objectives of medication are to reduce mortality, to prevent ongoing debilitating effects of the disease and to alleviate suffering and discomfort. In commercial poultry production the objective is to ensure that the costs associated with medicines and medication are recovered by the reduction in disease-related losses and improved productivity.

PHYSIOLOGICAL, PATHOLOGICAL AND MANAGEMENT FACTORS AFFECTING THE OUTCOME OF MEDICATION

Individual medication of poultry is occasionally practised, either on its own or in addition to flock medication. This strategy is used for severe localized problems, for instance eye and wound infections. Given the labour cost associated with individual medication it is more likely to be used in stock of relatively high unitary value, typically breeding stock. As the market for such use is very limited, there are few products specifically approved for individual application in poultry. However, individual medication is to be encouraged when practical, effective and possible without resulting in residues in any resulting food products.

In most other situations all birds in an affected group are medicated. The beneficial effects of such usage are well documented in controlled trials (e.g. Glisson et al 2004). There are a number of approved products and indications for use in group medication in most countries. For less numerous poultry species (turkeys, ducks, geese, game birds) there are generally fewer products with specific approvals than there are for chickens.

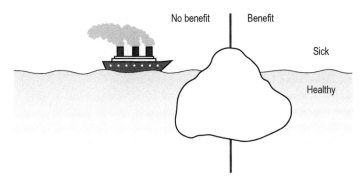

Fig. 6.1 The 'Iceberg effect'. Not all of the apparently sick birds benefit from medication, some apparently healthy birds do.

There are a number of sound reasons that dictate that flock-based medication will nearly always be the method of choice. The main one we might describe as the 'iceberg effect'. A poultry flock suffering a disease challenge is analogous to an iceberg, as shown in Figure 6.1. Sick birds may be detectable on cursory or careful inspection but apparently healthy birds will often have lesions if culled for post-mortem examination. There may be no direct correlation between discernible sickness at the individual bird level and benefit from medication. In some cases the birds that are clinically ill respond poorly to medication. This may be because of the advanced state of their illness or because of poor feed and water intake. Others, which are sick but have not yet developed clinical signs, often benefit from prompt, effective medication. In other words, every sick flock may be divided into a 2 × 2 contingency table similar to Figure 6.1. The greater the number of birds in the two right-hand quadrants of this table the more likely it is that medication is required. Although the actual number of birds in each quadrant is always unknown, an experienced poultry veterinarian will use all available data (such as post-mortem examination, results of microbiological examination, mortality and culling trends, previous site history, etc.) to estimate the benefit of medication in a particular situation.

Other benefits may be cited for flock medication. As there is intimate contact between large numbers of individuals in a poultry flock, control of infection (as distinct from disease) may benefit by reducing the exposure of flockmates. It should be kept in mind that the number of bird-to-bird routes of infection (RI) rises exponentially as the number of susceptible birds increases (one version of the formula is RI $= n \times (n - 1)$ where n is the population size). For a typical-sized commercial poultry flock the number of routes will be in the range of 10 million to 1 billion, assuming that all are susceptible. A further major benefit of flock-based medication compared to individual medication is that it avoids the need to bring large numbers of temporary staff into contact with a flock suffering from disease. This reduces stress on the flock and decreases the risk of a new disease or spreading the disease being treated to other flocks.

Drinking water or feed usually serves as the carrier for distributing and administering products used in the medication of poultry flocks. Although water intake closely follows eating patterns in healthy subjects, water medication is often desirable in sick flocks because disease affects water consumption less than feed intake. Water medication may, in addition, be implemented more rapidly in most circumstances. For these reasons this chapter concentrates on aspects of water medication. Administration of medicines via feed is used to extend the period of medication after initial water medication and for prophylactic treatment. Availability of dual feed bins enhances the control of in-feed medication because they can be used to avoid mixing medicated and unmedicated feed in the bin, so helping to ensure that the correct dose is administered.

Feed medication may also be preferable in flocks of ducks or geese held under free-range conditions or game birds in release pens because of the difficulty of medicating all sources of drinking water. Even for waterfowl in confined housing, water spillage results in considerable wastage (typically up to 50%) and this should be taken into account when calculating dosage. Nipple drinkers are used in modern systems and reduce water wastage.

Proper therapy in water requires adequate dosage and this must take into account both the dose and the duration of treatment. The dose of medicines has often been expressed as concentration of the active ingredient (usually parts per million, ppm). However, water consumption, irrespective of health status, varies widely according to bird species, age and ambient temperature. For example, 3-week-old broilers, adult breeder hens and breeder turkeys given a compound at 200 ppm in water, will, at normal ambient temperature, be dosed with approximately 40, 20 and 10 mg of active agent per kg body weight (BW) per day respectively. Relative water consumption and subsequent intake of the active ingredient decrease with age, being about half the quantity in adults compared to young birds. Within the temperature comfort zone (15–25°C) water consumption per unit BW mass and the ratio water/feed intake remain fairly stable. However, they increase abruptly once the heat stress threshold (typically 27°C for well-feathered birds) is exceeded. Hence in tropical climates the drug dose can be two to three times higher than under temperate conditions, at a given ppm dosage in water. For these reasons it is usually preferable to express the dosage as mg active agent per unit BW. The possible exception would be treatment for intestinal disease, where the aim is to achieve an effective concentration in the intestinal contents. When the concentration of active agent in water is converted into dose per kg metabolic weight ($BW^{0.75}$), the relationship between concentration and dose per kg is constant, regardless of age. With most antimicrobial drugs, however, the serum concentrations are proportional to drug intake per kg real BW within a specific age range. Data sheet recommendations for medicines in poultry are now more likely to show dosages on the basis of BW as opposed to those based on concentration in drinking water.

Lighting schedules, feeding programmes and disease strongly influence water consumption patterns. Broilers in controlled-environment houses, if given continuous light, eat and drink intermittently with little or no difference between day and night. Broilers and growing turkeys are now commonly managed under lighting programmes (with a dark period) that are likely to influence water consumption. Layer hens consume two-thirds of their total daily water and feed during the last 4–6 h of the light period. Maximal water intake in replacement breeders under feed restriction occurs during a few hours following feeding. Kidney disease may also increase water intake because of associated water losses.

For all the above-mentioned reasons administering medicines on the basis of a straightforward concentration of active ingredient in the water can lead to highly inaccurate dosing and should be avoided.

APPROACHES TO MEDICATION UNDER FIELD CONDITIONS

The risk of epidemic (or, more correctly, epizootic) spread of infectious agents, both poultry pathogens and zoonotic organisms, is ever-present on poultry farms. This risk is higher in large, integrated poultry companies with common chick and feed supplies, particularly in geographical areas of high poultry density. This has made technical advisory staff ever more vigilant with respect to the use of medicinal products in a timely fashion. In the classical approach, medicines are used in situations where a clinical cure for diseased flocks is required (therapy). Sometimes disease is so predictable that preventive or prophylactic medication is required. The term 'metaphylaxis' has been coined for the application of medicines to birds or flocks likely to be infected (and so exposed to an imminent disease risk). Medication is usually applied as soon as premonitory disease signs appear in just a few subjects of the group. Such strategic medication in anticipation of major disease damage is justifiable under conditions of good farm management, timely availability of flock health information, adequate diagnostic support and professional veterinary supervision.

Oral treatment requires sufficient stability and good solubility or homogeneous distribution of the product in water or feed. Freshly medicated solutions should be prepared every day. Water treatment medicines are commonly administered via bulk water tanks (typically 500–1000 L capacity) under low pressure or via water proportioners that meter the active ingredient into the water system at the appropriate dosage. Attention should be paid to less soluble inert fillers or precipitation due to unusual pH or hardness of drinking water, which may block drinking nipples and valves in water distribution equipment. The daily dose can be calculated on the basis of the weight of a bird sample. Alternatively, and in many instances, the total live mass to be treated can be calculated by multiplying the normal standard BW found in the manual guide by the flock size. As growth is usually linear, the actual BW can be interpolated between weekly weights. The total daily amount of drinking water needed by the flock can be derived from the daily total feed intake and the ratio of water consumption to feed intake, which is fairly constant for a given bird species in the temperature comfort zone. The ratio of water consumption to feed consumption is often taken to be 1.8–2 in chickens and turkeys and 3 in domestic ducks. In well-managed farms that have water flow measuring devices installed in every poultry house, the total daily water consumption can be assessed precisely.

ADVERSE REACTIONS AND SIDE EFFECTS

Drug toxicity is usually associated with incorrect treatment programmes or accidental overdosage. Medicines with a narrow therapeutic margin (lethal dose/effective dose, LD_{50}/ED_{50}) that have been used in the past in poultry medicine are dihydrostreptomycin, furazolidone and nonpotentiated sulphonamides but these are rarely used today (and furazolidone is prohibited in most countries). Specific examples are discussed in some detail in Chapter 40, and in Reece (1988). The occurrence and degree of adverse effects are very dependent on dose and length of treatment. Within the same product category even slight changes of the chemical structure of a compound can substantially modify target animal safety. Impaired palatability of the drug in feed or water may also indirectly affect bird health and performance by reducing feed or water intake. Turkeys are more taste-sensitive than chickens. Dehydration can occur in young poults subsequent to refusal of medicated water.

Certain narrow-spectrum Gram-positive antibiotics have been shown to disturb the inherent *Salmonella* colonization resistance of the avian indigenous gut flora in a dose-dependent way. More research is needed to clarify the capability of antimicrobials to disrupt components of the intestinal flora that are protective against colonization of pathogenic enterobacteria. Use of normal caecal flora ('competitive exclusion' products) may play a role in minimizing this effect. Antibiotic use may also mask the occurrence of infections subject to routine monitoring by preventing their detection with the tests normally used. Official disease control programmes may restrict antibiotic use in particular circumstances to avoid this effect, as is being planned for the monitoring of *Salmonella* in chicken breeders in the EU.

In case of doubt about drug compatibility, information must be obtained from the manufacturers. The same holds for possible detrimental effects of antimicrobials or their diluents on Marek's disease vaccine virus in solutions for parenteral injection. Adverse reactions may include suspected adverse reaction in the user or unexpected lack of efficacy. When suspected adverse reactions do occur, most countries have a formal system for recording and investigating them. Both end users and veterinarians are encouraged to report such occurrences.

Table 6.1 Pharmacodynamic properties of antimicrobial medicines and common indications of different acute compounds

GROUP ACTIVE	RESTING	PROLIFERATING	MECHANISM	COLIBACILLOSIS	MYCOPLASMOSIS NON-COMPLICATED	MYCOPLASMOSIS COMPLICATED (E. COLI)	SALMONELLOSIS	PASTEURELLOSIS	STAPHYLOCOCCOSIS	NECROTIC ENTERITIS	INFECTIOUS CORYZA	ERYSIPELAS INFECTION	YOLK SAC INFECTIONS
Aminocyclitol Apramycin	Bactericidal	Bactericidal	Inhibition of protein synthesis	✓			✓						Inj. ✓
Aminoglycosides Gentamicin Neomycin Spectinomycin Streptomycin	Bactericidal	Bactericidal	Inhibition of protein synthesis	✓	✓	✓	✓ ✓	✓ ✓	✓		✓ ✓		✓ Inj.
Beta lactam Amoxicillin Ceftiofur Penicillin V		Bactericidal	Inhibition of cell wall synthesis	✓			✓	✓	✓ ✓	✓ ✓		✓ ✓	✓
Fluoroquinolones Danofloxacin Difloxacin Enrofloxacin Flumequine	Bactericidal	Bactericidal	Inhibition of DNA replication	✓ ✓	✓ ✓ ✓	✓ ✓ ✓	✓ ✓ ✓ ✓	✓ ✓ ✓ ✓	✓ ✓ ✓		✓ ✓ ✓ ✓	✓	✓

Group	Drug	Type	Mode of action											
Folate inhibitors	Sulphonamides	Bacteristatic	Modification of bacterial energy mechanisms	✓		✓	✓	✓			✓			✓
	Trimethoprim			✓		✓	✓	✓			✓			✓
Lincosamides	Lincomycin	Bacteristatic	Inhibition of protein synthesis	✓				✓	✓					
Macrolides	Erythromycin	Bacteristatic	Inhibition of protein synthesis	✓		✓		✓	✓					
	Aivlosin®			✓										
	Spiramycin			✓										
	Tilmicosin			✓										
	Tylosin			✓	✓				✓					
Polypeptide	Colistin	Bactericidal	Inhibition of cytoplasmic membrane synthesis	✓i		✓		✓			✓			
	Polymyxin B				✓i									
Quinolones	Oxolinic acid	Bactericidal	Inhibition of DNA replication	✓		✓		✓	✓			✓		
Tetracyclines	Chlortetracycline	Bacteristatic	Inhibition of protein synthesis	✓	✓	✓		✓	✓	✓		✓		✓
	Doxycycline			✓	✓	✓		✓	✓	✓		✓		✓
	Oxytetracycline			✓	✓	✓		✓	✓	✓		✓		✓
	Tetracycline			✓	✓	✓		✓	✓	✓		✓		✓
Tiamulin	Tiamulin	Bacteristatic	Inhibition of protein synthesis		✓									

Inj., Day-old injection; i, intestinal activity only

✓ indicates a compound which commonly has an indication for the condition

CLASSES OF MEDICINES USED IN POULTRY

Miscellaneous products

Soluble multivitamins are used for treatment of specific deficiencies, such as rickets. However, poultry suffering a range of disease challenges tend to benefit from additional supplementation because of a number of factors:

- Damaged intestines can reduce absorption of vitamins
- Damage of any tissues may increase requirement because of the reparative mechanisms
- Activation of the immune response mechanisms may also increase requirement
- Damage to the liver can reduce storage and mobilization of vitamins
- Reduced feed intake due to disease tends to reduce the availability of vitamins when demand is increasing.

The water-soluble vitamins (sometimes called B complex) are not stored in the body, so any deficit of these tends quickly to have an effect. The fat-soluble vitamins (A, D, E and K) are usually well stored in the liver so daily intake is less critical. In some countries maximum daily intakes of vitamins A and D are intended to avoid excessive levels accumulating in livers. Water-soluble supplements are a convenient and effective way of improving intake of important vitamins at particular times of increased demand. Balanced salt or electrolyte solutions may also be of benefit in diseases characterized by abnormal intestinal or respiratory function.

Analgesic and anti-inflammatory products are approved in some countries. Usually these are based on aspirin or soluble aspirin. These treatments have the potential to provide symptomatic relief in a variety of diseases characterized by acute inflammation and help improve the ability of affected birds to maintain adequate feed and water intake.

Antiparasitics

Prophylactic medication for coccidiosis is commonly practised in commercial chickens and turkeys reared on litter, while for both turkeys and game birds, control of *Histomonas* and flagellates may also be required but is not currently available in the EU (see Table 39.2). Anticoccidial medication (or vaccination) occasionally fails, so medication for treatment of these diseases is also required. Prophylactic medication for worms is sometimes required, especially for long-lived birds and those allowed access to range.

Antiviral products

In spite of the fact that most primary disease in commercial poultry is caused by viruses, antiviral compounds have not been marketed or developed for use in poultry in Europe, although there are reports of their use in some other areas of the world. Some use of natural antiviral proteins produced by the immune system, known as cytokines, has been made experimentally. Antiseptics and disinfectants approved for spraying in poultry houses and for sanitizing drinking water may help to reduce viral challenge at the flock level by reducing bird-to-bird transmission.

Antimicrobials

A review of options for antimicrobial treatment in domestic poultry is shown in Table 6.1. The information included is based on package inserts and published scientific data but is provided for general guidance only. In vitro sensitivity and local conditions of approval should be checked prior to treatment. Not all antimicrobials listed are authorized by the regulatory agencies in all countries for use in poultry.

PHARMACOLOGICAL CONSIDERATIONS OF PARTICULAR RELEVANCE TO ANTIMICROBIALS

To ensure clinical efficacy, antibiotic activity must be available at the site of infection during a sufficient time of exposure. The outcome of antibacterial medication is a result of many interacting factors, such as pharmacodynamics (drug interaction with the bacterial cell), pharmacokinetics (drug absorption, distribution and excretion) and host defence mechanisms. The pharmacological characteristics of antibacterials commonly used in poultry medicine are listed in Table 6.1. Antimicrobials are categorized according to their chemical group (compound category), their spectrum of activity and their mode of action (bactericidal or bacteristatic). The form of a specific antimicrobial product (active ingredients and diluents or other complementary ingredients) may markedly affect absorption and serum kinetics. At therapeutically achievable concentrations, bacteristatic compounds inhibit or slow down bacterial multiplication whereas bactericidal drugs kill bacteria in a time-dependent and/or concentration-dependent way. With bactericidal drugs, which possess rapid killing effects on replicating bacteria (e.g. fluoroquinolones), the bird is less dependent on its immune system to make a quick recovery from disease. In general terms and under *in vitro* circumstances, combinations of bacteristatic and bactericidal compounds are antagonistic, whereas associations of either bactericidal or bacteristatic substances are not. Bactericidal agents of different compound categories can potentiate one another or act synergistically. Synergism between drugs in the test-tube, however, does not necessarily reflect better clinical cure in the host. Combinations are best avoided unless specifically approved. Sulphonamides and trimethoprim, both bacteristatic agents, are bactericidal when used in combination. The combination of lincomycin and spectinomycin is synergistic against mycoplasmas.

The activity or potency of an antibacterial compound against a microorganism is expressed as the minimal concentration (MIC) that is inhibitory to bacterial multiplication after 24 h of in vitro exposure. In order to be efficacious, the concentration of antibiotic activity in serum (systemic bioavailability) and target tissues is expected to exceed the MIC of the relevant microorganisms during the stationary phase or during logarithmic growth of the bacteria. Setting the breakpoint between susceptibility and resistance in vitro is based on the availability of the drug *in vivo*, in relation to the MICs of the disease pathogens. Hence sensitivity and resistance are relative terms because within the same bird species a microorganism may be susceptible at a specific organ location but not susceptible in another body compartment. Pharmacokinetic data measured in mammals are not directly applicable to poultry because the avian species have a higher metabolic rate, a shorter alimentary tract passage and a lower plasma half-life.

The practice of administering the total daily dose of the drug as a pulse during a few hours in the morning ('breakfast therapy') is suitable for bactericidal antimicrobials only. When medicating ducks or geese in the water it is especially beneficial to administer medicines as a 'pulse' dose. For maximum uniformity of intake this should be administered shortly after feeding. The majority of antibiotics also exert antimicrobial effects at concentrations below the MIC during a few hours following termination of medication (postantibiotic effect, PAE). This PAE is of less significance for continuous medication in water or feed over several days. Improved phagocytosis and other immunomodulating effects of antimicrobials in response to the immune system can contribute to clinical cure. Medication of breeder stock may hinder or delay the development of specific antibody to *Mycoplasma* or *Salmonella* and this effect should be taken into account in eradication programmes.

THE ASSESSMENT OF ANTIMICROBIALS IN CLINICAL SETTINGS

Unfortunately, sensitivity/resistance breakpoints used in veterinary medicine are not uniform worldwide and still often rely on standards set in human medicine. Standards for drug suscepti-bility testing for veterinary purposes have been published in the USA (Anon 1999). Prescott & Baggot (1985) consider in detail the interpretation of sensitivity test data for use in veterinary medicine. Although in vitro and in vivo models are important laboratory instruments to eluci-date pharmacodynamic/pharmacokinetic relationships, the cure of disease by an anti-infective agent in a clinical setting or field situation is the main guide in establishing the dosage and the usage label directions. The main criterion to monitor success of treatment under field condi-tions is the reduction of mortality. Other important parameters of health improvement are less conspicuous, for example return to regular feed intake and growth, clearance of internal inflam-matory lesions (abattoir condemnations) and the degree of reduction of bacterial shedding. Particularly with bacteristatic compounds, the lag time between onset of treatment and visible flock health improvement may expand to 24–48 h. Even when mortality returns to normal very rapidly and the birds behave thriftily again, medication must be maintained for the complete recommended length of treatment in order to avoid disease relapse. Treatment periods of 3–7 days are common. Relapses following treatment are most often encountered in chronic diseases where the causative organism persists, such as staphylococcal synovitis–arthritis, mycoplasmo-sis or chronic fowl cholera. Although, for the treatment of immunocompromised birds, bac-tericidal drugs are to be preferred over bacteristatic ones, clinical success is hampered with any antimicrobial in flocks having concomitant virus-induced immunodeficiency disease (Marek's disease, infectious bursal disease, infectious anaemia, reticuloendotheliosis).

Respiratory colibacillosis is a major area for the use of antibacterial products and in vitro resistance is more prevalent than with other pathogens. Frequent and improper use of anti-bacterials should be avoided, for example in cases presumably not responsive to antimicrobial medication (failures in climate control, early stages of viral multiplication). For *Escherichia coli* sensitivity testing, mixed strain inocula (e.g. 20–50 colonies), encompassing the variation of drug sensitivity within the multiplying bacteria population, are recommended. Published resistance rates are indicative of possible emergence of resistance in the field but have limited predictive value for drug prescription on a case-by-case basis. In drug sensitivity surveys, post-treatment isolates from problem farms and cases of therapy failure may be strongly represented and the calculated averages do not account for farm-to-farm variability. On the contrary, the on-site availability of historical drug sensitivity records is extremely useful for a prompt inter-vention when laboratory results are awaited.

Egg dipping, a technique whereby an antimicrobial compound is transferred by pressure dif-ferential from a dip bath into the interior egg compartments, is principally aimed for the control of egg-transmitted *Mycoplasma* infections (e.g. *M. gallisepticum* in chickens and *M. iowae* in tur-keys). Egg dipping with antimicrobials must be seen as a transitory measure to decrease the infec-tion pressure in the production chain before a top-down eradication programme can be put in place. Contamination of dip solutions with opportunistic pathogens (e.g. *Pseudomonas* spp.) must be carefully controlled. The physical process of egg dipping, even when carried out correctly, can result in a decline in hatchability. As the uptake of active agent by the hatching egg can be very irregular during dipping, individual egg injection with accurate delivery of the proper dose is preferred in elite and grandparent breeding stock. Automated systems for in ovo drug administration before hatch have been developed; however injection at transfer to the hatcher is too late for optimal control of vertical transmission of most infections. Specific solutions of ceftiofur and gentamicin for the injection of day-old chicks or turkey poults are approved in some countries. The main indication of such parenteral treatment is to reduce neonatal mortality caused by hatchery infections associated with vaccine contamination or yolk sac infection. These are usually administered along with Marek's disease vaccine.

Antibacterial treatment will not usually eliminate all infecting microorganisms from treated subjects; however, it can be a supplementary tool in sanitation or eradication programmes. Intensive use of antibiotics in an eradication programme in a small number of birds in the higher levels of the breeding pyramid can reduce total antibiotic usage. Where the target of such programmes is a potential zoonosis, or where such usage could result in incidental exposure of zoonotic organisms to antibiotics, then the resistance profile of the zoonotic organisms needs to be carefully monitored. It has been shown that use of certain antibiotics in *Salmonella*-infected parents, if followed by the administration of 'competitive exclusion flora', can substantially reduce or eliminate vertical transmission for considerable periods. This is not permitted in all countries and under the EU zoonoses regulations is permitted only with certain serotypes and with the approval of the veterinary authorities. In any case, it should not be regarded as a routine procedure, rather as an interim measure to improve infection status while other required actions are implemented.

RESPONSIBLE AND PRUDENT USE OF ANTIMICROBIAL PRODUCTS

Much has been said and written on the potential impact of use of growth-promoting and therapeutic antimicrobials on resistance patterns. Bywater (2004) summarized the arguments and presented the results of extensive European surveys on this topic. Rational antibacterial therapy is based on a combination of clinical judgement, laboratory diagnosis, medical knowledge and information about the flock to be treated ('good veterinary practice'). A major constraint on the use of antimicrobials in agriculture is that the cost of a product and its administration must be outweighed by the benefit obtained. A broad range of organizations have recently published responsible- or prudent-use guidelines and others are in development (see Further reading). Poultry veterinarians and other professionals with an interest in poultry health are encouraged to both contribute to and be fully aware of the content of such documents. With all use of antimicrobials, the prescriber and user have responsibilities to the poultry, the owners of the poultry, consumers of products derived from poultry, and society. A fundamental principle common to most guidelines is that the usage of antimicrobials can never replace fundamental shortcomings in husbandry, biosecurity measures and prophylactic hygiene on the premises. Effective preventive medicine and good management reduce but may not eliminate the need for antimicrobials.

Sensitivity testing of the causative microorganisms in a representative bird sample (typically ill subjects, recent deaths) prior to or concurrently with the commencement of medication is commonly practised in poultry medicine. Whereas for monitoring and epidemiological studies MIC testing is advocated, the disk diffusion test (Kirby–Bauer, antibiogram) is a quick, practical and reliable tool to determine susceptibility of pathogenic bacteria isolated from necropsy specimens. Routine surveillance of resistance patterns of poultry pathogens can help guide treatment decisions, particularly for diseases associated with pathogens of variable resistance profiles. Resistant organisms can spread within production systems even in the absence of anti-microbial medication so special care in infection control is indicated where highly resistant organisms are identified.

As a general rule different antimicrobial products should not be mixed or administered simultaneously as they may interfere with solubility, absorption and potency (drug antagonism). Multiple drug therapy is no substitute for deficiencies in diagnosis. Consecutive use of the same compound category within the same production cycle should be avoided, unless preceding in vitro testing has shown satisfactory susceptibility of the microorganisms involved.

Meat must be withheld from human consumption until residues are depleted below the tolerance limits set by the competent authorities. These maximum residue limits relate to the acceptable daily intake that poses no risk for the consumer. As commercial layer farms cannot afford to destroy table eggs, layer flocks are compulsorily excluded from treatment with anti-infectives that result in egg residues over the maximum residue limit.

In order to demonstrate responsible use of antimicrobials, timely, accurate records of medicine usage and the reasons for usage are a basic requirement. Increasingly food retailers, and others, expect to be able to audit such records and monitor trends in antibiotic use.

New veterinary medicines and feed additive regulations

The EU legislation regulating veterinary medicines was 'recast' into a new veterinary medicines Directive 2001/82/EC, which was further amended, following a review of community law, by Directive 2004/28/EC. As with all EU directives it is given effect under national law in each member state. The UK legislation implementing the new directive are the Veterinary Medicines Regulations 2005 and came into effect in October 2005. The main change implemented is the classification of all veterinary medicines for food animals as 'prescription-only'. This applies to veterinary vaccines and medicines applied by any route, including in-feed. The only vaccines excluded from these regulations are those made from pathogens or antigens isolated from specific animals or farms – often referred to as 'emergency' vaccines. In making the change to prescription-only status it was accepted that not all products required prescription of the same type. In the UK the medicines used in poultry are classified mainly as either POM-V (requiring prescription by a veterinary surgeon) or POM-VPS, which may be prescribed by a veterinary surgeon, pharmacist or 'suitably qualified person'. The previous options for the licensing of veterinary medicines are retained – this may be by a centralized procedure with the European Medicines Evaluation Agency, in each individual company with the appropriate national regulatory body or by mutual recognition of products approved in another member state. The Directive also makes it clear that, where a suitable locally approved product is not available, a suitable product approved in another member state may be used as part of the 'prescribing cascade'. In the UK this provision is given effect by a system of special import licensing in which the veterinary surgeon applies to the Veterinary Medicines Directorate for permission to do this.

There has been a separate process of review of the feed additives regulations that culminated in the approval of EU regulation 1831/2003. EU regulations apply in member states without further national legislation. Approval of feed additives is carried out centrally and managed by the European Food Safety Authority. This regulation required that all use of growth-promoting antimicrobials cease in poultry production by 31 December 2005. Anticoccidials used for prevention of the disease and administered through feed remain classified as feed additives, although a review of their regulation is being conducted by the EU.

REFERENCES

Anon 1999 Performance standards for antimicrobial disk and dilution susceptibility tests for bacteria isolated from animals. Approved Standard M31-A. National Committee for Clinical Laboratory Standards, London. Details on line at www.nccls.org

Bywater R J 2004 Veterinary use of antimicrobials and emergence of resistance in zoonotic and sentinel bacteria in the EU. J Vet Med B Infect Dis Vet Public Health 51: 361–363

Glisson J R, Hofacre C L, Mathis G F 2004 Comparative efficacy of enrofloxacin, oxytetracycline, and sulfadimethoxine for the control of morbidity and mortality caused by *Escherichia coli* in broiler chickens. Avian Dis 48: 658–662

Prescott J F, Baggot J D 1985 Antimicrobial susceptibility testing and antimicrobial drug dosages. J Am Vet Med Assoc 187: 363–368

Reece R C 1988 Review of adverse effects of chemotherapeutic agents in poultry. WPSA J 44: 193–196

FURTHER READING

Anon 1998 Antimicrobial guidelines. British Veterinary Poultry Association. Available on line at www.bvpa.org.uk/medicine/amicguid.htm

Anon 2005 The responsible use of antimicrobials in poultry production. The RUMA Alliance. Available on line at www.ruma.org.uk – full guidelines at www.ruma.org.uk/guidelines/RUMA%20Poultry%20Guidelines%20Long%20(2005).pdf

Anon 1999 Prudent use of antibiotics: global basic principles WVA/COMISA/IFAP. Available on line at: http://www.poultry-health.com/library/antimicrobials/wvacoifa.htm

Anon 2005 Veterinary medicines guidance notes. Available on line at www.vmd.gov.uk/Publications/VMGNotes/VMGNotes.htm

Bell I 1986 Rational chemotherapeutics. The Postgraduate Committee in Veterinary Science of the University of Sydney in Association with the Australian Veterinary Poultry Association, Proceedings No. 92. Poult Health 429–467

Langston V C, Davis L E 1989 Factors to consider in the selection of antimicrobial drugs for therapy. Compendium 11: 355–363

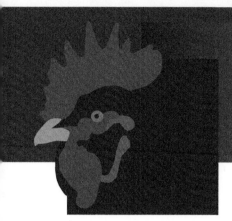

Sue Haslam

Legislation and poultry welfare

Interest in the welfare of food-producing animals throughout the European Union (EU) continues to increase and the perceived 'welfare status' of the animal from which food is produced is now seen as part of product quality. This has resulted in the enactment of a body of animal welfare legislation under the direction of the EU and, concurrently, the development of Welfare Assurance Schemes by retail companies, charitable organizations and food production industry bodies. Both legislation and Welfare Assurance Schemes controlling welfare are evolving relatively rapidly, informed by the findings of work in the field of animal welfare science: this is an equally rapidly expanding discipline and one in which major methodological and conceptual advances have been achieved in recent years.

Consensus is building that, for accurate, representative assessment of the welfare of an animal or group of animals, a combination of several welfare indicators should be measured, rather than a single measure, and that animal-based indicators, i.e. those which take measurements directly from the animal rather than measures of resources provided for the animal, should be used where possible. Indicators of welfare include physiological, pathological, biochemical, behavioural and 'fitness' measures, these last being measures of growth rate, longevity and reproductive success. Furthermore, for the purposes of welfare audit, indicators of welfare should be: feasible, in that they are practical to measure in the field; valid, in that they reflect animal welfare; and reliable, in that they give a consistent measure between observers and observations. However, consensus is lacking on how different indicators of welfare should be weighed against each other or integrated to give an overall assessment of animal or bird in order to facilitate comparison of welfare between individual animals, groups of animals or animals produced in different husbandry systems.

Infectious disease is a major, but not sole, cause of poor bird welfare. Prevention of infectious disease in poultry is of considerable importance to the poultry industry, and much of this book is devoted to the subject and extensive measures are taken routinely to control disease, including vaccination protocols, biosecurity measures, disease monitoring and rapid treatment. However, injury, fear and distress caused by social stress or frustration due to husbandry systems that do not provide sufficient space or resources to permit performance of normal behaviour may also be a cause of poor welfare. Additionally, genotypes that have been developed for high production may predispose birds to noninfectious diseases that cause pain and/or distress, such as lameness in broiler chickens or osteoporosis and subsequent bone fractures in laying hens.

In this chapter measurement systems that have been developed for the assessment of poultry welfare are first discussed. The principal welfare issues that are not related to infectious disease but cause poor welfare in poultry, as well as causing economic loss to the industry, and that arise from husbandry system specifications or bird genotype are briefly outlined and practical methods for assessing these are described. The provisions of statutory instruments that regulate bird welfare in EU Member States, and those in the process of consultation or implementation, are then discussed.

ASSESSMENT OF BIRD WELFARE

Current assurance schemes used by retail companies, such as the RSPCA Freedom Foods Scheme operated by the Royal Society for the Prevention of Cruelty to Animals and the Assured British Chicken scheme in the UK, are invariably based on a checklist that is completed on farm by independent, trained auditors during an audit that takes between 1 and 4 h. The checklists are based on the resources available to the birds, such as the capacity of the ventilation system, the length of feed track or number of nipples per bird and the length of dark periods in the lighting regimen. The level above which each of these measures is considered to be compliant is informed by scientific findings but is essentially arbitrary and tends to be pragmatic. However, there is some evidence that such assessment systems may not accurately reflect welfare for some species.

A welfare assessment system based on output measures of bird welfare and known as the Bristol Welfare Assurance Programme has been developed at the University of Bristol for laying hens and is being trialled in the UK by the Soil Association, which regulates some organic farmers. Details can be found at www.vetschool.bris.ac.uk/animalwelfare. Additionally, a system that amalgamates weighted measures to give an overall assessment of broiler welfare, expressed numerically as a percentage, has been developed and successfully evaluated in the field using alternative, more complex, measures of welfare that it would not be feasible to use in a routine welfare audit, details of which have been published (Haslam 2004). These systems are based primarily on animal-based measures of welfare, such as percentage mortality, percentage of birds that are lame, percentage with foot pad lesions, percentage with damaged plumage, pale combs and respiratory symptoms.

The use of animal-based assessment is being adopted throughout the EU. The Committee of Senior Officials for Scientific and Technical Research (COST) initiative no. 846 group entitled 'Measuring and monitoring farm animal welfare', funded by the EU, seeks to find consensus between experts in poultry behaviour and welfare from across the EU on measures to include in a Welfare Assessment System (Blokhuis 2006) and the associated Welfare Quality scheme aims to develop reliable on-farm monitoring systems, product information systems and practical species-specific strategies to improve animal welfare. Details of these initiatives can be found on line at www.cost846.unina.it/ and www.welfarequality.net/everyone, respectively. In the USA, welfare audit systems based on the Hazard Analysis Critical Control Point system, originally developed to ensure food safety, are in use by some US retail companies. The system, designed to assess and monitor welfare in poultry slaughter plants, for example that designed by Temple Grandin, can be seen at www.grandin.com/poultry.audit.html and www.grandin.com/welfare.audit.using.haccp.html. This system identifies points in the processing of birds at which welfare is most at risk and requires welfare measures to be made at these points, which have pass/fail levels. This system largely uses bird-based welfare measures, such as the percentage of birds shackled by one leg, percentage with broken or dislocated wings and the number of birds going into the scald tank in a conscious condition.

Such Welfare Assessment Schemes can only allow comparison between production units and cannot address underlying problems that arise from bird genotype, housing specification or transport and handling systems. For such problems the comparison will be, for example, between farms with a 'bad percentage' of laying hens with bone breaks and those with a 'very bad percentage'. Much of the remainder of this chapter is now devoted to a brief review of the principal welfare problems inherent to the poultry industry and the legislation in place to monitor and control welfare.

CONTACT DERMATITIS

Ulceration of the skin over the plantar surface of the feet (foot pad dermatitis), the caudal intertarsal joint (hock burn) and the sternum (breast burn) may occur in any class of poultry that is raised on deep litter. This condition may cause pain directly, and may also reflect environmental conditions in bird houses, such as poor litter and air quality. Hock burn and possibly breast burn may result from pressure necrosis when birds spend excessive amounts of time sitting down because of illness or lameness (discussed below).

The incidence of contact dermatitis lesions is customarily measured at the processing plant. Lesions are readily assessed on the processing line, immediately after defeathering, when birds are clean. If these data are collected with reference to a visual scale, rather than being recorded as 'present' or 'absent', both the prevalence and severity of the problem may be determined. Where the prevalence and/or severity of contact dermatitis in flocks is found to be high, producers may take remedial action to improve the quality of litter in subsequent flocks. Litter may be improved by increasing ventilation rates, raising house temperatures, repairing leaking drinkers or reducing water pressure, reducing stocking rate, i.e. the number of chicks placed per square metre of house floor area, or adding additional litter during the flock cycle.

LAMENESS IN BROILERS

There is evidence that a high proportion of broilers show gait abnormalities: the level of birds with severe lameness was found in one study, carried out in the UK 15 years ago, to be 26%. A more recent Danish survey of commercial birds found that 30.1% of birds were severely lame, which is in agreement with a recent UK study, which found nearly 28% of birds to be in this category. For both these studies, a significant proportion of the abnormalities were so severe as to prevent the bird from reaching food or water. Lameness in broilers is conventionally assessed on a six-point scale – 0, completely normal gait, to 5, not able to walk – known as the Bristol Gait Score. However, other assessment systems have been described, including the Latency to Lie (LTL) test, a more objective indicator, which measures the time birds take to lie down after the introduction of a small amount of tepid water to the pen. The LTL test was modified by Berg and Sanotra to enable faster testing of individual broilers.

There is some evidence that birds with a gait score of 3 experience pain but it is unclear to what extent the degree to which birds with gait scores other than 3 experience pain, if at all. Leg problems may be divided into those caused by developmental abnormalities, those caused by infectious agents and those caused by nutritional imbalances. There is evidence that bird genotype, gender, age, growth rate and weight, as well as length of the dark period in the lighting programme, affect levels of lameness in broilers. Older, heavier, male birds that are growing rapidly tend to have greater levels of leg abnormality, especially when subject to shorter dark periods, than younger, slower-growing, female birds. The incidence of leg problems may be reduced by the use of restricted feeding programmes and longer dark periods, especially in weeks 2 and 3 of the flock cycle. There is also some indication that feeding whole/cracked wheat early in the flock cycle (weeks 2–3), using poorly pelleted or dusty feed, reducing bird stocking densities and using genotypes that are less prone to leg problems may reduce the incidence of leg health problems in broilers. Many of these factors may be protective of leg health by reducing growth rate. Although the use of antibiotics has been found to result in a lower incidence of leg problems, this is not a satisfactory way forward given current concern about the overuse of antibiotics in livestock production.

FEATHER PECKING, CANNIBALISM AND AGGRESSIVE PECKING IN LAYING HENS

Feather pecking activity in hens has been classified into five main categories: gentle pecking, severe pecking, vent pecking, cannibalism and aggressive pecking. Gentle and severe feather pecking seem to be redirected ground pecking behaviour and may progress to cannibalism. Vent pecking, the onset of which usually occurs as egg laying begins, is directed at the prolapsed cloaca: it may start as investigative behaviour which may then progress to cannibalism. Cannibalism involves ingestion of part of other conspecifics, including skin, tissue and organs. Injuries are frequently of such severity that death follows, thus constituting a severe welfare problem: this problem has been reviewed by Newberry (2004). Cannibalistic attacks are usually made by groups of hens on one individual; pecks are usually delivered from behind or from the side of the victim and are delivered in a foraging posture with head and neck lowered. Cannibalism has been reported in all systems but outbreaks are often more severe in large flocks of free-range or aviary birds, as a cannibalistic bird in these systems has contact with many more birds and so can affect more individuals than a cannibalistic bird in a small group; up to 30% of the flock may be affected during an outbreak. Currently, beak trimming and reduced lighting are used to control cannibalism, although beak trimming has been shown to cause chronic pain due to neuroma formation, reduction in light levels may cause eye pathology and light restriction is not possible in free-range systems. Cannibalism may be reduced by: selecting less cannibalistic strains of bird; avoiding early onset of lay; ensuring an adequate diet; providing attractive foraging materials; removing individuals that have bleeding injuries and that are diseased or slow growing; providing high perches from an early age; providing nests that minimize visibility of the cloaca during laying.

Aggressive pecking is distinct from feather pecking and cannibalism in form and underlying motivation. Aggressive pecking is always directed at the head, with the aggressor in an upright posture with the two birds facing each other and it is thought to be a means of establishing social order. Many factors may be involved in the development of these complex pecking behaviour patterns, including colony size, stocking density, nutrition and lighting regime.

Experimentally, several protocols have been used to assess levels of feather pecking in laying hens, some of which use numerical rating scales to assess the levels of feather cover and skin damage on different parts of the birds, including head, neck, wing, breast and vent. However, these systems are currently time-consuming and so not practical to use in a welfare audit.

The development of a single, simplified system for the assessment of feather cover and skin damage would be necessary if this aspect of bird welfare were to be assessed routinely. Levels of cannibalism are reflected to some extent by the level of mortality, as many victims die from their injuries. However, not all dead birds are found as they may be consumed by other birds.

BONE FRACTURES IN HENS

A recent study found that the number of birds with old bone fractures that occurred during the laying cycle in commercial layers in a barn system was approximately 60%. This represents the high end of the spectrum of prevalence of bone fractures in hens: prevalence of old fractures has been found to be around 10% at end of lay in several other studies of caged birds. However, it is clear that bone fractures that occur during the flock cycle are a very serious welfare problem for laying hens; this problem has been reviewed by Webster (2004). Bone fractures occur as a result of high production levels, for which birds have been genetically selected: the calcium requirement to produce over 300 eggs per year, in comparison to between 140 and 160 in broiler breeders and 10–15 in wild jungle fowl, from which domestic hens originated, results in osteoporosis. There is evidence that bone strength may be genetically determined and that different strains of bird have different susceptibilities to bone fractures. Although bone strength in hens tends to be greater in free-range and aviary systems than in either conventional or enriched cages, the incidence of fractures is higher in free-range or aviary birds because of collisions with house furniture and equipment. A method of assessing the incidence of fractures in a live flock, by palpation of the keel bone, has been described by Wilkins et al (2004).

HANDLING AND TRANSPORT OF POULTRY

Few poultry kept commercially, whether broilers or layers, are handled after placement until collected for slaughter. There is a considerable body of evidence, in both layers and broilers, that the welfare of these birds may be severely compromised during this process (reviewed by Kettlewell and Mitchell (2004)). The principal welfare problems arise from trauma and fear due to manual handling of birds, both at the farm and the slaughter plant, and heat or cold stress during transport.

Traditional methods of harvesting broilers involve catching teams who capture birds by one leg, invert them and carry as many as five birds in each hand to transport crates: this predisposes to trauma, fear and distress, which may lead to death through haemorrhage or circulatory failure. A recent study in the UK found that the level of birds dead on arrival (DoAs) at the factory was 0.05%, ranging from 0.01% to 0.1%: this is very low in comparison with levels of DoA reported by studies from 15 years ago of between 0.21% and 1.14% of total birds. This may be due to improved handling and transport practices in the industry, including the widespread use of modular transport, which replaces side-loading vehicles. Poultry harvesting machines are in use in some countries, including the UK and Australia, which have one type of system and the USA, which has five systems. The evidence for improved bird welfare due to mechanical, rather than manual harvesting is equivocal.

The percentage of birds with new fractures after the harvesting of end-of-lay hens may be up to 50% of the flock. The welfare of end of lay hens during handling and transport has been reviewed by Knowles (1998). As discussed above, laying birds suffer from osteoporosis and bone fractures occur as a result of trauma either suffered during removal from cages in caged systems or due to collision with house furniture while attempting to avoid capture in aviary or free-range

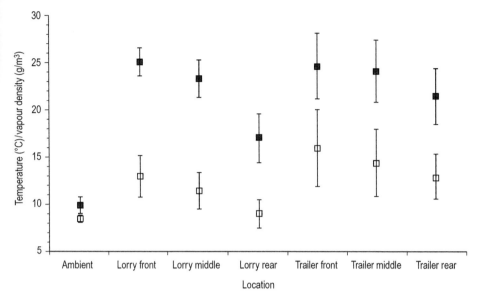

Fig. 7.1 Spatial distribution of temperature (closed boxes) and vapour density (open boxes) in a passively ventilated broiler transport vehicle. The vehicle is comprised of two components, lorry and drawbar trailer. (With permission from Kettlewell and Mitchell 2000.)

systems (birds are housed for depopulation in free-range systems). Perches in percheries or furnished cages may exacerbate this problem, although there is no experimental evidence to support this supposition. Care in removal of birds from cages reduces trauma and removing birds from the cages by two legs significantly reduces the chances of birds acquiring fractures. A wheeled modular system has been developed for depopulating caged birds, which is positioned next to the cages, so minimizing the duration of human contact: it is based on the Whurr module used to transport pullets. End-of-lay hens have a very low economic value because of the high level of bone fragments in the meat and a system for killing birds in house would avoid the considerable welfare problems arising from handling and transportation prior to slaughter. The incidence of bone fractures in end-of-lay hens may be assessed immediately after slaughter using the keel palpation method designed for live birds.

There are inherent difficulties in designing transporters to carry large numbers of poultry that can adequately protect bird welfare in changing environmental conditions. For example, poultry in crates on the outside of an open lorry trailer may be subjected to severe cold exposure when the vehicle is moving at speed, while at rest there may be difficulties in providing adequate fresh air to crates positioned centrally. Broilers have a very high metabolic rate and so are susceptible to heat stress in hot weather, and end-of-lay hens, which may have lost a considerable amount of feather cover during the laying cycle, are susceptible to cold stress. Heat stress in broilers and cold stress in end-of-lay hens are major causes of bird death during transport in periods of either hot or cold weather, especially where journey times are prolonged or in the event of vehicle breakdown. Figure 7.1 shows the spacial distribution of temperature and vapour density in a conventional broiler transport vehicle. High temperature and humidity at the front of the vehicle pose a severe risk to birds at this site. A climate-controlled poultry transporter has been developed that is available commercially and would eliminate these severe welfare problems if used more widely; further information about this vehicle is available in Kettlewell and Mitchell (2004).

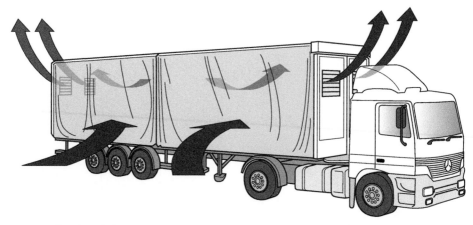

Fig. 7.2 Air flow through the Concept 2000 mechanically ventilated broiler transport vehicle. Hot air is extracted through the fans at the front and rear and cold air enters through the perforated side curtains, ensuring controlled airflow over all the birds. (Redrawn with permission from Kettlewell and Mitchell 2000.)

Figure 7.2 is a diagram of the Concept 2000 vehicle for broiler transport, showing air flow through the vehicle when fans are in operation. Hot air is extracted through fans at the front of the lorry and the back of the draw bar trailer and cold air enters through perforations in the side curtains, ensuring controlled airflow over all the birds, even when the vehicle is stationary; this is only effective when side curtains are in place, which is therefore essential even in hot weather.

COMPULSORY SLAUGHTER FOR NOTIFIABLE DISEASE

On-farm slaughter because of an outbreak of a notifiable disease may present a particular problem for poultry because of the large numbers involved in a single outbreak on large production units on which hundreds of thousands of birds may be housed. The various methods available for killing poultry on farm have recently been reviewed by the Animal Health and Welfare Panel of the European Food Safety Authority. These included: lethal injection; neck dislocation; concussive humane killers; gas stunning, either in sealed containers or by sealing the house; and mobile killing lines. The method selected may depend on the numbers and type of birds involved, the number of trained staff, the design of housing and feasibility of sealing the house, and the amount of gas or percussion killing equipment available. The method chosen may also depend on the risk of disease spread likely to occur because of the method, the risk of offending public sensibilities and the danger posed to operators involved in killing birds. For example, mobile killing lines were effectively used during the Dutch avian influenza outbreak of 2003 but, where they can only be set up outside, may spread disease in dust emissions and may offend the public if in public view. Carbon monoxide at 4–6% is a more humane method of killing birds than carbon dioxide, which is very aversive, but is more dangerous to human operatives. Similarly, nitrogen and argon are humane methods of gaseous euthanasia but only work where the oxygen content of the chamber can be reduced to less than 2%, which is difficult to achieve either in houses, because of leaks, or in containers, because of air held under birds' wings. Gas killing of ducks is problematic from a welfare standpoint, as they are adapted for breath holding and so require protracted exposure for killing. Intravenous lethal injection is an ideal method of euthanasia from a welfare point of view but is not feasible for flocks of over a few hundred birds and requires a number of skilled operatives. Euthanasia by ventilation shutdown is the cessation of natural or mechanical ventilation of air in a building in which birds are housed with or without any action taken to raise the air temperature in the building. The use of ventilation shut down, only on the written authority of the Secretary of State and when no other method of killing is considered practicable, has recently been permitted under the auspices of the Welfare of Animals (Slaughter or Killing) (Amendment) (England) Regulations 2006 in England. This method causes death through hyperthermia and is of considerable welfare concern. In order to ensure that the most humane method of euthanasia is employed that is feasible, given the number of birds, the equipment and the personnel available, and is least likely to spread disease or pose a risk to operators, it is essential that an advance plan is developed for each poultry production site and that steps are taken to make this plan immediately and effectively operational in the event of diagnosis of a notifiable disease at that site.

INTRODUCTION TO THE LEGISLATIVE FRAMEWORK IN THE EUROPEAN UNION

In the EU, the Council of Europe Convention for the Protection of Animals Kept for Farming Purposes provides for a Standing Committee to adopt recommendations on welfare requirements for specific farm animal species and systems. The European Commission (EC) may use these recommendations as the basis for European legislation. Additionally, the European Parliament's Intergroup on Animal Welfare and Conservation, a cross-party group of members of the European Parliament who discuss European and international animal welfare issues, takes initiatives that seek to promote the enactment of European legislation. The Scientific Committee on Animal Health and Animal Welfare (SCAHAW) is an independent scientific committee, made up of scientists from Member States, that gives the EC scientific advice on animal health and animal welfare issues. The Committee considers all available and up-to-date scientific data and evidence and provides the EC with a sound scientific basis for the drafting of legislation and other proposals. The Animal Health and Welfare (AHAW) panel of the European Food Safety Authority (EFSA), comprised of scientists from the Member States, also provides opinions and reports on aspects of animal health and animal welfare relating to food-producing animals, when required.

The EC may produce either European Regulations, which are directly applicable in each member state, or European Directives, which are implemented by all member states through enactment of national legislation, which must reflect the Directive but may be interpreted by each Member State. The EU legislation controlling poultry welfare is largely in the form of Directives. The principal Directives that control poultry welfare are: Council Directive 98/58/EC, which has general provisions for the keeping of farm livestock; Council Directive 1999/74/EC, which lays out minimum standards for laying hens; Council Directive 91/628/EEC, which controls animal transport; and Council Directive 93/119/EEC, which controls stunning and slaughter.

Directives are enacted under national legislation in each member state. For example, Council Directive 98/58/EC on the protection of animals kept for farming purposes, which gives general rules for the protection of animals of all species kept for the production of food, is enacted under the Welfare of Farmed Animals (England) Regulations 2000 (SI 2000 no. 1870) in England but under alternative legislation in the delegated regions of the UK and in other Member States. In areas where Directives appear not to be effective, EU Regulations may be enacted, the provisions of which are immediately applicable in all member states. In the field of animal welfare, Regulations have recently been enacted in order to improve implementation of the Animal Transport Directive.

General animal welfare legislation

Council Directive 98/58/EC requires member states to make provision to ensure that all owners and keepers take reasonable steps to ensure the welfare of animals under their care and to ensure that these are not caused any unnecessary pain, suffering or injury. This Directive makes provisions on staffing, record keeping, freedom of movement of animals, buildings and accommodation, feed, water and other substances, mutilations and breeding procedures.

Legislation specific to laying hens

Council Directive 1999/74/EC recognizes three types of rearing systems for laying hens:
- **Enriched cages,** where laying hens have at least 750 cm^2 of cage area per hen
- **Un-enriched cage systems,** where hens have at least 550 cm^2 of cage area per hen. Such cages may no longer be built or used for the first time. By January 2012, this system will be prohibited
- **Noncage systems** with nests (at least one for every seven hens) and adequate perches and where the stocking density does not exceed nine laying hens/m^2 usable area.

This Directive requires that hens kept in the enriched cage systems and the noncage systems must have a nest, perching space of 15 cm per hen, litter to allow pecking and scratching and unrestricted access to a feed trough measuring at least 12 cm per hen in the cage. Article 7 of the Directive provides that all egg production units must be registered with the competent authorities in member states and must each have a unique number which ensures traceability of eggs to individual holdings. The arrangements for registrations are detailed in Commission Directive 2002/4/EC.

Article 10 of the Directive provides that the Commission shall submit to the Council a report on the different systems of keeping laying hens. This will take into account inter alia an EFSA opinion on this subject and the findings of a socioeconomic study that indicates that costs to the industry would be likely to rise by up to 20% and egg imports would increase by approximately 3–4%.

The Commission's report is due to be submitted to the Council in the second half of 2007 in order to take account of the final results of a Community-funded research project ('LAYWEL'), which is currently investigating the welfare implications of changes in production systems for laying hens. The scientific evidence available at the time of writing suggests that furnished cages have the potential to improve hen welfare, in comparison with that of birds kept in either conventional cages or in some noncage systems, allowing a greater degree of freedom to carry out normal behaviour while, in many cases, reducing the incidence of feather pecking and subsequent fear and distress associated with noncage systems. However, the results of studies vary with the design and numbers of hens per cage and there is currently insufficient evidence to indicate which design or group size is ideal with respect to hen welfare. The Commission's Food and Veterinary Office (FVO) has also published a report, based on a series of visits to production units in 2004, which found that most hens in the EU are still kept in unfurnished cages and that compliance with the Directive in many states is poor.

Legislation specific to poultry transport

The welfare of poultry during transport is controlled by Council Directive 91/628/EEC. A consolidated text of this Directive with various amending Directives and Regulations can be seen at europa.eu.int/eur-lex/en/consleg/pdf/1991/en_1991L0628_do_001.pdf. Apart from the general provision that animals must not be transported in a way likely to cause injury or undue suffering, as well as details of how this should be achieved, this Directive lays out the maximum journey time birds may travel without food and water, which is 12 h (disregarding loading and unloading times). As it is practically impossible to provide food and water on a commercial poultry transporter, 12 h is actually the maximum period for which commercial birds may be transported. The legislation also limits journey times for chicks: transport should be completed in less than 72 h after hatching and last less than 24 h. Prescribed space allowances during transport for birds of different weights are detailed in this Directive.

Legislation specific to stunning and slaughter

The welfare of poultry during stunning and slaughter is controlled by Council Directive 93/119/EEC. It provides that an animal shall be spared any avoidable pain, suffering or excitement during movement, lairaging, restraint, stunning, slaughter or killing. This Directive requires that equipment and fittings are designed, constructed, maintained and used in such a way as to be rapid and effective and that these be subject to inspection by the competent authority. It requires that slaughter personnel have the knowledge and skill to perform the task humanely and effectively. Authorities must have free access to all parts of the slaughterhouse. It makes provision for inspection of slaughterhouses, both within the EU and in third countries wishing to export meat to the EU, by Commission experts. Slaughterhouses are required to have suitable unloading facilities, birds must be unloaded as soon as possible after arrival at the slaughter plant, protected from adverse weather, provided with ventilation, inspected regularly and immediately slaughtered if they have experienced pain or suffering during transport. The Directive lists permitted methods of killing, including carbon dioxide gas, electronarcosis and, where authorized by the competent authority, decapitation, dislocation of the neck or the use of a vacuum chamber. Specific requirements for each method of killing are detailed. An animal must not be stunned unless it can be immediately killed and current levels in water baths must be adequate to ensure that all the birds remain stunned. Manual back-up is required where birds are killed by automatic neck cutters. The Directive specifies permitted methods for killing chicks at hatcheries, although other methods may be permitted by the competent authority: the concentration of carbon dioxide in apparatus for killing chicks using carbon dioxide must be 100%.

Legislation specific to broiler chicken

At the time of writing, the Council of the European Union has agreed on the provisions of a Directive on the conditions of keeping for broiler chickens (Council Directive 2007/43/EC: Council of the European Union 2007), to come into force in Member States, under national legislation, by June 2010. These provisions will apply to flocks of 500 or more birds and will limit the stocking density of broiler chicken to 33 kg/m^2 with derogation to stock at 39 kg/m^2 where certain specified conditions are met: these conditions are defined in Annex II to the Annex of the Directive. For houses where very high levels of welfare standards are met, as outlined in Annex V to the Annex of the Directive, stocking densities will be permitted of up to 42 kg/m^2. The Directive sets out training and Certification requirements for all keepers of intensively produced broiler chickens although experience before 2010 will be accepted as equivalent to a training course, and certificates issued for such experience. Details of the content of the training are detailed in Annex IV to the Annex of the Directive.

The Directive details general requirements, including requirements for feeders, drinkers, litter, ventilation and heating, noise, light, inspection of birds, record keeping and surgical interventions. Specifically, minimum light levels will be 20 lux at bird level over at least 80% of the useable area of the house and a dark period of at least 6 h must be provided in a 24-h lighting cycle, of which 4 h must be continuous: this will apply from within 7 days of bird placement until 3 days from expected slaughter date. Fresh litter must be permanently available, birds must be inspected twice daily and sick or injured birds must be immediately culled or treated. Starving of birds prior to expected slaughter time will be limited to less than 12 h. Details of records to be kept are specified, which include the number of birds placed, house floor area, bird genotype, number of birds found dead or culled, recorded by cause, and number of birds remaining after thinning. All surgical interventions are prohibited except those carried out for therapeutic or diagnostic purposes: Member States may authorise beak trimming or castration by trained personnel and, in the case of castration, under veterinary supervision.

Establishments intending to stock at the higher stocking density of 39 kg/m^2 will be required to notify the competent authority and provide specific technical details of their establishment and equipment, including house plans, feeder and drinker locations, details of ventilation, cooling and heating systems and air flow patterns, details of alarm and back up systems and floor and litter types used. Levels of ammonia in the house will be limited to a maximum of 20 ppm and levels of carbon dioxide to a maximum of 3000 ppm. The building will be required to be constructed so as to hold the internal temperature at no more than 3°C above the external temperature when that temperature exceeded 30°C and the relative humidity will be required to be a maximum of 70% during 48 h when outside temperature are less than 10°C.

For a house to stock at 42 kg/m^2, no deficiencies with respect to the Directive must have been found during inspections within the previous two years, monitoring of bird health and welfare must be carried out using guides to good management and mortality levels during the flock cycle must be less than a given level (1% of birds placed plus 0.07% multiplied by the age of the flock in days) over the previous seven consecutive flock cycles. Allowance may be made for exceptional circumstances.

The Directive requires Member States to enact national legislation which will provide for regular monitoring of premises stocking at the higher densities and will empower the Competent Authority to take appropriate enforcement actions, subject to certain mitigating circumstances, where non-compliances are found to have occurred. Annex III to the Annex of the Directive requires the documentation accompanying the flock to the slaughterhouse to include daily and cumulative mortality and bird genotype. The Official Veterinarian at the slaughter house is required to supervise collection of records of birds 'DoA' and results of post mortem examination for each flock, including contact dermatitis, parasite infestation and disease. Where bird welfare during the flock cycle appears, from the mortality and post mortem results, to have been poor, the Official Veterinarian will inform the farmer and, if necessary the Competent Authority, which may take appropriate action. An annual report on the findings of farm inspections, slaughterhouse data and enforcement actions taken will be required to be submitted to the Commission.

Some provisions of this draft Directive remain controversial. In particular, the inclusion of culled birds in the recorded mortality level may tend to discourage farmers from adequately culling sick or injured birds, resulting in poor welfare. Additionally, the requirement for 6 h darkness until 3 days prior to slaughter may have the effect of increasing bird damage at depopulation.

The Directive gives the Commission a mandate to look into further welfare provisions for broiler chickens in the future. Member States will be required to collect scientifically based welfare assessment data over a period of 1 year and submit it to the Commission, which will prepare a report based on these data as well as bird welfare, socio-economic and administrative effects of the Directive, by June 2012. On the basis of this report, the Commission will determine whether additional measures for improving broiler chicken welfare would be beneficial. The Directive also invites the Commission to prepare a report on the possible introduction of a specific welfare labelling scheme for chicken meat with the aim of providing incentives to producers to improve bird welfare, for submission by December 2009. A report on the influence of genetic factors on welfare problems in broiler chicken is due to be submitted by December 2010. Member States are required to lay down rules for penalties for infringements of national provisions made to enact the provisions of the Directive and to notify the Commission of these before June 2010.

CONCLUSION

Methods of assessing bird welfare on farm and during transport and slaughter have developed over the last few years and several comprehensive methods are available that are based on output measures and are feasible, reliable and valid. Such measures are likely to replace existing resource-based assessment systems, which are widely used in current farm assurance schemes but may not be effective in improving bird welfare. Modern intensive poultry farming systems give rise to a number of very serious welfare concerns, some of which are inherent to the bird genotypes and husbandry systems used and may not be readily amenable to improvement through legislation. Such concerns range from contact dermatitis in birds on litter to lameness in broilers to cannibalism and bone fractures in laying hens. The tendency for large numbers of birds to be housed on a single unit gives rise to inherent welfare problems during handling and transport and, in the event of the outbreak of notifiable disease, during euthanasia on farm. Technological developments have led to the production of automatic harvesting systems, modular handling systems and mechanically ventilated poultry transport vehicles, which are available commercially and some of which have been shown to effectively improve bird welfare during these operations, although all may not be currently in wide use because of economic constraints. There is a wide range of methods available for the humane euthanasia of birds during disease outbreaks and it is essential that, for each poultry production site, advanced planning takes place, taking into consideration the size and type of husbandry system, to ensure that the most humane, effective and safe method of euthanasia is available.

Persistent public pressure to improve farm animal welfare in the EU has led to the enactment of EU Directives controlling the keeping of animals on farm, including specific statutes for broilers and laying hens and for transport and slaughter. The provisions of the current draft broiler Directive reflect recent developments in animal welfare science in that this Directive advocates the use of multiple, bird-based measures of welfare as welfare indicators rather than simply prescribing resources to be provided for the birds. However, it is essential that the Directive provisions are based on good welfare science or they may inadvertently result in a negative effect on welfare by discouraging culling of diseased and injured birds, reducing chick viability after placement, increasing injury during catching prior to slaughter and, possibly, increasing levels of leg abnormalities and DoAs during transport. In order to avoid the law of unintended consequences, by which measures put in place to improve bird welfare may paradoxically cause poorer welfare, we must ensure that the measures selected holistically reflect bird welfare as established by scientific evidence. The Laying Hen Directive provides for the gradual removal of conventional cages from use in egg production systems in the EU, to be complete by 2012, and the poultry transport Directives and legislation limit stocking densities in transport crates and restrict journey times to a maximum of 12 h.

While the draft EU animal welfare Directives will improve bird welfare, if adequately enforced and enacted rigorously throughout the EU and, in the case of the Broiler Directive, suitably amended, they are unlikely to address some inherent welfare problems. These can only be ameliorated by improvements to bird genotype, the development of husbandry systems that are more suited to the behavioural needs of the birds and increased use of technology available for poultry handling and transport. Some of these measures may increase costs to the industry and consumers: if consumers really wish to improve poultry welfare in the EU, they must be prepared to pay a premium for EU-produced poultry products produced to higher welfare standards. Additionally, political negotiation with the World Trade Organization to exempt farmed livestock from trade rules that prevent discrimination of products on the grounds of 'process and production' criteria, are imperative in order to allow EU producers to take measures to improve bird welfare that may otherwise affect productivity and profitability adversely. High-welfare husbandry systems should not be in direct competition with poultry products produced in low-welfare systems in developing countries, which would result ultimately in the reduction, or even the disappearance, of the EU poultry production industry: this would do nothing to improve bird welfare.

There is evidence that, at least in some European countries, the poultry industry is prepared to modify husbandry and other practices in order to improve bird welfare and that, in some cases, the consumer is prepared to pay more for animal products from higher-welfare systems. There has been a massive expansion in the proportion of eggs sold from free-range flocks in the UK, from in the order of 4% in the 1980s to around 35% today, as consumers are prepared to pay a premium for eggs from a perceived higher-welfare husbandry system, although some would argue that increased feather pecking and cannibalism, and so mortality, in free-range flocks outweighs the increased freedom to carry out normal behaviour.

Parts of the broiler industry are taking the problem of bird welfare, and especially leg and cardiovascular health problems, seriously. In the last few years there has been a rapid rise in higher-profit-margin, organic and free-range producers, many of which are using slower-growing genotypes that are much less prone to lameness and cardiovascular health problems. At least one of the four major breeding companies that produce conventional, intensively reared genotypes also recognizes that leg abnormalities and cardiovascular health problems are serious issues with regard to bird health and welfare and is including leg and cardiovascular health in heritability calculations in elite bird selection programmes. The use of such breeding strategies has resulted in a dramatic fall in mortality resulting from lameness culls and cardiovascular failure: a recent study at the University of Bristol found that mean flock mortality in traditional, intensively reared, UK broiler flocks was approximately 2%, in comparison with 6–7% reported in studies of 15–20 years ago. The recent considerable reduction in the numbers of broiler chickens dying because of trauma and stress during harvesting and transport in the UK, due to improved harvesting and transport systems and improved bird cardiovascular health, has been discussed earlier.

However, there is also some evidence that, for some broiler breeding companies, it is 'business as usual': continued selection for ever-increasing growth rates and breast yields and pay lip service to welfare imperatives. This is not an acceptable policy in the current climate in the EU, as shown by the proposed provisions of the Broiler Directive: commercial producers would be well advised to steer clear of genotypes from breeding companies that persist in such policies.

Notably, for some specific cases, real or perceived bird welfare improvements have been accompanied over the past few years by increased profitability for producers: the challenge is to continue these very promising trends, to extend them to other classes of poultry and to take all, not just part, of the industry forward. The poultry industry, consumers, marketing companies, politicians, scientists and veterinary surgeons all have a role to play in escalating the pace of improvement in bird welfare, for all types of poultry production, in Europe and, ultimately, world-wide. As Mahatma Gandhi once said: 'The civilization of a nation may be judged by the way in which it treats its animals'.

REFERENCES

Blokhuis H 2006 COST 846 – Measuring and monitoring farm animal welfare. Available on line at: www. cost846.unina.it. Accessed 2 March 2007

Council of the European Union 2007 Council Directive 2007/43/EC. Laying down minimum rules for the protection of chickens kept for meat production. OJ L 182/19, 12.7.2007

Haslam S 2004 Compare welfare between different systems. In: Weeks C, Butterworth A, eds. Measuring and auditing broiler welfare. CABI Publishing, Wallingford, p 183–196

Kettlewell P J, Mitchell M A 2000 Mechanical ventilation: improving the welfare of broilers during transport. Silsoe Research Institute, Bedford

Knowles T G 1998 The problem of broken bones during the handling of laying hens – a review. Poult Sci 77: 1798–1802

Mitchell M A, Kettlewell P J 2004 Transport and handling. In: Weeks C, Butterworth A, eds. Measuring and auditing broiler welfare. CABI Publishing, Wallingford, p 145–160

Newberry R C 2004 Cannibalism. In: Perry G C, ed Welfare of the laying hen. CABI Publishing, Wallingford, p 239–258

Webster A B 2004 Welfare implications of avian osteoporosis. Poult Sci 83: 184–192

Wilkins L J, Brown S N, Zimmerman P H et al 2004 Investigation of palpation as a method for determining the prevalence of keel and furculum damage in laying hens. Vet Rec 155: 635–635

FURTHER READING

Assured Chicken Production 2005 Assured Chicken Production Standards. Assured Chicken Production Ltd, Cobham, Surrey. Available on line at: www.assuredchicken.org.uk/_code/common/item. asp?id=4033512. Accessed 2 March 2007

Baylis P A, Hinton M H 1990 Transportation of broilers with special reference to mortality rates. Appl Anim Behav Sci 28: 93

Berg C, Sanotra G S 2003 Can a modified latency-to-lie test be used to validate gait-scoring results in commercial broiler flocks? Anim Welfare 12: 655–659

Danbury T C 2000 Self-selection of the analgesic drug carprofen by lame broiler chickens.Vet Rec 146: 307

Ekstrand C 1997 Rearing conditions and foot-pad dermatitis in Swedish turkey poults. Acta Vet Scand 38: 167–174

Ekstrand C 1997 Rearing conditions and foot-pad dermatitis in Swedish broiler chickens. Prev Vet Med 31: 167–174

European Food Safety Authority 2005 Animal health and welfare aspects of avian influenza. Annex. EFSA J 266: 1–21

Haslam S 2005 Report to DEFRA: Associations between abattoir data and leg health and welfare of chickens. University of Bristol, Bristol

Haslam S, Brown S N, Wilkins L J et al 2006 A preliminary study to examine the utility of using foot burn or hock burn to assess aspects of housing conditions for broiler chicken. Br Poult Sci 47: 13–18

Haslam S M, Knowles T G, Brown S N, Wilkins L J, Kestin S C, Warriss P D, Nicol C J 2007 Factors affecting the prevalence of foot pad dermatitis, hock burn and breast burn in broiler chicken. Br Poult Sci 48: 264–275

Kestin S C 1999 Different commercial broiler crosses have different susceptibilities to leg weakness. Poult Sci 78: 1085–1090

Kestin S C 2001 Relationships in broiler chickens between lameness, liveweight, growth rate and age. Vet Rec 148: 195–197

Kestin S C, Knowles T G, Tinch A E, Gregory N G 1992 Prevalence of leg weakness in broiler chickens and its relationship with genotype. Vet Rec 131: 190–194

Knowles T G, Haslam S, Warriss P D et al 2006 The effect of aspects of flock husbandry on the prevalence of lameness in broiler chicken. Report to DEFRA. University of Bristol, Bristol

McGeown D 1999 Effect of carprofen on lameness in broiler chickens. Vet Rec 144: 668–671

Main D C J 2003 Effect of the RSPCA Freedom Food scheme on the welfare of dairy cattle. Vet Rec 153: 227–231

Offner 2003 Application of methods of on-farm welfare assessment. Anim Welf 12: 523–578

Royal Society for the Prevention of Cruelty to Animals 2002 Freedom Food welfare standards for chickens. RSPCA, Horsham, Sussex

Sanotra G S 2001 Monitoring leg problems in broilers: a survey of commercial broiler production in Denmark. World Poult Sci J 57: 55–69

Sorensen P 1999 The effect of photoperiod:scotoperiod on leg weakness in broiler chickens. Poult Sci 78: 336–342

Su G 1999 Meal feeding is more effective than early feed restriction at reducing the prevalence of leg weakness in broiler chickens. Poult Sci 78: 949–955

Weeks C A 2000 The behaviour of broiler chickens and its modification by lameness. Appl Anim Behav Sci 67: 111–125

Weeks C A 2002 New method for objectively assessing lameness in broiler chickens. Vet Rec 151: 762–764

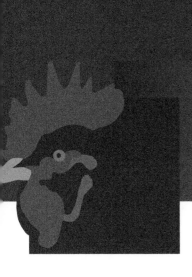

Janet M. Bradbury

BACTERIAL DISEASES

Chapter **8**	*Enterobacteriaceae*	**110**
Chapter **9**	Infections caused by species of *Pasteurellaceae*, *Ornithobacterium* and *Riemerella*: an introduction	**146**
Chapter **10**	Fowl cholera	**149**
Chapter **11**	Infectious coryza and related diseases	**155**
Chapter **12**	*Gallibacterium* infections and other avian *Pasteurellaceae*	**160**
Chapter **13**	*Ornithobacterium rhinotracheale*	**164**
Chapter **14**	*Riemerella* infections	**172**
Chapter **15**	Avian bordetellosis (turkey coryza)	**176**
Chapter **16**	*Campylobacter*	**181**
Chapter **17**	Staphylococci, streptococci and enterococci	**191**
Chapter **18**	Clostridia	**200**
Chapter **19**	*Erysipelothrix rhusiopathiae* – erysipelas	**215**
Chapter **20**	Avian mycoplasmas	**220**
Chapter **21**	Avian chlamydophilosis (chlamydiosis/ psittacosis/ornithosis)	**235**
Chapter **22**	Some other bacterial diseases	**243**

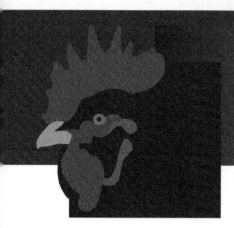

Stephen A. Lister and Paul Barrow*

Enterobacteriaceae

The family *Enterobacteriaceae* consists of Gram-negative aerobic or facultatively anaerobic, asporogenous, rod-shaped bacteria that grow well on artificial media. Motile species are peritrichously flagellated and nonmotile variants may occur. Some species are nonmotile. Glucose is utilized fermentatively with formation of acid or of acid and gas. The oxidase test is negative and with a few exceptions catalase is produced. Nitrates are reduced to nitrites.

The family comprises a large number of antigenically related and biochemically similar bacteria that include the genera *Salmonella*, *Escherichia*, *Shigella*, *Citrobacter*, *Klebsiella* and *Proteus*. More recently *Yersinia* has been taxonomically grouped within the *Enterobacteriaceae*. Some of these bacteria are primarily intestinal parasites of animals and are widespread in the environment and commonly found in farm effluents, human sewage and any material subject to faecal contamination. A number of important diseases of poultry are caused by members of the *Salmonella* and *Escherichia* genera.

The classification of the members of the genus *Salmonella* has been controversial for many years. According to the latest nomenclature, which reflects recent advances in taxonomy, the genus consists of only two species: *Salmonella enterica* and *Salmonella bongori*. The former is divided into six subspecies, which are distinguishable by certain biochemical characteristics and some of which correspond to previous subgenera. These subspecies are listed in Table 8.1. For the 17 serovars of *S. bongori*, the V was retained to avoid confusion with the serovar name of *S. enterica* subsp. *enterica*. Thus the full name would be *S. enterica* subsp. *enterica* serovar Typhimurium. Since this is cumbersome, it is proposed to follow the suggestion of Old (1992) and use italic for the genus name *Salmonella* and roman for the serovar, e.g. *Salmonella* Typhimurium. In veterinary literature a distinction is usually made between infections caused by the two host-adapted serovars of *S.* Pullorum (pullorum disease), *S.* Gallinarum (fowl typhoid), the Arizonae subspecies of *Salmonella* (arizonosis) and the remainder of the salmonella infections (salmonellosis, paratyphoid infection).

The Kauffmann–White scheme still forms the basis for classification of *Salmonella* serovars and essentially involves serological grouping by means of the somatic O antigens and flagellar H

*The authors wish to acknowledge the contribution of Clifford Wray and Robert Davies, coauthors of this chapter in the 5th edition.

Table 8.1	Subspecies of *Salmonella enterica*
Subspecies I	*enterica*
Subspecies II	*salamae*
Subspecies IIIa	*arizonae*
Subspecies IIIb	*diarizonae*
Subspecies IV	*houtenae*
Subspecies VI	*indica*

antigens. The host-adapted serovars *S.* Pullorum and *S.* Gallinarum are nonmotile and do not express H antigens.

SALMONELLOSIS – PARATYPHOID

Infections caused by the motile *Salmonella* serovars were reported in poultry at least as early as 1899 and have been extensively investigated as they are important zoonoses and agents of major clinical disease. Infections, generally subclinical, are common in all species of domestic poultry and game birds throughout most of the world and have also been reported in many different species of wild bird. Many different serovars have been identified in domestic poultry and one serovar may be the predominant isolate in a country for a number of years before it is replaced by another. Thus, in 1943, *S.* Thompson appeared in the UK poultry flock and within 2 years it was the most frequent serovar isolated from poultry. More recently, *S.* Agona was introduced into the country in imported Peruvian fishmeal and became widespread in poultry and subsequently in humans. Similarly, *S.* Hadar was cause for concern to the turkey industry because it caused disease in table birds that led to foodborne illness in humans. In countries where the major part of the poultry industry is concentrated within a small number of larger companies, problems with *Salmonella* in their specific integrated breeding flocks or feed mills may have a substantial effect on the national prevalence of specific *Salmonella* strains.

Efforts to control *Salmonella* infections in domestic poultry are, with the exception of a few serovars, driven by public health concerns rather than by expectations of securing important improvements in production efficiency. *Salmonella* infections are among the most frequent foodborne infections in humans and contaminated poultry products are one of the major sources of infection. In the UK, the commonest serovars in man are currently *S.* Enteritidis and *S.* Typhimurium.

S. Enteritidis was seldom isolated before 1987 and its prevalence increased markedly in subsequent years. In the UK this increase was largely associated with the emergence of phage type 4 (PT4). A corresponding increase occurred in humans and many food-poisoning outbreaks were attributed to shell eggs and particularly to products such as mayonnaise made with raw or lightly cooked eggs, in addition to the more usual source of poultry meat. A similar increase in the prevalence of *S.* Enteritidis in both humans and poultry was observed in many countries, although in some instances it was caused by phage types other than PT4 (e.g. PT13a in the USA); other countries, such as Australia, appear to have remained free of endemic infection. To safeguard public health, national control measures, often including legislation, have been implemented in many countries. As a consequence, in the UK the prevalence of *S.* Enteritidis, especially PT4, has declined dramatically over recent years. More recently *S.* Typhimurium DT104 was isolated with increasing frequency from poultry, especially turkeys, in the UK and caused some concern because isolates showed resistance to five or more antibacterial drugs. This isolation trend, however, now seems to be reducing. In the EU, Europe-wide monitoring and control programmes are continuing based on target reduction schemes for the 'Top 10' human *Salmonella* serovars.

EPIDEMIOLOGY

Cause

Members of the genus *Salmonella* are Gram-negative, nonsporing rods (2–4 $\times$ 0.5 µm) that do not have capsules. They are usually motile and have long flagella, although occasional nonmotile variants may occur. (NB. The species-specific *S.* Pullorum and *S.* Gallinarum are always nonmotile when grown under normal laboratory conditions.) Salmonellas grow readily on ordinary media, forming large, thick, greyish-white, dome-shaped colonies. All ferment glucose but not lactose, all reduce nitrates to nitrites and all can survive for several months away from the host.

About 2500 different *Salmonella* serovars have been described and reported.

Hosts

The paratyphoid group of salmonellas has a very wide host range in birds and mammals. Some have also been isolated from reptiles, fish and insects. While all members of the species are considered to be potentially pathogenic, different serovars differ widely in their host range and the pathogenic syndromes that they produce.

Spread

When poultry over 4 weeks of age are infected with salmonellas the organism may colonize the intestine but almost all such chickens free themselves of infection within 60 days. However, a small percentage of infected birds will excrete the organism either continuously or intermittently for long periods. Stress, such as coming into lay, may also reactivate infection and excretion. Although the large majority of infected birds carry *Salmonella* species for only short periods, the conditions in intensive poultry units allow considerable scope for infection to recycle from bird to bird.

The modes of spread of the non-host-specific salmonellas are very complex and, since knowledge of these is an integral part of control, the details of this are discussed in the section on Control.

DISEASE

Pathogenesis

Paratyphoid *S. enterica* serovars are ubiquitous in the environment and as such are easily introduced into poultry farms through rodents, insects, birds or fomites. Infection of newly hatched chicks results in rapid and massive multiplication within the alimentary tract in the absence of a competing, complex gut flora. This results in extensive faecal shedding for a number of weeks, with cross-contamination within the house or hatchery. Infection of older birds that have acquired a mature gut flora results in shedding of reduced numbers of bacteria for shorter periods of time. If the infecting strain is virulent for birds a strong inflammatory response occurs in the intestine with tissue damage and a typhlitis. Invasion to the spleen may result in systemic spread and multiplication where immunity is reduced, as in very young or old birds or at onset of lay. Mortality may ensue depending on the degree of virulence and host genetic background. Spread of certain strains, especially certain phage types of *S.* Enteritidis to the reproductive tract, particularly the oviduct, may result in vertical transmission. Transmission between birds is largely faecal–oral, although respiratory infection is also thought to be important, particularly in establishment of systemic infection of the reproductive tract.

Clinical signs

Disease caused by non-host-specific *Salmonella* infections is uncommon in poultry and is usually seen in chicks, poults or ducklings under 2 weeks of age and rarely in birds over 4 weeks of age. The morbidity and mortality varies considerably and deaths are usually less than 10% of the affected group but in exceptional cases can approach 100%. The clinical signs are not specific and are similar whichever *Salmonella* serovar is involved. In an outbreak with clinical signs affected birds are depressed, reluctant to move and huddle dejectedly together with their eyes closed and with ruffled feathers and drooping wings. Diarrhoea with pasting of the feathers around the vent is commonly seen and in some outbreaks visual impairment, due to corneal opacity or caseous plaques in the eyeball, has been reported. In ducklings additional signs may be trembling, swollen eyelids and sudden death. An unusual feature of the initial outbreaks of *S.* Enteritidis in broilers is the appearance of clinical signs of disease in birds over 4 weeks of age. Affected birds become uneven, stunted and badly feathered. Clinical signs are also sometimes seen in laying hens and mortality rates of up to 1.6% per month have been described, associated with decreased egg production.

Lesions

These vary considerably, from the complete absence of visible lesions to a septicaemic carcass with the lungs, liver, spleen and kidneys swollen and congested. When baby chicks are affected an inflamed, unabsorbed yolk sac is a common feature. Discrete necrotic lesions in the lungs, liver and heart, peritonitis and haemorrhagic enteritis may be seen in birds that do not die in the acute septicaemic phase of the disease. The most characteristic post-mortem finding, seen in approximately one-third of birds dying of salmonellosis, is typhlitis, with the caeca distended by hard, white, necrotic cores. This may be exacerbated by necrosis and bleeding when *Eimeria* infection is also present. In broilers with salmonellosis caused by *S.* Enteritidis there are usually gross post-mortem findings of polyserositis manifested as pericarditis and perihepatitis. The pericarditis may be distinctive and, in addition to thickening and increased vascularity of the pericardium, the pericardial sac is typically distended with a considerable quantity of turbid fluid containing large numbers of organisms. Ovarian lesions of intense blood vessel congestion and deformed shrunken ovules have also been associated with *S.* Enteritidis infection in laying birds.

DIAGNOSIS

When infection is suspected, confirmation of the diagnosis requires the isolation and identification of the causal agent, preferably to the specific serovar. *Salmonella* organisms are readily isolated from infected tissues of clinically affected birds by direct culture; thus, in chicks dying of septicaemia, direct isolations can be made from the liver, gall bladder or yolk sac. In severely affected flocks salmonellas may be isolated from pericardial sac or affected ovaries. In older birds they are often confined to the intestine, with the caeca being the most likely site for isolation.

Methods used for identifying infection in large populations must take into account the frequency of a very low incidence of infection. Several methods have been developed to collect samples from the environment as an indirect indication of flock infection. These methods include samples from nest or floor litter, dust accumulations or samples collected by dragging modified Moore's swabs (drag swabs) over a large surface area of floor litter or dropping pit. More recently, absorbent overshoes worn over the stockperson's boots have been used for extensive sampling of the litter environment of the poultry house. It is also important to take samples of the environment for bacteriological culture after cleaning and disinfection following depopulation, and also to confirm that mice are not acting as a reservoir of infection on the site.

Isolation

Numerous techniques and methods have been described for the isolation of *Salmonella* strains from different types of specimens and consequently it is not possible to recommend a particular technique because of the lack of comparative data on the efficacy of the various media. Clearly, any techniques used should be audited, assessed and where possible accredited by independent bodies.

Pre-enrichment is used for culturing samples where *Salmonella* organisms are sublethally damaged, as may occur during feed manufacture, and in dry samples and environmental samples in which the number of organisms is low (e.g. dust) or where disinfectants have been used. Buffered peptone water is normally the medium of choice. Three different selective enrichments or families of enrichment are in common use: selenite, tetrathionate and Rappaport–Vassiliadis (RV) medium. It is not possible to recommend one as the best for all purposes. They may be made more selective by the addition of antibiotics such as novobiocin or dyes such as brilliant green. Enrichment broths are used for culture of samples that are likely to be contaminated with high numbers of other bacteria (e.g. faeces, cloacal swabs, environmental samples or subculture from pre-enrichment). Selenite broth should not be used for selective enrichment after pre-enrichment because its selectivity is easily reduced by excessive contamination. RV medium has been shown to work very efficiently after the sample has been pre-enriched and subcultured to give a sample:RV broth ratio of 1:100. Most enrichment broths are usually incubated at 41–42°C because the higher incubation temperature helps to inhibit enteric bacteria other than salmonellas. There is currently much interest in semisolid media (e.g. modified semisolid RV medium – MSRV), which are considered to be more suited to isolation of motile *Salmonella* species, particularly serovars Enteritidis and Typhimurium, when low numbers are present in faecal and environmental samples.

A large number of plating media have been formulated for the isolation of *Salmonella* species. Various selective and differential agents have been incorporated to facilitate isolation from samples contaminated with other bacteria and to distinguish the salmonella colonies from those of other bacteria. It is recommended that at least two selective and two plating media should be used for optimal isolation, although increasing the number of samples tested with a single effective medium will further increase the accuracy of the test. Plating media in common use include MacConkey agar, desoxycholate citrate agar (DCA), on which salmonella colonies appear colourless, and brilliant green agar and its modifications, on which the colonies are red. Other media include xylose lysine desoxycholate agar (XLD) and its modifications and chromogenic media such as Rambach and 'Salmonella detection and identification medium' (SM ID) agar.

Identification

Salmonella organisms can be identified by their colonial characteristics on selective media, supported by biochemical and serological tests. Suspect colonies should first be tested by a slide agglutination test using polyvalent O and H sera and also normal saline. Those colonies that react with either both or one of these sera and do not aggregate in normal saline are then subjected to further biochemical and serological tests to identify the serovar. The main biochemical tests for most *Salmonella* species are the production of H_2S, but not indole, in peptone water after incubation, together with certain sugar reactions. These latter comprise fermentation of glucose, mannitol, maltose and dulcitol and failure to ferment lactose, sucrose and salicin. These biochemical reactions can be conveniently carried out in the composite media now available for bacterial identification such as Kohn's or triple sugar iron (TSI) agar. Cultures that give the biochemical reactions characteristic of *Salmonella* species are then tested with the appropriate O and H sera until the group and serovar are identified. The biochemical tests for identification of salmonellas can be combined to form an identification test. A number of these, such as the API 20E or Enterotube II systems, are currently available for purchase.

Further subdivision for epidemiological purposes can be achieved by phage typing schemes, antibiograms, various molecular genetic techniques such as plasmid profile analysis and biotyping of the isolate.

Serological diagnosis

The value of serological tests for diagnosis depends to some extent on the *Salmonella* serovar involved. As described later, *S.* Pullorum and *S.* Gallinarum do not colonize the digestive tract but readily infect the rest of the bird's body. This stimulates the production of antibodies, which can be detected by serological tests. Other *Salmonella* serovars colonize the alimentary tract but do not readily invade the tissues and thus may not stimulate the production of antibodies. Infection with other serovars that are invasive, including *S.* Enteritidis and *S.* Typhimurium, is also detectable by serology.

Serological methods should be used to identify infected flocks rather than to identify infected individual birds, and bacteriological confirmation should always be sought. It is well recognized that some poultry with a positive serological response may no longer be infected with salmonella organisms. Similarly, poultry that are actively excreting salmonellas in the early stages of infection may be serologically negative for a period of up to 2 weeks or so. If immunization is used to control salmonella infections in the flock, it may not be possible to differentiate the vaccine response from that of actual infection. Newly hatched chicks are immunologically immature and do not respond serologically to the somatic lipopolysaccharide (LPS) antigen until 2–3 weeks of age. Chicks may, however, acquire *Salmonella* antibodies passively from their parents via the yolk, which may indicate an infected or a vaccinated parent flock. Egg yolk may also be tested for immunoglobulins to *Salmonella*, and this may provide an easy method of screening nonvaccinated laying flocks for *S.* Enteritidis.

A number of serological tests have been developed for the diagnosis of *Salmonella* infections in poultry. The whole blood test (WBT), which uses a stained antigen, and the serum agglutination test (SAT) have been used successfully for more than 50 years for the identification of flocks infected with *S.* Pullorum/Gallinarum. As *S.* Enteritidis possesses the same group D somatic antigen as *S.* Pullorum, the WBT and related tests can be used for the diagnosis of infection with this serovar. The WBT is fully described later in the section on pullorum disease.

In recent years other tests, such as enzyme-linked immunosorbent assay (ELISA), have been developed for the identification of *S.* Enteritidis- or *S.* Typhimurium-infected flocks and a number of test kits are commercially available and used in many countries.

Two main basic systems are used for the detection of *S.* Enteritidis-infected flocks, the indirect ELISA and the competitive 'sandwich' ELISA. The indirect ELISA involves the use of a detecting antigen coated on to the wells of a microtitre plate. After the application of a blocking reagent to reduce nonspecific binding, test samples are applied to the wells. Specifically bound antibody in the sample is detected by an antibody-enzyme conjugate. A variety of antigens, including LPS, flagella, SEF14 fimbriae, outer membrane proteins and crude antigen preparations, have been used. The competitive 'sandwich' ELISA employs a specific monoclonal antibody for coating antigen to wells. This is then followed by a pure or crude antigen preparation. Test serum samples are then applied, followed by conjugated monoclonal antibody, which will not bind to the antigen if the serum sample contained specific antibodies. The assay time can be shortened by adding both test sample and conjugate together.

There are advantages and disadvantages to both systems. The indirect assay is simpler and reagents are available for all *Salmonella* serovars for chickens, turkeys, ducks and mammalian hosts. The competitive ELISA can be applied to all animal species and in general shows higher specificity; however, reagents are not commercially available for all serovars. There are also some affinity problems and it may be less sensitive than the indirect assays. In the field both systems have produced false-positive reactions and a careful interpretation of the overall results from the whole sampled population must be made.

Both types of assay may be used with serum, yolk or reconstituted dried blood, which may be treated with some antibacterial agents with minimal loss of antibody titre. Some cross-reaction occurs between groups B and D and further work is needed to overcome this problem. The optimal method for choosing a 'cut-off' absorbance value, above which sera are designated as having come from a *S.* Enteritidis-infected flock, has not yet been universally agreed because of the difficulties in assessing the infection status of naturally infected flocks used to evaluate the test and the practical consequences of false-positive reactions in breeding flocks.

ELISAs are readily adapted to automation and hence to large-scale testing programmes. A major problem is that expensive equipment is necessary and many of the reagents are also expensive. However, they may be adapted for use without equipment and may be read by eye. Both systems are now commercially available.

CONTROL

Treatment

A number of antibacterials are useful in limiting morbidity and mortality within a flock, although the prime aim must be the use of an effective biosecurity programme to prevent infection in the first place. Where treatment is necessary a variety of drugs may be effective, including amoxicillin, tetracyclines, potentiated sulphonamides, spectinomycin, enrofloxacin and other fluoroquinolones. None, however, is capable of totally eliminating infection from a flock. If it is decided to treat an outbreak of salmonellosis, this should always be on the basis of pretreatment sensitivity testing of the organism involved by laboratory tests. Where a breeder flock is known to be contaminated it may be necessary to keep this flock in production and therefore treat the breeder flock in question. It may also be considered appropriate to treat progeny from such a flock for several days after hatching for serovars suspected as being transmitted vertically either in ovo or by surface shell contamination. Although treatment might seem to be effective, a number of birds may become carriers and furthermore antibiotic-resistant *Salmonella* strains or *Escherichia coli* might appear.

Monitoring

Monitoring either by culture or serology should be carried out at all stages of the production cycle. The World Health Organization (WHO) *Guidelines on detection and monitoring of salmonella-infected poultry flocks with particular reference to* Salmonella *Enteritidis* provide a comprehensive account of a practical programme. Monitoring for *Salmonella* is an important consideration in a hazard analysis and critical control point (HACCP) (see Ch. 4) approach for poultry units and the EU Directive (Regulation 2160/2003) gives minimal requirements for sampling.

At the hatchery, fluff from the interior surfaces of the hatchers and broken eggshells from the hatcher trays should be cultured every 2 weeks. Other samples such as macerated waste, meconium, surface swabs from different parts of the hatchery and dead-in-shell and cull chicks should assist checking for the presence of *Salmonella* organisms as well as the effectiveness of routine hygiene measures. Any positive samples should be traced to individual supply flocks.

At the rearing site, the presence of *Salmonella* organisms in newly arrived replacement birds can be checked by culture of chick box liners or swabs from the bottom of the boxes, chicks dead on arrival and those culled or dying within a few days of arrival. During the rearing period bulked litter or faeces samples, boot or drag swabs and dust from various sites (e.g. exhaust fans) provide the most convenient method of monitoring. When breeders are in lay the most reliable samples are nest box floor swabs, nest box litter, dust from internal feed hoppers and swabs from egg sorting tables and corridors; for elite birds and grandparents, more frequent sampling is desirable. Laying flocks may be sampled by using dust samples, swabs of the manure scraper and spilled debris from the egg collection belt. In the case of barn layers, litter, dust and nest boxes should be sampled. At the processing plant, samples such as pieces of neck skin and swabs from different sites throughout the factory should be cultured.

The method adopted for *Salmonella* monitoring will be determined by the staff and laboratory facilities available, and the cost. Whatever method is adopted it should be carried out regularly and methodically according to an appropriate programme. In this way trends over time and the impact of hazard reduction measures may be assessed.

Houses and buildings should be designed to facilitate cleansing and disinfection and should be thoroughly cleaned and disinfected between flocks of birds, and fresh, clean litter used. When cleansing and disinfection has been carried out, buildings should be checked for the persistence of salmonellas and it is pertinent to point out that inadequate procedures may disseminate pathogens widely and possibly exacerbate problems. Samples should include scrapings or drag swabs of earth floor surfaces or floor sweepings from concrete floors, swabs from cracks in the floor and lower walls, nest box floors, slave feed hoppers, beams and pipes and electric fittings. In laying flocks, additional samples include sweepings or swabs of the egg store area, egg sorting equipment, egg handling room floor and, if rodents are numerous, these should be trapped and examined.

Origins of infection

Once a *Salmonella* serovar with an affinity for poultry has become established in a primary breeding flock, it can infect poultry in other units by movement of eggs and equipment via hatcheries by both vertical and lateral spread. This can have far-ranging and serious effects on the health of both poultry and humans. It is thus of considerable importance to identify the specific risk factors for the primary introduction of *Salmonella* into individual poultry operations (Fig. 8.1) in order to identify the critical control points that form the basis of a HACCP approach. It is essential that, in establishing HACCP, the plan is designed for the particular circumstances pertaining to that enterprise and that the efficacy of the control measures is independently checked by bacteriological tests as well as record audits.

If a breeding flock is infected with *Salmonella* organisms, a cycle can be established in which the organism passes via the egg to the progeny and even to chicks hatched from eggs laid by these

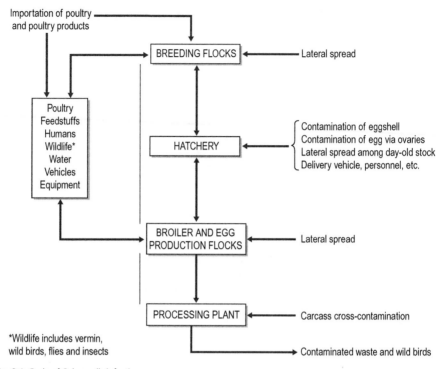

Importation of poultry and poultry products

BREEDING FLOCKS ← Lateral spread

Poultry
Feedstuffs
Humans
Wildlife*
Water
Vehicles
Equipment

HATCHERY ← { Contamination of eggshell
Contamination of egg via ovaries
Lateral spread among day-old stock
Delivery vehicle, personnel, etc.

BROILER AND EGG
PRODUCTION FLOCKS ← Lateral spread

PROCESSING PLANT ← Carcass cross-contamination

*Wildlife includes vermin,
wild birds, flies and insects

→ Contaminated waste and wild birds

Fig. 8.1 Cycle of *Salmonella* infection.

infected progeny. This cycle can occur by true ovarian transmission, as is the case in Pullorum disease and *S.* Enteritidis. However, it is much more likely to happen through faecal contamination of the surface of the egg. When the egg passes through the cloaca, *Salmonella* organisms in faeces attach themselves to the warm, wet surface of the shell and may be drawn inside as it cools. Penetration of the shell by the bacteria will occur more readily if the eggs are stored at above room temperature or are washed. When chicks hatch from infected eggs, there is ample opportunity for lateral spread to contact chicks in hatcheries and brooding and rearing units. *Salmonella* serovars are thus commonly introduced into a unit with purchased poultry and can also be introduced into a country with imports of live poultry or hatching eggs.

Humans, rodents, wild birds, insects, water and feed can all introduce infection into a poultry unit and salmonellas can spread from unit to unit through movement of vehicles, equipment and utensils, including contaminated hatchery egg trays and trolleys. Control of salmonellosis from such sources can be attained only by maintaining a high standard of flock management and adopting the discipline of a good flock biosecurity programme. See below and Chapter 4.

Biosecurity

Staff on a poultry farm can carry *Salmonella* organisms mechanically from one unit to another on contaminated footwear, clothing and hands. It is also possible for humans in this way to transmit infection from poultry to cattle, sheep, pigs, dogs, cats and horses on the same farm. By the same token, *Salmonella* infection can be introduced into a poultry flock from other infected animals on the site by movement of staff. Infected humans may also be excreters of the organism and thus infect poultry in their charge. For the above reasons visitors to poultry units should be restricted to those on essential business and adequate protective clothing should be provided and hygienic procedures adhered to. Staff looking after poultry should not attend other animals on the farm.

The farm should be located away from other poultry holdings, where circumstances permit, and visitors should park away from the buildings, preferably outside the holding.

Litter

Young chicks or poults often contaminate litter with faeces containing salmonellas and such contaminated litter is an important source and means of transmission. Poultry often ingest large numbers of organisms by picking at droppings from pen mates and the infection may spread rapidly within a group. Salmonellas spread more rapidly when chicks are on litter than when in wire cages. In fresh litter the bacteria may survive for long periods and a positive relationship has been described between the moisture content of litter and the level of *Salmonella* contamination.

Rodents, wild birds, insects and water

Rats and mice are a well-documented source of paratyphoid *Salmonella* serovars and are attracted to poultry houses by the abundance of easily accessible food. Mice have been shown to be important vectors of *S.* Enteritidis; they become infected during the life of a flock, move outside the house at depopulation of the flock, then re-enter and infect the next crop of chickens. Strict attention should be paid to control and, if possible, eradication of such vermin from poultry sites. It has become increasingly clear in recent years that wild birds can also be infected with *Salmonella* serovars and can also mechanically carry material contaminated with bacteria on their feet. This may lead to the contamination of walkways and equipment outside the poultry houses. Although controlled environment houses should be bird-proof, poultry kept on free range or in naturally ventilated housing could come into direct contact with wild birds. Domestic flies and beetles are both capable of transmitting salmonellas and infection can persist through the contamination of their eggs and larvae.

Although mains water is unlikely to be a source of salmonellas, care should be taken to ensure that storage and header tanks do not become contaminated via wild birds, rats and mice, and chlorination is desirable for borehole water. Nipple drinkers are less likely to transmit *Salmonella* infection through flocks than bell or cup drinkers.

Role of feedstuffs

Contaminated feedstuffs are undoubtedly a common and important route by which a poultry flock may become infected with *Salmonella*. Animal protein may be included in the ration in the form of fishmeal, or various meat and bone meals, where these are permitted. Surveys of such raw materials used in poultry feeds have revealed that they are occasionally contaminated. Similarly, vegetable proteins may become contaminated either before or during processing.

Heat treatment of poultry feed in the pelleting process may eliminate the organism but in many cases insufficient temperatures and conditioning times merely reduce the number of organisms. Treating feed with chemicals such as formic or propionic acid, or formaldehyde has also been shown to reduce the level of salmonellas in feed. In the UK, the Animal By-Products Order introduced by the Ministry of Agriculture in 1999 requires any home-produced material of animal or fish origin intended for incorporation in poultry feed to be processed and as far as possible rendered free of salmonellas. The materials are tested by a standard method in an approved laboratory. The 1981 Importation of Processed Animal Protein Order prohibits the landing of processed animal protein from countries outside the EU except under the authority of a licence from the Ministry of Agriculture (in 2001 the Ministry of Agriculture became the Department for Environment, Food and Rural Affairs (DEFRA)). Both the above orders are aimed at reducing the likelihood of poultry feed being contaminated with *Salmonella* organisms.

Hatching egg hygiene

Effective prevention of wide dissemination of salmonellas requires that breeding stock be free of infection to prevent vertical transmission through the egg to progeny. Exposure must be prevented in the hatchery and throughout the life of the flock by high standards of management and flock biosecurity.

Preventing transmission of *Salmonella* infection from infected parent birds via the hatchery to chicks following contamination of the outside of the eggshell is an important factor in control. Eggs from flocks infected with the paratyphoid *Salmonella* serovars are usually sterile when laid and most contamination occurs in the nest box from contact with faeces. Strict attention should be paid to management of nest boxes and adequate clean, dry litter should always be available and regularly changed and topped up. Paraformaldehyde prills may be added to each nest box every 2 weeks, but regular removal of litter and using an appropriate disinfectant may be more effective. Eggs should be collected as frequently as possible and never less than three times each day. Cracked, dirty and floor eggs should not be used for hatching and should be kept well separate from clean eggs. Lightly soiled eggs may be cleaned by gentle buffing so that the cuticle is not damaged. Alternatively, such eggs can be washed in a bactericidal solution used at the concentration and temperature recommended by the manufacturer. However, this must be done in strict accordance with these recommendations, as poor egg washing or sanitization can increase contamination rates. All eggs used for hatching should be disinfected on the farm as soon as possible after collection and cleaning. Products with proven efficacy for this procedure must be used, and applied at the correct dilution rates. The eggs should then be stored and transported correctly. They should be kept in a clean, dry vermin-proof area at a temperature of 13–16°C and 75% relative humidity. They should be packed firmly and correctly in suitable containers to prevent damage during transit to the hatchery.

The hatchery

Salmonellas are normally introduced into a hatchery by incubation of unidentified infected eggs or by equipment from infected premises. Measures to prevent this are difficult because infection of the supply flocks may not be discovered before infected eggs are produced. Controlling dissemination of salmonellas within, and leaving, the hatchery is of the utmost importance as the hatchery receives eggs from all supply flocks and delivers chicks to all broiler farms. An effective hatchery hygiene code of practice should be formulated for each site. This would include procedures for spatial or temporal segregation of high-risk flocks, a one-way system for the flow of eggs, chicks, trolleys and trays and identification of critical control points within the hatchery. A good programme of general hygiene control within a hatchery has a beneficial influence on chick quality and control of salmonellas may be closely related, although visibly clean surfaces may still harbour the organisms if an effective disinfectant is not used. The ventilation system should be designed so that air flow is from clean to dirty areas and contaminated air exhausts are sited away from air inlets and other clean areas of the hatchery. Recontamination of cleaned and disinfected trolleys and trays to be returned to breeder units should be prevented. A high volume of waste potentially infected with salmonella organisms is produced during normal operations, and the difficulty in handling such waste to prevent further spread via wildlife or aerosols should not be underestimated. All waste should be enclosed in a secure pest-proof area in an enclosed container. The hatchery is therefore one of the most important critical control points in poultry production for control of *Salmonella*.

Cleansing and disinfection

Complete and effective cleansing and disinfection of poultry houses and the surrounding environment and equipment is crucial to prevent any carry over of salmonellas to the new flock. Guidelines on cleaning, disinfection and vector control in *Salmonella*-infected poultry flocks, with special reference to *S*. Enteritidis, have been produced by the WHO.

After a poultry building has been depopulated all manure should be removed and the building should be thoroughly cleaned before disinfection. The disinfectant should be a product that has a high activity against *Salmonella* organisms and it should be applied thoroughly at a suitable application rate. *Salmonella* organisms are sensitive to most disinfectants although the efficacy can be profoundly affected by the presence of organic matter. A large amount of useful information is available from the manufacturers of these products.

If the depleting flock is suspected or known to be *Salmonella*-positive, it is important to plan sufficient time to achieve effective terminal disinfection. The ease of cleansing and disinfection obviously depends on the design of the building and problems may be encountered with caged layer units where the only realistic option is the use of fogging and/or fumigation. Ideally buildings should be soaked with detergent/sanitizer and then power washed. All surfaces should be left to dry completely before applying disinfectant, which is then allowed to dry. Finally the house and equipment should be fogged with formaldehyde solution, which may also be repeated after placing the litter.

Competitive exclusion

Competitive exclusion (CE) is the term used for the early application of the natural phenomenon in which the developing gut flora of newly hatched chicks can limit intestinal colonization by several enteric pathogens including salmonellas. Since poultry are usually hatched and reared in an environment that precludes their early access to the range of bacteria necessary for protection, commercial products have been developed that contain defined or undefined bacterial flora to aid active colonization of the intestine of very young chicks. They may also be used in older birds after antibiotic treatment. If chicks are provided with this microflora, usually derived from the caecal contents, a highly stable protection develops within 32 h, which effectively reduces the prevalence of *Salmonella* infection within the flock. CE works against heavy continuous environmental exposure and may prevent infection completely when low levels of *Salmonella* contamination are present. CE must be applied as soon as possible at the hatchery or the farm before the birds are exposed to *Salmonella* serovars and administration is either by using a coarse sprayer or an automatic spray cabinet that delivers droplets of at least 1 mm. Some consider the use of CE in the hatchery to be illogical because large numbers of microorganisms are released into an environment that has to be kept sterile. Despite this, no adverse effects have been demonstrated. Alternatively, CE can be applied in the drinking water when the young birds are on the farm but this may be too late to achieve maximum protection if they have already been exposed to enteric pathogens.

In older birds in *Salmonella*-infected flocks, prior antibiotic treatment to suppress intestinal flora and *Salmonella* organisms, followed by treatment with CE mixture before movement to clean premises, has been used to eliminate infection from breeder birds. However routine or continuous use of antibiotics may lead to the development of resistant bacteria. A similar regimen in layer birds has not been as successful because of the impossibility of moving the birds to clean premises.

A number of CE preparations are commercially available, although undefined products have been found to be more effective than specific mixtures of organisms. Probiotics, which include *Lactobacillus*, *Enterococcus*, *Pediococcus*, *Saccharomyces* spp. and some other bacteria, have also been used for control of *Salmonella*. Several of these products have recently been approved by the EU for use as feed additives.

Vaccination

The general consensus is that live vaccines are more protective than inactivated vaccines as a result of the more prolonged exposure and the stimulation of both cellular and humoral arms of the adaptive immune system. In addition, live vaccines, if administered orally, stimulate the innate immune response through heterophil infiltration and activation and defensin production. Killed vaccines are probably mainly effective through the induction of high titres of circulating specific IgG.

Colonization of the gut by live vaccine strains also induces a form of competitive exclusion of other *Salmonella* strains. However, current live vaccines have undefined mutations and there is continuing concern over the use of genetic manipulation to produce more precise mutations. Live vaccines also require high standards of husbandry to ensure that all birds drink and receive a full vaccinal dose.

A variety of vaccines is now commercially available for control of *S.* Enteritidis and *S.* Typhimurium infection. Live vaccines for administration via the drinking water are available for both these serovars. They may be used in breeders or layers as a course of two or three administrations to give protection from rearing and throughout lay. Alternatively, live vaccines can be used as primers for injectable inactivated vaccines. A course of two inactivated injections can be very effective in protecting laying flocks throughout the laying period, either where live vaccines cannot be licensed for use in food animals or if passive yolk antibodies are required for progeny expected to meet early challenge. Live vaccines have generally been prepared from the homologous serovar. However, there is some experimental and field evidence that the 9R vaccine developed for use against *S.* Gallinarum also protects against *S.* Enteritidis by virtue of their antigenic similarity.

Other biological approaches

Chickens vary considerably in their susceptibility to both systemic and intestinal infection by different *Salmonella* serovars. This has not been exploited practically but there is potential to increase resistance through selection for the responsible genetic locus and to use increased genetic resistance alone or in combination with other approaches such as inactivated vaccines.

Colonization of the alimentary tract can be reduced by incorporation of selected short-chain fatty acids (SCFA) in the feed such that they are antibacterial in the crop. The most effective SCFA has been shown to be formic acid, although others also have some effect in reducing colonization under experimental conditions.

Bacteriophages have been explored as a means for control. Although they seem to be less than effective at controlling *Salmonella* infection in the caeca they are more effective at reducing levels of contamination on the carcass.

Statutory aspects of the control of *Salmonella* infections in poultry in the UK

Legislation to deal with *Salmonella* infections in livestock was originally introduced in 1975 following a case of *S.* Paratyphi B in cattle. The reporting procedures introduced by this legislation enabled trends in *Salmonella* isolations from poultry to be monitored and indicated the increase in *S.* Enteritidis that paralleled the increase in human cases and culminated in the 'salmonella in eggs' crisis in 1988.

In 1989, a new Zoonoses Order replaced and broadened the scope of the 1975 Order and is presently the legislation under which any action is taken when a *Salmonella* organism is isolated. Its main provisions are the requirement to report the results of tests that identify the presence of the organism, the provision of a culture to the Ministry of Agriculture, Fisheries and Food (MAFF), now DEFRA, the taking of live birds and other samples for diagnostic purposes, imposition of movement restrictions and isolation requirements, and a requirement for the cleansing and disinfection of premises and vehicles. The Order also applies the provision of the Animal Health Act 1981 with regard to compulsory slaughter and compensation.

The Poultry Breeding Flocks and Hatcheries (Registration and Testing) Order 1989 was introduced with the objective of reducing the vertical transmission of salmonellas so that birds placed at the commercial generation level do not take the infection to premises with them. In 1993 this was replaced by a new Poultry Breeding Flocks and Hatcheries Order, which enacted in the legislation of the UK the provision of EC Directive 92/117 on Zoonoses which, since 1 January 1994, has been the main European legislation for the control of *Salmonella* infections in poultry. This Order only applies to domestic fowls and requires regular monitoring of breeding flocks and hatcheries following a prescribed programme using methods laid down in the Order. A new EU Zoonoses Directive (2003/99) Regulation (2160/2003) is now being implemented in which the minimum requirements for sampling are laid down and breeding and rearing flocks will be monitored for all *Salmonella* serovars. In addition, commercial layer and broiler flocks, turkeys and ducks will also be monitored for *Salmonella* serovars of public health significance.

Feedstuffs have always been a potential source of *Salmonella* infection for poultry and in the UK, as well as replacing the Diseases of Animals (Processed Protein) Order 1981, the Processed Animal Protein Order 1989 considerably strengthened its provisions. This has now been replaced by the Animal By-Products Order (1999); it requires those who process animal protein to be registered with DEFRA and for them to test each day's consignment for salmonellas at an authorized laboratory. If a salmonella is isolated, the processor is required to ensure that no contaminated material is consigned from a store for incorporation into animal feedstuffs. This is in addition to any subsequent action that might be taken by the Ministry under the Zoonoses Order 1989. A number of voluntary codes of practice covering several sectors of the animal feedstuffs industry have been introduced relating to the production, handling and storage of material ranging from raw ingredients to finished feeds. Tighter controls on the importation of animal and fish protein were introduced at the same time so that consignments from overseas countries could be categorized according to the likely risk of being contaminated with *Salmonella* and dealt with appropriately.

These statutory measures reflect the complexity of *Salmonella* infections in poultry and the fact that no single measure is sufficient to solve the problem, which is essentially one of human public health rather than poultry health.

CONCLUSIONS

In general, in the UK salmonellosis has not been a disease of major economic importance (apart from the cost of monitoring and control schemes) or a significant cause of mortality in the National Poultry Flock, with the exception of pullorum disease and fowl typhoid in earlier years. However, more recently epidemics of *S.* Enteritidis have given cause for concern to the industry because of the loss of consumer confidence and ensuing legislation as a result of public health significance. Efforts to control paratyphoid infections in poultry are driven by public health considerations rather than expectations of securing improvements in production efficiency.

The substantial cost of meeting the conditions necessary for effective prevention of infection leads to questions of cost-effectiveness but there is little doubt that effective prevention is possible. A national programme in Sweden has reduced *Salmonella*-infected chicken flocks to a very low level and in the UK improved hygiene and biosecurity, combined with vaccination, has led to a substantial reduction in the prevalence of *Salmonella* in poultry flocks. Effective flock monitoring at all levels of production is necessary to detect infections and to institute appropriate control measures. The industry must therefore be constantly vigilant to maintain the highest standards of management and disease security at breeding farms, hatcheries, rearing farms, feed mills and processing plants in order to prevent the introduction and spread of salmonellosis, both from established serovars but also from new or emerging strains.

REFERENCE

Old D C 1992 Nomenclature of *Salmonella*. J Med Microbiol 37: 361–363

FURTHER READING

Comprehensive

Wray C, Wray A (eds) 2000 *Salmonella* in domestic animals. CABI, Wallingford, Oxfordshire

Taxonomy

Ewing W H (ed) 1986 Edwards & Ewing's identification of Enterobacteriaceae, 4th edn. Elsevier, New York
Le Minor L, Popoff M Y 1987 Request for an opinion. Designation of *Salmonella enterica* sp. nov., nom rev. as the type and only species of the genus *Salmonella*. Int J Syst Bacteriol 37: 465–468
Reeves M W, Ewins G M, Heiba A A et al 1989 Clonal nature of *Salmonella typhi* and its genetic relatedness to other salmonella as shown by multilocus enzyme electrophoresis and proposal of *Salmonella bongori* comb. nov. J Clin Microbiol 27: 313–320

Salmonellosis in poultry

Barrow P A 2000 The paratyphoid salmonellae. In: Beard C W, McNulty M S (eds) Diseases of poultry: world trade and public health implications. Rev Sci Tech 19: 351–374
Gast R K 2003 *Salmonella* infections. In: Saif Y (ed) Diseases of poultry, 11th edn. Iowa State University Press, Ames, p 567–568
Gast R K 2003 Paratyphoid infections. In: Saif Y (ed) Diseases of poultry, 11th edn. Iowa State University Press, Ames, p 583–613
Snoeyenbos G H 1994 Avian salmonellosis. In: Beran G W (ed) Handbook of zoonoses, 2nd edn. CRC Press, Boca Raton, p 303–310

Diagnosis

Barrow P A, Wray C (eds) 2006 ELISA for serological diagnosis of salmonella infection in poultry. Working Document. European Commission, Directorate General for Agriculture, Brussels

Davies R H, Wray C 1994 Evaluation of a rapid cultural method for identification of salmonellas in naturally contaminated veterinary samples. J Appl Bacteriol 77: 237–241

Harvey R W S, Price T H 1974 Isolation of salmonellas. Public Health Laboratory Service Monograph Series No. 8. HMSO, London

Mallinson E T, Snoeyenbos G H. Salmonellosis 1989 In: Purchase H L et al (eds) A laboratory manual for the isolation and identification of avian pathogens, 3rd edn. Kendall/Hunt Publishing, Dubuque, p 3–11

Office international des epizooties 1992 Salmonellosis: *S.* Typhimurium and *S.* Enteritidis. In: Manual of standards for diagnostic tests and vaccines. OIE, Paris, p 418–423

Van Zijderveld F G, Van Zijderveld-Van Bemmel A M, Anakotta J 1992 Comparison of four different enzyme-linked immunosorbent assays for serological diagnosis of *Salmonella* Enteritidis infections in experimentally infected chickens. J Clin Microbiol 30: 2560–2566

Wray C, Davies R H (eds) 1994 Guidelines on detection and monitoring of salmonella-infected poultry flocks with particular reference to *Salmonella* Enteritidis. WHO, Geneva

Control

Barrow P A 1996 Immunity to salmonella and other bacteria. In: Davison T F, Morris T R, Payne L N (eds) Poultry immunology. Poultry Science Symposium Series 24. Carfax, Abingdon, Oxfordshire, p 243–263

Barrow P A, Mead G C, Wray C, Duchet-Suchaux M 2003 Control of food-poisoning salmonella in poultry – biological options. Worlds Poult Sci J 59: 349–359

Cooper G L 1994 Salmonellosis: infections in man and chicken: pathogenesis and the development of live vaccines – a review. Vet Bull 64: 123–143

Davies R H, Wray C 1994 An approach to reduction of salmonella infection in broiler chicken flocks through intensive sampling and identification of cross-contamination in commercial hatcheries. Int J Food Microbiol 24: 147–160

Davies R H, Wray C 1995 Observations on disinfection regimens used on *Salmonella* Enteritidis infected poultry units. Poult Sci 74: 638–647

Nagaraja K V, Kim C J, Kumar M C et al 1991 Is vaccination a feasible approach for the control of *Salmonella*? In: Blankenship L C (ed) Colonisation control of human bacterial enteropathogens in poultry. Academic Press, San Diego, p 243–258

Van Immerseel F, Methner U, Rychlik I et al 2005 Vaccination and early protection against non host-specific *Salmonella* serotypes in poultry; exploitation of innate immunity and microbial activity. Epidemiol Infect 133: 959–978

World Health Organization 1994 Guidelines on cleaning, disinfection and vector control in salmonella infected poultry flocks. WHO, Geneva

Competitive exclusion

Goren E, de Jong W A, Doornenbal P et al 1988 Reduction of salmonella infection of broilers by spray application of intestinal microflora, a longitudinal study. Vet Q 10: 249–255

Mead G C Developments in competitive exclusion to control salmonella in poultry. In: Blankenship L C (ed) Colonisation control of human bacterial enteropathogens in poultry. Academic Press, San Diego, p 91–104

PULLORUM DISEASE

The causal agent was first described by Rettger in 1899; in 1909 he gave it the name *Bacterium pullorum* and later changed it to *Salmonella pullorum*. The disease had been previously known as bacillary white diarrhoea, or BWD, but as white diarrhoea was not always a clinical feature it became better known as pullorum disease. By 1930 the cycle of infection had been worked out, the key role of transmission of infection via the ovaries of carrier birds had been recognized and the value of the agglutination test in detecting carrier birds was established.

EPIDEMIOLOGY

Cause

S. Pullorum is a Gram-negative bacillus (0.3–0.5 $\times$ 1.25 μm), and under normal laboratory conditions is nonmotile and does not express flagellar or H antigens. More recently it has been reported that motility can be induced in some isolates of *S.* Pullorum under specialized laboratory conditions. Its somatic antigenic structure is 1, 9, 12 and it is in group D of the Kauffmann–White classification scheme. The 12 antigens can further be differentiated into 12_1, 12_2 and 12_3 and different strains of *S.* Pullorum contain different proportions of the 12_2 and 12_3 antigen factors.

Hosts

While all avian species can be infected with *S.* Pullorum, reports of clinical disease in species other than chickens, turkeys and pheasants are rare. Waterfowl are more resistant to this organism and there also seem to be varying degrees of resistance among different breeds of chicken.

Spread

The most important method by which pullorum disease infects any group of birds is from an infected parent bird via the ovary to the newly hatched chick. A proportion of infected birds become adult carriers with *S.* Pullorum infection persisting in the spleen until the birds become sexually mature, when the capacity to respond to infection is inhibited as a result of the presence of high concentrations of female sex hormones, resulting in the infection spreading to the reproductive tract, including the ovaries and ova. Such infected hens are not likely to be prolific egg layers and only a small percentage of the eggs laid are likely to be infected. The fertility and hatchability of infected eggs are also likely to be below average. However, viable chicks can hatch from such infected eggs and become a source of infection. Fluff from such chicks is likely to be heavily contaminated with *S.* Pullorum and, as it dries, the bacteria are rapidly disseminated through the incubator or brooder. Thus pullorum disease is passed from hen to chick by vertical transmission and then there is rapid lateral spread from chick to chick in hatcheries and rearing units. The organism can survive outside the body for many months.

The immunological basis for the carrier state is unclear but it is known that the bacteria persist within macrophages in the spleen and that secreted proteins associated with *Salmonella* pathogenicity island 2 are essential.

In recent years *S.* Pullorum has been detected on occasion in pheasants in the UK, which may pose a threat to free-range poultry flocks.

DISEASE

Clinical signs

Pullorum disease is seen predominantly in chicks under 3 weeks of age and the first indication is usually excessive numbers of dead-in-shell chicks and deaths shortly after hatching. Affected birds show variable and nonspecific signs, including depression with tendency to huddle, respiratory distress, lack of appetite and white, viscous droppings that adhere to the feathers around the vent. The mortality varies considerably and in extreme cases can be 100%.

A subacute form with lameness and swollen hock joints may be seen in growing birds and result in poor growth rates. Older birds may appear listless and have pale and shrunken combs. Reduced egg production with lowered fertility and hatchability may be the only sign of the disease when adult birds are affected. The condition, however, is rare in adult birds.

Lesions

Chicks that die shortly after hatching are likely to have peritonitis with an inflamed, unabsorbed yolk sac. The lungs may be congested and the liver dark and swollen with haemorrhages visible on the surface. Sometimes, in chicks that die in the acute phase of the disease there are no specific lesions, or only those of a septicaemia with the liver congested and the subcutaneous blood vessels dilated and prominent. In chicks that die after showing signs of disease for 1–2 days, there is likely to be typhlitis: the caeca are enlarged and distended with casts of hard, dry, necrotic material. Discrete, small, white, necrotic foci are also often found in the liver, lungs, myocardium and gizzard wall. In growers affected with arthritis, the hock and wing joints are usually enlarged because of the presence of excess lemon- or orange-coloured gelatinous material around the joints. In general, the lesions are neither characteristic nor constant.

In adult birds, the characteristic lesion is an abnormal ovary with the ova irregular, cystic, misshapen, discoloured and pedunculated with prominent thickened stalks (Fig. 8.2). There may also be peritonitis, arthritis and pericarditis. In some infected adult hens the ovary is inactive with the ova small, pale and undeveloped.

DIAGNOSIS

The clinical signs and post-mortem findings in pullorum disease are variable and not sufficiently characteristic to make a firm diagnosis. Therefore disease is diagnosed in the chick by isolating the causal organism following cultural examination of viscera. S. Pullorum grows readily on blood agar as small, discrete, round, transparent, glistening colonies. Growth on selective media is variable, when the organism forms small, round colonies. Selenite broth and tetrathionate are the enrichment media of choice for isolation of the organism; however, the organism will usually grow on direct culture on MacConkey agar as pale, non-lactose-fermenting colonies. S. Pullorum differs from S. Gallinarum in its inability to ferment dulcitol and maltose.

Serological tests can be used to detect S. Pullorum antibodies in infected older birds. Antibodies take several days to appear and maximum production may not occur until several months after initial infection. They may not be reliably detectable, therefore, until the bird has reached immunological maturity at 16 weeks of age. A number of tests are available to detect the antibodies but the two that have been most frequently used are the rapid plate agglutination test on whole blood, using a stained antigen, and a tube agglutination test carried out

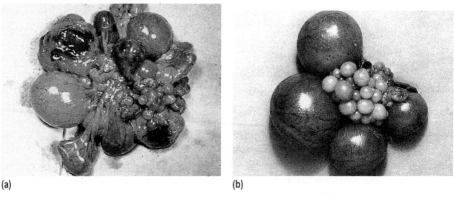

(a)   (b)

Fig. 8.2 The lesions in the ovary in pullorum disease (a) compared with a normal ovary (b).

on serum. In addition, indirect ELISA is able to detect infection and, by combining LPS and flagella antigens, can be used to differentiate infection with *S.* Enteritidis from *S.* Pullorum/Gallinarum.

The rapid plate agglutination test or WBT is carried out as described below. Reactions in most cases occur immediately on mixing of blood with antigen, and are nearly always complete within 30 s. If fine, pinpoint blue granules appear, either throughout the mixture or only at the margins, the result is interpreted as doubtful. Any reaction that occurs between 1 and 2 min must also be regarded as doubtful, while reactions occurring after 2 min are considered to be negative. When turkeys, geese, ducks, guinea-fowl, pheasants, partridges and quails are tested the above procedure for reading and interpreting the test results should be followed but the level of false-positive reactions is likely to be much higher than in chickens.

Flock testing

For flock testing the rapid plate test using whole blood is quick and easy to perform and reactor birds can be identified at one handling and do not have to be leg- or wing-banded. Labour is thus reduced to a minimum and delays in transit, leaking and broken tubes and errors in identifying samples are eliminated. This test can also be used on serum in the laboratory. The tube test, however, has the advantage of being quantitative, with a result expressed as a specific dilution, and is a useful back-up check for the plate test.

Two consecutive clear tests, 1 month apart, are necessary before a flock can be considered with confidence to be free of pullorum disease. When the tube test is used serum titres may fluctuate and in both types of test environmental contamination or carrier birds in the early stages of infection may cause reinfection immediately after a clear test. There is no significant difference in accuracy between the two tests on a flock basis, although the WBT is not satisfactory for testing turkeys.

In the early stages of a pullorum eradication scheme, where the disease is still widespread or where there is a recent flock history of the disease, the test should be interpreted strictly. All doubtful and positive reactors should be culled. As a check on the rapid plate test, blood samples should be taken from a proportion of the reactors and subjected to the tube agglutination test; the birds should then be killed and the viscera cultured in an attempt to isolate *S.* Pullorum. In the later stages of an eradication scheme occasional reactor birds may be found, and these should be submitted for bacteriological examination. It is possible for false-positive serological reactions to occur, usually because of cross-agglutination by other organisms such as coliforms and streptococci.

Two simple and effective tools for carrying out the rapid plate test are a needle/wire 10 cm in length, with the blunt end bent to form a loop 5 mm in diameter, and a white porcelain plate 15 × 12 cm in size divided into 12 equal squares. The needle is held by the operator and the brachial vein is pricked where it passes over the elbow joint. The needle is then reversed and a 0.02 mL drop of blood is picked up in the loop. This is mixed with 0.04 mL polyvalent crystal-violet-stained antigen on the porcelain plate. Between birds the needle is washed in saline, and after 12 tests have been completed the plate is washed in saline and wiped dry. The test should be carried out in a cool, dust-free atmosphere in good natural light. It should not be carried out in bright sunlight; in the open, a shaded area is best. A skilled operator supported by experienced helpers on a well-managed unit can test up to 200 birds an hour. A limit of 1000 birds a day for one operator is sensible in order to avoid fatigue and error.

For the rapid slide agglutination test in the laboratory 0.02 mL serum is mixed with 0.02 mL stained antigen. The interpretation of results is the same as for the WBT.

CONTROL

A number of antibacterial agents will reduce the morbidity and mortality if used to treat birds infected with *S.* Pullorum. However, no treatment is likely to eliminate all carriers from an infected flock. In most cases treatment is not recommended and control should be by repeated blood testing and elimination of reactor birds. In the event of disease in a small backyard flock the owner should be advised to slaughter the whole flock and restock on new ground with clean, tested, pullorum-free birds. Breeding from such small infected flocks should be strongly discouraged.

After the epidemiology of *S.* Pullorum infection had been worked out and a reliable test to detect carrier birds was available, many countries embarked on programmes to control the disease by eradication. Such programmes are based on repeated blood tests on birds in breeding flocks and removal of reactors, thereby reducing persistently infected birds and the associated risk of vertical transmission. This is combined with high flock management standards and hatchery discipline. Birds are usually tested between 16 weeks and point of lay, and two consecutive clear tests 1 month apart followed by an annual clear test provide the accepted evidence that a flock is pullorum-free. Replacement birds must be purchased only from flocks known to be free of the disease, or kept isolated until they have been tested and found to be pullorum-free. Eggs from pullorum-free flocks should be incubated and hatched only in hatcheries receiving eggs exclusively from clean flocks.

On a national basis, breeding flocks and hatcheries are usually grouped together in a scheme administered and supervised by government authority.

In the UK such a scheme (the Accredited Poultry Breeding Stations Scheme) was started in 1933 and offered free annual blood testing for detection of pullorum disease. In 1935 this was supplemented by the Accredited Hatcheries Scheme, which provided supervision of hatcheries by government inspectors, and in 1948 the two schemes were combined as the Poultry Stock Improvement Plan. Later this became the Poultry Health Scheme. Initially the tube agglutination test was used but in 1942 the rapid whole blood plate test was introduced. Between 1943 and 1963 the prevalence of infected flocks was reduced from 30% to 4%. However, it was not until 1972 that all flocks in the Poultry Health Scheme become free of *S.* Pullorum infection.

Eradication was complicated by the appearance in the late 1950s of a variant strain of S. Pullorum. Birds infected with this strain gave doubtful or negative reactions to the test. The problem was solved by using a polyvalent antigen that included both standard and variant strains.

When all flocks in the Poultry Health Scheme became free of pullorum disease the annual testing regimen was relaxed and, currently, parent breeding flocks are not normally tested. Testing is confined to grandparent flocks and only 25% of the adult birds are blood-tested each year.

The normal breeding pyramid in a country with a modern poultry industry is for a small number of primary or grandparent breeding flocks to supply breeding birds to parent or multiplier flocks. The commercial egg production hens and broilers are then supplied from these parent flocks. As pullorum disease spreads mainly by vertical transmission, if the grandparent flocks are pullorum-free, the parent and commercial birds should also be free of disease, if in a clean environment.

There are still a few flocks in the UK outside the Poultry Health Scheme that are infected with S. Pullorum. These are flocks of original pure breeds. Infection is unlikely to spread from such flocks to the breeding flocks in the scheme unless the rules are broken and a member is unwise enough to introduce untested birds into his main flock. Anyone wishing to buy old and rare breeds of poultry for flocks outside the Poultry Health Scheme should ensure that the birds are tested for pullorum disease before purchase.

FOWL TYPHOID (*SALMONELLA* GALLINARUM INFECTION)

Towards the end of the 19th century, an infectious enteritis causing heavy mortality in chickens was described in Europe and North America. In 1902 it was given the name fowl typhoid and recognized as a clinical entity distinct from fowl cholera. The causal organism was a non-motile, Gram-negative bacillus that eventually became known as *Salmonella* Gallinarum. For many years fowl typhoid was a major problem in poultry flocks throughout the world but in the UK and other countries with an advanced poultry industry it is now rare and seldom isolated. However, it has increased dramatically in recent years in South America and other parts of the world and constitutes a serious poultry health problem.

EPIDEMIOLOGY

Cause

S. Gallinarum is a short bacillus ($1.0–2.0 \times 1.5\,\mu m$) that does not possess flagella. It has the somatic antigen structure O1, 9, 12 and is thus classified within group D of the Kauffmann–White scheme. S. Gallinarum ferments glucose, mannitol, maltose and dulcitol but does not ferment lactose, sucrose and salicin.

Hosts

Almost all outbreaks in the UK have been in chickens but in some countries, notably the USA, serious incidents with heavy mortality have occurred in turkey flocks. Fowl typhoid has also been reported in ducks, pheasants, guinea fowl, peafowl, grouse and quail. The disease differs from other avian *Salmonella* infections in that clinical disease is usually seen in growers or adult birds, although chicks can be affected. Certainly under experimental conditions chickens of any age are susceptible, whereas S. Pullorum produces severe clinical disease only in very young chicks.

Spread

The causal agent is passed out by infected birds in the droppings and lateral spread is by the ingestion of such material in contaminated food or water. *S*. Gallinarum will persist in faeces for at least a month, and in infected carcasses for much longer periods. In the UK, fowl typhoid was a disease of flocks kept extensively and was often, but not always, associated with poor management. Rats, dogs, foxes and wild birds may carry parts of infected carcasses from flock to flock under these conditions and infected carcasses may also contaminate ponds and streams. Recovered birds frequently remain carriers for long periods, and it is axiomatic that the movement of such birds could readily be a means by which the disease spreads. Egg transmission also occurs, with the opportunity for lateral spread of infection to contact birds in the hatchery or rearing units. Similarly, attendants, visitors, etc. may carry infection from one farm to another, or house to house, unless appropriate disinfection procedures are in place.

DISEASE

Clinical signs

In acute outbreaks, the first sign of disease is likely to be an increase in mortality followed by a drop in food consumption and, if the birds are in lay, a drop in egg production. Depression, with affected birds standing still with ruffled feathers and their eyes closed, is a common feature. Respiratory distress with rapid breathing can occur but the most characteristic clinical sign is a watery to mucoid yellow diarrhoea. In birds that do not die within 2 or 3 days of developing these signs, a chronic phase follows. There is progressive loss of condition and an intense anaemia develops, which produces shrunken, pale combs and wattles. The incubation period is short, usually between 4 and 6 days; the disease will spread rapidly through the flock and, if untreated, can result in losses of 50% or more.

Subacute outbreaks of disease may result in sporadic mortality over a long period. Egg transmission is not a regular feature of the disease but can occur and leads to an increase in dead-in-shell embryos and small, weak, moribund or dead chicks on the hatching trays. When young chicks are affected, the signs are nonspecific and similar to those seen in pullorum disease or salmonellosis. Weakness, reluctance to move, a tendency to huddle and a drop in food consumption all occur. Yellow, pasty droppings, which adhere to the feathers around the vent, are also seen. Sometimes there is respiratory distress with rapid breathing and gasping.

Lesions

The carcasses of birds dying in the acute phase of the disease have a septicaemic, jaundiced appearance, with the subcutaneous blood vessels injected and prominent, and the skeletal muscles congested and dark in colour. A consistent finding is a swollen friable liver that is dark red or almost black, and the surface has a distinctive coppery bronze sheen after exposure to the air for a short period. The spleen may also be enlarged and a catarrhal enteritis, particularly involving the small intestine, is usually present. The intestines typically contain viscous, slimy, bile-stained material. Necrotic lesions in the small intestine may be visible through the wall of the intestine. A characteristic additional feature is dark-brown bone marrow. Emaciation and an intensely anaemic carcass with focal necrosis in the heart, intestines, pancreas and liver are found in birds dying in the chronic phase of fowl typhoid. Greyish-white necrotic foci are also seen in the myocardium, the mucosa and submucosa of the first part of the intestines, and the pancreas. A pericarditis, with turbid yellow fluid in the pericardial sac and fibrin attached to the surface of the heart, is a feature of chronic fowl typhoid. In young chicks, additional findings may be discrete necrotic foci in the lungs and gizzard. Well-defined necrotic foci in the testicles have been reported in cockerels affected with the disease. In laying birds there may be retained yolks, which may subsequently rupture.

DIAGNOSIS

S. Gallinarum grows on blood agar as well-defined, opaque, glistening colonies and will grow readily on MacConkey agar as pale, non-lactose-fermenting colonies and also on DCA and brilliant green agar (BGA). *S.* Gallinarum will also grow in selective enrichment media and, of these, selenite and tetrathionate are the most frequently used for its isolation. *S.* Gallinarum and *S.* Pullorum have many similar biochemical, cultural and serological properties. However, *S.* Gallinarum grows more readily on solid media and produces larger colonies and, in contrast to *S.* Pullorum, ferments maltose and dulcitol and does not decarboxylate ornithine. A further difference is that variant forms of *S.* Gallinarum do not occur. Like *S.* Pullorum, this bacterium can survive outside the host's body for many months.

As *S.* Gallinarum has the same antigenic structure as *S.* Pullorum the rapid plate agglutination test or whole blood, using the stained *S.* Pullorum antigen, can be used to detect carriers of *S.* Gallinarum. ELISA has also been demonstrated to be of use as a flock test.

CONTROL

Treatment

Therapy with a number of antibacterial agents will reduce clinical signs and mortality in a flock affected with fowl typhoid. Furazolidone given continuously in the feed for 10 days at a level of 0.04% was generally considered to be the best treatment regimen (furazolidone is no longer available in EU countries). Treatment is unlikely to eliminate *S.* Gallinarum infection completely and chronically infected carrier birds are likely to remain even after treatment. Reinfection of susceptible birds with the development of clinical disease may also occur, with the disease recycling in the flock. Treatment should therefore always be accompanied by culling of chronically affected birds and reactors to a blood test and the prompt removal and incineration of all carcasses. Prolonged and extensive use of treatment in some countries has resulted in increasing resistance, manifest by increasing minimum inhibitory concentration (MIC) values. Such resistance is not readily detected by disc diffusion tests.

Vaccination

When fowl typhoid was widespread in the UK between 1950 and 1960, a vaccine was developed that was used successfully in many flocks. It was a live attenuated rough strain of *S.* Gallinarum known as vaccine 9R. After subcutaneous injection into chickens between 10 and 18 weeks of age it usually gave solid, long-lasting immunity. Vaccination reduces mortality in flocks challenged with *S.* Gallinarum and does not depress egg production when used in flocks free of the disease. There is evidence, however, that immunity varies with the age and genetic susceptibility of the bird. Vaccinated birds can carry and excrete the rough strain of *S.* Gallinarum for long periods, and it can also be transmitted through the eggs laid by vaccinated birds, but there is no evidence of reversion to virulence. Some vaccinated birds develop hepatic and splenic lesions without mortality but the vaccine has the advantage that few birds produce antibodies detectable by the WBT. In countries where fowl typhoid remains a major problem vaccination still has a place and, if an early diagnosis of fowl typhoid is made, treatment with a suitable antimicrobial followed by vaccination after the effect of the drug has lapsed is a useful control procedure.

Genetic resistance and other approaches

Experimental work has indicated enormous differences in inbred White Leghorn lines in resistance to *S.* Gallinarum as a result of inheritance of a single genetic locus. Mapping is under way to establish the identity of the gene(s) involved.

Experimental work has also indicated the value of using formic acid incorporation in the feed to reduce horizontal transmission.

Blood testing

Serological testing can be used to monitor flocks and positive birds can then be culled from the flock. The blood test thus supports a treatment and vaccination control programme. On a national basis, systematic blood testing of breeding flocks for *S.* Pullorum disease with removal of reactors has undoubtedly been the main reason why fowl typhoid has been virtually eradicated from most countries with a progressive poultry industry.

FURTHER READING

Harbourne J F, Williams B M, Fincham I H 1963 The prevention of fowl typhoid in the field using a freeze-dried 9R vaccine. Vet Rec 75: 858–861

Shivaprasad H L 2003 Pullorum disease and fowl typhoid. In: Saif Y (ed) Diseases of poultry, 11th edn. Iowa State University Press, Ames, p 568–582

Silva E W, Snoeyenbos G H, Weinack O M, Smyser C F 1980 Studies on the use of 9R strain of Salmonella Gallinarum as a vaccine in chickens. Avian Dis 25: 38–52

ARIZONOSIS

In 1939, a Gram-negative bacterium was isolated from a lizard carcass in Arizona and tentatively identified as *Salmonella* var. *arizonae*. In the next few years other organisms with similar biochemical and cultural characteristics were reported from many different parts of the world. It was felt that they had certain common properties that distinguished them from *Salmonella* strains, and they became known as paracolons or arizonas. However, in 1982, members of the International Subcommittee on Taxonomy of *Enterobacteriaceae* decided that members of the Arizona group of bacteria should be classed in two subspecies of the genus *Salmonella* because their DNA was closely related to other *Salmonella* species. More than 300 antigenically distinct Arizona serovars have now been identified and have been incorporated into the Kauffmann–White scheme as *S. enterica* subspecies IIIa (*arizonae*) and IIIb (*diarizonae*).

Although the organisms were frequently isolated from diseased snakes on farms where there was a high mortality in infected turkey poults, it was suggested that Arizona organisms were opportunists that had spread from reptiles to turkeys. However, it was later shown that the infection was endemic in many turkey flocks in North America and spread occurred mainly by vertical transmission via the hatching egg. The types of Arizona organisms causing disease in turkeys were also found to be distinct from those affecting reptiles and the disease proved to be of considerable economic importance to the turkey industry in North America and certain other parts of the world.

EPIDEMIOLOGY

Cause

Arizonae organisms are Gram-negative, flagellated bacilli that do not form spores. They grow on ordinary liquid and solid media at 37°C in a similar way to other *Salmonella* organisms. However, unlike other salmonellas, in media containing lactose many Arizonae will ferment this sugar if incubated for several days. Arizonae grow on bismuth sulphite agar and the colonies have a distinctive black sheen. They can be differentiated biochemically from other *Salmonella* subspecies by their reactions on malonate, dulcite and *O*-nitrophenyl-β-galactopyranoside (ONPG). The basic serological identification procedures are similar to those used for other *Salmonella*. Thirty-four somatic O and 43 flagellar H antigens have been demonstrated; a colon is used to separate the O and H antigens when writing the formula for an isolate. Two serovars, $O18:z_4:z_{32}$ and $O18:z_4:z_{23}$, are the ones most frequently isolated from poultry in North America, and $O18:z_4:z_{32}$ was the strain that caused the outbreaks of disease in the UK in 1967.

Hosts

Turkeys appear to be the most susceptible avian host. Disease caused by Arizonae infection has been described in chicks and ducklings but outbreaks in poultry other than turkeys are not common.

Arizonae organisms have been isolated from a large number of different species of birds and mammals, including sheep, where they have produced occasional enteric problems, and probably all species can be transiently infected.

Spread

The organisms are widely distributed in the environment but poultry and reptiles probably provide the main reservoir of infection. Rodents and wild birds have also been blamed for introducing Arizonae into a previously clean poultry unit or carrying infection from one flock to another.

If an adult turkey is infected, the organism may localize in the intestine and such a bird may then become a carrier and excrete Arizonae organisms for long periods. It has also been shown that, after a female poult has recovered from systemic infection, the organism can localize in the ovary and from there be transmitted to progeny via the egg. However, it is generally agreed that transmission via the egg occurs most frequently following contamination of the shell with infected faeces. It has been shown that the Arizonae bacillus can readily penetrate the shell and shell membranes at 37°C. Once an embryo or poult is infected, lateral transmission can readily occur in the hatcher or hatchery by aerosol and in the brooder by direct contact and via contaminated food and water.

DISEASE

Clinical signs

The signs shown by poults with arizonosis are similar to those shown by chicks with salmonellosis but eye abnormalities are seen more frequently and nervous signs are a regular additional feature. Affected birds are listless, tend to huddle, look dejected and have pasty faeces, which stick to the vent feathers. Various nervous signs, including ataxia, trembling, leg paralysis, torticollis and convulsions, have been described. A characteristic finding is visual impairment, with a white opacity that can be seen deep in the eye when looking directly into the pupil. As with salmonellosis, clinical signs are virtually confined to poults less than 5 weeks of age. Morbidity and mortality vary, but losses of up to 90% in a group of poults have been reported. Adult birds generally show no clinical signs of disease but can be carriers and excrete the organisms for long periods.

Lesions

Poults dying of arizonosis are likely to have a septicaemic carcass with generalized peritonitis. The yolk sacs are frequently inflamed and the air sacs thickened with opaque white to yellow, cheesy, caseous deposits adhering. The livers may be swollen and discoloured (yellow) and discrete necrotic foci are sometimes found throughout the substance of the liver. Commonly there is an enteritis and a distinctive finding, as with salmonellosis, is typhlitis with white caseous casts filling the caecal lumen. Eye lesions are a characteristic feature, with retinitis and a thick exudate covering the back inner surface of the eyeball. Sometimes this varies and appears as a hard, circular white disc of inspissated caseous material. Changes are seen in the central nervous system and striking lesions may be seen histologically.

DIAGNOSIS

The clinical signs and post-mortem findings in birds affected with arizonosis are not specific and cannot be differentiated from other forms of salmonellosis. However, if there are any poults with incoordination and eye abnormalities, arizonosis should be strongly suspected.

Confirmation of the diagnosis is by isolation and identification of the causal agent. When dead poults are examined, retained yolk sac material, liver, retinal exudate, air sacs and caecal contents are suitable specimens for culture. If dead-in-shell or infertile eggs are available, the shell and shell membranes are the most rewarding specimens to examine. When examining the carcasses of adult birds to determine whether or not they are carriers, the ovaries should always be cultured. Direct cultural examination on MacConkey agar, after overnight incubation at 37°C and also after incubation for 24 and 48 h in selenite F broth before subculture on to MacConkey agar and DCA, is an effective standard routine for isolation of Arizonae organisms. In addition, it is advisable to culture onto bismuth sulphite agar, allowing the plate to remain for 4 days at 40°C to overcome excessive inhibitory properties. Arizonae will grow as black colonies on bismuth sulphite agar and as late or non-lactose-fermenting colonies on DCA. Such colonies are then stabbed into the butt of a lysine iron agar slope and streaked on to the slant. Colonies can be conveniently identified as *S.* Arizonae if a black streak appears on the butt of the media with no other media colour change after overnight incubation. Arizona colonies can then be differentiated from other *Salmonella* serovars by their reactions in malonate, dulcite and ONPG broth. Organisms that comply with the above biochemical reactions to indicate Arizonae are then checked for O and H Arizonae antigens by slide and tube agglutination tests using specific Arizonae O and H antisera.

Serological tests

Birds infected with Arizonae do not always produce detectable antibodies in their serum or the production may be transient. Adult female carriers may not have had detectable antibodies during their growing period but a rise in antibody level sometimes occurs at point of lay. Antibodies to the O antigen can be detected by either tube agglutination or rapid plate agglutination tests using an antigen comprising the Arizonae bacillus in buffered formal saline, 10% glycerine and 1% of a 3% alcoholic solution of crystal violet. The H antibodies can be detected only by tube agglutination tests using a formalinized motile broth culture. The rapid plate agglutination test is a useful field-screening test but needs to be supported by the O tube agglutination testing in a control programme. An ELISA using outer membrane proteins as the antigen has been recently used successfully for the detection of infected poultry.

CONTROL

Treatment of affected birds with certain sulphonamides, furazolidone (if available), furaltadone and fluoroquinolones may reduce losses in acute outbreaks. It is possible that treated birds may remain carriers or that treatment may prolong the length of time that carriers excrete the organism. At best, treatment should only be used to prevent spread of disease in commercial flocks.

As is the case with salmonellosis, the best way to control arizonosis is to start a flock with birds from a known clean source and then make every effort to prevent introduction of infection. This can be achieved only by maintaining sensible flock biosecurity and high management standards. Egg transmission plays an important role in disease spread and high standards of hatching egg hygiene are therefore vital. Frequent egg collection, keeping nest boxes scrupulously clean, avoiding incubation of floor or badly contaminated eggs and fumigation of eggs as soon as possible after collection are essential practices. Proper storage and handling of eggs is also necessary. Injection of hatching eggs with antibacterials has also been used but this is not recommended because of the risk of producing resistant organisms.

If a turkey breeding flock becomes infected with Arizonae, eradication is always difficult and sometimes impossible. Several types of vaccine have been applied to turkey breeding stock and shown to protect against systemic infection and reduce faecal shedding, and thus prevent egg transmission. By using an oil-adjuvant vaccine in turkey breeding flocks, it was possible to obtain Arizona-free progeny from vaccinated breeder flocks held in infected environments.

Experience in the UK has shown that the eradication of Arizonae infection from breeding turkey flocks is possible. In 1968 clinical arizonosis in turkeys was diagnosed in the UK in five widely separated flocks. All the affected birds originated from one breeding flock comprising birds that had been imported as day-olds from California. These had been in quarantine for 6 months without showing clinical or post-mortem evidence of arizonosis. The imported flock was slaughtered and infection in the progeny was eradicated by a programme of repeated serological testing of the breeding birds and cultural examination of infertile eggs, dead-in-shell embryos and cull poults. This was backed up by a system of management practices that included keeping the breeding birds isolated in small pens and slaughtering all the birds in a pen if one serological or cultural examination was positive. This control programme was effective and Arizonae infection was eliminated from the turkey industry in the UK. This illustrates that Arizonae infection can be eliminated from breeding flocks by a thorough and painstaking programme of testing and good management discipline. It also emphasizes how important it is for a country free of the infection to be constantly vigilant to ensure that arizonosis is not introduced with imported birds or hatchery eggs.

FURTHER READING

Gast R K 2003 Paratyphoid infections. In: Saif Y (ed) Diseases of poultry, 11th edn. Iowa State University Press, Ames, p 583–613

Greenfield J, Bigland C H, Dukes T W 1971 The genus *Arizona* with special reference to Arizona disease in turkeys. Vet Bull 41: 605–611

Jordan F T W, Lamont P H, Timms L, Grattan D A P 1976 The eradication of *Arizona* 7:1,7.8 from a turkey breeding flock. Vet Rec 99: 413–417

COLIBACILLOSIS

Bacteria of the species *Escherichia coli* are normal inhabitants of the digestive tract of mammals and birds and most strains are nonpathogenic. Certain serovars, however, can cause disease in all species of poultry and yolk sac infection, coligranuloma (Hjärre's disease), egg peritonitis and colisepticaemia are well-recognized results of *E. coli* infection. These conditions can be conveniently grouped together under the heading colibacillosis.

COLISEPTICAEMIA

Colisepticaemia is the most serious manifestation of colibacillosis and the disease rose to prominence with the development of the broiler industry. When the broiler industry expanded, large numbers of birds were kept intensively at high stocking rates in poorly ventilated houses. As conditions in the broiler industry improved, the incidence of the disease fell.

EPIDEMIOLOGY

Cause

Members of the genus *Escherichia* are Gram-negative, flagellated rods (2–3 $\times$ 0.6 μm). They grow readily on plain or blood agar as convex, circular, smooth, grey colonies. Most avian pathogenic serovars are nonhaemolytic on blood agar. They ferment glucose, mannitol and lactose but do not ferment inositol, liquefy gelatin or produce H_2S in Kligler's medium. The Eijkman test provides a useful screening procedure for identification and an organism producing acid and gas at 44°C in MacConkey's lactose bile broth can be tentatively regarded as *E. coli*.

Serovars are usually identified and referred to by only their O or somatic antigen, although the full antigenic formula also includes a K or capsular antigen and the H antigen. Usually, but not invariably, the O, K and H antigens occur in the same combination. The K antigen can be identified by a rapid slide agglutination test and gives an indication of which O antigen is likely to be in combination. To identify the O antigen it is necessary to remove the heat-labile K antigen and then carry out a tube agglutination test.

Most of the pathogenic *E. coli* belong to a small range of serogroups that includes O1:K1, O2:K1 and O78:K80. The O1 carbohydrate capsule has been identified as an important virulence determinant that inhibits phagocytosis.

Hosts

Chickens, turkeys, ducks and pheasants can all be affected with colisepticaemia but the disease is most commonly seen in young chickens.

Spread

E. coli organisms, including the pathogenic serotypes, may inhabit the intestinal tracts of poultry and wild birds and be shed in the faeces, sometimes in high numbers. *E. coli* will persist for long periods outside the bird's body in dry, dusty conditions and it has been shown that wetting the litter can reduce the incidence of colisepticaemia. *E. coli* challenges are contributed to or spread by bacterial load from contaminated drinking water. Faecal contamination of the egg may result in the penetration of *E. coli* through the shell and it has been estimated that in some cases 0.5–6% of eggs may contain the organism. *E. coli* may spread to other chickens during hatch and is often associated with high mortality rates, or it may give rise to yolk sac infections.

Influencing factors

Mycoplasma gallisepticum and certain viral infections predispose to or exacerbate colisepticaemia. Thus, Newcastle disease or infectious bronchitis (IB) and IB variants, even in live vaccine form, *Avian pneumovirus* (APV), infectious bursal disease (IBD), coccidiosis and nutritional deficiencies all increase susceptibility. In turkey poults bacterial and viral rhinotracheitis, haemorrhagic enteritis and aspergillosis predispose to colisepticaemia. Environmental stress (e.g. lack of feed/water, too high a temperature) may also predispose birds to this disease.

DISEASE

Pathogenesis

E. coli are always found in the digestive tracts of poultry and in particularly large numbers in the lower part of the small intestine and caecum. The serovars most frequently causing colisepticaemia are also likely to be found in the throat and upper trachea following inhalation of dust containing *E. coli*. These pathogenic *E. coli* probably invade the bird's body from the respiratory tract following infection with other respiratory pathogens to produce the characteristic condition. Experimental infections are most easily established following infection with respiratory viruses such as coronavirus or rhinotracheitis virus. However *E. coli* may also act as a primary pathogen when the bird's resistance is lowered by environmental stress and poor air quality (especially dust or high ammonia levels). Clinical colisepticaemia can be produced experimentally by parenteral injection or intratracheal administration of these pathogenic *E. coli* serovars into pathogen-free chickens, probably through avoiding respiratory tract defence mechanisms. The organism may also infect skin wounds or lesions leading to significant subcutaneous infections.

Clinical signs

Birds between 2 and 12 weeks of age are usually affected, with most losses occurring around 4 and 9 weeks. The first sign is likely to be a drop in food consumption, which is followed by the birds appearing listless and standing about dejectedly with ruffled feathers. The head and neck of affected birds may be drawn into their bodies. Affected birds develop laboured rapid breathing, gasping or other signs of respiratory distress. Morbidity and mortality are variable and losses are usually less than 5% of the group, but morbidity can be over 50%. After clinical signs have subsided, the affected groups are left uneven and commercially unsatisfactory and give rise to a high proportion of carcasses downgraded after slaughter. Lameness due to joint infections may also be seen.

Lesions

The gross lesions are striking and characteristic, and represent a generalized polyserositis with various combinations of pericarditis, perihepatitis, air sacculitis and peritonitis. The basic finding is a dark, dehydrated and septicaemic carcass with the liver, spleen, lungs and kidneys dark and congested. The air sacs are thickened, opaque and white with adherent caseous deposits. A fibrinous pericarditis, with the pericardial sac thickened, white and adhering to the surface of the heart, is a characteristic finding. A skin of fibrinous material almost always covers the surface of the liver.

DIAGNOSIS

Diagnosis can be confirmed by isolating a profuse pure growth of *E. coli* on direct culture from heart blood, the liver, lungs and air sacs.

CONTROL

The best method of controlling colisepticaemia is to maintain the highest standards of flock management and obtain chicks only from disease-free, well-managed breeding flocks and hatcheries. Pathogenic *E. coli* serovars can be transmitted via the hatchery following faecal contamination of hatching eggs. Chicks should be the progeny of mycoplasma-free stock that have also been vaccinated against IBD, IB, Newcastle disease and any other disease that is a local threat. Good litter management and properly ventilated houses are also vital factors in control of colisepticaemia. The litter should be dry but not dusty and the airflow through the houses should be controlled to avoid pockets of stagnant air or a build-up of ammonia fumes.

Open 'bell' drinkers are to be avoided and a move by the industry to closed nipple systems was a significant factor in the reduction of colisepticaemia outbreaks. However, the most important influencing factors have been the eradication of *M. gallisepticum* and more effective control of IB in broiler breeders. These factors, together with general improvements in housing, feeding and ventilation, have helped reduce the incidence of the disease. Nevertheless, it is still a major threat to poultry in the UK, particularly if management standards are not maintained at a high level.

Colisepticaemia can be treated with a number of antibacterial agents. The logical approach to treatment is to isolate the causal *E. coli* serovar and carry out a sensitivity test to choose the most suitable form of therapy prior to the start of treatment. However, in the face of disease it may be necessary to start treatment earlier, and the choice of antibacterial agent may be based on past experience. Data should be collected over time to assess changes in antimicrobial sensitivity to aid the efficient and strategic use of available medications.

There have been encouraging reports of successful trials with oil-emulsified multivalent vaccines and other types of vaccine. These can protect birds against mortality and active respiratory disease following challenge with pathogenic *E. coli* serovars, and are now commercially available.

It seems likely that they might have a role in control of colibacillosis in future, both in vaccinated birds and their progeny.

Under experimental conditions parenteral administration of lytic bacteriophages which attach to the K1 capsule can be highly effective since any mutants that develop are K1-negative and thereby less virulent.

EGG PERITONITIS

It is convenient to describe a number of reproductive disorders of poultry, including peritonitis, salpingitis and impaction of the oviduct, as egg peritonitis.

EPIDEMIOLOGY

Cause

Avian pathogenic *E. coli* serovars are involved as causative agents in all birds (layers and broiler breeders, turkeys, ducks and geese) that are sexually mature. The method of spread to the reproductive tract is unknown but is thought to be haematogenous and from the air sacs or by ascending infection from the vent.

Influencing factors

A variety of stressors can precipitate egg peritonitis ranging from internal and external parasites (e.g. worms, red mite), systemic infectious disease (e.g. pasteurellosis), viral infections disrupting oviduct activity (e.g. IB) to physical effects such as adverse weather conditions or contact with foxes.

DISEASE

Clinical signs

Affected birds may die suddenly or cease laying and become dull and emaciated. Eggs laid during illness are likely to be deformed and show shell defects. In any flock of laying birds there will be a small number of deaths, which is usually considered to be unavoidable. A high proportion of this background mortality will be due to various types of egg peritonitis. However, egg peritonitis can occur as a greater flock problem and when it does it is usually associated with some type of stressor that has an adverse effect on egg passage and the normal peristaltic movement of eggs along the oviduct. Flock peritonitis outbreaks are often linked to cannibalism or vent pecking.

Lesions

Post-mortem examination may reveal yolk debris, inspissated yolk, caseous material or milky fluid in the abdominal cavity, together with inflammation and distortion of the ovaries and salpingitis. This may be localized around the ovary or oviduct, or present as an abdomen distended with an offensive-smelling mass of caseous material. Alternatively, the oviduct may be obstructed by a core of inspissated inflammatory debris, which may sometimes result in rupture of the oviduct wall. A whole or partly formed egg may be impacted in the oviduct.

DIAGNOSIS

Almost invariably a profuse pure growth of *E. coli* can be isolated from the oviduct and caseous inspissated material in such cases. Unless the carcass is examined immediately after death the significance of *E. coli* may be difficult to determine because the organism is a frequent and rapid post-mortem invader.

CONTROL

Treatment can be difficult due to the unavailability of antimicrobials with a nil egg withdrawal period. Control measures are therefore aimed at controlling the many trigger factors associated with egg peritonitis. Again, the availability of fresh potable drinking water and preventing free-range flocks drinking from dirty puddles on range will reduce the birds' bacterial load.

YOLK SAC INFECTION (MUSHY CHICK DISEASE, OMPHALITIS)

This condition is one of the most common causes of mortality in chicks during the first week after hatching. *E. coli* can be involved either as the primary and sole causal agent or as a secondary opportunist. Yolk sac infection can be associated with a thickened inflamed navel, where the route of infection is via the unhealed navel, or bacteria can multiply in the hatching egg following faecal contamination of the shell. Yolk sac infection can cause 100% mortality in a batch of chicks in the first week of life but deaths are usually between 5% and 10%. Other bacteria, such as *Bacillus cereus*, staphylococci, *Pseudomonas aeruginosa*, *Proteus* spp. and clostridia, can also cause yolk sac infection, either on their own or, more commonly, together with *E. coli*. *E. coli* multiplies rapidly in the intestines of newly hatched chicks and infection spreads rapidly from chick to chick in the hatchery and brooders. A hatching environment that is not sufficiently humid is often associated with a high incidence of yolk sac infection.

DISEASE

Clinical signs

Affected chicks appear depressed and have distended abdomens and a tendency to huddle. Sometimes the navel is visibly thickened, prominent and necrotic. Mortality in brooding surrounds can be considerable.

Lesions

Affected carcasses may show a distinctive, putrefying smell. Post-mortem examination reveals a septicaemic carcass with the subcutaneous and yolk sac blood vessels engorged and dilated. The lungs are usually congested and the liver and kidneys dark and swollen. The striking finding is an inflamed unabsorbed yolk sac with the yolk abnormal in colour and consistency. The yolk may be yellow and inspissated or brownish green and watery, and is often fetid. Peritonitis with haemorrhages in the serosal surfaces of the intestines is a regular feature.

DIAGNOSIS

A profuse pure growth of nonhaemolytic *E. coli* may be recovered from the abdominal viscera and particularly the yolk sac on direct culture.

CONTROL

Treatment is not recommended as, although antibiotic therapy may appear to reduce the mortality, the recovered chicks will be uneven and will not become a viable commercial proposition. Control is best achieved by providing the best possible brooding conditions and ensuring that only healthy chicks from well-managed breeding flocks and hatcheries are purchased. The most important aspects are good hatching egg hygiene on the breeder farm and effective cleansing and disinfection in the hatchery.

COLIGRANULOMA (HJÄRRE'S DISEASE)

This condition usually occurs as the cause of sporadic death in adult hens. The clinical signs are nonspecific and affected birds are usually found dead or die after depression and loss of condition. Post-mortem examination typically shows hard, yellow, nodular granulomas in the mesentery and wall of the intestine, and particularly the caecum. Sometimes the liver is similarly affected and is hard, blotchy, discoloured and swollen. There is no effective method of control or treatment but the condition almost always presents as a pathological curiosity rather than a flock problem. Poor environmental conditions in small flocks are a frequent trigger.

SWOLLEN HEAD SYNDROME

Swollen head syndrome is characterized by an oedematous swelling over the eye of broilers, broiler breeders and commercial layers. The lesions consist of gelatinous oedema involving the facial skin and periorbital tissues, and a caseous exudate in the conjunctival sac, facial subcutaneous tissues and lachrymal gland. *E. coli* can be isolated from the lesions, although disease appears to require previous coronavirus or APV infection. Other viruses have been suggested as predisposing to *E. coli* infection and causing the syndrome. Antibacterial medication has been reported to control the disease.

CELLULITIS

Cellulitis (sometimes called necrotic dermatitis) of the lower abdomen adjacent to the vent region or over the thighs of broilers, and occasionally ducks (where it is often referred to as 'cherry hip'), results in considerable economic loss through condemnation or downgrading of carcasses. A related condition known as skin necrosis or infectious process leads to subcutaneous lesions in the same areas. *E. coli*, which may belong to serogroups O1, O2 and O78, are usually the most consistently isolated bacteria but other bacteria are sometimes recovered as well. Superficial skin scratches, especially in birds whose immune system may be compromised (e.g. following early subclinical Gumboro disease challenge) may allow introduction of *E. coli* organisms, although they may arise via haematogenous spread. There is anecdotal evidence that sanitization of drinking water in the last 2 weeks of production can reduce incidence at processing.

OTHER CONDITIONS

E. coli has also been incriminated in a number of other clinical conditions, including synovitis, arthritis, tracheitis, air sacculitis, panophthalmitis and localized abscesses. The organism is undoubtedly a great opportunist, but probably rarely causes disease in the field unless there is a precipitating management fault or some other underlying pathogen.

There have been recent reports of scouring in turkeys associated with reduced activity and huddling resulting in mortality both in the USA and the UK. This is caused by a combined infection with turkey coronavirus or astrovirus and secondary infection with an entero-pathogenic strain of *E. coli*, which has the capacity to produce attaching-effacing lesions but does not elaborate Shiga toxin.

FURTHER READING

Barnes H J, Vaillancourt J-P, Gross W B 2003 Colibacillosis. In: Saif Y (ed) Diseases of poultry, 11th edn. IA Iowa State University Press, Ames, p 631–656

Culver F, Dziva, F, Cavanagh D, Stevens M P 2006 Poult enteritis and mortality syndrome in turkeys in Great Britain. Vet Rec 159: 209–210

Dho-Moulin M, Fairbrother J M 1999 Avian pathogenic *Escherichia coli* (APEC). Vet Res 30: 299–316

Gross W G 1994 Diseases due to *Escherichia coli* in poultry. In: Gyles C L (ed) *Escherichia coli* in domestic animals and humans. CABI, Wallingford, p 237–259

Guy J S, Smith L G, Breslin J J et al 2000 High mortality and growth depression experimentally produced in young turkeys by dual infection with enteropathogenic *Escherichia coli* and turkey coronavirus. Avian Dis 44: 105–113

Harry E G 1964 A study of 119 outbreaks of colisepticaemia in broiler flocks. Vet Rec 76: 443–449

Harry E G 1965 The association between the presence of septicaemia strains of *Escherichia coli* in the respiratory and intestinal tracts of chickens and the occurrence of colisepticaemia. Vet Rec 77: 35–40

Sojka W J, Carnaghan R B A 1961 *Escherichia coli* infections in poultry. Res Vet Sci 2: 340–352

Wray C, Woodward M J 1994 Laboratory diagnosis of *Escherichia coli* infections. In: Gyles C L (ed) *Escherichia coli* in domestic animals and humans. CABI, Wallingford, p 595–628

YERSINIA PSEUDOTUBERCULOSIS INFECTION (YERSINIOSIS, PSEUDOTUBERCULOSIS)

EPIDEMIOLOGY

Yersinia pseudotuberculosis has a worldwide distribution, affecting the various species of domestic poultry and a variety of wild and caged birds and rodents throughout the world. Clinical cases of pseudotuberculosis in commercial poultry are uncommon and usually result from faecal contamination of the birds' environment or feed. It has been reported in humans but is not an important zoonosis. Human infection often appears to be related to consumption of food contaminated from avian or rodent sources.

EPIDEMIOLOGY

Cause

The causal organism is a Gram-negative coccobacillus; there are variations in its virulence and its survival outside the body is similar to that of *Pasteurella multocida*.

Hosts

Amongst domestic poultry the turkey has historically been the most frequently affected and, although reports of extensive outbreaks are scanty, flock mortality of 80% has been recorded. Young birds of 4–10 weeks are most susceptible. More recently, cases have been detected in free-range layers.

Spread

Infection is probably spread by contamination of food by an infected host; it is suggested that the organism gains entry through the intestinal mucosa or occasionally through breaks in the skin. *Y. pseudotuberculosis* can be a normal gut inhabitant of a variety of migratory avian species and this may be relevant to the introduction of pseudotuberculosis into a region.

DISEASE

Clinical signs

Signs of pseudotuberculosis are not very specific. Birds usually show no premonitory signs and can just be found dead. Alternatively, and less commonly, more chronic cases may occur where the picture is often of persistent diarrhoea, weakness, ruffled feathers, lameness and progressive emaciation.

Lesions

The gross lesions in acute cases include enlargement of the liver and spleen, sometimes with a mottled or speckled appearance of affected organs. In the more chronic form there are multiple caseous tubercle-like lesions of varying size in the liver, the spleen and sometimes the lungs. Severe enteritis may be observed.

DIAGNOSIS

The clinical signs and gross lesions are helpful in diagnosis but evidence of infection depends upon isolation and identification of the organism from the blood in acute cases and from lesions in chronic cases. Histopathological confirmation on affected liver and spleen may be helpful. It may be readily differentiated from *P. multocida* and *S.* Pullorum, with which it shares a number of antigenic similarities, in that *Y. pseudotuberculosis* is nonmotile at 37°C but motile when grown in semisolid medium at 20°C. Fermentation of sugars is also different.

CONTROL

Treatment may be of benefit for at-risk birds within a flock in which disease has been diagnosed. Such treatment must be administered without delay and therefore preferably via the drinking water. Wherever possible this should be on the basis of pretreatment sensitivity testing. A number of antibiotics may be effective, especially the tetracycline group or sulfadiazine/trimethoprim, initially via drinking water but possibly with follow-up in feed medication where there is a risk of chronic infection. Prevention depends upon high standards of hygiene and management. Specific measures should include reducing direct contact with wild birds or rodents and avoiding contamination of feed and environment with faeces from such sources.

FURTHER READING

Rhoades K R, Rimler R B 1989 Fowl cholera. In: Adlam C, Rutter J M (eds) Pasteurella and pasteurellosis. Academic Press, London, p 95–113

Rimler R B, Sandhu T S, Glisson J R 1998 Pasteurellosis, infectious serositis, and pseudotuberculosis. In: Swayne D E, Glisson J R, Jackwood M W et al (eds) Isolation and identification of avian pathogens, 4th edn. American Association of Avian Pathologists, Kennett Square, p 17–25

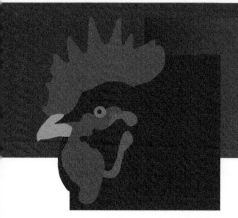

CHAPTER 9

Magne Bisgaard,
A. Miki Bojesen and
Jens P. Christensen

Infections caused by species of *Pasteurellaceae, Ornithobacterium* and *Riemerella*: an introduction

At present the family *Pasteurellaceae* contains 11 genera, which include *Pasteurella, Avibacterium* and *Gallibacterium*. There are 60 named species in the family and numerous taxa that are not yet named. In addition, the number of genomospecies representing genotypically distinct species but without sufficient phenotypic diversity to allow separation and naming, has increased. The genera *Ornithobacterium* and *Riemerella*, which are in the family *Flavobacteriaceae*, include only one and two species respectively.

Serious problems are associated with isolation and identification of these organisms because of difficulty in growing and characterizing them, which often results in weak or false-negative test results, just as the use of different media and indicators prevents comparison of results. In addition, commercial diagnostic kits may give rise to unreliable results. For the above reasons several examples of misidentification have been reported and therefore the use of reference strains and molecular methods is strongly recommended for identification. The key phenotypic characters used for differentiation of species are shown in Table 9.1.

The epidemiology of most species remains unclear. However, host specificity has been reported for several species, while others seem to be associated with a broad range of hosts. Surprisingly, recent observations with species obtained from several different host species seem to indicate the existence of host-related subclones.

Table 9.1 Important characters used to differentiate between taxa of *Pasteurellaceae* and other taxa causing differential diagnostic problems

	P. MULTOCIDA	AV. GALLINARUM	AV. AVIUM	AV. VOLANTIUM	AV. PARAGALLINARUM	G. ANATIS	O. RHINOTRACHEALE	R. ANATIPESTIFER
Symbiotic growth	−	−	+	+	d	−	−	−
Haemolysis	−	−	−	−	−	d**	−	−
Nitrate reduction	+	+	+	+	+	+	−	−
Urease	−	−	−	−	−	−	+	d
Arginine dihydrolase	−	−	−	−	−	−	−	(+)
Ornithine decarboxylase	+	−	−	d	−	−	−	−
Indole	+	−	−	+	−	+	−	−
D(−) Mannitol	+	−	−	+	+	+	−	−
D(−) Sorbitol	d*	−	−	d	+	d	−	−
D(+) Galactose	+	+	+	+	−	+	(+)	−
Maltose	−	+	+	+	d	d***	(+)	−
Trehalose	d*	+	+	+	−	d	−	−
Dextrin	−	+	+	+	−	+***	(+)	−
α-Galactosidase	−	−	−	−	−	−	+	+
α-Glucosidase (PNPG)	d*	+	+	+	−	+	+	+

+, 90% or more of the strains positive within 1–2 days; (+), 90% or more of the strains positive within 3–14 days; −, 90% or more of the strains negative; d, 11–89% of isolates investigated are positive for the character stated; *, character used for separation of subspecies of *P. multocida*; **, biovar *haemolytica* positive, biovar *anatis* negative; ***, biovar *haemolytica* mostly positive, biovar *anatis* negative.
PNPG, *p*-nitrophenyl-α-D-glucoside; AV., *Avibacterium*; G., *Gallibacterium*; O., *Ornithobacterium*; P., *Pasteurella*; R., *Riemerella*.

The genus *Pasteurella* has been reclassified and at present includes only four named species, of which only *Pasteurella multocida* is regarded as a major pathogen for birds.

A new genus, *Avibacterium*, has been proposed for species that are well known to veterinary bacteriologists as *[Haemophilus] paragallinarum*, *[Pasteurella] gallinarum*, *[Pasteurella] avium*, *[Pasteurella] volantium* and the unnamed *[Pasteurella]* sp. A. While all the species named are routinely encountered in investigation of upper respiratory tract disease of birds, only *Avibacterium paragallinarum* is regarded as a primary pathogen, being the causative agent of infectious coryza, an economically important disease of chickens.

A new genus, *Gallibacterium*, which incorporates organisms formerly known as avian *Pasteurella haemolytica*, *Actinobacillus salpingitidis* and *Pasteurella anatis* has recently been proposed and includes *Gallibacterium anatis* and two genomospecies.

Organisms isolated from fowl-cholera-like lesions in turkeys and misclassified as *P. multocida* were subsequently reclassified as *Ornithobacterium rhinotracheale*, thus underlining the difficulties associated with proper identification of these organisms.

As with species of Pasteurellaceae and *O. rhinotracheale*, organisms classified with *Riemerella* are difficult to grow and characterize because of their specific growth requirements and the absence of specific phenotypic characters. In addition, lesions are difficult to distinguish from those associated with *Escherichia coli*.

Although the above-mentioned groups of bacteria are phylogenetically different, the associated clinical signs and gross lesions may have common characteristics. For these reasons a safe and unambiguous diagnosis depends on phenotypic as well as genotypic characterization.

FURTHER READING

Bisgaard M, Christensen H, Bojesen A M, Christensen J P 2005 Avian infections caused by *Pasteurellaceae*, an update. In: 14th World Veterinary Poultry Congress, August 2005, Istanbul, Turkey. Final Program & Abstract Book, p 110–117

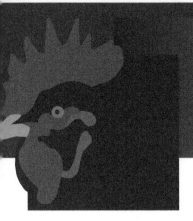

CHAPTER

10

Jens P. Christensen,
A. Miki Bojesen and
Magne Bisgaard

Fowl cholera

Pasteurella multocida is the causative agent of fowl cholera, a contagious disease affecting domesticated and wild birds. Fowl cholera occurs globally with a wide variety of manifestations ranging from peracute/acute systemic disease dominated by high mortality to relatively mild, chronic localized infections. The disease is considered to be of economic significance to most types of poultry and control of fowl cholera throughout the world depends mainly on appropriate biosecurity and vaccination. *Pasteurella multocida* subspecies *multocida* is the most common cause of disease, but the subspecies *septica* and *gallicida* can also cause fowl cholera-like disease. However, the importance of these subspecies needs to be investigated further.

EPIDEMIOLOGY

Cause

P. multocida is the causative agent of fowl cholera. The organism is a Gram-negative, nonmotile, non-spore-forming, rod-shaped bacterium. The species *P. multocida* includes the subspecies *multocida, septica* and *gallicida*. Information on the relationships between these subspecies and the serovars of *P. multocida* obtained by conventional serotyping systems has not been published. For many years a passive haemagglutination test was used for detection of capsule antigens, whereas tube agglutination and gel diffusion precipitin tests have been used to detect somatic antigens. A highly specific multiplex capsular polymerase chain reaction (PCR) assay has subsequently been developed and five capsular (A, B, D, E and F) and 16 somatic (1–16) serovars of *P. multocida* are currently recognized. All but serotypes 8 and 13 have been isolated from avian hosts, as have capsular types A, B, D and F. However, subspecies *multocida* and serovar A appear to be the most frequently isolated subspecies and serogroup from cases of severe fowl cholera. Several of the 16 somatic serovars have been demonstrated among serovar A isolates, just as somatic serotype variation has been shown to occur within serovars B, D and F. Isolates that have multiple somatic antigens are often encountered. Although the somatic antigen combination 1,3 and

3,4 within serovar A apparently dominate among strains isolated from fowl cholera in England and the USA, there is no particular serovar or antigen combination that appears to be more or less virulent than others. It has been demonstrated that different isolates of the common antigen combination A:3,4 vary greatly in virulence. Virulence properties of the different subspecies for different avian hosts are also unclear.

Hosts

All types of poultry are probably susceptible to infection with *P. multocida*. However, major differences in susceptibility to the infection have been documented. Among domestic poultry, turkeys are one of the most susceptible species, in addition to waterfowl. Chickens are considered to be relatively resistant to infection, although mortality may be high during outbreaks caused by some isolates under certain exaggerated conditions (accumulated mortalities up to 60% in organic layers have been observed in Denmark). Partridges and pheasants are also highly susceptible. Age markedly influences the outcome of the infection in chickens; in particular, birds less than 16 weeks of age appear fairly resistant. In turkeys this effect is not as pronounced, since 100% mortality may be observed following experimental infection of 3-week-old poults.

Spread

Newer molecular typing methods such as restriction endonuclease analysis (REA), ribotyping, pulsed field gel electrophoresis (PFGE), PCR typing and amplified fragment length polymorphism (AFLP) have in recent years added significantly to our understanding of the epidemiology of fowl cholera. These methods have been essential in this context as serotyping in many cases does not provide sufficiently detailed information because of genotypic variation within serotypes. However, basic information concerning, for example, the introduction of *P. multocida* to a flock or farm is still scarce.

It has been documented that wild birds carrying isolates of *P. multocida* may represent a source of infection for domestic poultry. In addition, it is generally accepted that carriers occur in flocks of domestic poultry previously affected by fowl cholera. Cloacal carriers may also be present in flocks of chickens and ducks with no previously recognized history of *P. multocida* infection. The significance of this finding for the epidemiology is unclear, as excretions from the mouth, nose and conjunctiva of diseased birds are generally believed to be the primary source of contamination of the environment. Rodents may also carry *P. multocida* but the role of these as a reservoir for isolates virulent for poultry has not been thoroughly investigated, although it has been suggested that dogs, cats and pigs may act as reservoirs for strains of *P. multocida* that are virulent for poultry. However, recent investigations seem to indicate that respiratory tract infections in different animal species are caused by different genetic subtypes of *P. multocida*.

Other potential sources of infection include cannibalism of sick or dead birds, and *P. multocida* is sufficiently resistant to spread via contaminated crates, feed bags, shoes, equipment and mechanically by insects. It has also been shown that *P. multocida* may survive in free-living amoeba in the environment. The infection does not seem to be egg-transmitted.

Although the reservoir of *P. multocida* appears complex and several sources may theoretically be responsible for introducing the infection to a flock of poultry, the most recent studies indicate that, in layer chickens at least, most fowl cholera outbreaks are caused by only one genetic subtype (clone). This suggests that only a few introductions actually take place during the production period or that once a certain clone has colonized the flock it is difficult for others to manifest themselves in the same flock. Outbreaks of *P. multocida* infection associated with a single clone have also been reported in wild birds involving different geographical regions.

Influencing factors

Many factors have been reported to influence the severity and incidence of fowl cholera including environmental factors such as crowding and climate in addition to concurrent infections and general stress.

DISEASE

Pathogenesis

The main site of infection for *P. multocida* is the respiratory tract. However, isolation of *P. multocida* from cases of salpingitis and peritonitis indicate that other mucosal membranes may serve as ports of entry. Furthermore, the organism may enter the host through cutaneous wounds. The ability of *P. multocida* to survive passage through the gastrointestinal tract remains to be investigated in more detail but, as *P. multocida* has been isolated from the cloacae of carrier birds, some strains may survive passage or may be taken up via cloacal pinocytosis. In addition, the observation that some strains of *P. multocida* can be virulent and immunogenic following oral administration (e.g. vaccine strains) suggests that intestinal invasion or some sort of interaction with the intestinal mucosa may occur. Following colonization of the upper respiratory tract pathogenic *P. multocida* strains may subsequently spread to the lungs, followed by invasion, bacteraemia and septicaemia. It has been suggested that some of the differences in host susceptibility to *P. multocida* infection may be due to differences in the host response expressed in the lung during the early phase of infection.

Clinical signs

With peracute/acute fowl cholera sudden, unexpected deaths of a large number of birds in a flock are often observed without any signs (web-footed birds in particular). Mortality often increases rapidly. In more protracted cases anorexia, ruffled feathers, mucous discharge from the mouth and nose, diarrhoea, cyanosis and general depression may be seen.

In chronic infections, signs are mainly due to localized infections of joints, abscesses of the head (cranial bones, infraorbital sinuses, subcutaneous tissue, comb and wattles), oviduct and the respiratory tract (dyspnoea and rales). Torticollis may be associated with infections of the cranial bones, middle ear and meninges. Dermal necrosis in turkeys may also be observed. The chronic infection may follow an acute infection or be caused by infection with an organism of low virulence.

Lesions

Lesions observed in peracute and acute forms of the disease are dominated by general septicaemic lesions, including vascular disturbances in the form of congestion throughout the carcass accompanied by enlargement of the liver and spleen. Often there are petechial and ecchymotic haemorrhages at sites such as the subepicardial fat of the heart, in mucous membranes, on the gizzard and in abdominal fat. In addition, acute oophoritis with hyperaemic follicles may be seen. Acute lesions develop as a result of disseminated intravascular coagulation. In subacute cases, pinpoint necrotic areas may be disseminated throughout the liver and spleen.

In chronic forms of fowl cholera suppurative lesions may be widely distributed, often involving the respiratory tract (in the form of pneumonia), the conjunctiva and adjacent tissues of the head. Caseous arthritis and productive inflammation of the peritoneal cavity and the oviduct are common in chronic infections. Lung lesions are commonly associated with fowl cholera and vary in nature from haemorrhages in peracute cases to fibrinonecrotic pneumonia and fibrinopurulent pleuritis in more protracted cases. Sequestered necrotic lung lesions in poultry should always arouse suspicion of cholera, as few microorganisms are capable of inducing such pathology.

A fibrinonecrotic dermatitis including caudal parts of dorsum, the abdomen and breast, involving cutis, subcutis and the underlying muscle, has been observed in turkeys and broilers.

DIAGNOSIS

Although the history, signs and lesions may be helpful in diagnosis, *P. multocida* should be isolated, characterized and identified for confirmation. As stated in the epidemiology section, subsequent molecular characterization is needed for epidemiological studies. Primary isolation can be accomplished using enriched media such as blood agar. *P. multocida* can be readily isolated from the viscera of birds dying from peracute/acute fowl cholera whereas isolation from suppurative lesions of chronic cholera may be more difficult. At necropsy, bipolar microorganisms may be demonstrated by the use of Wright's or Giemsa stain of impression smears obtained from the liver in the case of acute cholera. In addition, in situ hybridization may be used to identify *P. multocida* in infected tissues and exudates.

Recently a PCR has been developed and used for the detection of *P. multocida* in pure and mixed cultures and clinical samples. Such methods may be helpful for establishing knowledge concerning carrier animals within flocks and may also overcome the complexities associated with the diagnosis of fowl cholera by conventional methods of isolation, identification and capsular serotyping. However, the specificity and sensitivity of these tests remain to be investigated in more detail.

The carrier status of a population of animals may also be investigated by the use of mouse inoculation. Selective media (including an enrichment step) have also been used as an alternative to mouse inoculation but the method appears to be less sensitive.

Following isolation, classical identification is based on the results of biochemical tests. However, simple diagnostic keys do not allow a firm diagnosis within the family *Pasteurellaceae*. For this reason, extended characterization, including the use of reference strains, is recommended. Further delineation of *P. multocida* into subspecies presently seems of limited value considering the amount of work and expertise needed for this approach. Serotyping is important in order to evaluate the relevance of the vaccine strains used in a certain area, but serotyping is mainly reserved for specialized laboratories.

Detection of antibodies can be achieved by agar diffusion tests and ELISA. Although serology may be used to evaluate vaccine responses it has very limited value for diagnostic purposes.

It should be emphasized that several bacterial infections may be confused with fowl cholera based solely on the gross lesions. Thus *Escherichia coli*, *Salmonella enterica*, *Ornithobacterium rhinotracheale*, Gram-positive cocci and *Erysipelothrix rhusiopathiae* (erysipelas) may all produce lesions that are difficult to distinguish from those caused by *P. multocida*.

CONTROL

A number of drugs will lower the mortality from fowl cholera but mortality may resume when treatment is discontinued, showing that treatment will not eliminate *P. multocida* from a flock. The drugs used to control cholera via food or water application include various sulpha drugs, semisynthetic penicillins, tetracyclines and erythromycin. In ducks it has been reported that a good effect may be achieved by the combined use of streptomycin and dihydrostreptomycin given by injection. More recently, the fluoroquinolone norfloxacin has been shown to be effective against fowl cholera in chickens and turkeys when administered via drinking water; it lowered mortality significantly during experimental infections without recognized side effects. Whenever medication is considered, sensitivity testing of the causative agent should be performed and it should be remembered that resistance to treatment may develop and cause serious future problems.

The use of vaccination during an outbreak may also improve the situation. However, in order to eradicate infection from premises the only rational approach is depopulation, cleaning and disinfection of buildings and equipment. Subsequently, the premises should be kept free of poultry for a few weeks.

In order to avoid infection of a flock, the focus should be on the application of appropriate biosecurity measures. Contact with the avifauna, rodents and pet animals should be avoided as they have all been shown to represent a potential risk of introducing *P. multocida* to the flock. In addition, proper handling of carcasses should be employed, as asymptomatic carriers may be present in flocks. Only young birds should be introduced as new stock and the birds should originate from flocks with a high level of biosecurity and preferably those that follow all-in/all-out principles in a confined environment.

Extensive production systems in many parts of the world may have problems in achieving an appropriate level of hygiene and biosecurity, in which case vaccination against fowl cholera should be considered. This includes free-range poultry production in the industrialized world, a production system that has become increasingly popular because of animal welfare concerns. Vaccines used against fowl cholera include inactivated bacterins and live attenuated vaccines. Bacterins are widely used but must be injected and only induce immunity to homologous serotypes. Autogenous vaccines of inactivated organisms may be helpful under certain circumstances. In contrast, live vaccines have been reported to confer immunity against heterologous serotypes but may revert to virulence as all the live vaccines currently in use are undefined attenuated strains. The principal live strains currently used, primarily in North America, are the Clemson University strain, which is a naturally occurring organism of low virulence, and its derivative the M-9 strain, both of which are of serotype A:3, 4. Both strains have been implicated in outbreaks of fowl cholera and, as a consequence, attempts have been made to further modify them. Live vaccines are normally given as wing web inoculations to chickens and via drinking water to turkeys.

LEGAL REQUIREMENTS/ZOONOTIC ASPECTS

The disease is notifiable in many countries because of its often virulent and highly contagious nature.

Disease in humans caused by *P. multocida* is not uncommon, and *P. multocida* may be considered a zoonotic organism. This is substantiated by the observation that the disease occurs mainly among farmers. However, there are no reports of direct transmission from poultry to humans or vice versa but the possibility for such infections cannot be excluded.

FURTHER READING

Blackall P J, Mifflin J K 2000 Identification and typing of *Pasteurella multocida*: a review. Avian Pathol 29: 271–287

Bojesen A M, Petersen K D, Nielsen O L et al 2004 *Pasteurella multocida* infection in heterophil-depleted chickens. Avian Dis 48: 463–470

Christensen, J, Bisgaard M 1998 Phenotypic and genotypic characters of isolates of *Pasteurella multocida* obtained from back-yard poultry and two outbreaks of avian cholera in the avifauna in Denmark. Avian Pathol 27: 373–381

Glisson J R, Hofacre C L, Christensen J P 2003 Fowl cholera. In: Saif Y M (ed) Diseases of poultry, 11th edn. Iowa State University Press, Ames, p 658–676

Petersen K D, Christensen J P, Permin A, Bisgaard M 2001 Virulence of *Pasteurella multocida* subsp. *multocida* isolated from outbreaks of fowl cholera in wild birds for domestic poultry and game birds. Avian Pathol 30: 27–31

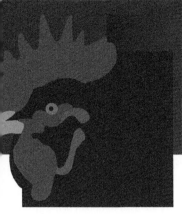

Par J. Blackall and
Karl-Heinz Hinz

CHAPTER 11

Infectious coryza and related diseases

Infectious coryza (also known as fowl coryza) is a disease caused by the bacterium *Avibacterium paragallinarum* (once known as *Haemophilus paragallinarum*). The genus *Avibacterium* also contains the species *Avibacterium gallinarum* (once known as *Pasteurella gallinarum*). There are reports of both acute and chronic disease conditions (fowl-cholera-like in nature) in chickens and turkeys that have been associated with *Av. gallinarum*.

AVIBACTERIUM PARAGALLINARUM INFECTION – INFECTIOUS CORYZA

Infectious coryza is highly contagious and presents typically as an acute disease of the upper respiratory tract of chickens. A chronic respiratory disease can develop when complicated by other pathogens. The disease occurs worldwide and causes economic losses due to an increased culling rate in meat chickens and significant reduction of egg production in laying and breeding fowl. The disease is limited to chickens and has no public health significance.

EPIDEMIOLOGY

Cause

There has been considerable confusion over the name that should be applied to the bacterium that causes infectious coryza. In the years from the 1930s to the 1960s, the agent was known as *Haemophilus gallinarum*, an organism that required both X (haemin) and V (nicotinamide adenine dinucleotide; NAD) factors for growth in vitro. From the 1960s to the 1980s, all isolates of the disease-producing agent were found to require only V factor and were termed *Haemophilus para-gallinarum*. V-factor-independent *H. paragallinarum* isolates have now been reported in both the Republic of South Africa and Mexico. An extensive taxonomic study has concluded that the species *H. paragallinarum* is not a member of the genus *Haemophilus* and is best assigned to a new genus, *Avibacterium*, along with several other chicken-associated members of the bacterial family *Pasteurellaceae*. These other members are *Av. gallinarum, Av. avium* and *Av. volantium* (all previously in the genus *Pasteurella*). Hence, the causal agent of infectious coryza is now called *Avibacterium paragallinarum,* an organism that can be either V-factor-dependent or V-factor-independent.

Av. paragallinarum is a Gram-negative, nonmotile, non-spore-forming and capsulated rod-shaped bacterium ($0.3–0.6 \times 1–3\,\mu m$) with a tendency to morphological degeneration after an incubation period of more than 24 h.

Complex media, microaerophilic conditions and high humidity are used to obtain dense growth on solid media. Chicken serum (1%) is required for the growth of some strains. Most strains require the presence of added V factor for growth in artificial media. *Av. paragallinarum* is organotrophic, mesophilic and facultatively anaerobic with pronounced microaerophilia. The main distinguishing properties of the bacterium are an ability to reduce nitrate to nitrite and to ferment D-glucose without formation of gas, the presence of phosphatase and phosphoamidase, and the inability to grow on MacConkey's agar. The organism does not produce indole, α-glucosidase, β-galactosidase, β-glucosaminidase, α-fucosidase, ornithine decarboxylase or arginine dihydrolase and does not hydrolyse urea, gelatin or aesculin. Acid is always produced from D-fructose and D-mannose, and in more than 90% of the strains also from mannitol, maltose and saccharose, whereas the reactions in D-sorbitol, D-xylose and dextrin are variable. Acid is not produced from arabinose, D-lactose, D-galactose, trehalose, L-sorbose, salicin, dulcitol, adonitol and mesoinositol.

Two different serotyping schemes, the Page and the Kume schemes, have been mainly used. The current nomenclature of the Kume scheme emphasizes the close immunological linkage between the well-established Page serovars A, B and C and the Kume serogroups A, B and C. Essentially, the Kume scheme recognizes subdivisions within Page serovars A and C. Thus, the nine currently recognized Kume serovars are termed A-1, A-2, A-3, A-4, B-1, C-1, C-2, C-3 and C-4.

Variation from very low to high virulence occurs. Little is known about virulence factors, although there is evidence that the presence of the capsule and specific haemagglutination antigens are necessary for the pathogenicity of *Av. paragallinarum*. The organism is a delicate bacterium, which dies quickly outside the host tissues. Survival outside the body under farm conditions is probably no more than 48 h at 18–24°C. Many drugs are known to have a more bacteriostatic than bactericidal effect on the organism.

Host

The disease is limited to chickens. There are reports of the organism being cultured from pheasants, Japanese quails and guinea fowls but these reports are not supported by detailed phenotypic or genotypic studies and should be regarded with caution. Chickens of all ages are susceptible but older birds tend to react more severely. While most literature reports on the disease in intensive production systems, there are also reports of the disease in village-type production systems.

Spread

The main source of infection is clinically affected and carrier birds, especially from replacement stock. As only a few viable organisms are necessary for the infection, it can be transmitted by drinking water contaminated by nasal discharge as well as by airborne means over a short distance.

Lateral transmission occurs readily by direct contact. Spread between batteries with nipple drinkers occurs more slowly.

Influencing factors

Factors that predispose to more severe and prolonged disease (chronic respiratory disease) include intercurrent infections with microorganisms such as infectious bronchitis virus, laryngotracheitis virus, *Mycoplasma gallisepticum*, *Escherichia coli* or *Pasteurella* spp. and unfavourable environmental conditions. The involvement of these additional pathogens may explain why *Av. paragallinarum* has been isolated from sites such as the hock in chickens in Argentina. As noted above, the age of the birds involved in an outbreak can be an important factor.

DISEASE

Pathogenesis

Adherence of the organism to the ciliated mucosa of the upper respiratory tract seems to be the first step of the infection. The capsule and the haemagglutination antigen play an important role in the colonization. Toxic substances released from the organism during proliferation are associated with production of lesions in the mucosa and appearance of the clinical signs. The capsule may act as a natural defence substance against the bactericidal power of complement through the alternative pathway.

Av. paragallinarum is a noninvasive bacterial agent with a strong tropism for ciliated cells and migrates into the lower respiratory tract (lungs, air sac) only after synergistic interaction with other infectious agents and/or if encouraged by immunosuppression.

Clinical signs

The disease in flocks on floor management is characterized by rapid spread, high morbidity and low mortality. The period of incubation is 1–3 days after contact infection and all susceptible birds in the flock will show signs within 7–10 days. If not complicated by other infections, the course of the disease is not more than about 10 days in the mild form and approximately 3 weeks in the more severe form. The first typical signs include seromucoid nasal and ocular discharge and facial oedema. In severe cases marked conjunctivitis with closed eyes, swollen wattles (wattle disease) and difficulty in breathing can been seen. Feed and water consumption is usually decreased resulting in a drop in egg production (10–40%) or an increase in the rate of culls. The disease can have a much greater impact than the relatively simple scenario described above. As an example, a recent outbreak of the disease in older layer birds in California, which was not associated with any other pathogen, caused a total mortality of 48% and a drop in egg production from 75% to 15.7% over a 3-week period.

If complicated with other infectious agents a more severe and prolonged disease may develop, with the clinical picture of a chronic respiratory disease. Swollen-head-like syndrome associated with *Av. paragallinarum* has been reported in the absence of *Avian pneumovirus* but in the presence of other pathogens such as virulent *E. coli*.

Lesions

Affected chickens have catarrhal to fibrinopurulent inflammation of the nasal passages and infraorbital sinus and conjunctivae. Subcutaneous oedema of the face and wattles is prominent.

The upper trachea may be involved but the lungs and air sacs are only affected in chronic complicated cases.

Histopathologically, marked loss of cilia and microvilli, cell oedema, degeneration and desquamation of mucosal and glandular epithelium, infiltration of leukocytes and deposition of mucopurulent substances can be seen and are followed by infiltration of mast cells into the lamina propria of the mucous membrane.

DIAGNOSIS

The history of a rapidly spreading disease and its clinical signs and lesions may allow a tentative diagnosis, which has to be confirmed by cultural isolation and identification of the causal agent. Culture should be attempted by swabbing from the infraorbital sinus of two to three acutely diseased chickens on to blood agar plates cross-streaked with a feeder organism such as *Staphylococcus epidermidis*. Fresh nasal exudate, expressed by pressing on the sinus, can also be sampled provided that care is taken in the sampling. The sampling is best done with a small sterile loop that just touches the surface of the fresh exudate and is then directly inoculated on to a blood agar plate and cross-streaked as described above. Swabs from the trachea and air sac may be taken, although *Av. paragallinarum* is less frequently isolated from these areas. After incubation for 24–48 h at 37°C in a candle jar or in an atmosphere of 5% CO_2, tiny translucent colonies of 0.3–1 mm in diameter appear on the culture plates adjacent to the feeder culture. The isolated organism can be identified by phenotypic tests (see Table 9.1) or by confirmatory polymerase chain reaction (PCR). The PCR can also be applied directly to nasal exudate. Another efficient diagnostic procedure is to inoculate exudate or culture suspensions into the sinuses of two or three susceptible chickens. If the organism is present in the inoculum clinical signs appear in 1–3 days.

A number of serological tests are used for the examination of sera for specific antibodies against *Av. paragallinarum*, including especially agglutination, haemagglutination inhibition and fluorescent antibody tests as well as a monoclonal antibody-based blocking enzyme-linked immunosorbent assay (ELISA).

CONTROL

Improved management measures such as depopulation, good sanitation, good biosecurity and avoidance of multiage farms may help to break the disease cycle. To eliminate the agent from a farm it is necessary to depopulate the infected or recovered flock because such birds remain a reservoir of the bacterial agent. After cleaning, disinfection and resting of the building for at least 1 week, new birds may be introduced. Only chickens that are known to be free from *Av. paragallinarum* should be used for the restocking. This may be impracticable on multiage farms.

Because of the difficulty of control by biosecurity and management, drug therapy and/or vaccination are used. Various sulphonamides and antibiotics are useful in alleviating the worst effects of the disease. After 5–7 days of treatment, the clinical signs very often disappear completely but relapse may occur after the treatment is discontinued. The reason for this is not the inefficiency of the drug itself but rather the fact that it is not capable of eliminating the agent in all birds of a large population as well as from the environment. The clinical signs do not disappear completely until a specific immunity has developed in most of the affected birds of the flock. Recovery of egg production takes longer than the recovery from clinical signs.

Vaccination using inactivated whole cells containing an adjuvant can protect chickens against the disease. Such a vaccine provides serogroup-specific immunity but no protection across serogroups; i.e. a vaccine containing Page serovar A (Kume serogroup A) will not protect against Page serovar C (Kume serogroup C). There is evidence that cross-protection within Page serovars B and C (equivalent to Kume serogroups B and C) may be limited, possibly requiring the use of more than one strain in the vaccine for these serogroups. If a commercial bacterin is unable to induce a protective immunity, an autogenous bacterin should be used. Appropriate vaccination is economically worthwhile, since it usually protects against the more severe falls in egg production. Two doses of vaccine, each of which must consist of at least 10^8 colony-forming units, are advocated, given subcutaneously 3–6 weeks apart. The timing of the vaccination doses is normally such that the first is given at about 12–16 weeks of age. The typical local epidemiology should be considered when creating a vaccination programme for a particular farm or operation. Controlled exposure is still practised in some endemic areas following vaccination with a bacterin.

AVIBACTERIUM GALLINARUM INFECTION

The traditional view is that *Av. gallinarum* is an opportunistic pathogen of chickens. Disease outbreaks are often thought to be associated with other viral and mycoplasmal agents. However, a close reading of the literature does indicate that this bacterium can play a significant role in infection. To date, infections associated with *Av. gallinarum* have been reported in chickens, turkeys and guinea fowl. However, only chicken and turkey isolates have been confirmed as *Av. gallinarum* by both phenotypic and genotypic methods. The lesions reported for the infections associated with *Av. gallinarum* are as diverse as those reported for *Pasteurella multocida* and include conjunctivitis, abscesses in the head and wattles, sinusitis, tracheitis, air sacculitis, hepatitis, endocarditis, salpingitis, oophoritis, peritonitis and synovitis. Severe mortality in a combined infection with *Mycoplasma synoviae* in broiler chickens has been reported. Careful evaluation of the potential role of *Av. gallinarum* is required and the organism should certainly not be dismissed as simply nonpathogenic. The identification of *Av. gallinarum* can be achieved using the tests shown in Table 9.1. A common characteristic of *Av. gallinarum* is improved growth in the presence of 5% carbon dioxide.

FURTHER READING

Bisgaard M, Christensen H, Behr K-P et al 2005 Investigations on the clonality of strains of *Pasteurella gallinarum* isolated from turkeys in Germany. Avian Pathol 34: 106–110

Blackall P J 1995 Vaccines against infectious coryza. World's Poult Sci J 51: 17–26

Blackall P J, Christensen H, Beckenham T et al 2005 Reclassification of *Pasteurella gallinarum*, [Haemophilus] paragallinarum, Pasteurella avium and Pasteurella volantium as *Avibacterium gallinarum* gen. nov., comb. nov., *Avibacterium paragallinarum* comb. nov., *Avibacterium avium* comb. nov. and *Avibacterium volantium* comb. nov. Int J Syst Evol Microbiol 55: 353–362

Chen X, Chen Q, Zhang P et al 1998 Evaluation of a PCR test for the detection of *Haemophilus paragallinarum* in China. Avian Pathol 27: 296–300

Shivaprasad H L, Droual R 2002 Pathology of an atypical strain of *Pasteurella gallinarum* infection in chickens. Avian Pathol 31: 399–406

Soriano V E, Longinos G M, Téllez G et al 2004 Cross-protection study of the nine serovars of *Haemophilus paragallinarum* in the Kume haemagglutinin scheme. Avian Pathol 33: 506–511

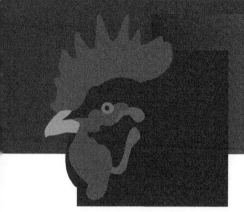

CHAPTER 12

A. Miki Bojesen,
Jens P. Christensen and
Magne Bisgaard

Gallibacterium infections and other avian *Pasteurellaceae*

Gallibacterium anatis is a common organism of the upper respiratory and lower genital tract of poultry. The bacterium has been reported worldwide from a broad host range among farmed and wild birds. The bacterium has no public health significance. It is potentially pathogenic for poultry and is mainly associated with lesions in the reproductive tract, including the ovary. Disease associated this microorganism is related to lowered egg production and occasionally an increase in mortality.

EPIDEMIOLOGY

Cause

Gallibacterium was previously reported as avian *Pasteurella haemolytica, Actinobacillus salpingitidis* or *Pasteurella anatis* but was recently established as an independent genus within the family *Pasteurellaceae* Pohl 1981. The genus contains one named species, *G. anatis*, and two genomo-species, 1 and 2. As the name implies, a genomospecies is a species defined by genotypic methods only. *G. anatis* contains two phenotypically distinct biovars, one which is haemolytic, biovar *haemolytica*, and one which is non-haemolytic, biovar *anatis*.

Isolates of *G. anatis* biovar *anatis* have been associated with lesions in the respiratory tract of ducks and geese but have not resulted in losses of economic importance and will not be discussed further.

Gallibacterium anatis is a Gram-negative, non-motile bacterium, which forms rod-shaped or pleomorphic cells occurring singly and in pairs. *G. anatis* forms greyish, smooth semitransparent colonies, butyrous in consistency, shiny and circular, slightly raised with an entire margin and a size of 1–2 mm in diameter after 24 h incubation at 37°C. In addition, haemolytic strains produce a wide β-haemolytic zone (1–2 mm). Twenty-four biovars based on differences in fermentation patterns of (+)-L-arabinose, (+)-D-xylose, *m*-inositol, (−)-D-sorbitol, maltose, trehalose and dextrin have been reported. Recent work has shown that V-factor-requiring strains exist within several species of the family *Pasteurellaceae*. However, although some isolates of biovar *haemolytica* are difficult to culture V-factor requirement has not yet been demonstrated for *G. anatis*.

Hosts and spread

G. anatis has been reported from many countries in Europe, Africa and Asia, and in Australia and American states, underlining its widespread occurrence. Although chickens have been suggested as the main host for haemolytic isolates *Gallibacterium* organisms do seem to have a wide host spectrum that also includes turkeys, geese, ducks, pheasants, partridges and various cage bird species in addition to wild birds.

The occurrence of haemolytic strains of *G. anatis* in commercial flocks has been investigated recently and it has been shown that these organisms are very common inhabitants of the upper respiratory and lower genital tract of healthy chickens. Furthermore the occurrence of *G. anatis* appeared to be highly influenced by farm biosecurity level such that only flocks kept under very high levels of biosecurity were likely to be free of *G. anatis*. In addition, once the microorganisms were present in a flock, nearly all individuals in the flock were infected.

Bird-to-bird transmission is considered to be the main mode of infection. Evidence for vertical transmission has not been shown so far.

DISEASE

Clinical signs and lesions

There is accumulated evidence of haemolytic isolates of *G. anatis* being able to act as a primary disease-causing agent. However, other factors possibly contribute to the clinical and pathological manifestations. The clinical signs are unspecific but will usually include depression, diarrhoea and pasting around the vent and reduced egg production around peak of lay. The lesions typically involve the reproductive tract and the ovary, exhibiting purulent salpingitis and oophoritis. Chronic cases tend to include local or generalized purulent peritonitis, often with simultaneous growth of *Escherichia coli*. Sudden mortality associated with acute septicaemia has occasionally been recorded from table-egg-producing flocks in good body condition from which *G. anatis* has been isolated in pure culture from various organs.

Clinical signs and pathological lesions have been reproduced experimentally in specific-pathogen-free birds as well as in conventional layers. The outcome of such infections varies and seems to depend strongly on the strain, the route of inoculation and secondary factors, including immune suppression. In addition, at onset, peak and late in the production period chickens appear more susceptible to infection. *G. anatis* seems to have different virulence factors influencing its pathogenicity. Recently, whole genome sequencing has revealed possession of a capsule locus, and the haemolytic phenotype appears to be encoded by a RTX-like toxin also known in other members of the family *Pasteurellaceae*. The direct role of these putative virulence factors in the pathogenesis remains to be demonstrated.

DIAGNOSIS

Signs and lesions cannot be used to distinguish infection by *G. anatis* from other bacterial infections affecting the salpinx, ovary and abdominal cavity. Furthermore, the fact that most birds carry haemolytic *G. anatis* as a part of their resident flora in the upper respiratory and lower genital tract makes careful identification and characterization crucial. The diagnosis should be confirmed by isolation and identification of the causal agent. This should be attempted by culture from the affected organs and, in the case of systemic disease, the liver and spleen. *G. anatis* grows readily on enriched media and in the case of the β-haemolytic biovar with a characteristic haemolysis zone following 24 h of incubation. Identification based on morphology and biochemical tests will give a good indication but this should be combined with one or more genotypic procedures. Recent work has demonstrated that a specific polymerase chain reaction (PCR) test, based on the internal transcribed spacer (ITS) separating the 16S and 23S rRNA genes, can be used as a confirmatory test following cultural isolation of *G. anatis* or directly on material from the affected bird. Another culture independent technique, fluorescence in situ hybridization (FISH) using a *Gallibacterium*-specific probe, similarly allows specific detection of the bacteria. Tools to determine genetic diversity have also been developed and include amplified fragment length polymorphism and pulsed field gel electrophoresis.

Currently, two serological tests based on latex agglutination and enzyme-linked immunosorbent assay (ELISA) are being developed and used for the examination of sera for specific antibodies against *G. anatis*. The number and prevalence of serotypes within *G. anatis* remains to be investigated in detail, in addition to cross-reactivity and cross-protection of serotypes.

CONTROL

The success of treating *Gallibacterium* infections with antibiotics depends highly on the practices used in the individual flocks. The level of acquired resistance in *G. anatis* seems limited under conditions of limited exposure to antibiotics, enabling the use of narrow-spectrum antibiotics, however, it is also evident that *G. anatis* readily acquires resistance. This has been demonstrated in a number of strains recovered from outbreaks in Mexican poultry flocks where the majority of the isolates were multiresistant to a broad range of antibiotics including penicillins, trimethoprim–sulfamethoxazole and fluoroquinolones. The antimicrobial sensitivity pattern should therefore always be established in relation to treatment.

Currently a commercial vaccine is available based on three of the more prevalent biovars, however, protection under field conditions remains to be investigated in further detail.

INFECTIONS CAUSED BY BACTERIA CLASSIFIED WITH THE TAXON 2 AND 3 COMPLEX OF *PASTEURELLACEAE*

Organisms classified with this complex represent a new genus-like structure containing several new species, most of which seem to be associated with specific hosts. In commercial poultry production these organisms are mainly associated with increased mortality due to salpingitis, oophoritis and peritonitis in ducks and geese. Although healthy carriers have been demonstrated, investigations of disease outbreaks have not allowed demonstration of other infectious agents or management faults.

Because the symptoms and lesions are similar to those associated with infections caused by *E. coli* and *P. multocida* in adult webfooted birds an unambiguous diagnosis depends on isolation and detailed characterization of the organisms, including the use of genotypic methods.

Principles used for treatment and prophylaxis of other species of *Pasteurellaceae* are also valid for infections caused by the taxon 2 and 3 complex.

FURTHER READING

Bisgaard M 1993 Ecology and significance of *Pasteurellaceae* in animals. Zentralbl Bakteriol 279: 7–26

Bojesen A M, Christensen H, Lerberg Nielsen O et al 2003 Detection of *Gallibacterium* spp. in chickens by fluorescent 16S rRNA *in situ* hybridization. J Clin Microbiol 41: 5167–5172

Bojesen A M, Torpdahl M, Christensen H et al 2003 Genetic diversity of *Gallibacterium anatis* in chicken flocks representing different production systems. J Clin Microbiol 41: 2737–2740

Bojesen A M, Saxmose Nielsen S, Bisgaard M 2003 Prevalence and transmission of haemolytic *Gallibacterium* species in chicken production systems with different biosecurity levels. Avian Pathol 32: 503–510

Bojesen A M, Nielsen, O L, Christensen J P, Bisgaard M 2004 *In vivo* studies of *Gallibacterium anatis* infections in chickens. Avian Pathol 33: 145–152

Bojesen A M, Christensen H, Nielsen S S, Bisgaard M 2007 Host specific bacterial lineages of the taxon 2 and 3 complex of *Pasteurellaceae*. Syst Appl Microbiol 30: 119–127

Christensen H, Bisgaard M, Bojesen A M et al 2003 Genetic relationships among strains of biovars of avian isolates classified as '*Pasteurella haemolytica*', '*Actinobacillus salpingitidis*' or *Pasteurella anatis* with proposal of *Gallibacterium anatis* gen. nov., sp. nov. Int J Syst Evol Microbiol 53: 275–287

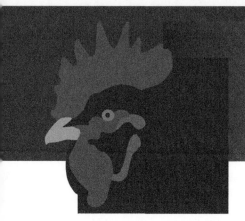

Paul van Empel

Ornithobacterium rhinotracheale

Ornithobacterium rhinotracheale is a relatively new bacterium associated with poultry diseases worldwide. The characteristic features of *O. rhinotracheale* infection include relatively mild respiratory signs in young broiler birds, which start with sneezing, a slightly increased mortality and poor performance. Lesions include air sacculitis and some pneumonia, which can lead to high condemnation (up to 50%) at slaughter. The infection can also cause sudden death in young birds, in the absence of respiratory signs, due to infection of the brain and skull. In older birds, for example turkeys of 12 weeks or more, *O. rhinotracheale* can cause acute pneumonia with high mortality, while another form of disease in older turkeys and chickens can cause lameness. Infection of layer and breeder birds can affect egg production and egg quality. The presence of *O. rhinotracheale* in commercial poultry and in wild birds has been shown to be worldwide, providing a broad potential reservoir. Maternally derived antibodies against *O. rhinotracheale* can be detected in eggs and day-old birds all over the world. Several surveys have shown that the majority of chicken and turkey flocks in Europe, Africa, North and South America and some Asian countries have been in contact with *O. rhinotracheale*. Up to now, *O. rhinotracheale* has not been found to be of public health significance.

EPIDEMIOLOGY

Investigation of the epidemiology of *O. rhinotracheale* is hampered by the difficulties in culturing from infected organs, the transience of the serological responses after infection and the complexity of the infections in which *O. rhinotracheale* can be involved. Moreover, most of the infections caused by *O. rhinotracheale* are not recognized as such, either because the causative agent cannot be isolated or because investigators are unaware of the possibility of *O. rhinotracheale* as a cause of infections other than the respiratory ones. Lately it has been shown that *O. rhinotracheale* infections are often overlooked or misinterpreted in the field and can sometimes only be recognized with the use of specific immunohistological techniques and/or polymerase chain reaction (PCR). Thus the details of the ecology of the infection and the importance of carriers in the epidemiology have yet to be evaluated.

Cause

O. rhinotracheale is a slow-growing, pleomorphic, Gram-negative, rod-shaped bacterium of the rRNA superfamily V. Initially, the bacterium was designated a *Pasteurella*-like, *Kingella*-like or pleomorphic Gram-negative rod (PGNR) and the name Taxon 28 was also used before 1994, when the name *Ornithobacterium rhinotracheale* gen. nov., sp. nov. was proposed for this species.

Optimal growth of *O. rhinotracheale* is obtained by incubation on 5–10% sheep blood agar for at least 48 h under microaerophilic conditions (5–10% CO_2) at 37°C. Under these conditions *O. rhinotracheale* develops small, circular, grey to grey-white colonies. The colonies sometimes have a reddish glow and always give off a distinct odour, similar to that of butyric acid. Because of their slow growth, *O. rhinotracheale* colonies can easily be overgrown and masked by faster-growing bacteria such as *Escherichia coli*, making isolation difficult. To reduce this problem, samples can be inoculated on sheep blood agar containing 5 μg/mL of gentamicin and polymyxin, because most *O. rhinotracheale* strains are resistant to both these antibiotics. On primary isolation, the colonies of most *O. rhinotracheale* cultures show great differences in size (1–3 mm after 48 h incubation) but when subcultured, the colony size becomes more uniform. In liquid media, *O. rhinotracheale* is pleomorphic, the thin (0.2–0.6 μm) cells being very variable in length (0.6–5 μm). Clusters are often formed that can contain up to thousands of cells but can be readily disrupted.

Biochemical test results can be very inconsistent because of the varied ability of *O. rhinotracheale* strains to grow in the liquid media that are normally used for identification. However, under optimal conditions the biochemical properties of *O. rhinotracheale* are fairly consistent: positive for oxidase, urease, β-galactosidase, arginine dihydrolase, α-glucosidase and acid production (without gas) from fructose, glucose, lactose and galactose and negative for catalase, gelatinase, indole production, nitrate reduction, motility, growth on MacConkey agar and acid production from fructose, maltose, ribose and sucrose.

For serological and biochemical identification of *O. rhinotracheale*, a combination of the agar gel precipitation test (AGP) with the API-20NE identification strip (bioMérieux, France) has been found to be useful, although the biochemical results may be different from those found when tests are performed under optimal conditions. A characteristic of *O. rhinotracheale* is that, when tested in the API-20NE strip at the recommended temperature of 30°C, the *p*-nitrophenyl-β-D-galactopyranoside test (for the presence of β-galactosidase) will become positive within 2–3 h. Test cultures showing the API 20NE result codes of 0/1-0/2-2-0-0-0-4 should be suspected as positive for *O. rhinotracheale* and should be tested by the AGP test and/or by PCR.

Using boiled extract antigens (BEAs) and monovalent antisera in the AGP test, 18 different serotypes of *O. rhinotracheale* can be distinguished (serotypes A–R). By using BEAs in an enzyme linked immunosorbent assay (ELISA), *O. rhinotracheale* can not only be serotyped but can also be distinguished from other relevant Gram-negative rods that are potentially pathogenic for fowl and it can be differentiated from other bacterial species with which it might be confused. Cross-reactions within the species *O. rhinotracheale* are encountered in the ELISA, mainly between the serotypes A, B, D, E, I and O.

Hosts

O. rhinotracheale has been isolated from chicken, chukar partridge, duck, goose, guinea fowl, gull, ostrich, partridge, pheasant, pigeon, quail, rook and turkey.

Spread

Transmission of *O. rhinotracheale* is possible both horizontally through aerosols and vertically through the egg and, because eggs are sent all over the world, this makes it easier to understand the relatively rapid worldwide spread of *O. rhinotracheale* infections in commercial poultry during recent decades.

Relationships are seen between the geographical origin of the *O. rhinotracheale* isolates and their serotype. From the 18 serotypes, serotype A is predominant among the chicken isolates (97%) and is also the most frequent isolate (61%) from turkeys, the isolates from which are more heterogeneous (Table 13.1). There is no explanation as yet for these differences in distribution but it has been shown that serotype A and C strains from chickens and serotype B, D and E strains from turkeys have a similar virulence for both chickens and turkeys, so there is no indication of any host specificity of the serotypes. A possible explanation could relate to different breeding practices in the chicken and turkey industries. In turkeys serotype A is almost always found at a young age while the other serotypes are mainly isolated in turkeys older than 8 weeks. These findings and the fact that the age of broiler chickens is normally restricted to 8 weeks may indicate a type of age-dependency for the occurrence of *O. rhinotracheale*.

The high similarity of biochemical reactions, pathogenicity, total-protein profiles, outer-membrane-protein profiles and 16S rRNA sequences among *O. rhinotracheale* strains from all over the world indicates a close relationship. However, genetic studies using the random amplified polymorphic DNA method or the amplified fragment length polymorphism method suggest that the genus *Ornithobacterium* should be subdivided into more species. Thus it is clear that more studies of the epidemiology and pathogenicity of *O. rhinotracheale* are needed to obtain final answers to the remaining questions about emerging *O. rhinotracheale* infections in poultry.

Influencing factors

Early experiments showed that the clinical disease could be induced by aerosol administration of *O. rhinotracheale* but only as a secondary infection after the administration of viral primers such as *Turkey rhinotracheitis virus* (TRTV), *Newcastle disease virus* (NDV) or infectious bronchitis virus. However, it has been demonstrated that aerosol or intravenous application of some strains of *O. rhinotracheale* can induce respiratory signs without priming. Nevertheless it is clear that some viruses have a strong aggravating effect on *O. rhinotracheale* infections and that bacteria such as *E. coli*, *Bordetella avium* or *Chlamydophila psittaci* can also trigger *O. rhinotracheale* to cause overt signs of disease. In fact, as with other respiratory infections in poultry, the outcome of *O. rhinotracheale* infection is influenced by a complex of factors such as stress, inadequate ventilation, poor hygiene, high ammonia levels and the type of secondary infection.

DISEASE

Clinical signs

The first signs in young broilers are sneezing and a slightly increased mortality and poor performance. *O. rhinotracheale* also can cause sudden death (up to 20% in a couple of days) in young birds through infections of the brains and skull, featuring totally weakened skull bones. This manifestation of *O. rhinotracheale* infection can be seen with or without the above-mentioned respiratory signs but is often not even noticed when mortality rates are low, since brains and skulls are not normally examined.

Table 13.1 Number of *O. rhinotracheale* isolates from 1991 to 2004 according to serotype and geographical location

COUNTRY	SEROTYPE																		TOTAL
	A	B	C	D	E	F	G	H	I	J	K	L	M	N	O	P	Q	NT	
Chicken isolates																			
Europe	882	8	5	2	6		1			2	4				2		2	4	918
South America	48									1									49
Africa	457		2								1				2	1			463
USA	608	2	4								3								617
Asia	22																		22
Total	2017	10	11	2	6	0	1	0	0	3	8	0	0	0	4	0	3	4	2069
Percentage	97	<1	<1	<1	<1	0	<1	0	0	<1	<1	0	0	0	<1	0	<1	<1	
Turkey isolates																			
Europe	1018	318	6	138	172	68	5	11				3	3			4		2	1748
USA	188	48	7		1				1										245
Africa	22	4																	26
Total	1228	370	13	138	173	68	5	11	1	0	0	3	3	0	0	4	0	2	2019
Percentage	61	18	<1	7	9	3	<1	<1	<1	0	0	<1	<1	0	0	<1	0	<1	

NT = Not typable with the presently available antisera. Serotypes N and R have not been found in chicken or turkey.
Update of previously published data (van Empel et al 1997, van Empel and Hafez 1999).

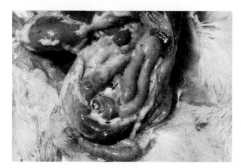

Fig. 13.1 Characteristic *Ornithobacterium rhinotracheale* infection in a broiler chicken featuring foamy, 'yoghurt like' exudate with clots of fibrin (arrows) in the abdominal air sacs.

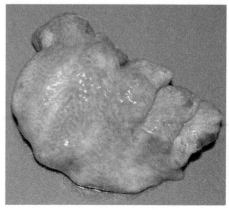

Fig. 13.2 Pneumonic lung from a broiler chicken infected with *O. rhinotracheale*, typically showing that only parts are affected.

Young turkeys appear less affected but when older birds are involved the economic losses due to *O. rhinotracheale* can be considerable. In turkeys of 12 weeks of age or more *O. rhinotracheale* can cause acute pneumonia, with mortality rates of up to 50%. Other signs of *O. rhinotracheale* infection in older turkeys and chickens can be lameness and paralysis due to arthritis, osteitis and osteomyelitis.

An *O. rhinotracheale* infection in layer and breeder birds leads to slightly increased mortality, a drop in egg production and a decrease in egg quality.

Lesions

At slaughter or post-mortem examination, young broilers with respiratory disease reveal foamy, white, 'yoghurt-like' exudate with clots of fibrin that can be seen in the (predominantly abdominal) air sacs (Fig. 13.1). This airsacculitis is commonly accompanied by unilateral pneumonia, typically showing only parts of the lung to be affected (Fig. 13.2). The lesions can lead to condemnation rates of up to 50% or more at slaughter of an affected flock.

Affected turkeys may show oedema in the lungs with fibrinous exudate on the pleura. When the turkeys are older the oedema can be markedly haemorrhagic.

In older turkeys and chickens with lameness and paralysis there is commonly a purulent, slimy exudate in the joints of the lame birds. Similar exudate can be found in young birds with brain and skull infections, with abundant exudate between the brain and the cranium and in the vacuoles of the bone structure, which normally only contain air.

DIAGNOSIS

The clinical signs and post-mortem lesions of the different manifestations of *O. rhinotracheale* infection are not sufficiently specific to be diagnostic and the respiratory signs can easily be confused with those caused by viral infections or by infections of *E. coli*, *Riemerella anatipestifer* and/or *Avibacterium paragallinarum* (formerly *Haemophilus paragallinarum*). Joint and brain infection caused by *O. rhinotracheale* can result in signs similar to those caused by other bacteria (e.g. *E. coli*, *Av. paragallinarum*, *Staphylococcus aureus* or *Streptococcus faecalis*).

Other factors also interfere with the diagnosis of *O. rhinotracheale* infections. For example, *O. rhinotracheale* can normally only be isolated at an early stage of the infection and attempts to recover it at a later stage will often fail. Another problem is that, after an *O. rhinotracheale* infection, several potential pathogenic bacteria can induce secondary infections. These bacteria will grow more readily than *O. rhinotracheale*, so they are often erroneously designated as the causal agent of the infection. In a field study, using a sensitive immunohistochemical staining technique for confirmation, it was found that *O. rhinotracheale* was the cause of 70% of cases with respiratory signs in broiler chickens, while through bacteriology and/or serology only 30% of the cases could be related to *O. rhinotracheale*.

Antibodies can be detected by an ELISA shortly after the start of a field infection and titres will peak between 1 and 4 weeks post-infection but, because titres then decline rapidly, serum samples for flock screening should be taken at frequent intervals. The serotype specificity of the ELISA is a disadvantage but commercial ELISAs are available with which most serotypes can be detected. A rapid serum agglutination (RSA) test has also been used for diagnostic purposes but it has several disadvantages, including the regular occurrence of strains that autoagglutinate and the fact that the test has a type of serotype-specificity that is not related to the AGP serotyping. Furthermore, closely related bacteria can cross-react in the RSA test.

Recently a commercial PCR test has been developed to identify *O. rhinotracheale*. The PCR amplifies a 784 bp fragment of the 16S rRNA gene of *O. rhinotracheale* and flocks can be screened by taking tracheal swabs. However, the presence of *O. rhinotracheale* does not always mean that infections seen are caused by this bacterium, since birds can be carriers without showing disease. The proof that a particular disease condition is caused by *O. rhinotracheale* is best accomplished by immunohistochemical staining, demonstrating that the bacterium is present in the infected tissue.

CONTROL

Treatment of *O. rhinotracheale* infections with antibiotics is very difficult because of the variable sensitivity of the strains. It has been shown that *O. rhinotracheale* easily acquires resistance to antibiotics such as doxycycline, enrofloxacin, flumequine, lincomycin, trimethoprim/sulphonamide and tylosin. The sensitivity pattern depends on the source of the strain and on the routine use of antibiotics in the poultry from which it is isolated. Successful antibiotic treatments of *O. rhinotracheale* infections through water medication were reported with chlortetracycline and/or amoxicillin. Injections of tetracyclines and/or penicillins were found to be effective in some cases. However, it should be emphasized that for successful treatment the sensitivity pattern of each isolate needs first to be established.

O. rhinotracheale bacteria can cycle and recycle from farm to farm and from house to house. The infections appear to become endemic and can affect newly introduced stock, especially in multiple-age farms and in areas of intensive poultry production. Therefore it is important to clean and disinfect houses thoroughly between flocks. Disinfectants that are based on different organic acids such as formic and glyoxylic acids and those that contain aldehydes were found to readily inactivate *O. rhinotracheale* in vitro.

Vaccination of meat turkeys with autogenous bacterins successfully reduced the number of outbreaks of *O. rhinotracheale* infections in the field. A problem in growing turkeys is that repeated infections caused by other serotypes regularly occur during the long rearing period. Antigens have been found that show cross-protection between serotypes of *O. rhinotracheale* but up to now no cross-protecting vaccines are available so, at present, vaccines given to turkeys should contain several serotypes and those vaccines with a long-lasting efficacy should be used. This last point also applies to autogenous vaccines.

Maternally derived antibodies, which can be found in almost all flocks, thwart the immunization of day-old birds against *O. rhinotracheale*. Vaccines in potent (oil) adjuvants are needed to break through this barrier but it is well known that the vaccination of day-old birds with this kind of vaccine can have negative effects on performance. The best results in broiler chickens are obtained by vaccination of the breeder flocks. This induces maternally derived antibody levels in the progeny that provide significant protection up to 3–4 weeks of age against experimental challenge. In field trials, the vaccination of breeders also significantly reduced the number of *O. rhinotracheale* isolates and outbreaks in their progeny and increased the production results of the progeny.

Live vaccination is feasible but up to now no nonvirulent strains of *O. rhinotracheale* have been found that could be used for this purpose.

FURTHER READING

Amonsin A, Wellehan L, Li L-L et al 1997 Molecular epidemiology of *Ornithobacterium rhinotracheale*. J Clin Microbiol 35: 2894–2898

Back A, Halvorson D, Rajashekara G, Nagaraja K V 1998 Development of a serum plate agglutination test to detect antibodies to *Ornithobacterium rhinotracheale*. J Vet Diagn Invest 10: 84–86

Back A, Rajashekara G, Jeremiah R B et al 1998 Tissue distribution of *Ornithobacterium rhinotracheale* in experimentally infected turkeys. Vet Rec 143: 52–53

Bock R R, Freidlin P J, Manoim M et al 1997 *Ornithobacterium rhinotracheale* (ORT) associated with a new turkey respiratory tract infectious agent in Israel. Proceedings of the 11th International Congress of the World Veterinary Poultry Association, Budapest, p 120

De Herdt P, Cauwerts K, Vervloesem J, Ducatelle R 2001 The relevance and efficacy of *Ornithobacterium rhinotracheale* control in chickens. World Poult 17: 32–33

Devriese L A, Hommez J, Vandamme P et al 1995 In vitro antibiotic sensitivity of *Ornithobacterium rhinotracheale* strains from poultry and wild birds. Vet Rec 137: 435–436

Goovaerts D, Vrijenhoek M, van Empel P 1998 Immuno-histochemical and bacteriological investigation of the pathogenesis of *Ornithobacterium rhinotracheale* infection in South Africa in chickens with osteitis and encephalitis syndrome. Proceedings of the 16th meeting of the European Society of Veterinary Pathology, Lillehammer, p 81

Moalic P Y 2005 Evaluation of a PCR test for *Ornithobacterium rhinotracheale* infections in birds. Proceedings of the 14th International Congress of the World Veterinary Poultry Association, Istanbul, p 197

Schuiffel D 2005 A strategic approach for immunity-based selection of cross-protective *Ornithobacterium rhinotracheale* antigens. PhD thesis, Faculty of Veterinary Medicine, University of Utrecht, Netherlands

Vandamme P, Segers P, Vancanneyt M 1994 Description of *Ornithobacterium rhinotracheale* gen. nov., sp. nov. isolated from the avian respiratory tract. Int J Syst Bacteriol 44: 24–37

Van Empel P, Hafez H 1999 *Ornithobacterium rhinotracheale*: a review. Avian Pathol 28: 217–227

Van Empel P, van den Bosch H 1998 Vaccination of chickens against *Ornithobacterium rhinotracheale* infection. Avian Dis 42: 572–578

Van Empel P, van den Bosch H, Goovaerts D, Storm P 1996 Experimental infection in turkeys and chickens with *Ornithobacterium rhinotracheale*. Avian Dis 40: 858–864

Van Empel P, van den Bosch H, Loeffen P, Storm P 1997 Identification and serotyping of *Ornithobacterium rhinotracheale*. J Clin Microbiol 35: 418–421

Van Empel P, Vrijenhoek M, Goovaerts D, van den Bosch H 1999 Immunohistochemical and serological investigation of experimental *Ornithobacterium rhinotracheale* infection in chickens. Avian Pathol 28: 187–193

Van Loock M, Geens T, De Smit L et al 2005 Key role of *Chlamydophila psittaci* on Belgian turkey farms in association with other respiratory pathogens. Vet Microbiol 107: 91–101

Van Veen L, van Empel P, Fabria T 2000 *Ornithobacterium rhinotracheale*, a primary pathogen in broilers. Avian Dis 44: 896–900

Van Veen L, Vrijenhoek M, van Empel P 2004 Studies of the transmission routes of *Ornithobacterium rhinotracheale* and immunoprophylaxis to prevent infection in young meat turkeys. Avian Dis 48: 233–237

Van Veen L, Nieuwenhuizen J, Mekkes D et al 2005 Diagnosis and incidence of *Ornithobacterium rhinotracheale* infections in commercial broiler chickens at slaughter. Vet Rec 156: 315–317

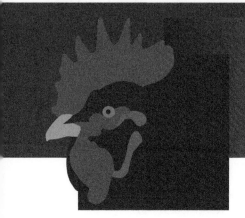

CHAPTER 14

Magne Bisgaard,
A. Miki Bojesen and
Jens P. Christensen

Riemerella infections

Riemerella anatipestifer infections mainly affect ducks, and less frequently geese and turkeys. However, sporadic infections have been reported in several domestic and wild avian species. The disease has been reported worldwide and most frequently affects young ducklings in intensive production systems, resulting in increased mortality, decreased weight gain, increased condemnations and downgrading at slaughter, and is estimated to cause substantial economic losses to the industry, with prevention and control programmes adding to the costs.

In typical cases infections caused by *R. anatipestifer* are characterized by an acute onset and development of polyserositis with lesions that are difficult to separate from those caused by *Escherichia coli*, *Coenonia anatina* and *Salmonella* spp. affecting the same age group.

EPIDEMIOLOGY

Cause

R. anatipestifer is Gram-negative, nonsporulating, catalase- and oxidase-positive and nonmotile. It grows microaerophilically in enriched media, and acid production from glucose in peptone-containing media is usually negative. *R. anatipestifer* is characterized more by the absence than the presence of specific phenotypic properties and for this reason isolation and identification procedures should be polyphasic. A definite diagnosis should include the use of genotypic methods.

A total of 21 serovars of *R. anatipestifer* have been reported so far. Multiple antigenic factors have been demonstrated within a single strain of *R. anatipestifer*, similar to the situation observed for *Pasteurella multocida*. Because immunity has been shown to be serovar-specific, knowledge generated by serotyping provides valuable information for the design of vaccines. However, together with biochemical characteristics they have contributed little to the understanding of the epidemiology of *R. anatipestifer* infections. DNA fingerprinting using *Hinf*I or *Dde*I for digestion of DNA has proved to be highly discriminatory, demonstrating 17 different profiles of serovar 1, the most common serovar in the USA. Using this method, considerable genetic diversity among strains isolated from a specific geographical region has also been demonstrated. Most strains of *R. anatipestifer* carry plasmids on which genes similar to virulence-associated genes of other bacteria have been demonstrated, but their importance remains to be further investigated.

Although some serovars seem more virulent than others the biological mechanisms behind this are not yet known.

Hosts

R. anatipestifer infections are primarily observed in web-footed birds; in particular, ducklings of 1–6 weeks of age are highly susceptible. Serious infections have also been reported in galliform birds, including turkeys, pheasants and partridges. Infections in pigeons are caused by a different species, *Riemerella columbina*, and isolates from avian species other than web-footed birds remain to be characterized genetically to verify they represent *R. anatipestifer sensu stricto*.

Spread

The mode of spread of *R. anatipestifer* is still debatable and due to lack of selective media very little is known about the importance of healthy carriers of *R. anatipestifer*. Lateral spread from the environment it thought to be by the respiratory route or through traumatic injury to the skin but no evidence has been published that indicates vertical infection. Once the infection is established on a farm it frequently becomes endemic.

The occurrence of multiple serovars in the same flock has been reported, just as change in predominant serovars from year to year seems common. The importance of persistence and multiple introductions of *Riemerella anatipestifer* should be investigated using molecular methods to improve our understanding of the epidemiology and of the possibilities for prevention of the infection.

Influencing factors

A seasonal occurrence has been reported underlining the possible importance of adverse environmental conditions or concomitant diseases predisposing infected birds to outbreaks of disease. The severity of the disease seems to depend on the serovar involved, the age of the host, the route of exposure and predisposing factors.

DISEASE

Pathogenesis

The exact route of infection remains unclear but it has been suggested that the ducklings are infected from the environment via the respiratory tract or through wounds, particularly of the feet. Strong variations of virulence as assessed by mortality and morbidity rates during outbreaks have been reported between serovars and within a given serovar, consistent with a high degree of genetic diversity among isolates.

Clinical signs

Clinical signs are usually observed after an incubation period of 2–5 days. Clinical signs and mortality can be seen as early as 24 hours post-infection after artificial infection of ducklings.

Signs most often include lethargy and listlessness, anorexia with ruffled feathers and the ducklings are hunched in appearance. Ocular and nasal discharge, mild coughing and sneezing, and greenish diarrhoea may develop subsequently, as well as ataxia and tremor of the neck and head. Affected ducklings often lie on their backs paddling their legs, unable to follow the flock. Morbidity is high and mortality may vary from 5% to 50%. Affected flocks become uneven.

Lesions

Gross lesions in affected birds include polyserositis with fibrinous exudates covering the serosal surfaces of the body cavity in addition to the hepatic capsule and pericardial sac. Various lesions may be observed in the respiratory tract, including fibrinous sinusitis, pneumonia and air sacculitis. Lesions in the brain primarily consist of a diffuse fibrinous meningitis. The spleen and liver are moderately to markedly enlarged. There may be moderate to marked multifocal to coalescing areas of lymphoid necrosis of the white pulp of the spleen and also varying degrees of lymphoid depletion and necrosis within the cortical and medullary regions of the bursa of Fabricius. A high proportion of affected birds also show a mucopurulent or caseous salpingitis and affected breeding stock should be slaughtered because of a high prevalence of blind layers that occurs subsequently. Chronic localized infections in the form of necrotic dermatitis on the lower back or around the vent may also be observed.

DIAGNOSIS

A presumptive diagnosis may be made from clinical signs and post-mortem findings provided that typical central nervous symptoms have developed. A definite diagnosis, however, depends on isolation and identification of *R. anatipestifer*. Suitable tissues for culture include the brain, bone marrow and the respiratory or reproductive tract. A PCR-based diagnostic test has been described but its specificity remains to be investigated in more detail. Different methods have been reported for serovar determination and, of these, plate agglutination is rapid and convenient. However, unless titrations are carried out, only absorbed antisera should be used because of the existence of multiple antigenic factors within a single strain.

Several ELISA tests have been reported for detection of antibodies, the sensitivity of which remains to be compared. Apart from their use in measuring the host response to vaccination, the practical value of these tests seems limited. Gross lesions indistinguishable from those caused by *R. anatipestifer* have been reported for *E. coli*, *C. anatina*, *S. enterica* and *P. multocida*. In turkeys the differential diagnosis of *R. anatipestifer* also includes chlamydiosis and infections with *Avibacterium gallinarum* and *Bordetella avium*.

CONTROL

In acute outbreaks antimicrobial susceptibility testing of fresh isolates of *R. anatipestifer* should be carried out. Enrofloxacin has been shown to be highly effective in preventing mortality in ducklings when given in the drinking water, while varying degrees of success have been obtained with other antibiotics and sulpha drugs. Inactivated bacterins are normally used to prevent or reduce mortality due to *R. anatipestifer*. Because of lack of cross-protection between serovars and the possible involvement of more than one serovar in an outbreak, several isolates should be taken over time for serotyping from an infected farm in order to allow design and production of an effective vaccine. Several types of bacterin have been reported, with oil-emulsion bacterins providing longer-lasting immunity in ducklings. A single inoculation of an oil-emulsified bacterin has been reported to protect ducklings until processing, although undesirable lesions may occur at the site of inoculation.

Where a farm is endemically infected, all-in all-out production should be implemented to control the infection and minimize losses. The most important aspects of prevention include a high level of biosecurity and good management and sanitation practices. This will include cleaning and disinfection between flocks and separation between flocks on multiple-age farms. Predisposing stress and intercurrent infections should be avoided.

The disease is of no public health significance.

FURTHER READING

Ryll M, Christensen H, Bisgaard M et al 2001 Studies on the prevalence of *Riemerella anatipestifer* in the upper respiratory tract of clinically healthy ducklings and characterization of untypable strains. J Vet Med B48: 537–546

Sarver, C F,. Morishita T Y, Nersessian B 2005 The effect of route of inoculation and challenge dose on *Riemerella anatipestifer* infection in Pekin ducks (*Anas platyrhynchos*). Avian Dis 49: 104–107

Subramaniam, S, Huang B, Loh H et al 2000 Characterization of a predominant immunogenic outer membrane protein of *Riemerella anatipestifer*. Clin Diagn Lab Immunol 7: 168–174

Vandamme R, Vancanneyt M, Segers P et al 1999 *Coenonia anatina* gen. nov., sp. nov., a novel bacterium associated with respiratory disease in ducks and geese. Int J Syst Bacteriol 49: 867–874

Weng S, Lin W, Chang Y, Chang C 1999 Identification of a virulence-associated protein homolog gene and IS Ra1 in a plasmid of *Riemerella anatipestifer*. FEMS Microbiol Lett 179: 9–11

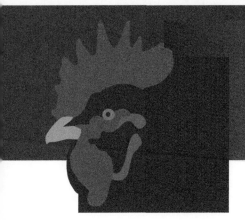

CHAPTER 15

Karl-Heinz Hinz*

Avian bordetellosis (turkey coryza)

Bordetella avium causes a highly contagious acute upper respiratory tract disease primarily in young turkeys and less frequently in young chickens, ducks and geese as well as in young birds of other species (e.g. psittacine birds, finches, quails, partridges). The disease causes economic losses in young turkeys due to impaired growth and slightly increased mortality and may result in high mortality when complicated by other pathogens. The disease was first described in 1967 in Canada and has been reported from the USA, Australia, Africa, Israel and most European countries. *B. avium* has been shown to have properties similar to those of other pathogenic bordetellas (e.g. *Bordetella pertussis*); however, there is no evidence that it can infect humans.

EPIDEMIOLOGY

Cause

B. avium is a strictly aerobic, capsulated and motile, Gram-negative, rod-shaped bacterium that is nonfermentative and nonsaccharolytic and therefore relatively inactive on biochemical tests. When grown on agar medium, most strains produce small (0.2–1 mm diameter), compact, pearl-like colonies with a smooth edge after 24 h incubation, which increase to 1–2 mm after 48 h incubation (these are called type I colonies). Another colony type (type II) is also smooth, circular and convex but is flatter and larger than type I colonies. A small percentage of strains dissociate into a rough colony type with a dry appearance and a serrated irregular edge (type III). Rough

* The author wishes to acknowledge the contribution of G. Philip Wilding, author of this chapter in the 5th edition.

colonies have been found to be apathogenic. Bordetella of the type I and II colonies are able to agglutinate guinea pig erythrocytes but the mean haemagglutination titre of the type I organisms is significantly higher than that of the intermediate type II organisms.

There appears to be considerable variation in virulence between strains. Avian *Bordetella* strains may differ in their adherence to the tracheal mucosa, toxin production, haemagglutination of guinea pig erythrocytes, plasmid profiles, antibiotic sensitivity, colony morphology and, last but not least, in their pathogenicity. Up to now the following virulence factors have been identified: surface structure for adhesion to cilia of tracheal mucosa, haemagglutinin, endotoxin, heat-labile dermonecrotic toxin (DNT), tracheal cytotoxin (TCT), osteotoxin and histamine-sensitizing factor.

B. avium survives best under the conditions of low temperature, low humidity and neutral pH. It was able to survive for 25–30 days within faeces and dust at 10°C and relative humidity of 32–58%. When the temperature was raised to 40°C survival of the bacteria was less than 2 days. It is susceptible to many disinfectants if used at the correct concentration.

Hosts

It should be emphasized that *B. avium* is not only a primary pathogen for turkey poults but also for Muscovy ducklings, quail chicks and cockatiel (*Nymphicus hollandicus*) chicks. It appears to be an opportunistic pathogen for chickens. There are also reports of *B. avium* isolations from numerous other species of bird but its role in these cases has been not clarified.

Spread

The main sources of infection are clinically affected birds, carrier birds and the contaminated environment. Only a few viable organisms are necessary for infection so it can be transmitted by drinking water or litter contaminated by nasal discharge and is spread readily by direct contact with infected poults. *B. avium* is widely distributed in populations of wild turkeys, ducks and geese, which act as a reservoir for the agent.

DISEASE

Pathogenesis

B. avium is a noninvasive bacterial agent with a strong tissue tropism for the ciliated cells of the respiratory tract. The first step in pathogenesis is the adhesion of the organisms to the ciliated nasal mucosa, followed by progressive colonization of the trachea down to the primary bronchi within 7–10 days. Toxic substances produced by the organisms during multiplication are associated with production of lesions via an apoptotic pathway, an inflammatory response and the appearance of clinical signs. Furthermore, virulent strains of *B. avium* are capable of inducing systemic pathophysiological effects (stress syndrome) that may be responsible for the more severe and prolonged disease process associated with intercurrent infections by other infectious agents, of which the most prominent is *Escherichia coli*.

In this connection it should be considered that differences in genetic susceptibility to bordetellosis may exist among species of bird and among commercial poultry lines. Recently published experimental research results indicate that turkeys of heavy lines are more susceptible than those of lighter lines. The lowered cellular immune response seems to be responsible for these differences.

Clinical signs

The uncomplicated disease in turkey flocks on floor management is characterized by rapid spread, high morbidity and low mortality. The onset of the disease is usually sudden and morbidity may approach 100% within 24–48 h. Bordetellosis usually occurs in 2–8-week-old birds, although clinical disease apparently due to this infection has been described in older birds.

Signs of bordetellosis result from local and systemic reactions caused by bacterial toxins, inflammatory response and physical obstructions of large airways. Signs include foamy conjunctivitis, sneezing and coughing, with moist tracheal rales. Some poults may also show 'mouth breathing' and the voice may become high-pitched. Submandibular oedema is commonly noted. Characteristically, excess mucus is seen in the nares, although in the early stages manual pressure across the beak may be necessary to make this visible. In the later stages the mucus becomes encrusted with dust.

Mortality rates vary widely but may be extremely high. This is probably influenced by the presence of intercurrent infections and is exacerbated by general management, especially inadequate ventilation and poor environmental conditions. *Escherichia coli* septicaemia appears to be one of the most common causes of death but other agents such as avian pneumovirus and *Ornithobacterium rhinotracheale* may be also involved. Levels of mortality that are higher than expected may continue for some weeks following bordetellosis. Infections have also been detected in older turkeys where the only clinical sign has been a dry cough.

Lesions

In the early stages the lesions are limited to excess mucus in the upper respiratory tract, which may become mucopurulent. Collapse of the trachea and/or bronchi associated with mucopurulent plugs has also been reported. Lower respiratory tract lesions are uncommon unless the disease is caused by a highly virulent strain of *B. avium* under stressful environmental conditions and/or complicated by other primary or secondary pathogens.

DIAGNOSIS

Bordetellosis is clinically indistinguishable from turkey rhinotracheitis caused by avian pneumovirus. Therefore, the history of a rapidly spreading disease and its clinical signs and lesions may allow only a tentative diagnosis that has to be confirmed by isolation and identification of the causal agent. *B. avium* grows slowly on MacConkey agar and may be easily overlooked after 24 h incubation; at 48 h small colonies of 1–2 mm diameter can be seen, which may have a brownish raised centre. Many rapidly growing bacterial species may also be present, which can overgrow *B. avium* colonies; it is therefore recommended that samples are taken early in the disease process before opportunistic bacteria colonize the respiratory tract. Samples should also be taken aseptically, the preferred method being at post-mortem examination by section of the infraorbital sinus and midtrachea as soon as possible after death.

The organisms should be identified by their macro- and micromorphology as well as by their biochemical properties. The reliability of *B. avium* identification can be enhanced by gas–liquid chromatographic analysis of whole-cell fatty acids using the MIDI system, a computer-assisted microbial identification system. Furthermore, the indirect fluorescent monoclonal antibody staining technique or a polymerase chain reaction (PCR)-based assay can also be used to detect the presence of the avian bordetellas in tissue samples. Specific attention should be given to differentiating *B. avium* from *O. rhinotracheale* and *Bordetella hinzii* in primary cultures.

Serological assays by microagglutination and enzyme-linked immunosorbent assay (ELISA) have been developed and may be used in diagnosis or epidemiological studies.

CONTROL

Avian bordetellosis is difficult to control on intensive turkey farms because environmental conditions are conducive to its perpetuation. Many disease outbreaks have occurred on continuous production farms or those where terminal hygiene procedures have been inadequate. Successful control depends upon rigorous routine hygiene procedures such as depopulation, complete removal of the litter and strict attention to cleaning and disinfection. Particular attention should be paid to disinfection of the food and water systems as well as the air ventilation system.

Numerous antimicrobial treatments have been used in affected flocks but with only limited success. In contrast, it has been reported that, after medication with sulphonamide/trimethoprim or enrofloxacin for 5 days in the drinking water, clinical signs disappeared almost completely; however, relapse occurred after the treatment was discontinued. The reason for this was not the inefficiency of the drug itself but rather the fact that the antimicrobials were not able to eliminate the agent in all birds of a large population as well as from the environment. Only if specific immunity has developed in most of the affected birds of the flock does the disease disappear completely. Nevertheless, treatment with chemotherapeutics can help to reduce losses in flocks with a severe, complicated form of bordetellosis.

Vaccines available commercially include a live temperature-sensitive mutant of *B. avium* and a whole-cell bacterin. The main problem is to induce a protective immunity early in life, because turkey poults of less than 3 weeks of age are unable to develop adequate protective immunity. However, it has been shown that poults derived from turkey hens vaccinated with an inactivated oil-adjuvant vaccine are protected within the first 2–3 weeks after hatching. Maternal antibodies of the IgG class may be responsible for the temporary passive immunity.

FURTHER READING

Hinz K-H, Glünder G 1985 Prevalence of *Bordetella avium* sp. nov. and *Bordetella bronchiseptica* in birds. Berl Münch Tierärztl Wschr 98: 369–373

Hinz K-H, Glünder G, Lüders H 1978 Acute respiratory disease in turkey poults caused by *Bordetella bronchiseptica*-like bacteria. Vet Rec 103: 262–263

Hinz K-H, Glünder G, Römer K J 1983 A comparative study of avian *Bordetella*-like strains, *Bordetella bronchiseptica*, *Alcaligenes faecalis* and other related nonfermentable bacteria. Avian Pathol 12: 263–276

Hopkins B A, Skeeles J K, Houghten G E, Story J D 1988 Development of an enzyme-linked immunoabsorbent assay for *Bordetella avium*. Avian Dis 32: 353–361

Jackwood M W, Saif Y M 2003 Bordetellosis. In: Saif Y M (ed) Diseases of poultry, 11th edn. Iowa State University Press, Ames, p 705–718

Kersters K, Hinz K-H, Hertle A et al 1984 *Bordetella avium* sp. nov., isolated from the respiratory tract of turkeys and other birds. Int J Syst Bacteriol 34: 56–70

Li Z, Nestor K E, Saif Y M 2001 A summary of the effect of selection for increased body weight in turkeys on the immune system. Special Circular No.184. Ohio Agricultural Research and Development Center, Wooster, p 21–28

Lister S A, Alexander D J 1986 Turkey rhinotracheitis: a review. Vet Bull 56: 637–663

Saif Y M, Moorhead P D, Dearth R N, Jackwood D J 1980 Observations on *Alcaligenes faecalis* infection in turkeys. Avian Dis 24: 665–684

Simmons D G, Rose L P, Grey J G 1980 Some physical, biochemic and pathologic properties of *Alcaligenes faecalis*, the bacterium causing rhinotracheitis (coryza) in turkey poults. Avian Dis 24: 82–90

Spears P A, Temple L M, Miyamoto D M et al 2003 Unexpected similarities between *Bordetella avium* and other pathogenic bordetellae. Infect Immun 71: 2591–2597

Vandamme P, Segers P, Vancanneyt M et al 1994 *Ornithobacterium rhinotracheale* gen. nov., sp. nov., isolated from the avian respiratory tract. Int J Syst Bacteriol 44: 24–37

Vandamme P, Hommez J, Vancanneyt M et al 1995 *Bordetella hinzii* sp. nov., isolated from poultry and humans. Int J Syst Bacteriol 45: 37–45

Varley J 1986 The characterisation of *Bordetella/Alcaligenes*-like organisms and their effects on turkey poults and chicks. Avian Pathol 15: 1–22

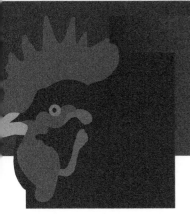

CHAPTER 16

Sarah Evans and
Laura Powell

Campylobacter

The genus *Campylobacter* derives its name from the Greek word for 'curved rod', because of the curved, spiral or S-shaped morphology of these bacteria. They are Gram-negative, flagellate bacteria with a characteristic darting motility. Most species are microaerophilic, requiring a reduced atmospheric oxygen tension for growth. There are many species of *Campylobacter* and in recent years the taxonomy has changed considerably. The bovine pathogen *Campylobacter fetus* (formerly *Vibrio fetus*) was recognized as a cause of ovine and bovine abortion as long ago as 1913. However, it was not until 1957 that Elizabeth King, on the basis of thermophilic characteristics (optimum microbial growth at high temperatures), identified a group of 'related vibrios' associated with human enteric disease. The importance of these thermophilic campylobacters as a major cause of human diarrhoeal disease was confirmed in the early 1970s following the development of selective isolation media for these fastidious organisms.

Thermophilic campylobacters are found in the intestinal tracts of a wide variety of animals and birds, often without causing disease. Unlike *C. fetus*, they are not major veterinary pathogens and their main significance lies in the ability of infected animals to serve as reservoirs of infection for human disease. The reasons for the differences in pathogenicity between animals and humans are not known. The three main species of thermophilic campylobacters of poultry are *Campylobacter jejuni*, *Campylobacter coli* and *Campylobacter lari* and they can be distinguished from others in the genus by their preferential growth at a temperature of 42–43°C.

All three species can be isolated from poultry but the main species is *C. jejuni*. Current evidence points to these bacteria existing in the intestinal tract of poultry as nonpathogenic commensals.

The purpose of controlling *Campylobacter* infection in poultry is to reduce the potential for foodborne transmission of the bacteria to humans. There is no evidence that campylobacteriosis in humans is attributable to the consumption of table eggs. Therefore, this review concentrates on the epidemiology and control of infection in broiler flocks because consumption or handling of chicken meat has been identified as a major source of *Campylobacter* infection for humans.

EPIDEMIOLOGY

Cause

Campylobacters have a typical Gram-negative cell wall, capsule and flagella and are slender, curved rods, measuring 0.2–0.5 µm by 0.5–5 µm. They are microaerophilic, requiring an atmosphere containing 3–15% oxygen and 3–5% carbon dioxide for growth. They do not ferment or oxidize carbohydrates and so biochemical tests used for *Enterobacteriaceae* cannot be used to differentiate between species. All three main species are catalase- and oxidase-positive and *C. jejuni* can be differentiated from *C. coli* by its ability to hydrolyse hippurate. *C. lari* is characterized by its resistance to nalidixic acid. There is a large diversity within species, particularly *C. jejuni* and *C. coli*, and the identification of individual strains has proved important in determining the extent of disease outbreaks and identifying the sources of the organism and modes of transmission.

In 2000 the genome sequence of *C. jejuni* NCTC11168 was published. The size of the chromosome (1 641 481 base pairs) is relatively small compared with other bacteria and consequently the number of genes is limited (around 1 600 compared with over 5 000 in *Salmonella* spp.).

The mechanisms by which these bacteria cause disease in humans are unknown but virulence has variably been associated with cytotoxin or enterotoxin production, adhesion and invasion, flagella and motility. Virulence differs between strains and there is a large reservoir of nonvirulent strains in the environment. There is evidence that the organism can enter a viable but nonculturable state in unfavourable conditions, although this may reflect the degenerative changes associated with a dying population. The potential for these cells to resuscitate and infect a host remains to be established. The immune status of the host is also important in determining the outcome of infection.

Campylobacters possess plasmids that can mediate resistance to tetracyclines. Resistance to other antibiotics, including kanamycin, erythromycin and recently ciprofloxacin, is also common. Resistance to fluoroquinolones has been shown to develop very rapidly and the incidence of resistant isolates has increased in humans in recent years, which has coincided with the approval of these drugs for veterinary use. Consequently, the use of these antibiotics in animal production systems may have serious implications for the treatment of human infections.

Hosts

Campylobacter bacteria are found in a wide range of warm-blooded animals but the preferred host for the thermophilic species, *C. jejuni*, appears to be poultry. Campylobacters are found wherever commercial poultry are kept and they have also been found in game birds, pigeons and various wild birds. As mentioned below, *C. jejuni* is also found in domestic and wild mammals on farms.

Prevalence of infection in broiler breeder flocks has been found to be as high as 80% but campylobacters are rarely isolated from hatcheries or newly hatched chicks. The prevalence reported in broiler flocks varies, possibly owing to variations in age, isolation technique or season. The prevalence also varies between countries. Sweden, Finland and Norway report relatively low rates of infection (5–20%) whereas the UK, other European countries and the USA appear to have higher levels of infection, with up to 90% of broiler flocks infected. *C. jejuni* is the most frequently isolated species from poultry but occasionally *C. coli* and *C. lari* are found. Comparisons between surveys should be made with caution because of a lack of standardization of surveillance methods. Flocks may be infected with more than one species of *Campylobacter* and within species multiple strains are commonly found in an infected flock, although there is a tendency for one strain to predominate.

Spread

Descriptive studies have shown that broiler flocks usually become infected, without showing clinical signs, when the chicks are 3–5 weeks old, but infection has been observed as early as 7 days of age. Within 3–7 days of initial infection, 80–100% of the flock become infected and remain carriers until slaughtered at 6–7 weeks of age. The transmission rate within a flock has recently been quantified at 1.04 new cases per colonized chick per day. Coprophagy may partially explain the rapid spread of infection within flocks and there is also evidence that transient palatine carriage may result in spread via communal drinking water systems. Extremely high numbers of campylobacters have been found in caecal contents once colonization is established and in the field the organism is usually isolated in large numbers from the majority of birds sampled. Experimentally, chicks have been shown to cease shedding the bacteria 3 months after challenge. However, the short life span of the broiler chick precludes this natural self-limitation of infection.

The reason for the delay in colonization of young chicks is not known. They are susceptible to infection at 1 day old in the laboratory yet organic flocks, which are frequently exposed to campylobacters in the environment, also show this so-called 'lag phase'; hence the delay is likely to be an inherent property of the chick. Recent studies have indicated that the lag phase may be related to maternally derived immunity.

Although vertical transmission of infection from breeder flocks seems unlikely to occur, there is continuing debate in this area. Campylobacters have been isolated from broilers within 1–2 days after hatching in a minority of flocks. The organisms have also been found in mature and immature ovarian follicles of broiler breeder hens and the semen of breeder cockerels, a finding that provides some support for vertical transmission. However, most research in the European setting has not supported this view and experimental studies have also shown that *C. jejuni* does not easily penetrate the eggshell. These findings suggest that control measures should be directed at limiting horizontal spread of infection to broilers by contact with infected animals or indirect transmission by vectors or other vehicles. Knowledge of the survival characteristics of *C. jejuni*, such as its sensitivity to oxygen and drying and its inability to multiply in feed, litter or water under ambient conditions, has helped to unravel the epidemiology of this infection.

As anticipated, feed samples taken from broiler houses have not been found to contain campylobacters because of the low moisture content of poultry feed. Drinking water may act as a vehicle of infection for growing broiler chicks. Campylobacters survive well in cold water and human waterborne outbreaks have been widely reported. Chlorination of the water supply has been shown to reduce the prevalence of *C. jejuni* in flocks supplied with water from a borehole but header tanks and drinkers must be kept clean, as organic matter rapidly inactivates chlorine. The use of a water sanitizer has also been shown to be protective.

Insects, including *Alphitobius* species, have been shown to be carriers of *C. jejuni*. It has been demonstrated in the laboratory that houseflies can transmit *C. jejuni* to chicks but it is not known how important this process is in the field. In a recent study 8.2% of flies caught outside a broiler shed in Denmark were contaminated and therefore had the potential to transmit *C. jejuni* to the chickens. It has been suggested that insects may be a contributing factor to the summer peak of infection, since their numbers are likely to be higher in the summer months. *C. jejuni* is also commonly carried by domestic and free-living animals found on farms, including cattle, pigs, dogs, rodents and wild birds. These species have been shown to carry similar

Campylobacter serotypes as poultry and research has found the presence of other farm animals on poultry farms to be a risk factor for *Campylobacter* infection. Rodent droppings may be particularly important sources of *Campylobacter* infection for flocks, especially if there is evidence of rodent access to poultry houses or food stores.

Because of the ubiquitous nature of campylobacters in the environment it is most likely that infection is introduced to flocks through environmental contamination from sources in the vicinity of the broiler sheds. Movement of personnel between broiler houses or farms may spread infection. In support of this view, campylobacters have been recovered from the boots of poultry farm workers and surface water near poultry houses. The risk of infection can be reduced by the use of effective boot dips or of house-dedicated boots. Thorough cleansing and disinfection of broiler sheds after depopulation is also very important to prevent carryover of infection.

The practice of 'thinning', i.e. reducing bird density within a broiler shed 1–2 weeks before slaughter age, is a common procedure in many European countries and is a major risk factor for the introduction of *C. jejuni* into the broiler shed. As well as campylobacters being recovered from the boots of personnel entering the sheds, the equipment and vehicles used at 'thinning' (crates, modules and forklift trucks) have been shown to carry *C. jejuni*. The potential risk of infection during transport to slaughter from *Campylobacter*-positive crates has also been highlighted. The main routes of transmission of *Campylobacter* infection in broiler flocks are summarized in Figure 16.1.

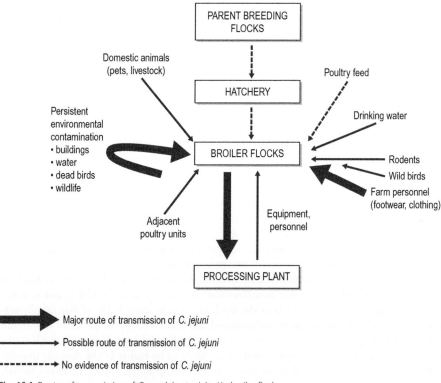

Fig. 16.1 Routes of transmission of *Campylobacter jejuni* in broiler flocks.

DISEASE

Large numbers of campylobacters can be present in the avian intestinal tract without any apparent gross pathology. There is no recognized clinical syndrome in poultry flocks attributed to infection with these bacteria. In the mid-1960s a new disease syndrome in laying flocks, called avian vibrionic hepatitis, was recognized and subsequently attributed to infection with thermophilic 'vibrio-like' organisms. This condition has since disappeared and there is now doubt as to whether campylobacters were the cause of the syndrome, as experimental studies have repeatedly failed to induce hepatopathy in chicks inoculated with *C. jejuni*.

DIAGNOSIS

Campylobacters are fragile, fastidious, slow-growing organisms. The principal niche for colonization in the bird is the caecum and caecal contents are the diagnostic sample of choice. However, cloacal swabs or fresh faecal samples are also suitable for the detection of infection as infected birds shed large numbers of campylobacters in their faeces. Samples should be sent to the laboratory without delay and stored at 4°C. A transport medium is beneficial if samples cannot be processed straight away or the specimen is likely to contain only a few organisms. Direct microbiological examination (smears) is not used routinely because it lacks sensitivity. However, polymerase-chain-reaction-based restriction fragment length polymorphism (PCR-RFLP) analysis of flagellar genes may prove useful for rapid detection and typing purposes in the future. Latex agglutination kits are also available but should only be used for confirmation purposes. A selective solid medium, containing antibiotics to inhibit unwanted organisms, is used routinely for isolation of the organisms. A pre-enrichment broth can be used to increase recovery, although the choice of enrichment medium can significantly affect the recovery of organisms. Currently there is no single method ideally suited to recovery of all species of *Campylobacter* from all sample types. Plates are incubated microaerophilically at 41.5 ± 1°C for 48–72 h to detect campylobacters from caecal/cloacal samples and plates can be incubated at 37°C to test the ability to grow under aerobic conditions. Environmental samples or samples exposed to the environment are normally incubated at 37°C for 48–72 h. Colonies are nonhaemolytic, round, smooth and greyish-white in colour.

Campylobacters should be speciated when possible. Despite their inability to ferment or oxidize carbohydrates, there are a number of recommended tests for the identification of *Campylobacter* species, including oxidase, catalase, nitrate and nitrite reduction, urease, H_2S production, hippurate hydrolysis, indoxyl acetate hydrolysis and testing for sensitivity to nalidixic acid and cefalothin.

Campylobacters are highly diverse phenotypically and genotypically. There are a number of different typing schemes that can be used to identify different strains within species but they are restricted to reference laboratories and there is no correlation between schemes. Currently, the most widely used scheme is serotyping and is based on either heat-stable (Penner scheme) or heat-labile (Lior scheme) antigens. However, serotyping is limited by the lack of availability of the large number of antisera required and the high level of nontypability. In recent years, molecular techniques, such as ribotyping, pulsed field gel electrophoresis (PFGE) and flagellin typing, have been developed. These are in use in a number of laboratories and can be highly discriminatory, especially when combined with serotyping. Recently, DNA sequencing methods such as multi-locus sequence typing (MLST) have been employed, which allow direct comparison between laboratories.

CONTROL

Campylobacters can survive routine poultry processing techniques. Superchlorination of the washing water, organic acid sprays, hot rinses and forced air chilling may reduce carcass contamination levels in the processing plant but are unlikely to achieve elimination. Post-harvest control is assisted by hazard analysis and critical control point (HACCP) protocols aimed at reducing the level of faecal contamination on the carcass and preventing cross-contamination. The organism is also very sensitive to irradiation but this is not an option in the UK at present because of public concerns over safety. Campylobacters are fragile organisms and are susceptible to drying (except when refrigerated), oxygen, direct sunlight and most disinfectants but they survive well in foods under refrigeration and can also survive in much lower numbers on frozen foods. Unlike salmonellas, campylobacters will not replicate in foods stored below 30°C. Thermal inactivation occurs at 48°C so they will not survive pasteurization or typical meat cooking procedures. However, consumer education and reinforcement of hygienic practices in catering establishments have so far been inadequate to prevent human campylobacteriosis.

Thus the control of poultry-associated infections in humans would appear to depend on the control of infections in broiler flocks. No commercial vaccine is available but there is the possibility to increase resistance by 'competitive exclusion'. This has been investigated as a method of preventing *Salmonella* and *Campylobacter* colonization of broiler chicks. However, the primary niche for *C. jejuni* colonization is the mucin layer of the caecum and it is therefore necessary to develop a culture that contains organisms to compete for this niche. Recently, competitive exclusion flora derived from this mucosal layer have shown some protective ability against both *Salmonella* and *C. jejuni* colonization. Research on reducing *C. jejuni* colonization of broiler chickens by bacteriophage therapy is also under way. Hygiene measures have been shown to be effective in reducing the risk of infection and the main recommendations are outlined in Table 16.1. The combination of enhanced biosecurity and the use of other preventive measures such as competitive exclusion is most likely to reduce the prevalence of *Campylobacter* colonization of broiler flocks.

Table 16.1	Prevention and control of *Campylobacter* in broiler flocks

- Maintain poultry buildings in a good state of repair
- Control rats and mice
- Thoroughly clean and disinfect poultry houses between flocks
- Supply birds with potable drinking water
- Dispose of dead birds promptly, away from the poultry farm
- Maintain strict disease security during the life of the flock:
  - Allow only essential visitors into poultry houses
  - Dip and change boots before entering each house
  - Replace boot dip at least twice a week using the correct amount of disinfectant
  - Add water sanitizer to the drinker system
- Carry out thinning only in association with proper crate washing and biosecurity

PUBLIC HEALTH CONSIDERATIONS

Campylobacter infection has become the most frequently implicated infectious cause of human gastroenteritis in the UK and other developed countries. All three species have been implicated but, in developed countries, *C. jejuni* is by far the most important and is isolated from 90% of cases of campylobacteriosis. An average annual rate of *Campylobacter* incidence in England and Wales was determined to be 78.4 ± 15.0 cases per 100 000 based on laboratory-confirmed cases between 1990 and 1999. However a study of infectious intestinal disease in England undertaken between 1993 and 1996 estimated that the rate of *Campylobacter* infection in the community was 870 per 100 000. The highest rates of infection are in children and young adults, particularly males. The numbers of reported infections reach a peak in May or June and then decline to less than 50% of this level in the winter months.

Most cases of campylobacteriosis are sporadic and large outbreaks of illness are relatively rare. Illness occurs 2–10 days after exposure and the presenting symptoms are watery and sometimes bloody diarrhoea accompanied by nausea, abdominal pain and sometimes fever. Campylobacterial enteritis does not usually require antibiotic therapy, as the disease is self-limiting, lasting about 5–7 days. Complications are uncommon (<1%) but can be serious. The most important manifestation is Guillain–Barré syndrome which is a postinfectious neurological disorder and can be fatal (approximately one-quarter of patients with Guillain–Barré syndrome have had a recent *C. jejuni* infection). Asymptomatic infection in developed countries is rare, as is person-to-person transmission. In contrast, in developing countries where human campylobacteriosis is hyperendemic, clinical illness in adults is rare (asymptomatic infection is the norm) because of the early acquisition of immunity by children persistently exposed to multiple strains of infection.

The precise role that infected animals and birds play in the human disease is not clearly defined. However, the majority of infections are foodborne and evidence has been accumulating that poultry are a major source of infection. Several studies have found high *C. jejuni* isolation rates in broiler farms and poultry processing plants. Campylobacters are commonly found in birds at slaughter and the caeca and intestines of infected birds have been shown to contain very large numbers of bacteria. Spillage of intestinal contents results in contamination of carcasses and the processing plant environment. The organism appears to survive the processing operation and cross-contamination during procedures such as scalding, plucking and evisceration and immersion chilling may even allow the prevalence of carcass contamination to exceed that of infection in the live bird. Retail surveys have shown that typically more than 50% of chicken carcasses are contaminated.

Serotyping has revealed similar strains in poultry and humans and case-control studies in the human population have attributed up to half of all cases to the consumption or handling of chicken. However, it is unlikely that all strains of *Campylobacter* carried by poultry are pathogenic to humans.

Campylobacters, being fragile organisms, are susceptible to most methods commonly used to eliminate enteropathogens from foods. However, the incidence of human enteritis is high. This may be due to a combination of factors, including the high numbers of organisms present on raw chicken, the low infective dose and cross-contamination during food preparation of utensils or foods that are not subsequently cooked. It has been shown that a small drop of raw chicken juice can be sufficient to provide an infective dose for humans.

However, there are other well-recognized sources of *Campylobacter* infection for humans, the importance of which has not been established. These include: red meats and shellfish; unpasteurized milk or contamination of milk delivered to the doorstep by wild birds pecking through the bottle tops; contaminated drinking or recreational water; and direct contact with infected animals, especially domestic pets; 10% of cases in the UK are attributed to foreign travel.

LEGAL REQUIREMENTS

There is no compulsory monitoring of poultry or reporting of *Campylobacter* infection in the UK and many other countries, although there is a substantial amount of voluntary testing within the poultry industry. Plans to implement a monitoring programme for *Campylobacter* spp. in the European Union are under discussion. In recent years Sweden, Denmark and the Netherlands have introduced *Campylobacter* control programmes in broiler production flocks that run alongside the *Salmonella* control programmes. In Norway, since implementing a specific action plan for broilers in 2001, there has been a considerable reduction in the prevalence of campylobacters.

FURTHER READING

Advisory Committee on the Microbiological Safety of Food 2005 Second report on *Campylobacter*. FSA/0986/0605. Food Standards Agency, London

Berndtson E, Emanuelson U, Engvall A, Danielsson-Tham M-L 1996 A 1-year epidemiological study of campylobacters in 18 Swedish chicken farms. Prev Vet Med 26: 167–185

Bouwknegt M, van de Giessen A W, Dam-Deisz W D et al 2004 Risk factors for the presence of *Campylobacter* spp. in Dutch broiler flocks. Prev Vet Med 62: 35–49

Cox N A, Stern N J, Hiett K L, Berrang M E 2002 Isolation of *Campylobacter* spp. from semen samples of commercial broiler breeder roosters. Avian Dis 46: 717–720

Cox N A, Bailey J S, Richardson L J et al 2005 Presence of naturally occurring *Campylobacter* and *Salmonella* in the mature and immature ovarian follicles of late-life broiler breeder hens. Avian Dis 49: 285–287

Dingle K E, Colles F M, Ure R et al 2002 Molecular characterization of *Campylobacter jejuni* clones: a basis for epidemiologic investigation. Emerg Infect Dis 8: 949–955

Evans S J 1992 Introduction and spread of thermophilic campylobacters in broiler flocks. Vet Rec 131: 574–576

Evans S J 1997 Epidemiological studies of salmonella and campylobacter in poultry: a cross-sectional survey of thermophilic campylobacter infection of broiler flocks in England and Wales. PhD Thesis, University of London

Evans S J, Sayers A R 2000 A longitudinal study of *Campylobacter* infection of broiler flocks in Great Britain. Prev Vet Med 46: 209–223

Genigeorgis C, Hassuneh M, Collins P 1986 *Campylobacter jejuni* infection on poultry farms and its effect on poultry meat contamination during slaughtering. J Food Prot 49: 895–903

Gibbens J C, Pascoe S J S, Evans S J et al 2000 A trial of biosecurity as a means to control *Campylobacter* infection of broiler chickens. Prev Vet Med 48: 85–99

Hakkinen M, Schneitz C 1999 Efficacy of a commercial competitive exclusion product against *Campylobacter jejuni*. Br Poult Sci 40: 619–621

Hald B, Wedderkopp A, Madsen M 2000 Thermophilic *Campylobacter* spp. in Danish broiler production: a cross-sectional survey and a retrospective analysis of risk factors for occurrence in broiler flocks. Avian Pathol 29: 123–131

Hald B, Skovgard H, Bang D D et al 2004 Flies and *Campylobacter* infection of broiler flocks. Emerg Infect Dis 10: 1490–1492

Hansson I, Engvall E O, Lindblad J et al 2004 Surveillance programme for *Campylobacter* species in Swedish broilers, July 2001 to June 2002. Vet Rec 155: 193–196

Hansson I, Ederoth M, Andersson L et al 2005 Transmission of *Campylobacter* spp. to chickens during transport to slaughter. J Appl Microbiol 99: 1149–1157

Harris N V, Weiss N S, Nolan C M 1986 The role of poultry and meats in the etiology of *Campylobacter jejuni/coli* enteritis. Am J Public Health 76: 407–411

Hofshagen M, Kruse H 2005 Reduction in flock prevalence of *Campylobacter* spp. in broilers in Norway after implementation of an action plan. J Food Prot 68: 2220–2223

Hood A M, Pearson A D, Shahamat M 1988 The extent of surface contamination of retailed chickens with *Campylobacter jejuni* serotypes. Epidemiol Infect 100: 17–25

Humphrey T J, Henley A, Lanning D G 1993 The colonisation of broiler chickens with *Campylobacter jejuni*: some epidemiological investigations. Epidemiol Infect 110: 601–607

Jacobs-Reitsma W F, van de Giessen A W, Bolder N M, Mulder R W 1995 Epidemiology of *Campylobacter* spp. at two Dutch broiler farms. Epidemiol Infect 114: 413–421

Kapperud G, Skjerve E, Vik L et al 1993 Epidemiological investigation of risk factors for campylobacter colonization in Norwegian broiler flocks. Epidemiol Infect 111: 245–255

Kramer J M, Frost J A, Bolton F J, Wareing D R A 2000 *Campylobacter* contamination of raw meat and poultry at retail sale: identification of multiple types and comparison with isolates from human infection. J Food Prot 63: 1654–1659

Loc Carrillo C, Atterbury R J, el-Shibiny A et al 2005 Bacteriophage therapy to reduce *Campylobacter jejuni* colonization of broiler chickens. Appl Environ Microbiol 71: 6554–6563

Louis V R, Gillespie I A, O'Brien S J et al 2005 Temperature-driven *Campylobacter* seasonality in England and Wales. Appl Environ Microbiol 71: 85–92

Mead G C, Hudson W R, Hinton M H 1995 Effects of changes in processing to improve hygiene control on contamination of poultry carcasses with campylobacter. Epidemiol Infect 115: 495–500

Nachamkin I, Blaser M J 2000 *Campylobacter*, 2nd edn. American Society for Microbiology, Washington, DC

Newell D G, Fearnley C 2003 Sources of *Campylobacter* colonization in broiler chickens. Appl Environ Microbiol 69: 4343–4351

Pearson AD, Greenwood M, Healing TD et al 1993 Colonization of broiler chickens by waterborne *Campylobacter jejuni*. Appl Environ Microbiol 59: 987–996

Ramabu S S, Boxall N S, Madie P, Fenwick S G 2004 Some potential sources for transmission of *Campylobacter jejuni* to broiler chickens. Lett Appl Microbiol 39: 252–256

Rollins D M, Colwell R 1986 Viable but non-culturable stage of *Campylobacter jejuni* and its role in survival in the natural aquatic environment. Appl Environ Microbiol 52: 531–538

Sahin O, Luo N, Huang S, Zhang Q 2003 Effect of *Campylobacter*-specific maternal antibodies on *Campylobacter jejuni* colonization in young chickens. Appl Environ Microbiol 69: 5372–5379

Shanker S, Lee A, Sorell T C 1986 *Campylobacter jejuni* in broilers: the role of vertical transmission. J Hyg 96: 153–159

Stern N J 1994 Mucosal competitive exclusion to diminish colonisation of chickens by *Campylobacter jejuni*. Poult Sci 73: 402–403

Thwaites R T, Frost J A 1999 Drug resistance in *Campylobacter jejuni*, *C. coli*, and *C. lari* isolated from humans in North West England and Wales, 1997. J Clin Pathol 52: 812–814

Van de Giessen A W, Bloemberg B P M, Ritmeester W S, Tilburg J J 1996 Epidemiological study on risk factors and risk reducing measures for campylobacter infections in Dutch broiler flocks. Epidemiol Infect 117: 245–250

Van de Giessen A W, Tilburg J J, Ritmeester W S, van der Plas J 1998 Reduction of campylobacter infections in broiler flocks by application of hygiene measures. Epidemiol Infect 121: 57–66

Van Gerwe T J, Bouma A, Jacobs-Reitsma W F et al 2005 Quantifying transmission of *Campylobacter* spp. among broilers. Appl Environ Microbiol 71: 5765–5770

Wagenaar J A, Van Bergen M A, Mueller M A et al 2005 Phage therapy reduces *Campylobacter jejuni* colonization in broilers. Vet Microbiol 109: 275–283

Wassenaar T M, Newell D G 2000 Genotyping and *Campylobacter* spp. Appl Environ Microbiol 66: 1–9

Wedderkopp A, Rattenborg E, Madsen M 2000 National surveillance of *Campylobacter* in broilers at slaughter in Denmark in 1998. Avian Dis 44: 993–999

Wheeler J G, Sethi D, Cowden J M et al 1999 Study of infectious intestinal disease in England: rates in the community, presenting to general practice, and reported to national surveillance. Br Med J 318: 1046–1050

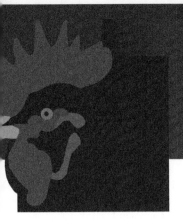

Joan A. Smyth and
Perpetua T. McNamee

Staphylococci, streptococci and enterococci

STAPHYLOCOCCI

Staphylococci are Gram-positive cocci belonging to the family *Micrococcaceae*, genus *Staphylococcus*. The genus continues to undergo revision, with seven new species accepted since 1997, and there are now 39 species listed in the genus. *Staphylococcus aureus* is the most common isolate from lesions in diseased birds but other staphylococcal species (both coagulase-positive and coagulase-negative) are sometimes involved. Staphylococci are associated with a wide variety of diseases in the chicken and turkey, and in other avian species. These include septicaemia, arthritis and tenosynovitis, bacterial chondronecrosis and osteomyelitis, gangrenous dermatitis, yolk sac infection, subdermal abscesses (bumble foot), comb necrosis and often with cellulitis, endocarditis and granulomas. Staphylococci have also been recovered from dead-in-shell embryos, blepharitis/conjunctivitis, salpingitis/salpingoperitonitis, a case of pneumonia in 3-day-old turkey poults and as a secondary infection in swollen head syndrome.

EPIDEMIOLOGY

Cause

Staphylococci are facultative anaerobes, catalase-positive and grow readily on blood agar. In contrast to mammalian strains, which are usually β-haemolytic, poultry strains of *S. aureus* usually show α- or δ-haemolysis. They grow in 6.5% NaCl supplemented media but not on MacConkey agar.

Capsular-typing, phage-typing, biotyping and more recently pulsed-field gel electrophoresis have been used for the recognition of *S. aureus* strains. Variation in virulence occurs among strains.

Hosts

Staphylococcal infections affect domestic poultry and many other avian species. They are common inhabitants of the skin and mucous membranes, and of the poultry environment.

Spread

Both pathogenic and nonpathogenic strains of staphylococci are ubiquitous and may be found on and in the bodies of birds and mammals, and are common in the environment of poultry. *S. aureus* can be found on the skin, in the nares and on the feet of apparently normal chickens and wild birds. They can also be found on hatchery fluff, work surfaces and in the air of hatcheries, and in the air and litter of poultry houses. More than one strain may be found in a flock but one often predominates. The organism can survive away from the host for many months, particularly under dry conditions.

Infection or contamination of hatching eggs and the environment are probably of most significance in the epidemiology and when disease exists staphylococci are more prevalent in the environment. Social and environmental 'stress' and simultaneous or earlier infections with other pathogens may lower resistance to this organism. For instance, staphylococcal arthritis can be a recurring problem in broiler breeders during rearing when feed restriction is maximal. Staphylococci have been recovered from semen.

DISEASES

Pathogenesis

Colonization of the upper respiratory tract in early life increases the likelihood of disease developing, particularly if birds are later infected with immunosuppressive viruses. Injury to the skin or mucous membrane may facilitate tissue invasion. The unhealed navel in chicks may also be a route for infection.

S. aureus is primarily an extracellular pathogen. It produces a range of cell surface factors and exotoxins that contribute to the virulence, during either attachment to host cells, evasion of host defences or while invading host tissues. During attachment, *S. aureus* can express cell surface factors known as microbial surface components recognizing adhesive matrix molecules (MSCRAMMs) that allow adherence to host tissues and initiate colonization. A study of 13 strains of *S. aureus*, recovered from infections in poultry, found that all strains harboured genes that encode for the virulence determinants protein-A, fibronectin-binding proteins (FnBp) A and B and clumping factors (Clf) A and B. However, only 20% of the 13 strains harboured the gene encoding for collagen adherence protein (CNA), which can bind to collagen present in bone and other tissues. In order to evade host defences, *S. aureus* can also produce an array of factors that interfere with the mechanisms of host immune systems for example protein-A, which can disrupt immunoglobulin-mediated opsonization and phagocytosis. Expression of capsular polysaccharide (CP) has also been shown to be important in the process of infection, by protecting *S. aureus* from the host immune response. In French and North American studies the majority of *S. aureus* isolates from poultry express either CP5 or CP8 serotype and CP5 is the predominant type.

To assist tissue invasion, *S. aureus* has the ability to produce a range of toxins and enzymes capable of breaking down host proteins, nucleic acids and lipids. Exotoxin production by isolates of *S. aureus* from humans has been the most extensively studied. At least 16 of the toxins are superantigens. Toxins produced include exfoliative toxin A or B, toxic shock syndrome toxin and several enterotoxins. Eighteen enterotoxin genes have been identified to date. The occurrence of genes for these exotoxins has been comparatively poorly studied in poultry isolates. Of 34 isolates from poultry in USA, only one contained a classical staphylococcal enterotoxin (SE). Of 15 isolates recovered from poultry in Northern Ireland, none contained a classical SE gene but 14 were positive for one or more of the more recently described SE genes. The same research showed that the frequency of occurrence of the genes varied markedly with geographical region. The contribution of enterotoxins to the pathogenicity of *S. aureus* in poultry is unknown.

Much remains to be learned about the occurrence of the various virulence factors in strains of *S. aureus* infecting poultry, and their role in poultry disease.

Clinical signs and lesions

Staphylococcal infection can lead to a wide variety of diseases. The main manifestations are described here.

Septicaemia

Birds may be found dead but commonly there are signs of lameness in the flock. The gross and histological lesions in birds dead from septicaemia are similar to those described below for streptococcal septicaemia. The lameness may be caused by arthritis and/or tenosynovitis in birds of any age, or in young birds it may be due also to bacterial chondronecrosis and osteomyelitis.

Arthritis and tenosynovitis

These conditions may occur in birds of any age. In broiler breeders, stress caused by uneven feed distribution or aggression may predispose to staphylococcal infection. The affected joints, usually the hocks, are hot, swollen and painful and affected birds are usually depressed, lame and reluctant to walk. In tenosynovitis, the synovial membranes of tendon sheaths (commonly in the region of the hock and feet) become thickened and oedematous, with fibrinous exudate within and around the tendon sheaths. The exudate may become caseous. *S. aureus* is the most common isolate, but other staphylococcal species, including *Staphylococcus epidermidis*, have been recovered.

Bacterial chondronecrosis and osteomyelitis

S. aureus is the most common isolate from bacterial chondronecrosis and osteomyelitis of chickens, turkeys, ducks and geese. *Staphylococcus hyicus* and less commonly other staphylococcal species have been recovered from bone lesions in both chickens and turkeys. *Escherichia coli* has also been recovered from such lesions, particularly in turkeys. This disease is the most common cause of lameness in broiler chickens accounting for 17.3% of lame male birds in the first 42 days of life and for 17.4% of mortalities in fattening turkeys from 16 weeks of age until slaughter. In turkeys, the disease is often associated with green discoloration of the liver. Although sometimes called femoral head necrosis, the proximal end of the tibiotarsus is also commonly affected (Fig. 17.1) and occasionally other bones including vertebrae may be affected. Since many lesions are not visible to the naked eye and may occur in one of several possible sites, the disease is likely underdiagnosed.

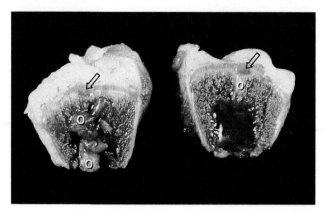

Fig. 17.1 Chondronecrosis (arrows) with osteomyelitis (o) in the proximal end of tibiotarsal bones. The osteomyelitis extends well into the marrow cavity in the left specimen.

Gangrenous dermatitis

This may occur in birds of all ages, but most commonly in broiler chickens. The wing tips and back are most frequently affected. The skin is dark and often moist or weeping, and the underlying tissue may be oedematous. Staphylococci have been recovered, commonly together with *Clostridium* spp. Experimentally, *S. aureus* isolates have had variable ability to produce gangrenous dermatitis, some strains only doing so when in combination with *Clostridium septicum*. The staphylococcal isolates from Japanese cases produce comparatively high levels of a thiol (cysteine) protease and produce dermatolysis when inoculated into chickens and mice. The gene encoding for this protease was not recognized in the tested bovine and porcine strains or low protease-producing avian strains.

Subdermal abscesses

Subdermal abscesses most commonly affect the feet (bumble foot) and sternal bursa. They occur most frequently in mature birds, particularly those of the heavy breeds. Caseous material accumulates and there may be swelling, heat and pain. In bumble foot, the undersurface of the foot is first involved but the whole foot may become affected.

Endocarditis and granuloma

Vegetative endocarditis may also be a sequel to septicaemic infection, and particularly affects the left atrioventricular valves. Small granulomatous lesions may occur in liver, and sometimes in spleen and kidney.

Pneumonia

There has been a recent report of *S. aureus* pneumonia in association with heavy contamination by *S. aureus* in the hatchery. Grossly, these lesions resembled aspergillosis, however, histologically, intralesional Gram-positive cocci but no fungi, were observed. *S. aureus* was recovered in pure culture.

DIAGNOSIS

The clinical history, signs and lesions may be helpful but other organisms, such as *Escherichia coli*, salmonellas, *Pasteurella multocida, Mycoplasma synoviae* and reoviruses, may cause some of the disease conditions described. Gram-stained smears of blood, liver and spleen may also be helpful but it is necessary to isolate and identify *S. aureus* to confirm diagnosis. For diagnosis of bacterial chondronecrosis and osteomyelitis the bones should be split longitudinally for examination.

CONTROL

Birds in the early stages of infection and disease may respond to treatment but those with well-established lesions are unlikely to respond. *S. aureus* is inherently a rather resistant organism. It is therefore important that antimicrobial sensitivity testing is carried out when faced with disease problems. Penicillin, streptomycin, tetracyclines, erythromycin, novobiocin, sulphona-mide, lincomycin, spectinomycin and fluoroquinolones have all been used with some success, but antibiotic resistance is common. *S. aureus* has intrinsic resistance to many antibiotics and can acquire resistance via mobile genetic elements encoding resistance mechanisms. *S. aureus* strains recovered from poultry flocks in Denmark have shown resistance to fluoroquinolones, tetracyclines and macrolides. There are a few reports of methicillin-resistant strains of *S. aureus* recovered from samples collected in poultry slaughterhouses. Methicillin-resistant coagulase-negative staphylococci have also been isolated from poultry in Japan.

Attempts to reduce staphylococcal contamination of the environment, particularly in the hatchery, are important. Effective control and prevention of exposure to immunosuppressive viruses and avoidance of stress and aggression are likely to be beneficial. Bacterial interference using *S. epidermidis* by aerosol has been effective in reducing staphylococcal infections in both chickens and turkeys.

FURTHER READING

Andreasen C B 2003 Staphylococcosis. In: Saif Y M (ed) Diseases of poultry, 11th edn. Iowa State University Press, Ames, p 798–804

Devriese L A 1980 Pathogenic staphylococci in poultry. World's Poult Sci J 36: 227–234

Dinges M M, Orwin P O, Schlievert P M 2000 Exotoxins of *Staphylococcus*. Clin Microbiol Rev 13: 16–34

McNamee P T, Smyth J A 2000 Bacterial chondronecrosis with osteomyelitis ('femoral head necrosis') of broiler chickens. Avian Pathol 29: 477–496

Nicoll T R, Jensen M M 1987 Staphylococcosis of turkeys. 5. Large scale control programs using bacterial interference. Avian Dis 31: 85–88

Quinn P J, Carter M E, Markey B K et al 1994 Clinical veterinary microbiology. Wolfe, London

Rodgers J 2003 An investigation into *Staphylococcus aureus* associated with chicken disease; charac-terisation, control measures and interactions with the chicken immune system. PhD thesis, Queens University, Belfast

Takeuchi, S, Matsunaga K, Inubushi S et al 2002 Structural gene and strain specificity of a novel cysteine protease produced by *Staphylococcus aureus* isolated from a diseased chicken. Vet Microbiol 89: 201–210

STREPTOCOCCI AND ENTEROCOCCI

Streptococci and enterococci are Gram-positive cocci. The enterococci were formerly classified as Lancefield's Group D streptococci, but they are now assigned to a separate genus within the family *Streptococcaceae*. These genera continue to undergo revision as the application of molecular techniques, in particular 16S rRNA gene sequencing, generates discriminating genetic information. Since 2000, several new species have been identified and currently more than 50 species of streptococci and at least 21 species of enterococci are recognized. In terms of poultry disease, the most noteworthy new species is *Streptococcus gallinaceus*, which has been associated with outbreaks of septicaemia and endocarditis in breeding birds. Organisms previously classified as *Streptococcus bovis* are now suggested to represent five different streptococcal species. Thus, isolates of *S. bovis* that can degrade gallate are now assigned to a new species, *Streptococcus gallolyticus*. Several isolates recovered from septicaemia in pigeons have now been shown to be *S. gallolyticus*. Older literature does not discriminate between these new species and *S. bovis*.

Among the streptococci, *Streptococcus zooepidemicus* (*Streptococcus equi* subsp. *zooepidemicus*) has most frequently been associated with disease in the past but *Streptococcus gallinaceus* has been identified in some disease outbreaks since 2000. In the last decade there have been an increased number of reports of disease associated with enterococci, particularly with *Enterococcus hirae*, *Enterococcus durans* and *Enterococcus faecalis*. Diseases associated with streptococci or enterococci in poultry, although worldwide in distribution, are relatively uncommon. However, it has recently been shown that early mortalities in flocks, which are likely to be attributed to 'poor chick quality', are in some cases due to enterococcal infections. Thus infections may currently be underdiagnosed. It has been suggested that the increased number of outbreaks seen in Denmark in recent years may be a consequence of the banning of antibiotic growth promoters. Septicaemic streptococcal infection is probably more common in ducks and pigeons than in other species. Such infections are mainly due to *Streptococcus bovis/gallolyticus* (note: gallate degrading strains of which are now assigned to the species *S. gallolyticus*). Streptococci and/or enterococci have been recovered from cases of yolk sac infection, cellulitis, blepharitis/conjunctivitis, endocarditis, arthritis, amyloid arthropathy, osteomyelitis and salpingitis/salpingoperitonitis in chickens and turkeys, and from dead-in-shell embryos.

EPIDEMIOLOGY

Cause

The organisms are Gram-positive facultative anaerobes, usually occurring in chains or in pairs when in broth culture or in tissues. They are usually catalase-negative and can be grown on blood agar, although they are more fastidious than staphylococci. Incubation in a CO_2-enriched (5–10%) atmosphere can enhance growth. Identification of species can be aided by the colonial morphology and the type of haemolysis produced. The enterococci can be grown in the presence of bile and thus they can grow on MacConkey agar plates, unlike staphylococci. Enterococci form a dark brown/black pigment in bile aesculin medium and are also heat-resistant (60°C/30 min).

Hosts

Streptococci and enterococci are intestinal inhabitants of birds and mammals. They have also been recovered from the surface of eggs, normal salt glands in ducklings and, in the case of streptococci, from semen. The organisms are not commonly recovered from other sites.

Spread

Enterococci and streptococci can be recovered from the environment of poultry, including hatchers and hatchery air samples. They are rather susceptible to the effects of drying. Spread is direct through the egg or indirect by the oral or respiratory routes and perhaps skin wounds. *S. zooepidemicus* affects mainly mature chickens while the enterococci can cause disease in birds of any age. Severity is always greater in embryos, young chicks and poults. Other factors probably influence disease associated with these infections. A recent study compared enterococci recovered from farms using antimicrobial feed additives with those where antimicrobials were not used and found that the resident population of enterococci was not affected, but other studies conclude that antimicrobials do affect resident populations.

A study of four outbreaks of enterococcal disease in broilers showed some degree of clonality of isolates within flocks in three outbreaks, with either one or two dominant pulsed-field gel electrophoresis (PFGE) types. However, different clones occurred between flocks. In a fourth outbreak isolates were spread across six PFGE types.

DISEASE

Streptococci and enterococci can cause both septicaemic and localized infections in chickens, turkeys, ducks, pigeons and other birds. Septicaemic streptococcal infection is probably more common in ducks and pigeons than in other species.

Septicaemia

In chickens, septicaemia is most common in adults but may occur at any age. Birds may be found dead. Usually there is marked depression with ruffled feathers, pallor or cyanosis of the face and comb and bloodstaining of feathers around the head. Mortality can vary but may reach 50%. Egg production may fall and, in hatching eggs, there is late-embryo mortality.

Gross lesions include carcass congestion, splenomegaly and, more variably, hepatomegaly. There may be serosanguineous fluid subcutaneously, in the pericardial sac or in the trachea. Small necrotic foci from pinpoint to 1 cm in diameter may be seen in the liver or occasionally in the kidney. In more chronic cases there may be fibrinous pericarditis, perihepatitis and pneumonia.

S. bovis/gallolyticus is a common cause of septicaemia in pigeons and *S. bovis* septicaemia has also been reported in ducks and occasionally in turkey flocks. It is possible that at least some of these cases may have been caused by *S. gallolyticus*. These streptococci are associated with increased mortality, enlarged mottled spleens and dark livers, which may have multifocal necrosis. *S. bovis (gallolyticus)* is common in the intestinal tract of pigeons but uncommon in other species. This may be of epidemiological significance.

Cellulitis

Cellulitis has become an important cause of carcass condemnations. Affected birds usually appear healthy, but when the feathers are removed, areas of skin may appear thickened or discoloured ('waffle skin'). Caseous plaques, which may be quite extensive, can be found under the skin. *Streptococcus dysgalactia* has been recovered from dermatitis/cellulitis lesions together with *E. coli* in both chickens and turkeys.

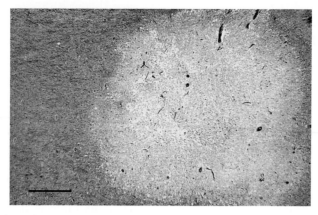

Fig. 17.2 Discrete focus of necrosis (malacia) associated with *Enterococcus hirae* infection in brainstem of a chicken. Bar = 625 μm.

Encephalomalacia

There have been several reports of mortalities due to encephalomalacia associated with *Enterococcus hirae* or *Enterococcus durans* infections. This occurs from 3–12 days of age and a morbidity rate of up to 4% has been reported. Affected chicks may be found dead or exhibit nervous signs (torticollis is common). Malacic lesions are found most commonly in the brainstem and lesions may be up to 5 mm in diameter (Fig. 17.2). There is a recent report describing for the first time, the presence of typical lesions and recovery of bacteria from the optic lobe and cerebral peduncles. Encephalomalacia suggestive of enterococcal infection accounted for 22% of all histologically diagnosed brain disorders of broilers in one US study.

Endocarditis

E. hirae has been recovered from lesions of vegetative endocarditis in young birds, while *Enterococcus faecalis* has been recovered from similar lesions in older birds. *S. gallinaceus, S. equi* subsp. *zooepidemicus, Enterococcus faecium* and *E. durans* have also been recovered from cases of endocarditis in chickens.

Bone and joint disorders

E. faecalis was commonly recovered from amyloidotic joints of chickens, and amyloid arthropathy has been reproduced experimentally by infecting with *E. faecalis. Enterococcus cecorum* has been recovered from a case of bacterial chondronecrosis with osteomyelitis in broiler chickens.

DIAGNOSIS

With the possible exception of *E. hirae*-associated encephalomalacia, the clinical signs and lesions are not specific for streptococcal or enterococcal infection. Congested carcasses with hepatomegaly and splenomegaly may suggest a septicaemic infection but other bacteria such as staphylococci, *Pasteurella, Erysipelothrix* and *E. coli* may produce similar signs and lesions.

Enterococcus-associated encephalomalacia must be differentiated from encephalomalacia associated with vitamin E deficiency. Cerebellar lesions are consistently present in the latter (often evident grossly) but are uncommon in the former.

Diagnosis is dependent on demonstration of the causal organism. Demonstration of Gram-positive cocci in smears from blood, liver, spleen or other lesions may be helpful but culture and identification of the organism is necessary to confirm a diagnosis. *S. equi* subsp. *zooepidemicus* is β-haemolytic while *S. bovis* is nonhaemolytic. Most grow in selective media containing 6.5% NaCl (*S. bovis* is an exception) and may then be distinguished from staphylococci by their negative catalase reaction.

CONTROL

A number of drugs, such as the quinolones, penicillins, macrolides and the tetracyclines, have been of value in treatment of the acute disease. Isolates should be subjected to sensitivity tests in support of treatment. In view of concerns about acquisition of antibiotic resistance by organisms causing disease in humans, there are many published studies examining resistance patterns (particularly to vancomycin) of enterococci recovered from food animals fed antimicrobial growth promoters.

A *S. gallolyticus* strain of low virulence failed to immunize pigeons against strains of high virulence of the same serotype, indicating that serotype-specific antigens do not induce a protective response.

FURTHER READING

Buxton J C 1952 Disease in poultry associated with *Streptococcus zooepidemicus*. Vet Rec 64: 221–222

Chadfield, M S, Christensen J P, Juhl-Hansen J et al 2005 Characterization of *Enterococcus hirae* outbreaks in broiler flocks demonstrating increased mortality because of septicemia and endocarditis and/or altered production parameters. Avian Dis 49: 16–23

Chamanza R, Fabri T H F, van Veen L, Dwars R M 1998 Enterococcus-associated encephalomalacia in one-week-old chicks. Vet Rec 143: 450–451

Devriese L A, Hommez J, Wijfels R, Haesebrouck F 1991 Composition of the enterococcal and streptococcal intestinal flora of poultry. J Appl Bacteriol 71: 46–50

Facklam R 2002 What happened to the streptococci: overview of taxonomic and nomenclature changes. Clin Microbiol Rev 15: 613–630

Facklam R R, Sahm D F 1995 Enterococcus. In: Murray P R et al (eds) Manual of clinical microbiology, 6th edn. ASM Press, Washington, DC, p 308–314

Peckham M C 1966 An outbreak of streptococcosis (apoplectiform septicaemia) in White Rock chickens. Avian Dis 10: 413–421

Quinn P J, Carter M E, Markey B K, Carter G R 1994 Clinical veterinary microbiology. Mosby Wolfe, London

Randall C J, Pearson D B 1991 Enterococcal endocarditis causing heart failure in broilers. Vet Rec 129: 535

Ruoff K L 1995 Streptococcus. In: Murray P R et al (eds) Manual of clinical microbiology, 6th edn. ASM Press, Washington, DC, p 299–307

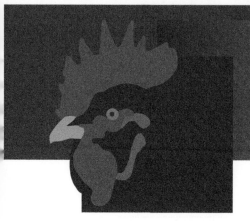

18

Magne Kaldhusdal and
Frank T. W. Jordan

Clostridia

Four disease conditions involving mainly one of four clostridial species (*Clostridium perfringens*, *Clostridium colinum*, *Clostridium botulinum* and *Clostridium septicum*) are described in this chapter. Although a number of other clostridia (*Clostridium chauvoei*, *Clostridium difficile*, *Clostridium fallax*, *Clostridium novyi*, *Clostridium sordelli* and *Clostridium sporogenes*) have been associated with disease in poultry, this chapter will focus on those conditions that are considered of major importance.

Clostridia are large, Gram-positive, rod-shaped, toxin-producing bacteria that are anaerobic and can produce endospores as a means of survival. They are ubiquitous worldwide, being found in soil, dust, animals and insect larvae. They are frequently found in low numbers in the intestinal tract of normal birds. Factors that predispose to outbreaks of disease in a flock are important. These factors include management, nutrition and environmental conditions. Overcrowding of birds kept on litter, predisposing feed factors and inadequate hygiene routines are the main issues.

Increasing restrictions on the use of in-feed antimicrobials in Europe and other regions has changed the status of *C. perfringens*-associated necrotic enteritis in poultry, especially broilers, from one of history to one of emerging importance. Developing a nonantibiotic preventive strategy against this disease is one of today's major challenges with regard to poultry health and welfare.

CLOSTRIDIUM PERFRINGENS (NECROTIC ENTERITIS AND HEPATIC DISEASE)

The two most well-known forms of *C. perfringens*-associated disease in poultry are necrotic enteritis and cholangiohepatitis.

Necrotic enteritis is found worldwide, and is a disease of increasing importance owing to ever-increasing restrictions on the preventive use of in-feed antimicrobials. Clinical disease may have devastating effects on production. Milder forms, including subclinical disease, are more common, and may exert a significantly negative impact on production.

The most common form of *C. perfringens*-associated liver disease is cholangiohepatitis. *C. perfringens* has also been implicated in wet litter problems and impaired production performance but without the detection of specific lesions.

EPIDEMIOLOGY

Cause

Toxin types A and C of *C. perfringens* have been associated with necrotic enteritis although most cases appear to be caused by type A. Although several molecular subtypes of *C. perfringens* may be present in healthy flocks and even in flocks with subclinical necrotic enteritis, only one or a few subtypes seem to proliferate in flocks affected by clinical disease.

Subtypes isolated from affected birds in different flocks may differ, and it has not yet been possible to relate any specific subtype to disease induction.

C. perfringens toxin type A has been isolated from livers of birds with cholangiohepatitis.

Hosts

Necrotic enteritis is most common in broiler chickens, young replacement broiler breeders and young meat turkeys. Broilers aged 2–5 weeks are most frequently affected. The disease is also regularly found in layers, mostly in pullets and young birds kept on litter.

Necrotic enteritis has been reported in farmed ostriches, captive capercaillies, wild geese and wild crows. It has also been reported in domestic geese and ducks but the involvement of *C. perfringens* has not been well documented. *C. perfringens*-associated liver disease has apparently only been reported in chickens.

In humans *C. perfringens* toxin type C-associated necrotizing enterocolitis mainly affects severely protein-deprived populations in poor countries or more rarely, susceptible individuals in the developed world. A few cases of toxin-type-A-associated necrotizing enterocolitis in previously healthy adults have been reported. See also section on Public health considerations.

Spread

C. perfringens type A is ubiquitous in nature. It is commonly found in intestinal contents of broiler chickens from 2 weeks of age and throughout the rearing period. It is also found in environmental samples from within and outside the chicken house before placement and during rearing, on cages used for transportation of birds to the slaughterhouse and in carcasses. This organism is able to grow faster than most other pathogenic bacteria if the conditions are optimal. An in vitro generation time of 7 min at 41°C has been reported. *C. perfringens* is spore-forming and therefore able to survive under variable environmental conditions for extended periods.

Horizontal transmission is assumed to be the significant means of dissemination but findings have been published suggesting that even vertical transmission is a possibility. Molecular subtyping of *C. perfringens* isolates suggests that organisms contaminating the processed product could originate from the poultry environment prior to grow out. Further, *C. perfringens* may be transmitted between facilities within an integrated broiler chicken operation. Spread within a flock kept on litter predominantly takes place via the faecal–oral route but flies are also suspected to be of importance as mechanical vectors. Another potential source of infection is feed, which may be contaminated despite pelleting and heat treatment. Fish meal is considered a particularly likely source of *C. perfringens* contamination.

The incidence of cholangiohepatitis shows a striking parallel with the incidence of necrotic enteritis, which suggests that this is another manifestation of clinical or subclinical necrotic enteritis and that the sources of infection are the same.

Influencing factors

The risk of necrotic enteritis is low when birds are kept on wire floors or other types of housing that minimizes their contact with faeces. However, if other predisposing factors are present, necrotic enteritis outbreaks occasionally appear even in birds kept on wire floors.

Data have been published suggesting that low-level maternal immunity against *C. perfringens* is associated with an increased risk of necrotic enteritis in broiler chickens. Birds are likely to be particularly susceptible during the time when maternal antibodies have waned and the level of actively produced specific antibodies is still low. Published data suggest that broiler offspring from young parent hens have lower levels of maternal antibodies against *C. perfringens* than chicks derived from older parents.

Commonly used dietary protein sources of animal origin (e.g. fish meal, meat and bone meal and feather meal) seem to be associated with a higher risk of necrotic enteritis than some relevant protein sources of plant origin (e.g. soy protein concentrate). These differences between feed ingredients have been correlated with dietary glycine levels, and experiments have established a direct causative link between dietary glycine level and *C. perfringens* counts, suggesting that high levels of glycine may be a predisposing factor for necrotic enteritis. High levels of crude dietary proteins may also be a risk factor.

Several studies indicate that maize-based diets may contribute to the prevention of necrotic enteritis, and that maize compares favourably with wheat, barley and rye in this respect. The mechanism behind the effect of cereal type on *C. perfringens* and necrotic enteritis is not established.

There is experimental evidence suggesting that dietary fat may be of importance. Intestinal counts of *C. perfringens* in soy-oil-fed broilers were lower than in broilers fed a mixture of lard and tallow. Feed structure may also be of significance. Whole-wheat feeding has been reported to lower the pH of gizzard contents and to reduce intestinal counts of *C. perfringens*.

Mucosal damage induced by coccidia, in particular *Eimeria* species that colonize the small intestine, is an important predisposing factor. Although *Eimeria tenella* does not induce lesions in the small intestine where necrotic enteritis lesions usually develop, caecal coccidiosis may increase the shedding of *C. perfringens* and consequently the contamination of the bird environment.

Management is assumed to be particularly important with regard to a multifactorial disease such as necrotic enteritis. Management is an integral part of an ill-defined factor often designated the 'farm effect'. This has been shown to be significantly associated with *C. perfringens*-associated health problems in commercial broilers. More work is needed to increase our knowledge of the effect of specific management factors on *C. perfringens* and necrotic enteritis.

DISEASE

Pathogenesis

The pathogenesis of necrotic enteritis is incompletely understood. The presence in the intestine of *C. perfringens* alone is not sufficient to induce necrotic enteritis. The following two requirements for induction of necrotic enteritis have been proposed: (1) the presence of some factor caus-ing damage to the intestinal mucosa, and (2) the presence of higher than normal numbers of intes-tinal *C. perfringens* organisms. If these two requirements are fulfilled, lesions may develop, often starting at the tips of the villi. Bacterial cells adhere to damaged epithelium and denuded lamina propria where they proliferate and induce coagulative necrosis. Attraction and lysis of heterophil granulocytes as well as further tissue necrosis and bacterial proliferation proceed rap-idly. The alpha toxin, a necrotizing toxin produced by all the toxin types, has been assumed to be an important virulence factor involved in this process. This toxin destroys cell membranes by recognition and hydrolysis of membrane phospholipids. Toxins may also enter the blood stream, causing systemic effects and death. The potential role of toxins other than alpha toxin has not been documented so far.

In the pathogenesis of cholangiohepatitis, which is poorly understood, it has been pro-posed that *C. perfringens* or its toxins may reach the liver via the portal blood or via the bile. Cholangiohepatitis, which is the most common form of *C. perfringens*-associated liver disease, has been reproduced experimentally by inoculation of *C. perfringens* into the hepatoenteric bile duct or by ligation of both bile ducts. These results suggest that *C. perfringens* organisms and/or toxins may reach the liver and lead to bile stasis and inflammation of the biliary tract.

Clinical signs

Clinical signs are variable and nonspecific. Acute necrotic enteritis is characterized by increased mortality but few visibly sick birds, indicating that affected birds die rapidly. Clinical signs in birds from outbreaks with a more protracted course include depression, decreased feed intake, reluctance to move, ruffled feathers and diarrhoea. The mildest form of necrotic enteritis induces no visible illness of the birds but is associated with temporarily reduced weight gain, impaired feed conversion ratio and increased condemnation rates at slaughter due to liver lesions.

Cholangiohepatitis is usually detected at slaughter or as an incidental finding during necropsy of birds collected during the rearing period. In each flock with a given number of birds affected by the disease, a much higher total number of birds have, most probably, been affected by sub-clinical and possibly clinical necrotic enteritis during the rearing period.

Lesions

Gross lesions

The characteristic gross lesion of necrotic enteritis is a pseudomembrane attached to the intes-tinal mucosa, primarily the small intestine. The mucosa of the caecal pouches are not changed but the caecal tonsils and adjoining narrow segments of the caeca may occasionally be affected. The extension of the pseudomembrane is variable, from barely visible spots affecting some villi to diffuse necrosis of the entire mucosa. The pseudomembrane may be partly or entirely detached from the viable mucosa, leaving behind a depression or a more extended smooth sur-face that on first sight may appear normal. Haemorrhage and hyperaemia may or may not be associated with the mucosal lesions. The pseudomembrane may be white, yellow, green, brown or red. A yellow or green discoloration is most commonly found. The affected gut segment may be dilated and soft with fluid contents, or the gut wall may appear turgid and rigid with dry and sparse luminal contents. A detached pseudomembrane is occasionally found in the gut lumen. The contents of the caecal pouches are often dark and dry.

Birds dying with necrotic enteritis often show a dark liver with dilated gall bladder, pale kidneys with prominent lobular outlines, and dark and dry pectoral musculature indicating dehydration.

The body condition depends on the course of disease. Birds dying with acute necrotic enteritis are in good bodily condition.

Three main types of liver lesion may be found. The most common and most characteristic is cholangiohepatitis. Livers with the second type of lesion show light, randomly localized nodules (focal necroses and granulomas) of the liver parenchyma, and the third and most rare type is massive liver necrosis causing a smaller or larger part of a liver lobe to be homogeneously discoloured.

Cholangiohepatitis may affect both the extrahepatic and intrahepatic segments of the biliary tract. The extrahepatic bile ducts may be swollen and discoloured. The gall bladder may be oedematous, necrotic and discoloured, and may contain discoloured and inspissated bile. Inflammation of the extrahepatic biliary tract may be transmural and affect adjoining serosal surfaces. Inflammation of the intrahepatic biliary tract may be associated with the appearance of small, light islets with an irregular outline surrounded by a more normally coloured liver parenchyma. These islets are visible beneath an unaffected capsule covering a smooth liver surface. The liver parenchyma is often swollen, with a slightly yellow appearance. The liver texture is often hardened. The carcass may show ascites and yellow discoloration of body fat.

Microscopic lesions

The characteristic microscopic lesion of necrotic enteritis is an aggregation of large, Gram-positive, rod-shaped bacteria surrounded by necrotic tissue delineated from viable tissue by a zone of granulocyte infiltration containing pyknotic cell nuclei. The lesions are usually located within the lamina propria of the gut mucosa. The least extensive lesions are limited to focal necroses comprising some epithelial and stromal cells on the villus tips. The deepest lesions may even affect the muscular wall of the gut.

The principal lesions of cholangiohepatitis are necrosis and inflammation mainly associated with the biliary tract. Acute changes include Gram-positive rods or bile-like pigments surrounded by necrotic tissue. Degenerative lesions are usually accompanied by periportal inflammatory cells, including cells inducing granulomas. Bile ductule proliferation is a prominent feature in subacute to chronic lesions.

DIAGNOSIS

The gross lesions of *C. perfringens*-associated necrotic enteritis are usually diagnostic. In case of doubt, the diagnosis may be supported by bacteriology (including examination for *C. colinum*; see differential diagnosis below), histopathology and examination for coccidia. Specimens should be collected from the intestinal lesions or (for bacteriology) from intestinal contents. On a routine basis examination for *C. perfringens* on blood agar plates is an adequate support of a presumptive diagnosis based on pathology. However, a positive identification of *C. perfringens* requires more specific methods.

If subclinical necrotic enteritis is suspected, quantitative examination of freshly voided faeces may be of value, but inspection of the intestinal mucosa of randomly sampled birds immediately after properly executed killing is the preferable method. Enumeration may be based on cultivation or DNA-based methods. Procedures for DNA-based quantification of *C. perfringens* in intestinal contents have been described. Intestinal contents and faeces from affected birds usually contain more than 1 million *C. perfringens* organisms per gram, and often as much as 100 million per gram.

The gross lesions of cholangiohepatitis are usually diagnostic and the diagnosis is supported by detection of *C. perfringens* in the gall bladder.

Differential diagnosis is essential. Coccidia are often involved in field cases, as evidenced by the presence of oocysts in smears prepared from the intestinal mucosa. In chickens, severe lesions induced by *Eimeria brunetti* are similar to those of necrotic enteritis. Gut lesions induced by other pathogenic *Eimeria* spp. in chickens are distinct from those of necrotic enteritis, although lesions induced by *E. acervulina* may at first glance appear similar to mild focal lesions induced by *C. perfringens*.

Ulcerative enteritis caused by *C. colinum* induces lesions in the caeca, liver and spleen, which are uncommon in birds with necrotic enteritis. Peritonitis, caused by transmural gut lesions, is another feature of ulcerative enteritis that is not found in birds with necrotic enteritis.

In turkeys, gross gut lesions of viral haemorrhagic enteritis may be similar to those of necrotic enteritis but the pale carcass and bloody gut contents commonly found in haemorrhagic enteritis are not typical of necrotic enteritis. Turkeys with haemorrhagic enteritis show splenic cells with intranuclear viral inclusions, which are not found in birds dying with necrotic enteritis.

Liver lesions caused by congestive heart failure may appear similar to those of cholangiohepatitis. Occasionally, cases with a regular pattern of pale lesions beneath the liver capsule are found in both conditions but with congestive heart failure there is usually a fine reticular pattern of pale bands differing from the pale islets seen in cases with cholangiohepatitis. The two conditions are in most cases easily distinguished by examination of the right ventricle of the bird's heart. In cases of doubt histopathology will help differentiate between lesions primarily associated with the biliary tract (cholangiohepatitis) and lesions located mainly to the periacinar zone of the liver (congestive heart failure).

CONTROL

The most important way of controlling necrotic enteritis is through prevention.

Up to now the use of in-feed antimicrobials has been the single most important preventive measure against necrotic enteritis. From a legislative point of view, this group of feed additives comprises two subgroups. These are antibiotic growth promoters and anticoccidials. From 2006 approval of antibiotic growth promoters for use as feed additives for poultry has been withdrawn by European Union legislation. However, in-feed anticoccidials are still in use and ionophorous anticoccidials remain an important preventive measure against necrotic enteritis.

Prevention of coccidiosis remains an important factor and may be achieved by use of in-feed anticoccidials or anticoccidial vaccination. If coccidiosis is implicated, a modified prevention method for coccidiosis should be considered. The ionophorous anticoccidials are generally very effective against *C. perfringens*. If resistance among the coccidia is of no concern, these anticoccidials are therefore a good alternative.

Increasing restrictions on the use of in-feed antimicrobials have promoted the interest in nonantibiotic measures against necrotic enteritis. Nonantibiotic feed additives and oral treatments that have been proposed as potential preventive measures include probiotics or competitive exclusion products (defined and undefined microbial cultures), plant-derived products, nondigestible compounds assumed to promote a healthy gut flora (prebiotics), supplementary enzymes and acids. Promising effects in terms of suppressing growth of *C. perfringens*, and in some cases also a preventive effect on necrotic enteritis, have been reported for products within all of these groups of oral treatments but so far no single alternative measure as effective as the in-feed antimicrobials has been found.

Management and hygienic precautions are likely to be of major importance but exact knowledge about the significance of specific measures is scarce. Wood shavings may be superior to straw as litter material and keeping the litter dry and soft is likely to be favourable. Nipple drinkers may reduce the risk of *C. perfringens* transmission. A period of restricted feed intake may be beneficial in birds at particular risk, for example birds with low levels of specific antibodies.

If possible, major feed ingredients and nutrient contents should be selected on the basis of known risk factors associated with the birds (age, immunity, strain), their environment (housing conditions, farm history) and management (feeding regimen, lighting programme, stocking density). Lowering in-feed inclusion rates of animal fats, certain cereals (e.g. wheat and barley) and proteins (in particular animal proteins, including fish meal) should be considered in flocks at particular risk. The use of whole grain (e.g. whole wheat instead of ground wheat) may exert a preventive effect. Avoiding excessive heat treatment during feed processing and checking feed ingredients for *C. perfringens* should be considered if problems with a particular feed mill are suspected.

Vaccines against necrotic enteritis in poultry are not yet available but experimental work suggests that vaccination may become a significant contribution to the preventive efforts.

Treatment

Patterns of resistance against antimicrobials may vary with time, region and even farm. The antimicrobials of choice for therapeutic treatment are the penicillins, including amoxicillin. According to a recent report from Belgium, all *C. perfringens* strains tested were also sensitive to tylosin. Variable degrees and frequencies of resistance to tetracyclines have been found.

PUBLIC HEALTH CONSIDERATIONS

C. perfringens type A food poisoning is, in most cases, caused by isolates carrying a chromosomal enterotoxin gene (*cpe*). This is the most common public health problem caused by *C. perfringens* and has been associated with the consumption of meat, including poultry, that has not been handled properly. Studies have shown that enterotoxigenic strains coexist in poultry meat in relatively low numbers with much higher numbers of nonenterotoxigenic *C. perfringens* type A strains. More work is needed to assess clearly the importance of poultry meat in *C. perfringens*-associated foodborne disease in humans. See also the section on Hosts, above.

CLOSTRIDIUM COLINUM (ULCERATIVE ENTERITIS)

Ulcerative enteritis occurs worldwide. The disease is of particular importance in quail and game birds in confinement. Ulcerative enteritis is not a commonly diagnosed disease in commercial chickens and turkeys in Europe today.

EPIDEMIOLOGY

Cause

The causal organism is *Clostridium colinum*, an anaerobic spore-forming bacterium with fastidious in vitro growth requirements.

Hosts

A wide range of avian species are affected. Quail, in particular bob-white quail, are among the most susceptible species. Chickens, turkeys, pheasants, partridges, grouse and pigeons are also affected. Broiler chickens and layers are susceptible. In chickens and turkey poults, birds 3–10 weeks of age are most commonly affected. Waterfowl do not seem to be affected and infection of humans has not been reported.

Spread

C. colinum is ubiquitous in nature and is excreted in large numbers in the faeces of affected stock, which are an important source of infection. The spores result in persistent contamination of premises after an outbreak.

Influencing factors

Influencing factors appear to play an important part in the production of disease. They include coccidiosis, immunosuppressive factors such as infectious bursal disease, chick anaemia virus and others, and overcrowding and inadequate hygiene. Keeping chickens on wire floors has been reported to be preventive.

DISEASE

Clinical signs

In acute disease there may be increased mortality without any obvious signs. In other cases signs may include depression, huddling with ruffled feathers, anorexia and watery droppings.

Lesions

Gross lesions

Birds dying with acute disease show good condition and may have feed in the crop. More protracted disease may lead to emaciation. The most important lesions are found in the intestine, liver and spleen.

There are small, circular to lenticular mucosal ulcers affecting the small intestine, caeca and upper large intestine. The ulcers may penetrate as deep as the serosa, which may become perforated and result in peritonitis. The ulcers may coalesce to form large areas with a pseudomembrane. Small ulcers have a haemorrhagic border, which may be seen on the serosal and mucosal surfaces. A haemorrhagic border is less frequently found in larger lesions. Lesions with raised edges may also be found. Quail with acute disease may show haemorrhagic enteritis of the duodenum, with small red spots visible on the serosal surface.

Liver lesions are yellow–grey and of varying size. The spleen is often enlarged and haemorrhagic.

Microscopic lesions

Intestinal ulcers consist of small haemorrhagic and necrotic areas, often with clumps of Gram-positive bacteria. The ulcers involve villi and extend into the submucosa. The ulcers sometimes reach as deep as the muscular coat and serosa. Affected tissue is surrounded by granulocytes and mononuclear inflammatory cells. Liver lesions consist of multifocal foci of coagulative necrosis that are often poorly demarcated and with minimal inflammatory reaction. Gram-positive bacteria are occasionally found within the necrotic foci.

DIAGNOSIS

Because of the fastidious in vitro growth requirements of *C. colinum*, intestinal and hepatic lesions often form the basis of a presumptive diagnosis. A definitive diagnosis requires detection of the bacterium in specimens from affected birds. The liver is the most suitable organ for isolating *C. colinum*. Slide smears of liver and spleen tissues may be Gram-stained for detection of Gram-positive bacilli, and subterminal and free spores. A direct fluorescent antibody test to demonstrate the presence of *C. colinum* in cryostat sections of liver and intestine from chickens has been published.

Differential diagnosis is important and *C. perfringens*-associated necrotic enteritis, coccidiosis and histomoniasis should be differentiated from ulcerative enteritis. Histomoniasis is also associated with lesions in the caeca and liver but does not induce small intestinal lesions. Histological examination of the caeca and liver will reveal histomonads.

Coccidiosis may precede ulcerative enteritis, or both conditions may occur simultaneously. Coccidiosis and ulcerative enteritis require different medications.

C. perfringens and *C. colinum* may be present concurrently in diseased birds. Necrotic and ulcerative enteritis have some similar intestinal lesions that may complicate the diagnosis, and the possibility that both organisms are of importance in an outbreak cannot be ruled out. But differentiation based on lesions will in most cases be possible (see Necrotic Enteritis, above).

CONTROL

Important preventive measures include avoiding coccidiosis, immunosuppressive viral diseases, overcrowding, and inadequate hygiene. Keeping birds on a wire floor may be beneficial, unless it is inadvisable for other reasons.

Outbreaks may be treated with numerous antibiotics added to the drinking water or feed, including penicillins, streptomycin and tylosin.

CLOSTRIDIUM BOTULINUM (BOTULISM, LIMBERNECK)

Botulism is a worldwide disease that can affect a variety of birds, including broiler chickens, and mammals, including humans. The disease is relatively rare in domestic poultry kept under good standards of hygiene. Poultry are a potential source of botulism in cattle. The public health significance of avian botulism outbreaks is considered minimal, but restrictions on sale of produce for human consumption from flocks experiencing an outbreak of botulism may be an advisable precautionary measure.

EPIDEMIOLOGY

Cause

Botulism is caused by toxins produced by the bacterium *Clostridium botulinum* and there are seven toxin types (A–G). Botulism in birds is caused by toxin types A, C, D and E, with type C the most common cause. *C. botulinum* type C produces the neurotoxin C_1 and the enterotoxin C_2, although recent findings suggest that the neurotoxin of avian type C is a mosaic of neurotoxins from types C and D. The genes encoding neurotoxins C_1 and toxins from type D are transmitted between bacterial strains by bacteriophages.

Hosts

Chickens, turkeys, pheasants and peafowl are susceptible to types A, B, C and E but not D or F. Ducks and pheasants are more susceptible to C_1 neurotoxin than chickens. Compared with other toxins, C_1 and C_2 are more easily absorbed by chickens when given orally. Ostriches and more than 100 wild avian species are susceptible to type C botulism, which may also affect pigs, cattle, dogs, horses, minks, ferrets, mice, farmed fish and a variety of zoo mammals. Poultry may carry *C. botulinum* type D without showing symptoms and may be a source of type C and D botulism for cattle.

For botulism in humans, see the section on Public health considerations, below.

Spread

C. botulinum type C is present globally wherever large populations of wild and domestic birds are found. Spread is favoured by the presence of the organisms in the gastrointestinal tract of wild and domestic birds and the presence of resistant spores. Feed, drinking water and unused litter do not seem to be important sources of infection or toxins for poultry, although *C. botulinum* type C was found in feed that had been given to an affected flock.

Faecal–oral transmission of bacteria and possibly toxins is an important means of spread within a flock. Insects feeding on faeces have also been suspected as vectors. Carcasses of affected animals have been implicated as a likely source of toxin within a flock. Toxic carcasses have also been implicated in cases of botulism in wild birds. Fly larvae feeding on carcasses of affected animals may transmit the disease as such maggots are devoured readily by chickens, pheasants and ducks. Experiments have shown that ingestion of a single larva is enough to kill a 3-week-old chicken.

Litter and faeces from infected flocks represent a potential source of infection for other domestic and wild birds and mammals. This is illustrated by the reports on botulism in cattle associated with the presence of contaminated poultry litter on pastures or in cattle feed.

Influencing factors

Predisposing factors are likely to be required for toxico-infectious (see Pathogenesis section, below) type C botulism to occur in broiler chickens. The risk of botulism is increased if the birds have access to faeces. In an experimental infection, birds kept on a wire floor remained healthy, whereas birds kept on litter became ill 3 days after challenge. Access to decaying carcasses is a significant risk factor. The bacterium is often present in the gut of healthy birds, and toxins may develop in carcasses. As broiler chickens age, they become less susceptible to C_1 toxin. Most outbreaks in broiler chickens occur between 2 and 8 weeks of age. Wound contamination in association with caponizing has been suspected as a contributory factor to botulism in broiler chickens up to 14 weeks of age. Outbreaks in poultry have been associated with increased levels of iron in drinking water and feed; *C. botulinum* is favoured by increased availability of iron.

DISEASE

Pathogenesis

Botulism can arise from ingestion of material containing preformed toxins or may be induced by in vivo production of toxins by *C. botulinum* (toxico-infection). A toxico-infection may arise from an infected wound or from a gastrointestinal infection. Intestinal toxico-infection is possibly the most common disease form in commercial poultry flocks. This assumption is supported by the facts that (1) a toxin-contaminated source is often difficult to identify during outbreaks; (2) the growth temperature for toxin types C is optimal in the chicken gut; and (3) higher numbers of *C. botulinum* spores have been found in litter from affected flocks compared with that from non-affected flocks. Experimental findings indicate that toxin production takes place in the caeca. In broiler chickens this toxin production is apparently not at levels sufficient to kill the birds; however, caecal droppings containing toxins may be ingested by birds with access to faeces. It has been proposed that disease may be induced through uptake of faecal toxins, which are activated and absorbed in the small intestine.

The neurotoxins of *C. botulinum* become toxic through cleavage by proteases. They are transported from the gut via the blood or lymph to peripheral tissues, where transmission of nerve impulses to musculature is blocked through interference with acetylcholine and paralysis is induced. Cardiac and respiratory failures are common causes of death.

Clinical signs

Clinical signs, which depend on the level of toxin, range from subclinical disease up to 40% mortality. Mortality may become very high in wild birds and in pheasants reared on game farms. Flaccid paralysis is a predominant sign. Paralysis progresses cranially from the legs to include wings, neck and eyelids. Reluctance to move and apparent lameness may be observed before the birds become recumbent. The birds may drop their head on the floor using the beak as support, or they may lie down with the extended and paralysed neck on the floor. Breathing difficulties, quivering of feathers and ruffled hackle feathers may be seen. There may be loss of neck feathers in chickens but not in turkeys. Bruised and reddish skin caused by feather picking may be seen, as well as trauma caused by other birds trampling on recumbent individuals. Broiler chickens may have diarrhoea with excess urates.

Lesions

There are no specific gross or microscopic lesions. Putrid ingesta, maggots or feathers may be found in the crop. Stained tail and vent feathers associated with diarrhoea may be observed.

DIAGNOSIS

A presumptive diagnosis is based on clinical signs and lack of organ lesions. Eyelid paralysis is a particularly useful sign but symptoms vary with the level of intoxication. A definitive diagnosis is achieved by detection and typing of toxin in serum, crop or intestinal washings from diseased birds. Serum is the preferred sample. Detection of toxin within tissues of dead birds does not confirm botulism. Toxin may be detected using in vivo testing in mice or chemical, immuno-logical or enzymatic methods. Sensitivity of the test method is a critical issue.

Isolation and characterization of *C. botulinum* from feed and environmental samples may provide useful epidemiological data, but is of limited diagnostic value.

Mild forms of botulism must be differentiated from other causes of leg problems and para-lytic symptoms, including other toxins (for example ionophorous poisoning).

CONTROL

Removal of potential sources of *C. botulinum* and its toxins from the environment is important. Dead and diseased birds should be removed from the house frequently and regularly, and disposed of in a way that denies access to carcasses by domestic or wild animals. Fly control is also of importance. Used litter should be removed between growouts and disposed of in a way that mini-mizes the access of domestic and wild animals to the litter. Pheasants have been successfully vac-cinated with bacterin-toxoids.

No simple and effective means of treatment of poultry has been well documented. Treatments with sodium selenite, vitamins A, D_3 and E and antibiotics in feed or water have been reported to be of benefit. Bacitracin, streptomycin, chlortetracycline and penicillin have been useful in some cases but lack of effect of antibiotics (penicillin) has also been reported. Type C antitoxin treatment has been used successfully in ostriches.

Although *C. botulinum* type C is thought to be common in poultry environments, thorough cleaning and disinfection efforts are recommended in affected premises. The spores are very resistant to heat but sodium hypochlorite, calcium hypochlorite, formaldehyde and iodophor disinfectants are reported to reduce their numbers. A procedure with repeated disinfections after cleaning may be useful. Attention should also be paid to outdoor areas as spores may be located outside the poultry house and may be transported back into the facility after cleaning and disinfection.

PUBLIC HEALTH CONSIDERATIONS

Humans are mainly affected by toxin types A, B, E and F. Although botulism caused by types A and E has been reported in poultry on rare occasions, these cases have generally been associ-ated with the consumption of spoiled human food products fed to backyard chicken flocks. A few cases of human disease associated with *C. botulinum* types C and D have been reported. At present it seems unlikely that poultry produce represents a significant cause of human botulism but a precautionary approach to food safety suggests that restrictions on the sale of such prod-ucts from flocks experiencing an outbreak of botulism may be advisable. It has been suggested that products from food animal herds/flocks exposed to botulism should be withheld from the food chain until 2 weeks have elapsed since the last clinical case.

GANGRENOUS DERMATITIS (MALIGNANT OEDEMA, CELLULITIS)

Gangrenous dermatitis occurs worldwide in chickens and turkeys. The syndrome is precipitated by various detrimental microbial, nutritional and environmental factors.

EPIDEMIOLOGY

Cause

The two clostridia most frequently implicated are *C. septicum* and *C. perfringens* type A. *Staphylococcus aureus*, either alone or as an additional pathogen, is involved in some outbreaks and, rarely, *C. novyi* (*oedematiens*) and other clostridial organisms. When *S. aureus* is present with a clostridial pathogen the disease is more severe than either alone.

Hosts

Gangrenous dermatitis affects chickens and turkeys and is most commonly seen in broilers of about 4–7 weeks.

Spread

The organisms involved are ubiquitous and may be found in the intestine, in litter, in soil and on the skin (*Staphylococcus* spp.).

Influencing factors

Gangrenous dermatitis is often precipitated by one or several of various predisposing factors. These include:

- Skin wounds
- Immunosuppressive agents such as infectious bursal disease, chicken infectious anaemia, reticuloendotheliosis, adenovirus infections, reovirus infection and Marek's disease
- Nutritional deficiencies
  - Inadequate nutrients (e.g. amino acids) for feather and skin growth
  - Insufficient vitamin E for immunity and as an antioxidant; rancid fat in the diet increases requirement for vitamin E
  - Inadequate salt, which exacerbates fighting and skin damage
- Mycotoxicosis, with increased susceptibility to bruising and immunosuppression
- Management deficiencies allowing an increasing concentration of pathogens in the poultry house and environment
  - High stocking density
  - Unhygienic housing and provision of feed and water
  - Inadequate handling of litter and carcasses
  - Inadequate cleaning and disinfection between flocks.

DISEASE

Clinical signs

The clinical signs include increased mortality, marked depression, incoordination of movement and death within a few hours. The carcasses decompose rapidly with a foul odour. Mortality varies from low to very high.

Gross lesions

The lesions are seen under the wings, between the thighs, over the ribs and flanks in the form of reddened moist skin and oedema and inflammation in subcutaneous tissue. There is extensive sloughing and red and swollen areas may be found on the feet, legs and occasionally around feather follicles of the wings. Underlying muscle is usually discoloured and oedematous, and gas is produced by the clostridial organisms. The kidney and liver are often congested and in some birds the lungs are congested and oedematous and can resemble a mass of dark-red jelly.

DIAGNOSIS

Diagnosis is based on the presence of gross lesions and the demonstration of the pathogen(s), which may include *S. aureus.* Diagnosis or determination of the underlying cause is desirable.

Squamous cell carcinoma of the skin of chickens may induce gross lesions similar to those of gangrenous dermatitis, and histopathology may be necessary to differentiate.

CONTROL

Important management measures include a high standard of hygiene, avoiding overcrowding of stock and the protection of the birds against immunosuppressive agents.

FURTHER READING

Critchley E M R 1991 A comparison of human and animal botulism – a review. J R Soc Med 84: 295–298

Dohms J E 2003 Botulism. In: Saif Y M (ed) Diseases of poultry, 11th edn. Iowa State University Press, Ames, p 785–791

Engström B, Kaldhusdal M, Pedersen K 2006 Enteritis and enterotoxaemia in birds. In: Mainil J et al (eds) Genus *Clostridium*. Clostridia in medical, veterinary and food microbiology. Diagnosing and typing. European Concerted Action QLK2-CT2001–01267. European Commission, Brussels, p 92–96

Holzhauer M 2004 Bovine botulism in the Netherlands. Tierarztl Umsch 59: 29–31

Kondo F, Tottori J, Soki K 1988 Ulcerative enteritis in broiler chickens caused by *Clostridium colinum* and *in vitro* activity of 19 antimicrobial agents in tests on isolates. Poult Sci 67: 1424–1430

Sharpe R I, Livesey C T 2005 Surveillance of suspect animal toxicoses with potential food safety implications in England and Wales between 1990 and 2002. Vet Rec 157: 465–469

Takeda M, Tsukamoto K, Kohd T et al 2005 Characterization of the neurotoxin produced by isolates associated with avian botulism. Avian Dis 49: 376–381

Van Immerseel F, De Buck J, Pasmans F et al 2004 *Clostridium perfringens* in poultry: an emerging threat for animal and public health. Avian Pathol 33: 537–549

Wages D P 2003 Ulcerative enteritis (Quail disease). In: Saif Y M (ed) Diseases of poultry, 11th edn. Iowa State University Press, Ames, p 776–781

Wages D P, Opengart K 2003 Necrotic enteritis. In: Saif Y M (ed) Diseases of poultry, 11th edn. Iowa State University Press, Ames, p 781–785

Wages D P, Opengart K 2003 Gangrenous dermatitis. In: Saif Y M (ed) Diseases of poultry, 11th edn. Iowa State University Press, Ames, p 791–795

Williams R B 2005 Intercurrent coccidiosis and necrotic enteritis of chickens: rational, integrated disease management by maintenance of gut integrity. Avian Pathol 34: 159–180

Wilson J, Tice G, Brash M L, St Hilaire S 2005 Manifestations of *Clostridium perfringens* and related bacterial enteritides in broiler chickens. Worlds Poult Sci J 61: 435–449

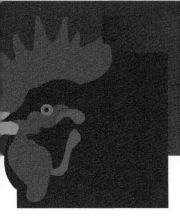
Frank T. W. Jordan and
Magne Bisgaard

Erysipelothrix rhusiopathiae – erysipelas

The disease caused by this ubiquitous bacterium is known as erysipelas except in human medicine, in which it is known as erysipeloid. A variety of vertebrate and nonvertebrate species are susceptible to infection and among domestic poultry its primary economic importance is as a disease of turkeys, which seem to be most frequently affected. However, as a result of animal welfare pressure in many European countries, table egg production in alternative production systems, including free-range and organic production, has increased. Because of a lack of biosecurity, disease problems have been increasingly reported for these systems including the re-emergence of classical poultry diseases such as erysipelas, blackhead, *Ascaridia galli* and *Dermanyssus gallinae* infections.

EPIDEMIOLOGY

Cause

The causal agent, *Erysipelothrix rhusiopathiae* (*insidiosa*), is a Gram-positive, slender, rod-shaped bacterium with a tendency to form long filaments. Although Gram-positive, the organisms decolorize easily and may appear Gram-negative. They are facultative anaerobes, growing between 5°C and 42°C. *Erysipelothrix* spp. are nonmotile, fermentative and catalase- and oxidase-negative. H_2S is formed in triple sugar iron agar. A characteristic 'pipe cleaner' type of growth is observed in gelatin stab cultures incubated at room temperature for 2–3 days. At least three species of *Erysipelothrix* have been reported of which only two have been named so far, *E. rhusiopathiae* and *Erysipelothrix tonsillarum*. However, only *E. rhusiopathiae* has been reported to be pathogenic for avian species. Although 26 serovars of *E. rhusiopathiae* have been described, the identification of other species of *Erysipelothrix* has led to confusion as to the correlation between serovars and species of *Erysipelothrix*. The majority of outbreaks, however, seem to be caused by *E. rhusiopathiae* serovars 1, 2 or 5.

The reservoir of *E. rhusiopathiae* seems to be domestic pigs but rodents, fish and birds are also frequently colonized. Sporadic problems also occur in sheep. *E. rhusiopathiae* is widely distributed in the soil and surface waters of farms and in the sewage effluent of abattoirs.

Before it was made obligatory in some countries to dispose of pig slurry by burying, disease outbreaks on turkey farms were reported subsequent to surface spreading of pig slurry, with possible associated aerosols. It is now generally accepted that the organism is not indigenous to the soil and that its presence reflects contamination by infected animals or slurry. *E. rhusiopathiae* is considered to be quite resistant to environmental influences.

Hosts

E. rhusiopathiae is ubiquitous in distribution and can infect a wide variety of vertebrate animals, including humans and other mammals, birds, fish, reptiles, amphibians and insects. It is also found subclinically in the mucoid slime of the scales of fish and in fish meal.

Although poultry of various ages can be infected the disease seems to be more common in the later growth stage and in mature stock and is most common in turkeys. However, serious losses have also been reported in chickens, ducks and geese following natural outbreaks of the disease.

Spread

In the spread of infection the source and portal of entry of the organism can be obscure but there may be a history of indirect contact with pigs or sheep. Breaks in the mucous membranes or skin have been suggested as portal of entry. Infection occurs more frequently in earth-floored houses than in concrete-floored ones. Recovered birds can be carriers for several weeks and shed the organism in their droppings. It is considered that some birds may be unaffected carriers. Contaminated fish and fish meal and carcasses of infected birds can be sources of infection. The role of vectors in transmission is unclear. It can also be spread during fighting among birds, through vaccination and to females, particularly turkeys, during artificial insemination. Spread from pen to pen may be very slow and adjacent pens may show no mortality.

Surprisingly, application of molecular methods for tracing sources of infection and investigation of genetic diversity among outbreak isolates has received little attention so far. Multilocus enzyme studies and pulsed field gel electrophoresis have clearly indicated that the same serovar represents enough diversity to allow these methods to be used in epidemiological studies.

Influencing factors

There seems to be little knowledge of influencing factors such as intercurrent infection with other pathogens or management problems in the precipitation of disease. However, adverse weather conditions and intestinal parasite injury have been coincidental in some outbreaks.

DISEASE

Pathogenesis

The route of infection is still unclear but infection from the environment through damage to the skin or mucosal membranes has been suggested. The demonstration of multiple serovars in the same flock seems to indicate that intercurrent infections or management faults may precipitate an outbreak. However, clonal outbreaks have also been observed and major differences in mortality during outbreaks between serovars and within a given serovar seem to indicate considerable variation in virulence, although the basis for the virulence of *E. rhusiopathiae* is not fully understood. Production of neuraminidase, which cleaves α-glycosidic linkages of sialic acid, a mucopolysaccharide on the surface of cells, has been suggested as a virulence factor in addition to possession of a capsule-like structure that confers resistance to phagocytosis. In addition, genes that express heat-shock proteins have been identified. The impact of genetic resistance remains to be investigated.

Susceptible avian species include wild birds, caged birds and domestic poultry consisting of turkeys, ducks, geese, chickens, pigeons, emus and game birds. Disease may be acute or chronic. Turkeys appear to be most susceptible but chickens may also be affected by the acute form, while the infection in web-footed birds is often sporadic, persisting in a flock for several months with individual or a few birds becoming affected at any one time.

Clinical signs

The onset of acute disease is sudden and birds are found dead or dying after a short, acute illness with depression and diarrhoea and sometimes an unsteady gait, and in some cases dark, thickened skin over any part of the body. In turkeys there is cyanosis of the head with the snood in males showing marked turgidity and being purple in colour. Ducks may show dark areas of congestion of the web between digits. Mortality in a flock can range from less than 1% to over 50%. Most sick birds die. Some recovered birds and those chronically affected may show gradual loss of condition, drop in egg production and chronic lameness.

Lesions

Apart from the skin lesions associated with clinical signs there is congestion of the whole carcass and especially the head and skin in turkeys. Internal lesions are those of a generalized septicaemia with congestion and petechial haemorrhages frequently in the myocardium, coronary fat, epicardium, gizzard serosa, mesentery, abdominal fat, liver and pleura. Enlarged, friable, mottled, congested livers, spleens and kidneys are frequently seen. Often, the whole liver is affected by coagulative necrosis. Enteritis is seen in some cases in which there is a marked catarrhal inflammation of the small intestine, dilatation and thickening of the walls of the proventriculus and gizzard, and ulceration of the walls of the caeca with small, round, yellow lesions. The lungs are normal in consistency but may be brown in colour. Chronic cases may show yellow, cauliflower-like, vegetative endocardial lesions and in lame birds a fibropurulent exudate in the joints. Peritonitis, perineal congestion and haemorrhage have been observed in female turkeys following insemination with contaminated material. In very acute cases there may be no gross lesions.

DIAGNOSIS

Diagnosis is based upon the history, signs and post-mortem picture, together with the isolation and identification of the causative organism. Smears for Gram staining and swabs for culture should be taken from tissue from several sites, including the liver, spleen, bone marrow and heart blood. *E. rhusiopathiae* can be difficult to grow and carcasses have proved better sources of the organisms than infected, live but sick birds. All inoculated plates should be left in the incubator for 48 h. A tentative diagnosis can be obtained by a Gram-stained smear of heart blood, liver or spleen, especially in peracute cases. Phenotypic identification is based upon cell and colonial morphology, growth characteristics in nutrient gelatin, catalase and oxidase test, hydrogen sulphide production in TSI and production of acid from carbohydrates. Differences in acid production from sucrose and whole-cell protein profiling can be used for separation of *E. rhusiopathiae* and *E. tonsillarum*. Several polymerase chain reaction (PCR) methods for detection have been reported. Comparison of specificity and sensitivity, however, remains to be carried out. Immunofluorescence may still be used in some laboratories. In differential diagnosis consideration should be given to such conditions as fowl cholera, peracute Newcastle disease, avian influenza and acute serohaemorrhagic colibacillosis.

CONTROL

Management

For prevention, the practice of a high standard of hygiene in management with and between flocks is essential and carcasses should be removed from flocks as soon as possible. The contact of poultry with pigs or sheep or infected poultry should be avoided, as should areas where these have recently been kept. Rats and mice should be controlled and attention should be paid to feed quality.

Vaccination

Vaccination of poultry species other than turkeys and free-range chickens is rarely practised. For turkeys, vaccination using either bacterin or live vaccine is advised for sites where infection is indigenous. For breeding turkeys at least two doses, at 4-week intervals, should be given before the birds are 14 weeks old, or 2 weeks prior to the age when an outbreak usually occurs on the premises. Replacement breeders may be given another dose just prior to onset of lay. For meat birds, one vaccination may be sufficient.

These vaccines may stimulate nonspecific reactions to *Mycoplasma gallisepticum* and *Mycoplasma meleagridis* serum plate agglutination tests; monitoring for these conditions should therefore be avoided within a few weeks of vaccination.

Treatment

Most strains of *E. rhusiopathiae* are resistant to sulphonamides, gentamicin, kanamycin, neomycin, vancomycin, novobiocin and polymyxins. The majority of isolates are very susceptible to penicillins, cephalosporins, erythromycin and clindamycin in vitro and penicillins are the drugs of choice for treatment. However, medication via the food or water usually fails to eliminate infection but can give temporary respite. If the birds are shortly to be slaughtered, subcutaneous injection into the back of the base of the neck with a mixture of procaine benzyl penicillin (procaine penicillin; rapid-acting) and benzathine penicillin (long-acting), quickly brings an outbreak under control. However, care must be taken to observe the required antibiotic withdrawal periods. In addition, catching and handling each bird may be impractical or even harmful. If there are more than 2 weeks before the birds are due for slaughter, they should simultaneously receive penicillin and a dose of inactivated erysipelas vaccine. Intramuscular injections should not be given to meat birds in order to avoid producing abscesses or other blemishes in the carcass musculature.

PUBLIC HEALTH CONSIDERATIONS

Human infections caused by *E. rhusiopathiae* may result in three distinct entities: erysipeloid, generalized cutaneous infection and septicaemia. The most common of these is erysipeloid, a localized infection usually on the fingers or hands. The septicaemic form, with or without endocarditis, is very rare in nonimmunosuppressed hosts. This form may occur with or without skin lesions. People at risk are those handling at-risk animals and animal products, and include veterinarians and veterinary students.

FURTHER READING

Adler H E, Spencer G R 1952 Immunization of turkeys and pigs with erysipelas bacteria. Cornell Vet 42: 238–296

Bisgaard M, Olsen P 1975 Erysipelas in egg-laying chickens. Clinical, pathological and bacteriological investigations. Avian Pathol 4: 59–71

Bisgaard M, Norrung V, Tornoe N 1980 Erysipelas in poultry. Prevalence of serotypes and epidemiological investigations. Avian Pathol 9: 355–362

Blackmore D K, Gallagher G L 1964 An outbreak of erysipelas in captive wild birds and mammals. Vet Rec 76: 1161–1164

Bricker J M, Saif Y M 2003 Erysipelas. In: Saif Y M et al Diseases of poultry, 11th edn. Iowa State University Press, Ames, p 812–826

Chirico J, Eriksson H, Fossum O, Jansson D 2003 The poultry red mite, *Dermanyssus gallinae*, a potential vector of *Erysipelothrix rhusiopathiae* causing erysipelas in hens. Med Vet Entomol 17: 232–234

Mazahari A, Lierz M, Hafez H M 2005 Investigations on the pathogenicity of *Erysipelothrix rhusiopathiae* in laying hens. Avian Dis 49: 574–576

Milne E M, Windsor R S, Rogerson F, Pennycott T W 1997 Concurrent infection with enteric protozoa and *Erysipelas rhusiopathiae* in chicken and pheasant flocks. Vet Rec 141: 340–341

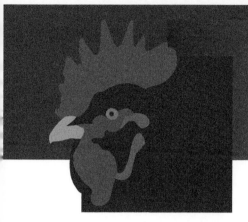

CHAPTER 20

Janet M. Bradbury and
Chris Morrow

Avian mycoplasmas

The mycoplasmas infecting birds belong almost exclusively to the genus *Mycoplasma*, although members of the genus *Acholeplasma* are sometimes isolated and an avian *Ureaplasma* species has been described. All belong to the class *Mollicutes*, which contains the smallest known prokaryotes able to replicate in cell-free medium. Although the trivial name 'mycoplasma' is still used for members of the class, the term 'mollicute' is considered more appropriate, with 'mycoplasma' being reserved for members of that genus.

The *Mollicutes* (Latin: *mollis* = soft, *cutis* = skin) are bounded by a thin membrane and lack a conventional bacterial cell wall and any evidence of peptidoglycan synthesis. These properties render them fragile in the environment but resistant to antibiotics such as penicillins and cephalosporins, which act on the cell wall. All mollicutes are readily killed by disinfectants and do not survive for prolonged periods outside the host. They are thought to have undergone reductive evolution, leaving them with a minimal complement of genes and considerable host dependency. A complex medium is usually needed for laboratory culture and traditionally serological reagents are needed for species identification.

As a group the avian *Mycoplasma* pathogens are responsible not only for clinical disease (usually respiratory or locomotory) but also for poor weight gain, reduced feed conversion efficiency, reduced hatchability and downgrading at slaughter. Although classed as primary pathogens, these mycoplasmas often cause greater damage when acting together with other pathogens or when infecting a debilitated host.

There are currently 23 recognized avian *Mycoplasma* species (Table 20.1) but only *Mycoplasma gallisepticum*, *Mycoplasma synoviae*, *Mycoplasma meleagridis* and *Mycoplasma iowae* have been associated with significant economic losses in domestic poultry. The importance of the other mollicutes, including those in the genera *Ureaplasma* and *Acholeplasma*, is less clear.

Table 20.1 | *Mycoplasma* species found in birds

SPECIES	MAIN HOSTS*
M. anatis	Duck, goose
M. anseris	Goose
M. buteonis	Buzzard
M. cloacale	Turkey, goose
M. columbinasale	Pigeon
M. columbinum	Pigeon
M. columborale	Pigeon
M. corogypsi	Vulture
M. falconis	Falcon
M. gallinaceum	Chicken, pheasant, partridge
M. gallinarum	Chicken, turkey
M. gallisepticum	Chicken, turkey, pheasant, partridge, songbirds[†]
M. gallopavonis	Turkey
M. glycophilum	Chicken, pheasant, partridge
M. gypis	Vulture
M. iners	Chicken, turkey, pheasant, partridge
M. iowae	Turkey, chicken
M. imitans	Goose, duck, partridge
M. lipofaciens	Chicken, turkey
M. meleagridis	Turkey
M. pullorum	Chicken, pheasant, partridge
M. sturni	Starling (European)
M. synoviae	Chicken, turkey

Several *Acholeplasma* spp. and *Ureaplasma gallorale* have been isolated from birds; their significance is unknown.

* Indicates more common host(s) but not current prevalence. † Several other species are isolated sporadically from songbirds.

MYCOPLASMA GALLISEPTICUM

Disease associated with *M. gallisepticum* has probably existed in chickens and turkeys for many years but intensive management synchronized and exacerbated the pathogenic effects and hastened its recognition. *M. gallisepticum* typically causes chronic respiratory disease in chickens and conjunctivitis and sinusitis in turkeys and game birds. The disease tends to run a long course and morbidity may be high, although without complicating factors mortality is low. *M. gallisepticum* has been recognized as a pathogen in North American finches and causes conjunctivitis, sinusitis and rhinitis.

M. gallisepticum probably occurs in all countries where poultry are kept, although the primary breeding companies maintain *M. gallisepticum*-free stock. In countries with well-developed poultry industries, most commercial breeding flocks are also *M. gallisepticum*-free and 'breaks' in such flocks are generally sporadic. The organism is more difficult to control on continuous production sites and remains a problem for some table egg producers. The infection in finches reached epidemic proportions, extending throughout the eastern USA and into Canada, but evidence of spread to or from poultry is lacking.

The economic impact of *M. gallisepticum* is widely acknowledged but figures are difficult to obtain. In addition to overt disease, the infection causes reduced feed conversion efficiency, downgrading of broilers and turkeys at slaughter and suboptimal egg production in layers. Infections during lay can cause egg production losses of between 10% and 20% in layers for periods of up to 1 month. Chronic infection without overt clinical disease may cause the loss of 5–20 eggs per hen. In breeders the infection may necessitate slaughter of valuable flocks and even suspicion of infection in such flocks may result in export restrictions for eggs and progeny. Other costs include treatment, laboratory diagnosis and control measures such as increased biosecurity or vaccination.

EPIDEMIOLOGY

Cause

M. gallisepticum is one of the 'flask-shaped' mycoplasmas, possessing a specialized tip structure by which it attaches to respiratory epithelium. Lipoproteins involved in attachment have been identified on the surface of *M. gallisepticum* that exhibit considerable variation in the expression of their surface antigens, a phenomenon that is believed to play an important role in the disease process (see below).

M. gallisepticum strains vary in virulence, a property that is readily lost by laboratory passage. Some strains may be poorly antigenic and they may also vary in tropism, although epithelial surfaces, especially the respiratory epithelium, are the main targets. Strains can be distinguished by molecular 'fingerprinting' of their DNA, sequencing specific genes or electrophoretic analysis of their proteins. Strain typing can be useful in epidemiological tracing but there are no markers yet for virulence. *M. gallisepticum* is sensitive to common disinfectants, to extremes of pH and temperature and to lysis by detergents. It is also susceptible to a number of antimicrobials, including macrolides, pleuromutilins, aminoglycosides and fluoroquinolones.

Hosts

Chickens, turkeys, pheasants and partridges can probably be infected by *M. gallisepticum* at any age, although the young or stressed bird seems more likely to develop clinical signs. *M. gallisepticum* has been isolated from natural infections of ducks and geese in contact with infected chickens, also guinea fowl, quail, peafowl, racing pigeons and an Amazon parrot. Budgerigars are susceptible experimentally. The situation in free-flying birds is less clear but *M. gallisepticum* has been isolated from tree sparrows in Japan, house sparrows in India and choughs in Scotland. The North American epidemic in finches also affected other songbirds.

Little information is available on the influence of host breed or gender on *M. gallisepticum* disease but male house finches are less likely to survive *M. gallisepticum* infection than females.

Spread

Spread of *M. gallisepticum* is both direct and indirect. It can be transmitted through the chicken or turkey hatching egg to the offspring and the proportion of infected eggs probably varies between individuals and with the stage of infection. Some infected embryos may die, especially if the *M. gallisepticum* strain is virulent, but enough may hatch to disseminate the infection among the progeny. Such transmission could occur in the hatchery. *M. gallisepticum* survives well in egg contents (allantoic fluid and yolk) highlighting the potential importance of egg debris as a mode of indirect spread in the hatchery. Egg transmission is also important for avian vaccine manufacturers using eggs or egg-derived cell cultures, since infection could contaminate live vaccines and be widely administered to poultry.

Spread of *M. gallisepticum* within a flock occurs through close contact, probably as the result of exhalation, coughing or sneezing of the organisms. It is therefore more likely to occur during the acute phase of disease when *M. gallisepticum* populations are highest and birds with damaged respiratory epithelium may provide a more favourable target for colonization. The rate of spread also depends on factors such as flock size, stocking density, numbers of organisms and perhaps the individual properties of the *M. gallisepticum* strain. There is evidence that *M. gallisepticum* may not always spread to birds in adjacent pens and that pen walls may act as a partial barrier against transmission.

The practice of introducing younger cockerels into breeding flocks ('spiking') should also be considered as a potential risk. Testing cockerels for *M. gallisepticum* and *M. synoviae* infections before transfer is a good precaution. Also, although not considered an important route, it is possible that venereal transmission might occur, since *M. gallisepticum* has been isolated from the oviduct and semen of chickens and turkeys.

Routes of indirect contact are difficult to define but there is circumstantial evidence that fomites, including windborne transmission, may play a role in spread of *M. gallisepticum* between flocks. It can survive on some materials up to a few days. Of several materials tested, *M. gallisepticum* survived best on feathers, human hair and cotton clothing. Thus humans and/or equipment moving between premises without adequate precautions are potential carriers of infection. Wild birds and vermin have not been conclusively incriminated.

Influencing factors

Much has been written on the role of other pathogens in *M. gallisepticum* disease. In the chicken the viruses of Newcastle disease and infectious bronchitis (even live vaccine strains) may exacerbate the disease. Other pathogens reported to act synergistically with *M. gallisepticum* in chickens are infectious laryngotracheitis virus, reo- and adenoviruses, *Infectious bursal disease virus* (IBDV) and *Haemophilus paragallinarum*. Less is known about the turkey but *Avian pneumovirus* (APV) can increase the severity and duration of *M. gallisepticum* infection and influenza A virus has been similarly incriminated. Of great importance in both hosts is the ability of pathogenic strains of *Escherichia coli* to act synergistically with *M. gallisepticum*.

Other influencing factors include increased environmental ammonia, high levels of dust, poor nutrition, immunosuppressive agents and social stresses associated with intensive management.

DISEASE

Pathogenesis

It is assumed that *M. gallisepticum* enters the respiratory tract by inhalation of aerosols or via the conjunctiva but it is unclear how it overcomes the bird's natural defences. Attachment to avian cell surface glycoproteins is probably the first step. *M. gallisepticum* attaches to mucosal cells by its terminal tip and motility may also play a part in colonization. The events that follow remain obscure but *M. gallisepticum* has ciliostatic properties and it is likely that other factors that impair ciliary activity, such as excessive ammonia or damage by other microorganisms, will assist colonization. Adherence to host cells may interfere with the cell's transport mechanisms, and furthermore *M. gallisepticum* is one of several mycoplasmas that secrete hydrogen peroxide, which may impose oxidative stress on the host cell membrane. Although traditionally regarded as pathogens of mucosal surfaces, recent evidence suggests that *M. gallisepticum*, like some other mycoplasmas, may be able to invade cells. This could allow it to evade the action of antibodies and some antimicrobials. One strain of *M. gallisepticum* (S6) can produce a neurotoxin, which causes arteritis in turkey brain, and neurological signs have been seen, albeit rarely, in natural infections.

It is now clear that *M. gallisepticum* has sophisticated ways of varying its surface antigens (phenotypic switching) and that these changes may permit subpopulations to avoid the immune response and persist in the host for long periods. Despite the very small number of genes, the proportion dedicated to antigenic cell surface variation in *M. gallisepticum* is large and suggests that phenotypic switching is important to its success as a pathogen.

Very little is known about the interactions of *M. gallisepticum* and the avian immune system but some mycoplasmas have immunomodulatory effects on the cells of the immune system and can suppress or stimulate B and T lymphocytes and the production of cytokines. They can also increase cytotoxicity of macrophages, natural killer cells and T cells and can activate the complement cascade.

There is thus insufficient information to explain how the lesions and clinical signs seen in *M. gallisepticum* evolve from the cellular and molecular effects although many of the lesions seem to result from the host immune and inflammatory response rather than direct effects of the mycoplasma.

Clinical signs

Except for very young poults and chicks, the development of clinical disease may depend upon the presence of other pathogens or stress factors, as indicated above. Uncomplicated infections frequently cause no clinical signs or mortality, especially in chickens. The most common clinical signs are respiratory in nature and may include nasal discharge, conjunctivitis, sneezing, moist rales and breathing through the partly open beak. Nasal discharge is less severe in chickens than in turkeys, in which sinusitis, with swelling of one or both infraorbital sinuses, may be sufficiently severe to cause complete closure of the eyes. Nasal exudation frequently accompanies sinusitis and the wing feathers of turkeys are often soiled where they have attempted to wipe away the discharge. This is rarely seen in chickens. In both chickens and turkeys mild conjunctivitis with frothy ocular exudate may be the only sign, or it may be the early stage of more severe disease. If the air sacs alone are affected there may be no respiratory signs. Lowered egg production may occur in layer chickens and turkeys. Other clinical signs are rare and include ataxia in the turkey and swelling of the hock and lameness in chickens.

Lesions

Gross lesions of the respiratory tract may be almost imperceptible or consist only of excess mucus or catarrhal exudate in the nares, trachea and lungs and oedema of the air sac walls. Caseous exudate may appear later within the air sacs or on their walls. Distension of the infraorbital sinuses, particularly in turkeys, is caused initially by excess mucus, which may be replaced later by caseous material. Where the disease is exacerbated by other pathogens the lesions are more severe and prolonged, giving rise to a chronic condition. With *E. coli* infection in young chickens of about 4–10 weeks old, especially those reared intensively, colisepticaemia may result, with pericarditis, perihepatitis and respiratory disease, including air sacculitis. In encephalopathy of turkeys there are no gross lesions and the rare instances of tenosynovitis and arthritis of chickens resemble the condition caused by *M. synoviae*. In salpingitis associated with *M. gallisepticum*, caseous exudate occurs in the oviduct.

DIAGNOSIS

Laboratory methods are essential since *M. gallisepticum* infection cannot be diagnosed by clinical signs or pathological lesions. The three approaches are: detection of specific antibodies, isolation and identification of the organism and detection of its DNA. Of these serological testing is most often used, particularly for regular screening of flocks.

The most commonly used test is probably rapid serum agglutination (RSA) using commercial stained antigen, although several enzyme-linked immunosorbent assay (ELISA) kits are now marketed. In the RSA test equal volumes of chicken or turkey serum and antigen are mixed at room temperature and examined at 2 min for clumping of the antigen by specific antibodies. It is most important that positive and negative control sera are included because antigens can vary in their sensitivity and specificity. Poor-quality sera, sera from birds recently vaccinated with oil-emulsion vaccines or birds recently infected with *M. synoviae* are just some of the causes of nonspecific agglutination of *M. gallisepticum* antigen.

Since there is no international standard for interpreting RSA tests, laboratories develop their own procedures to follow up suspect positive sera. One approach is to heat the sera at 56°C for 30 min. If they still react, particularly after dilution to 1:5 or more, the flock should be investigated further, which may mean a retest after 2–4 weeks. The flock and its progeny may need to be placed in quarantine until a negative retest is obtained. The RSA test has never been validated for use with serum from other avian species; neither is it suitable for detecting egg yolk antibodies or maternally derived antibodies in young poultry because such antibodies are mainly IgG and the test detects mainly IgM antibodies. Sera from day-old chicks or poults may give more nonspecific positive reactions than serum from older birds.

Other serological tests are the haemagglutination inhibition test and the ELISA. Some diagnostic laboratories prefer the former but should be aware that this test is strain-specific and therefore may be relatively insensitive. Several commercial ELISA kits are marketed and some are approved by the United States Department of Agriculture for use in the National Poultry Improvement Plan (NPIP). Some ELISAs appear to have similar problems to the RSA test with regard to specificity and sensitivity. Kits designed for detecting chicken antibodies should be validated before using with turkey sera. One kit is a blocking ELISA using a monoclonal antibody and should be usable with sera from any avian host.

The number of birds sampled will influence the accuracy of the results but in reality will depend upon factors such as company policy, the type and value of the flock, export requirements and financial constraints. The European Union Directive 90/539/EEC, which governs intra-Community trade in, and imports from third countries of, poultry and hatching eggs, states that screening tests must be performed on a representative sample just before the onset of lay and every 3 months thereafter. In order to detect infection at a prevalence of 5% with 95% confidence 60 birds should be tested in flocks exceeding 5000 birds. At this prevalence, 90 birds should be tested for 99% confidence of detection. A flock should be considered as birds housed within a single airspace and testing should select birds randomly from all areas.

Flocks with clearcut positive sera might not be further investigated; however, for flocks with dubious serological results or for valuable breeding flocks, attempts will be made to isolate *M. gallisepticum* or to detect its DNA. Samples for culture can be taken from live birds, fresh carcasses, dead-in-shell embryos or chicks or poults that have broken the shell but failed to hatch (pipped embryos). Swabs may be taken from the choanal cleft, oropharynx, oesophagus, trachea, cloaca and phallus of live or dead birds and exudates may be aspirated from the infraorbital sinuses and joints. After death samples may also be taken from the nasal cavity, air sacs and lungs. Samples from embryonated eggs include the inner surface of the vitelline membrane and oropharynx and air sacs of the embryo. It is helpful to dip swabs before use in *Mycoplasma* broth as a transport medium, and it is imperative that samples are kept chilled and sent to the laboratory by the fastest route. If mycoplasmas are isolated *M. gallisepticum* can be identified by a variety of tests using specific antisera. Immunofluorescence, immunoperoxidase and growth inhibition tests are most commonly used for this purpose.

Detection of *M. gallisepticum* DNA is normally carried out by polymerase chain reaction (PCR) on tracheal swabs. Several PCRs have been described using different primers and commercial kits are available. At present PCR tests tend to be conducted in specialized laboratories but they should be carefully validated before use. It is also now possible to carry out strain typing which may help in tracing the source of the *M. gallisepticum*.

CONTROL

The *M. gallisepticum* control strategy of many countries is based on maintaining *Mycoplasma*-free breeding stock. *M. gallisepticum*-free stock became available some years ago following eradication programmes by the primary chicken and turkey breeding companies. However, despite the high level of biosecurity practised by many commercial breeding companies, it has not always proved possible to maintain freedom from *Mycoplasma* at the multiplier level. *M. gallisepticum* infections are even less easily controlled in broilers and table egg layers, particularly on continuous production sites. Therefore other measures such as antimicrobial treatment are widely used and vaccination is practised in some countries. Thus there are several approaches to control, depending on the type and value of the flock and the local circumstances (Table 20.2). However, the practice of good management and hygiene is pivotal in all circumstances.

Eradication

Primary breeding companies successfully eradicated *M. gallisepticum* many years ago. This was achieved by reducing egg transmission using either antimicrobial or heat treatment of eggs prior to incubation. Heat treatment (to an internal temperature of 46°C over 11–14h) caused some embryo mortality, particularly in turkeys. Antimicrobials were administered either by injection or by 'dipping' using temperature or pressure differential. Since none of these treatments was guaranteed to kill all mycoplasmas, the hatched birds were reared in small groups under strict biosecurity, monitored regularly for infection and discarded from the programme if found to be positive.

Routine control measures

M. gallisepticum-free primary breeding flocks are kept under very strict biosecurity and closely monitored for early serological evidence of 'breaks'. Some breeding companies ensure a 3-day break between visiting an infected flock and contacting other poultry. Infected flocks are slaughtered immediately and hatching eggs are withdrawn for disposal. *M. gallisepticum* infection at the commercial breeder level may also be controlled by slaughter in some companies, although antimicrobial treatment may be chosen by others. This will alleviate clinical problems but is likely to allow some egg transmission, with consequent problems in the progeny.

Table 20.2 | Producer strategies for *Mycoplasma* infection

STRATEGY	ADVANTAGES	DISADVANTAGES	COMMENTS
Mycoplasma-free	Low input costs	Constant concern about introducing infection; higher capital costs. Danger from neighbouring poultry industries. Cost of monitoring programme	Good biosecurity needed; may be possible to move from positive to negative status with vaccination. Need to decide which mycoplasmas will be controlled and actions to be taken on *Mycoplasma* breaks
Live vaccination of parents	No clinical signs in parents and reduced risk	Possible positive antibody and/or PCR status may be incompatible with export; may limit therapeutic options around vaccination	Must vaccinate before field challenge. *M. gallisepticum* and *M. synoviae* vaccines do not cross-protect
Killed vaccination of parents	No clinical signs in parents; only need to vaccinate before onset of lay	Danger of silent infection in parents being passed horizontally to offspring	*M. gallisepticum* and *M. synoviae* vaccines do not cross-protect
Strategic medication	Low input costs	High cost of medication and potential development of resistance. Cost of monitoring programme	Parents, eggs and offspring may need medication. Multiple *Mycoplasma* species usually controlled
Do nothing		High mortality and poor performance in offspring; increased condemnation in broilers	Uncompetitive performance

PCR, polymerase chain reaction.

Antimicrobials used for *M. gallisepticum* infections include tetracyclines, macrolides, aminoglycosides, fluoroquinolones and tiamulin. These may be given by injection, in the drinking water or in feed as appropriate, but should be capable of delivering suitable doses to these mucosally located organisms. Antimicrobials that have additional activity against other bacteria may be a good choice in some circumstances. Nevertheless it should be appreciated that treatment will not eliminate all mycoplasmas and overuse may encourage emergence of resistant strains.

Vaccination

The failure to control *M. gallisepticum* infection on continuous production sites has led to the development of a number of vaccines, although vaccination is recommended only where field exposure is considered to be inevitable. It is important to vaccinate before field challenge is likely to occur. Live and killed vaccines are marketed and, despite the antigenic variation seen among *M. gallisepticum* strains, vaccination with a single strain seems to be effective. Killed oil-adjuvanted vaccines ('bacterins') have proved of value in protecting against egg production losses in layers although they do not prevent infection. Two subcutaneous or intramuscular doses are usually given to pullets for best efficacy. Bacterins have also been given to breeder pullets to reduce the level of egg transmission.

The live vaccines, ts-11 and 6/85, have been introduced more recently. The former is a temperature-sensitive mutant vaccine, which is given by eye drop. The latter is given by aerosol and both have proved effective, although in a dose-dependent manner. The ts-11 vaccine persists in the chicken for long periods and can be used in combination with respiratory virus vaccines. Strain 6/85 vaccine does not persist and may be difficult to recover after a few weeks. Neither vaccine produces a consistent serological response but this should not be interpreted as lack of protection. Currently no vaccines are marketed for turkeys or broilers.

MYCOPLASMA SYNOVIAE

M. synoviae disease was first described as 'infectious synovitis' in chickens and turkeys in the USA, although nowadays *M. synoviae* tends to cause subclinical upper respiratory infection. It may cause overt respiratory disease and air sacculitis if exacerbated by other respiratory pathogens. There is some debate about its effects on egg production. *M. synoviae* has been reported from many countries. The primary breeding stock is *M. synoviae*-free but infections are seen from time to time in commercial chicken and turkey breeding stock and appear to be particularly widespread in commercial layers.

The economic importance of *M. synoviae* is not properly established because documented evidence is lacking. Infected breeders are usually asymptomatic, although there are sometimes reports of considerable impact on broilers. Its importance in layers is unclear, with descriptions ranging from no effects to egg production losses of 5–10%. *M. synoviae* was not included in the control measures stipulated by the European Community's Directive 90/539/EEC, although it is now included in the Office International des Épizooties (OIE) list of notifiable diseases.

EPIDEMIOLOGY

Cause

M. synoviae shares many characteristics with *M. gallisepticum* although there is little evidence for an attachment organelle in *M. synoviae* and adherence probably occurs by some other mechanism. Haemagglutination is an inconsistent property of *M. synoviae* and may be explained by the high-frequency, phase-variable expression of its lipoprotein haemagglutinins. The means of generating diversity in the haemagglutinin gene family appears to be different from that in *M. gallisepticum* and more complex. Strains may vary in virulence and tropism and the haemagglutinin-positive phenotype has been shown to induce experimental synovitis in chickens more readily than the negative phenotype. Molecular methods have been developed to distinguish between strains of *M. synoviae*.

M. synoviae resembles *M. gallisepticum* in having a relatively short survival time outside the host and in its susceptibility to detergents and disinfectants. It is also sensitive to a similar range of antimicrobials but rather less so than *M. gallisepticum*.

Hosts

The main hosts are chickens and turkeys but natural infection has been reported in guinea fowl, ducks, geese, pigeons, quail, pheasants and red-legged partridges. All ages of bird appear susceptible. *M. synoviae* has also been isolated from house sparrows on infected farms in Spain.

Spread

M. synoviae spreads vertically and horizontally as described for *M. gallisepticum*. Egg transmission rates are unpredictable and probably vary with strain and with the age at infection. Spread within a flock is via the respiratory tract and is thought to be more rapid than *M. gallisepticum*, although *M. synoviae* strains of low transmissibility have been reported. It seems likely that factors which aid the spread of *M. gallisepticum* affect *M. synoviae* similarly. Routes of indirect spread between flocks are largely unknown and may involve windborne and fomite transmission as well as intermediate hosts.

Influencing factors

Although less studied in *M. synoviae* than *M. gallisepticum*, available evidence indicates that similar predisposing factors play an important role in exacerbating disease, especially of the respiratory system.

DISEASE

Pathogenesis

M. synoviae enters via the respiratory tract and some strains appear to cause ciliostasis. As with *M. gallisepticum* little is known of the events that follow but a multigene family is responsible for variation in the size and expression of membrane antigens and may help *M. synoviae* to evade the immune response and persist for long periods. Haematogenous spread can occur, leading to infection of the joints, and experimental work indicates that thymus-dependent lymphocytes are necessary for the development of macroscopic joint lesions.

Clinical signs

M. synoviae infections in chickens and turkeys frequently occur without clinical signs. When signs are seen they may be respiratory or arthritic but these are not mutually exclusive. The incubation period may be relatively short in young birds and the respiratory tract of every bird may become infected although the morbidity is very variable in the arthritic form. Infected chickens may show slight tracheal rales and coryza while in turkeys there may be swelling of the infraorbital sinuses. In the acute arthritic form there is marked depression, pale comb, retarded growth and rapid loss of condition accompanied by swelling of the joints and consequent lameness. Sternal bursitis ('breast blister') may also occur. The disease may progress to a chronic form or it may remain in this form and synovitis may persist for the life of the flock.

Lesions

Gross lesions in respiratory disease are similar to those in *M. gallisepticum* infection but may be milder. Lesions in affected joints include oedema and thickening of the periarticular tissues, especially the synovial membranes. The tendon sheaths become swollen and erosion of the articular cartilage may be seen. The foot and hock joints are most frequently involved and an exudate occurs that at first is clear but then becomes creamy. In the chicken it may become caseous and orange or brown in colour. In sternal bursitis there is enlargement of the bursa and accumulation of exudate. Some chickens may exhibit enlarged spleens and livers and the kidneys are swollen, pale and mottled.

DIAGNOSIS

As with *M. gallisepticum* the signs and lesions are not pathognomonic and diagnosis requires demonstration of specific antibodies or detection of the organism or its DNA. For serology the RSA test and ELISAs are commonly used. Isolation and PCR methods are generally similar to those used for *M. gallisepticum* although culture medium must contain a nicotinamide adenine dinucleotide supplement. *M. synoviae* is very susceptible to acid pH and cultures may die if allowed to become too acidic. The trachea is the best site for detection of *M. synoviae* and its DNA. It can rarely be found in affected joints.

CONTROL

Methods and strategies are similar to those for *M. gallisepticum* (Table 20.2), bearing in mind that *M. synoviae* is considered less pathogenic than *M. gallisepticum* but more resistant to antimicrobials. Routine administration of chlortetracycline in feed is widely used in infected table egg layers but the loss of zero withdrawal periods for such treatments will see this phased out in many areas. A live temperature-sensitive mutant vaccine MS-H is available in some countries for use in breeders and commercial layers and this has helped to reduce routine antibiotic treatments. The more variable approach to *M. synoviae* control in different poultry sectors appears to make control more difficult than *M. gallisepticum* control, possibly because sectors not controlling *M. synoviae* are a reservoir for infection of other sectors. Other factors may also influence control including the apparent ability of *M. synoviae* to spread between farms over greater distances than *M. gallisepticum*, possibly because of the higher tracheal populations in chronically infected birds.

MYCOPLASMA MELEAGRIDIS

M. meleagridis is a specific pathogen of turkeys, causing an egg-transmitted disease in which the main lesion is air sacculitis. It also causes poor growth and skeletal disorders in young poults.

M. meleagridis was eradicated by the primary turkey breeders but the infection still occurs sporadically.

Before eradication it was responsible for considerable economic loss but is now of much less significance. Control measures for *M. meleagridis* are included in European Community Directive 90/539/EEC and the NPIP of the USA, although it is not included the OIE list of notifiable diseases.

EPIDEMIOLOGY

Cause

M. meleagridis is a typical member of the genus in many properties. It agglutinates erythrocytes less readily than *M. gallisepticum* or *M. synoviae* and haemagglutination does not appear to be essential for virulence. Little comparison of *M. meleagridis* strains has been attempted but variation is seen in protein profiles.

Hosts

M. meleagridis was thought to infect only turkeys but recently it has been isolated from several clinically normal birds of prey in Germany.

Spread

In addition to egg transmission and horizontal transmission between birds by the respiratory route, *M. meleagridis* can also spread venereally. The organism may be harboured in the respiratory tract for months in mature turkeys and it is possible that infected air sacs may be the source of contamination of the oviduct. After egg transmission the cloaca and bursa of Fabricius of embryos and poults may be colonized with *M. meleagridis*, which can later ascend to infect the reproductive tracts of hens. The phallus of the male also harbours *M. meleagridis* and the hen can be infected by insemination with contaminated semen. This is considered to be an important means of sustaining infection in the female. Eggs laid early and late in the laying cycle are less likely to be infected. Indirect transmission of *M. meleagridis* can occur by handlers during artificial insemination procedures and at the hatchery during sexing.

Influencing factors

Pathogenic strains of *E. coli* can exacerbate respiratory disease with *M. meleagridis*, as can coinfection with *M. iowae*. *M. meleagridis* and *M. synoviae* together can act synergistically in causing sinusitis. Environmental factors probably exacerbate respiratory disease as for *M. gallisepticum*.

DISEASE

Pathogenesis

Lesions occur only in young poults, where the organism gains access either congenitally or through the respiratory tract. It has been suggested that the osteodystrophic form of disease (TS-65) results from reduction of nutrient supply, in particular biotin, to the growth plates of the long bones. However, the exact mechanism of disease production is not known for this or the respiratory form. There are also reports that *M. meleagridis* may cause immunosuppression in young poults.

Clinical signs

Mature birds do not show signs but there may be reduced egg hatchability. Young poults do not necessarily show clinical disease but in some flocks morbidity may exceed 10%, with poor growth and skeletal abnormalities.

Lesions

Skeletal lesions include osteodystrophy, with shortening, bowing and torsion of the tarsometatarsus and abnormalities of the cervical vertebrae. Wing feathers may protrude (helicopter feathering). Air sacculitis, which can result in condemnation at slaughter, usually affects only the thoracic air sacs initially but may spread later to other air sacs.

DIAGNOSIS

Clinical signs and lesions are not specific for *M. meleagridis* although those described above are suggestive. Confirmation is by serology, isolation of the *Mycoplasma* or demonstration of its DNA by PCR. Serology is usually by RSA test or ELISA and some ELISAs are produced specifically for use with turkey sera. Isolation can be attempted from respiratory tract, cloaca and bursa of Fabricius of poults and from the cloaca, oviduct, phallus or semen of mature birds. Many strains will grow well on mycoplasma agar but poorly in broth.

CONTROL

Control methods, including eradication, are as outlined for *M. gallisepticum* but heating of hatching eggs is not effective for killing *M. meleagridis* and causes unacceptably high embryo mortality. During eradication programmes pipped embryos and day-old culls are examined for *M. meleagridis* and all birds are examined at about 12 weeks. The phallus of males should be monitored by culture for *M. meleagridis* contamination during the prebreeding period of increased lighting. The oviducts of hens should also be swabbed and monitoring should continue for both sexes during the breeding period. Hygienic precautions are similar to those practised in other eradication programmes but, because of the importance of venereal transmission, extra care should be taken at artificial insemination and at the sexing of day-old poults.

MYCOPLASMA IOWAE

Some strains of *M. iowae* can cause turkey embryo mortality and poor-quality poults but successful eradication programmes have been conducted. Before eradication *M. iowae* was estimated to cause a 2–5% reduction in hatchability in UK commercial turkeys. Although the *M. iowae* status of many countries is unknown, it is now rarely encountered in commercial poultry in Europe.

EPIDEMIOLOGY

Cause

There appears to be more antigenic diversity within this species than in others and it was earlier divided into six serovars (I, J, K, N, Q and R). These groups are not supported by molecular studies. Virulence varies among strains and haemagglutination is an unstable property. *M. iowae* strains differ from other avian mycoplasmas in surviving longer in the environment, being more resistant to bile salts and having a predilection for the gastrointestinal tract and a relative resistance to many antimicrobials.

Hosts

The turkey is the favoured host for *M. iowae* but chickens are susceptible and it has been isolated from several species of free-flying bird.

Spread

The organism probably enters the egg via infected oviducts and is transmitted laterally after hatch. Venereal spread from contaminated males is also significant. Eggs laid late in the laying season are less likely to be infected.

Influencing factors

Concurrent infection with *M. meleagridis* increases the frequency and severity of air sacculitis but little is known about the influence of other infections or the environment.

DISEASE

Pathogenesis

There is little information available on the disease process. Proteins involved in cytadherence have been identified but no attachment organelle has been reported. *M. iowae* may cause transient immunosuppression in young poults.

Clinical signs

The only abnormality in mature birds is reduced hatchability of their eggs. Embryos usually die in the last stages of incubation and are stunted and congested. If any poults hatch with the infection they may be of poor quality with suboptimal growth and poor feathering. Experimental infection of embryos and day-old poults can cause a generalized disease with reduced growth, abnormal feathering, twisted leg, chondrodystrophy and some mortality. This is rarely seen under commercial conditions.

DIAGNOSIS

Reduced hatchability is a nonspecific sign and laboratory diagnosis should be attempted. *M. iowae* does not produce a reliable humoral antibody response so culture or PCR methods should be used. The organism can be found in the oropharynx, cloaca and air sacs of embryos and of very young poults and in the oviduct, cloaca and phallus of mature turkeys.

CONTROL

Eradication of *M. iowae* followed the same lines as *M. meleagridis* except that the effective drugs were limited to tiamulin and some quinolones. Other control methods are also as for *M. meleagridis*.

FURTHER READING

Bradbury J M 1998 Recovery of mycoplasmas from birds. In: Miles R J, Nicholas R A J (eds) Methods in molecular microbiology: mycoplasma protocols, vol 104. Humana Press, Totowa, p 45–51

Bradbury J M, Kleven S H 2003 *Mycoplasma iowae* infection. In: Saif Y M (ed) Diseases of poultry, 11th edn. Iowa State University Press, Ames, p 766–771

Chin R P, Ghazikhanian G Y, Kempf I 2003 *Mycoplasma meleagridis* infection. In: Saif Y M (ed) Diseases of poultry, 11th edn. Iowa State University Press, Ames, p 744–756

Christensen N H, Yavari C A, McBain A J, Bradbury J M 1994 Investigations into the survival of *Mycoplasma gallisepticum*, *Mycoplasma synoviae* and *Mycoplasma iowae* on materials found in the poultry house environment. Avian Pathol 23: 127–143

Ferguson N M, Hepp D, Sun S et al 2005 Use of molecular diversity of *Mycoplasma gallisepticum* by gene-targeted sequencing (GTS) and random amplified polymorphic DNA (RAPD) analysis for epidemiological studies. Microbiology 151: 1883–1893

Hong Y, García M, Leiting L et al 2004 Specific detection and typing of *Mycoplasma synoviae* strains in poultry with PCR and DNA sequence analysis targeting the hemagglutinin encoding gene *vlhA*. Avian Dis 48: 606–616

Jordan F T W 1981 Avian mycoplasmas. In: Tully J G, Whitcomb R (eds) The mycoplasmas, vol II. Academic Press, New York, p 1–18

Kempf I 1998 DNA amplification methods for diagnosis and epidemiological investigations of avian mycoplasmosis. Avian Pathol 27: 7–14

Kleven S H 2003 *Mycoplasma synoviae* infection. In: Saif Y M (ed) Diseases of poultry, 11th edn. Iowa State University Press, Ames, p 756–766

Kleven S H, Bradbury J M 2007 Avian mycoplasmosis (*Mycoplasma gallisepticum*, *Mycoplasma synoviae*). In: OIE Manual of diagnostic tests and vaccines for terrestrial animals (mammals, birds and bees), 6th edn. OIE, Paris, in press

Kleven S H, Levisohn S 1995 Mycoplasma infections of poultry. In: Razin S, Tully J G (eds) Molecular and diagnostic procedures in mycoplasmology, vol II. Academic Press, New York, p 283–292

Lauerman L H 1998 Nucleic acid amplification assays for diagnosis of animal diseases. American Association of Veterinary Laboratory Diagnosticians, Turlock

Levisohn S, Kleven S H 2000 Avian mycoplasmosis (*Mycoplasma gallisepticum*). Rev Sci Techn 19: 425–442

Ley D H 2003 *Mycoplasma gallisepticum* infection. In: Saif Y M (ed) Diseases of poultry, 11th edn. Iowa State University Press, Ames, IA, p 722–744

Naylor C J, Al-Ankari A R, Al-Afaleq A et al 1992 Exacerbation of *Mycoplasma gallisepticum* infection in turkeys by rhinotracheitis virus. Avian Pathol 21: 295–305

Stipkovits L, Kempf I 1996 Animal mycoplasmoses and control: mycoplasmoses in poultry. Rev Sci Techn 15: 1495–1525

Whithear K G 1996 Animal mycoplasmoses and control: control of avian mycoplasmoses by vaccination. Rev Sci Techn 15: 1527–1553

Workshop of European Mycoplasma Specialists 2005 Diagnostic problems associated with testing day old birds. Worlds Poult Sci J 61: 355–357

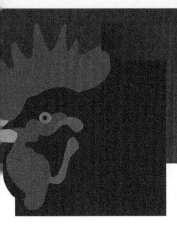

CHAPTER
21

Zerai Woldehiwet

Avian chlamydophilosis (chlamydiosis/psittacosis/ornithosis)

Avian chlamydophilosis (chlamydiosis) in humans and birds was originally called psittacosis because the disease was first recognized in parrots and other psittacine birds and in humans associated with psittacine birds. The term ornithosis was introduced later to describe the disease in other birds, including poultry. The rationale for separating these disease syndromes was based on the assumption that infections acquired from psittacine birds caused a more severe disease in humans than those contracted from other birds. As the organisms are known to affect humans and a wider range of avian hosts with variable degrees of severity, the term avian chlamydophilosis (chlamydiosis) is more appropriate. It is worldwide in prevalence but only occasional epidemics occur in poultry. Because of increasing evidence of its great genetic diversity, and the recent gene sequence analysis, the taxonomy of the family *Chlamydiaceae* has been revised recently. Thus the genus *Chlamydia* was retained and divided into three species and a new genus, *Chlamydophila*, with five new species, was created. All the human biovars associated with trachoma and other syndromes continue to be called *Chlamydia trachomatis*, whereas the hamster and mouse isolates were renamed *Chlamydia muridarum* and porcine isolates were renamed *Chlamydia suis*. The organisms formerly known as *Chlamydia pecorum* and *Chlamydia pneumoniae* were designated *Chlamydophila pecorum* and *Chlamydophila pneumoniae* respectively. The bacteria previously known as various serotypes of *Chlamydia psittaci* were assigned to four new species in the new genus *Chlamydophila*. The strains that cause avian chlamydiosis (psittacosis/ornithosis) belong to the new species *Chlamydophila psittaci* and the strains that cause abortion in ruminants, formerly *Chlamydia psittaci* serovar 1, were renamed *Chlamydophila abortus*. Strains of *Chlamydia psittaci* that affect cats and guinea pigs were renamed *Chlamydophila felis* and *Chlamydophila caviae* respectively. However, this new taxonomy has not yet gained general acceptance and papers using the old and new classification continue to appear in scientific journals.

EPIDEMIOLOGY

Cause

The chlamydias are Gram-negative, coccoid bacteria that depend on an intracellular environment for their multiplication. They differ from other intracellular bacteria mainly by their unique developmental cycle within the host cell. They also appear to lack peptidoglycan in their cell walls, which confers structural rigidity to other Gram-negative bacteria. Infection of host cells is initiated by endocytosis of the elementary bodies (EBs), which are small in size (250–300 nm diameter) and characteristically dense, with a rigid cell wall designed to withstand the rigours of the environment and transit between cells. Once these infectious EBs are enclosed within intracytoplasmic vacuoles, they are transformed into the larger (400–600 nm diameter), noninfectious reticulate bodies (RBs). The RBs have permeable and flexible walls which enable them to be metabolically active. Their primary role is the production of more progeny by binary fission before their transformation into EBs. The development cycle within the host, which takes about 30 h, is completed by daughter RBs reorganizing into EBs (Figs 21.1 and 21.2).

Avian strains have been classified into highly virulent ones causing acute epizootic infections and strains of low virulence causing slow spread of infection. However, some strains that are of low virulence in some birds may be more pathogenic to others and this variation in virulence may be seen between wild birds and domestic poultry and even between birds and humans.

Spread

Chlamydophila psittaci infection is endemic in parrots and other psittacine birds and natural infection also occurs in domestic poultry and free-living birds, including seagulls, wild and feral pigeons, house sparrows and blackbirds. Over 100 avian species have been shown to be infected. In many cases naturally infected birds show no clinical signs, remaining as carriers of infection for prolonged periods. Because of the broad range of hosts for *C. psittaci*, the reservoir of infection is very large. Infected birds are the main sources of infection for susceptible poultry,

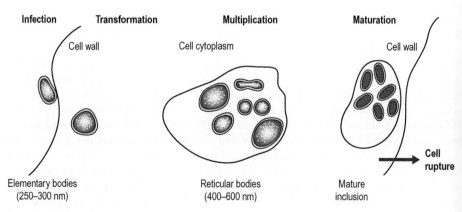

Fig. 21.1 Development cycle of chlamydia. Time from infection to release is 28–32 h.

with mammalian hosts playing a less significant role. The main sources of infection are birds in the prepatent stage of infection, birds with acute infections, carriers and contaminated inanimate material. Faeces and respiratory excretions from infected birds are particularly rich in EBs. Susceptible birds get infected mainly through the ingestion or inhalation of dust containing

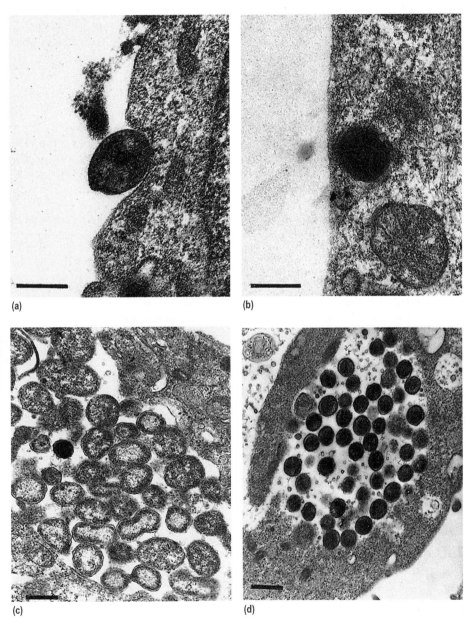

(a)

(b)

(c)

(d)

Fig. 21.2 (a) Elementary body attached to cell membrane ($\times$ 45 000; bar = 250 nm). (b) Elementary body within cell cytoplasm ($\times$ 45 000; bar = 250 nm). (c) Dividing reticular bodies in cytoplasmic vesicle ($\times$ 14 000; bar = 500 nm). (d) Elementary bodies in mature inclusion prior to rupture ($\times$ 14 500; bar = 500 nm).

EBs from dried faeces and other discharges, as the EBs are sufficiently resistant to survive the extracellular environment for days or even months. Infection also occurs by direct contact when birds are in close contact with acutely infected birds or carriers and indirectly through fomites and perhaps biting insects, mites and lice. Free-ranging domestic poultry are likely to acquire infection from infected migratory birds. Vertical transmission through the egg has not been demonstrated but the young are often infected from the exudates and faecal contamination of the parent and the general contamination of the nest in free-living birds. Although the EBs are highly resistant outside the host and can survive in dried excrement for many months within the carcass, they may not survive putrefaction.

Hosts

Among domestic poultry, turkeys are more susceptible than ducks and pigeons while chickens are rarely affected. Clinical disease is more common in young birds than in mature birds.

The main source of human infections is pet caged birds, with owners of parrots and other psittacine birds, owners of pet shops and those with regular contact with pigeons being at a higher risk, followed by other people who may come in contact with psittacine birds and pigeons professionally such as veterinarians, quarantine station workers, laboratory technicians and zoo workers.

However, serious infections could also be acquired from domestic poultry, particularly turkeys and ducks, with farmers, animal attendants and those working in processing plants being at a higher risk.

Influencing factors

Factors that may contribute to precipitation of disease or increase its severity include stress due to movement of birds, overcrowding, change of diet or environment and concurrent infections with other organisms such as salmonellas or *Pasteurella multocida*. Many of these influencing factors are of particular significance in recently imported psittacines.

DISEASE

Pathogenesis

After entry into the body, mainly by inhalation, the organisms multiply in the lungs, air sacs and pericardium and by haematogenous spread reach the liver, spleen and kidneys where further replication occurs and the production of RBs and EBs. In turkeys the organism is reported to reach the abdominal air sacs within 4 h and there is massive multiplication in the lungs within 24 h. After 48 h the organisms are released from the lungs and the air sacs into the blood, spleen, the liver, kidneys and into the environment via the nasal and intestinal secretions.

Clinical signs

Strains of *C. psittaci* that cause avian chlamydiosis may be highly virulent, causing a disease that spreads rapidly and with a mortality rate of 5–30%. When acute epidemics occur, up to 90% of the flock may be affected by the time clinical signs are noticed. When less virulent strains are involved, the disease spreads slowly, with mortality rates of less than 5%.

The incubation period is influenced by a number of factors including the virulence of the organism, the number of *Chlamydia* inhaled, the species and age of the host and other influencing factors. For example, in young turkeys infected with a virulent strain the incubation period may be as short as 5–10 days whereas in adult birds naturally infected with a less virulent strain the incubation period could be as long as 60 days. In some birds there may be no clinical signs at all and birds that have recovered from infection may carry the infection without apparent clinical disease. However, overt clinical signs may develop or the birds may die suddenly following environmental stress or other infections. In humans the incubation period of avian chlamydiosis is usually 5–14 days but longer incubation periods have also been described.

In turkeys, ducks and pigeons the clinical signs may be absent, mild or severe. At the peak of an acute clinical disease affected turkeys, ducks and pigeons are usually depressed, with ruffled feathers, anorexia, purulent nasal exudate and conjunctivitis. Sometimes there are obvious signs of respiratory disease characterized by rales and grey-green, gelatinous diarrhoea that may contain blood. The disease may also be manifested by nervous signs, with trembling and an unbalanced gait in ducklings and occasional transient ataxia in pigeons. In a flock the disease may be sporadic or a number of birds may be affected at the same time. Chickens, although susceptible, are rarely affected with clinical disease. However, sometimes affected birds may be characterized by growth retardation, weight loss and the reduction or end of egg-laying. Often, psittacine birds harbour infection without apparent clinical disease but typical clinical signs of anorexia, depression, diarrhoea and nasal and ocular discharge usually develop following stress of transport or after a change of diet or environment. Some birds may die suddenly following the rupture of the enlarged liver and spleen in chronically infected birds.

Lesions

The gross lesions vary according to the susceptibility of the host and the severity and duration of the disease. The lesions caused by the less virulent strains are less severe and extensive. In acutely infected turkeys and ducks the serosal surfaces are usually covered by serofibrinous exudate; there is pericarditis, congestion of the lungs, clouding of air sac walls and enlargement of the liver and spleen, both of which may be softer than normal and may show small necrotic foci and petechiae. Myocarditis and pneumonia may be present in turkeys with chlamydiosis. In pigeons and other birds with chronic infection splenomegaly and hepatomegaly may lead to the rupture of these organs and the acute fibrinous lesions of the air sacs may develop into granulomatous lesions. In psittacine birds the gross lesions are usually limited to the spleen, liver and the air sacs.

The histopathology is characterized by proliferative and necrotic changes in the affected organs, with tracheitis, pneumonitis and focal necrosis of the liver, particularly in parrots.

DIAGNOSIS

Clinical signs and gross lesions are helpful but definitive confirmation requires the demonstration of *Chlamydia*, chlamydial antigens or specific nucleic acids in infected tissues or body secretions or serological evidence of recent infection. However, because of the zoonotic nature of *C. psittaci*, tests that require the growth of the organisms are carried out only in specialist laboratories.

It is important that great care is taken when handling birds or carcasses suspected of being infected with *C. psittaci*, and this includes the wrapping of carcasses for dispatch to a specialist laboratory. Pathologists and laboratory workers should take special care when handling infected carcasses or live birds as they shed large quantities of infectious EBs. Dead birds should be immersed in effective disinfectants before post-mortem examinations are carried out. All procedures must be carried out under Class III containment to avoid the generation of dangerous aerosols.

Microscopic examination of stained smears

The demonstration of EBs in impression smears prepared from exudates, affected serosal surfaces, the liver, spleen or the lungs is a powerful and simple method of diagnosis. Fluids can be applied directly to slides or the cells from these fluids can be concentrated by centrifugation, washed and applied on to slides. The cytological preparations are then fixed with methanol, Zenker's or Bouin's fixative for better preservation before staining with the modified Ziehl–Neelsen, Machiavello or Gimenez method. EBs stand out as single or clusters of red particles. The direct examination of smears using stains that are specific to EBs may not be suitable for the demonstration of inclusion bodies of chlamydia grown in embryonated eggs, cell cultures or tissues of inoculated mice. Therefore, for these, other staining methods such as Giemsa should be employed.

Demonstration of antigens

When inclusion bodies suggestive of *C. psittaci* have been demonstrated in smears stained by modified Ziehl–Neelsen or other methods, it may be necessary to verify their identity by testing for specific antigens. Smears from affected tissues are fixed and then processed for fluorescent antibody or immunoperoxidase staining using monoclonal or polyclonal antibodies. Tests should include positive and negative controls for antigen and positive and negative sera. These methods can also be used to establish the identity of *C. psittaci* isolated in embryonated eggs or cell cultures.

Demonstration of specific DNA

DNA probes and the polymerase chain reaction (PCR) can be used to demonstrate specific DNA. It is now possible to design specific primers for the 16S ribosomal RNA to allow differentiation of *C. psittaci* from other similar agents, including *C. pecorum, C. trachomatis* and *C. pneumoniae*. Once the PCR has been used to identify an avian or human isolate as *C. psittaci*, it is also possible to differentiate it from nonavian strains of *C. psittaci* by restriction enzyme analysis of the nucleotide sequence generated by PCR.

Isolation and identification

The most definitive method of diagnosis involves the isolation of organisms in cell culture systems or embryonated hens' eggs.

To reduce bacterial contamination, ground tissues, exudate, other fluids or faeces are suspended in buffer or tissue culture fluid containing vancomycin, streptomycin, gentamicin or other antibiotics to give a final 10% concentration. The suspension is centrifuged at $2000\,g$ for 15–20 min to remove debris and tissue fragments and the supernatant used as inoculum for cell cultures or embryonated hens' eggs. The isolation of *C. psittaci* in continuous cell lines such as 'L' cells, McCoy cells or primary chick embryo cells can be enhanced by centrifuging the inoculum on to the monolayer of cells at $2000\,g$ for 30 min and by adding cycloheximide to the maintenance medium. The organism can also be isolated following the inoculation of the yolk sac of 5–7-day-old chicken embryos. It is important that fertile eggs are obtained from a flock receiving no antibiotics. Embryos are candled daily for evidence of loss of motility or death.

To detect the presence of *C. psittaci*, 'L' cells, McCoy cells, other cells or impression smears prepared from the yolk sac membrane are stained with Giemsa or other stains and the cells are examined for the presence of typical cytoplasmic inclusion bodies. The identity of the organisms can be confirmed by the demonstration of specific antigens by the complement fixation tests (CFT) or the enzyme-linked immunosorbent assay (ELISA) using monoclonal or polyclonal antibodies. Alternatively, the identity of the isolates can be established by PCR using species- and type-specific primers and restriction enzymes.

Laboratory mice and guinea pigs are susceptible to infection but are rarely used for diagnostic purposes. Mice are infected when they are 3–5 weeks old by injecting not more than 200 μL of the inoculum by the intraperitoneal route or by putting several drops of the inoculum into the nasal cavity of lightly anaesthetized mice.

Serology

Serological tests can be used to demonstrate current or past infections but diagnosis of recent infection depends on the demonstration of a rise in antibody titre by the examination of 'paired' serum samples. Serological methods of detecting and measuring antibodies include CFT, ELISA, immunofluorescence, latex agglutination and gel diffusion. The standard or direct CFT is widely used for the detection and assay of antibodies against *C. psittaci* in a wide range of hosts because it is sensitive and the procedures are well standardized. However, direct CFT cannot be used in some avian species, such as budgerigars and poultry, because of false-negative results. In these cases a modified (indirect) CFT or other serological method such as immunofluorescence can be used. Because of the tedious and complicated nature of the CFT, most laboratories are adopting the ELISA as a standard method for the detection and assay of antibodies against *C. psittaci*. The latex agglutination test has the advantage of being simple and rapid and, because it detects IgM, a positive reaction indicates current infection; however, it is less sensitive, resulting in more false-negative results. The agar gel precipitation test is slow and relatively insensitive.

CONTROL

The organisms are susceptible to a number of antimicrobials. Treatment of infected and in-contact birds with broad-spectrum antibiotics for several weeks is effective in reducing infection and may eliminate it in some cases. Chlortetracycline has been most commonly used and for turkeys a dose of 200–800 g/tonne in the food or 0.2–0.4 g/L (1–2 g/gallon) in the drinking water is recommended. The lower doses are effective against severe disease but the higher doses are necessary for attempted elimination of the organism. For either, treatment should be continued for up to 45 days.

Doxycycline, a semisynthetic tetracycline derivative, is also recommended. It is rapidly and almost completely absorbed from the gastrointestinal tract and its absorption is less adversely affected by calcium than chlortetracycline. It has a longer serum half-life and provides greater tissue concentrations. Quinolones are also effective against *C. psittaci* infections in avian species. Exotic birds can be treated by incorporating the antimicrobial in seed or syrup.

Hygienic precautions are essential to minimize spread of infection to other birds and human attendants. These include restriction on movement of stock and people, quarantine, cleaning and the use of appropriate disinfectants such as iodophors or formaldehyde. In particular, attention should be paid to minimizing the spread of infected dust.

Live and inactivated vaccines (bacterins) have been found to be protective. However, the former may result in carriers and several inoculations of the latter are necessary. There are no vaccines commercially available in Europe for the protection of poultry against chlamydiosis.

LEGAL REQUIREMENTS AND PUBLIC HEALTH SIGNIFICANCE

Several countries have import and export controls and quarantine regulations on psittacine birds. In the USA several states have regulations that make it mandatory to report all cases of chlamydiosis and the Surgeon General of the USA may declare an area 'infected' with chlamydiosis if persons or psittacine birds are considered to have been infected with *C. psittaci*. In the UK the disease is not notifiable but is subject to control measures stipulated in the Psittacosis/Ornithosis Order 1953. This provides for the detention and isolation of affected or suspect birds and for other measures to prevent spread, such as cleaning and disinfection. All birds, including poultry, imported into the UK are subject to quarantine for a period of 35 days.

FURTHER READING

Andersen A A, Vanrompay D 2003 Avian chlamydiosis (psittacosis, ornithosis). In: Saif Y M (ed) Diseases of poultry, 11th edn. Iowa State University Press, Ames, p 863–879

Anon 1989 Reports from the Symposium on Avian Chlamydiosis. 125th Annual American Veterinary Medical Association Meeting, Portland, Oregon, USA, 1988. J Am Vet Med Assoc 195: 1501–1575

Bevan B J, Cullen G A, Read W M F 1978 Isolation of *Chlamydia psittaci* from avian sources using growth in cell culture. Avian Pathol 7: 203–211

Brumfield H P, Benson H N, Pomeroy B S 1961 Procedures for modified complement fixation test with turkey, duck and chicken serum antibody. Avian Dis 5: 270–282

Everett K D, Bush R M, Anderson A A 1999 Emended description of the order Chlamydiales, proposal of Parachlamydiaceae fam. nov. and Simkaniaceae fam. nov., each containing one monotypic genus, revised taxonomy of the family Chlamydiaceae, including a new genus and five new species, and standards for the identification of organisms. Int J Syst Bacteriol 49: 415–440

Flammer K, Trogdon H N, Papich M 2003 Assessment of plasma concentrations of doxycycline in budgerigars fed medicated seed or water, duck and chicken serum antibody. J Am Vet Med Assoc 223: 993–998

Hewinson R G, Rankin S E S, Bevan B J et al 1991 Detection of *Chlamydia psittaci* from avian field samples using PCR. Vet Rec 128: 129–130

Sheehy N, Markey B, Quinn J P 1997 Analysis of partial rRNA nucleotide sequences of *Chlamydia pecorum* and *C. psittaci*. FEMS Immunol Med Microbiol 17: 201–205

Smith K A, Bradley K K, Stobierski M G, Tengelsen L A 2005 Compendium of measures to control *Chlamydophila psittaci* (formerly *Chlamydia psittaci*) infection among humans (psittacosis) and pet birds. Am J Vet Res 226: 532–539

Spencer W N, Johnson F W A 1983 A simple transport medium for the isolation of chlamydia from clinical material. Vet Rec 113: 535–536

Treharne J D, Darouger S, Jones B R 1977 Modification of the micro-immunofluorescence test to provide a routine serological test for chlamydial infection. J Clin Pathol 30: 510–517

Woldehiwet Z, Scott G R 1993 Public health significance of animal rickettsiae and chlamydiae: In: Woldehiwet Z, Ristic M (eds) Rickettsial and chlamydial diseases of animals. Pergamon, Oxford, p 395–412

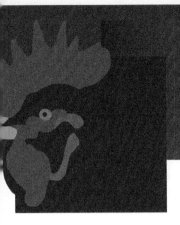

CHAPTER

22

Frank T. W. Jordan and
David J. Hampson

Some other bacterial diseases

AEROMONAS HYDROPHILA AND *AEROMONAS FORMICANS*

Aeromonas bacilli appear to be opportunist pathogens of poultry, with *Aeromonas hydrophila* occasionally causing diarrhoea in chickens and turkeys, cellulitis in turkeys and salpingitis, air sacculitis and septicaemia in ducks. *Aeromonas formicans* has been isolated from arthritic lesions in ducks and inflammation of the penis in geese. These organisms are motile, Gram-negative, aerobic or facultative anaerobes that are present in fresh and brackish water and in seawater, sewage and soil. Diagnosis is associated with signs, lesions and the isolation of the organism. *A. hydrophila* is of public health significance, usually through poultry meat, causing human gastroenteritis and diarrhoea.

FURTHER READING

Barnes H J 2003 Aeromonas. In: Saif Y M (ed) Diseases of poultry, 11th edn. Iowa State University Press, Ames, p 846

BRACHYSPIRA SPP. – INTESTINAL SPIROCHAETOSIS

Avian intestinal spirochaetosis (AIS) is a disease complex that has been reported mainly in laying hens and in broiler breeder hens and is associated with chronic diarrhoea and/or reduced egg production. Where it has been specifically investigated, infection with *Brachyspira* species has been found to be remarkably common. Between 30% and 70% of laying hen and broiler breeder hen

243

farms in different regions have been found to be infected with intestinal spirochaetes, although obvious signs of AIS are not always present in these farms. AIS is known to occur in Europe, the USA and Australia, and is almost certainly under-reported and endemic worldwide.

EPIDEMIOLOGY

Cause

AIS results from colonization of the caeca and rectum with one or more species of anaerobic intestinal spirochaete of the genus *Brachyspira*. The genus currently contains seven species and several possible species. Previously some of these species were classified in the genus *Treponema*, or more recently in the genus *Serpulina*. The two most commonly reported pathogenic species in poultry are *Brachyspira intermedia* and *Brachyspira pilosicoli*, with a third, *Brachyspira alvinipulli*, to date having been reported as a pathogen in two laying hen flocks in the USA and in two goose flocks in Hungary. The porcine pathogen *Brachyspira hyodysenteriae* (the cause of swine dysentery) has been reported as a cause of necrotizing typhlocolitis in captive rheas (*Rhea americana*) and has been isolated from feral mallards and laying hens but is not currently thought to be a major problem in commercial poultry. The proposed species '*Brachyspira pulli*' is widespread in poultry and may be mildly pathogenic under certain circumstances. Other *Brachyspira* species that are sometimes isolated from poultry are assumed to be commensals, although further work is required to confirm this. The existence of such morphologically similar commensal species can complicate the diagnosis of AIS.

Brachyspiras are anaerobic, Gram-negative helical bacteria. They have multiple periplasmic flagella running along the length of the cells under the outer envelope, which confer to them a corkscrew-like motility. The organisms can be examined by dark-field or phase-contrast microscopy and can be stained with Wright–Giemsa stain.

Hosts

B. intermedia infection is mainly confined to pigs and poultry. This species is closely related to the important pig pathogen *B. hyodysenteriae* and has occasionally been suspected to cause colitis in pigs.

B. pilosicoli colonizes the large intestines of many species of domestic and feral animals and birds, as well as humans (particularly in developing countries). It is considered to be a common and important enteric pathogen of pigs.

In addition to layer hens and broiler-breeders, turkeys, geese and game birds may also be affected. *B. intermedia*, *B. pilosicoli* and *B. alvinipulli* have all been used under experimental conditions to induce disease in commercial adult hens, including increasing faecal water content and reducing egg production. Disease was not as severe as sometimes reported in the field, presumably because the experimental hens were less crowded and stressed than their counterparts in commercial conditions. Young birds (broilers) are also susceptible to these three species, as well as to other species such as *B. hyodysenteriae* and '*B. pulli*' but do not appear to be exposed to infections with *Brachyspira* species under normal conditions and therefore natural infection of broiler chickens has not been recorded.

Spread

Colonization with *Brachyspira* species is rarely found before birds are 15 weeks of age; hence, the hatchery or rearing flocks appear unlikely to be the major source of infection for laying hen or breeder flocks. The *Brachyspira* species involved in AIS only survive for a few hours to days in chicken faeces and are highly susceptible to most commonly used disinfectants. Hence, provided that newly stocked sheds have been cleaned, disinfected and rested, birds are unlikely to acquire infection from the local environment. Feral birds, rodents and animals such as dogs may carry intestinal spirochaetes and could potentially introduce infection into a flock. Faecal contamination of drinking water, for example from ducks visiting dams or ponds, is another possible means of introduction. The most likely source of infection, however, is from other adult birds in older flocks on a site, with contaminated faeces being transmitted to new flocks via movement of staff and equipment.

Once a new flock becomes infected, the spirochaetes are readily transmitted in faeces and probably also by aerosol. Consequently, the prevalence of infection within flocks increases with increasing age, with up to 100% of birds being colonized in older flocks. Mixed infections with more than one pathogenic *Brachyspira* species, as well as other commensal species, can occur, with multiple different strains of each pathogenic species potentially being present.

Influencing factors

As indicated, infection is more common in older flocks. Housing multiple hens in cages in close proximity is likely to facilitate transmission. Disease is more common during stressful periods such as moulting or onset of lay. Infection of outdoor flocks is common. Dietary influences on AIS have been demonstrated. In particular, diets based on wheat seem to predispose hens to infection with *Brachyspira* species.

DISEASE

Pathogenesis of *B. pilosicoli* and *B. intermedia*

The pathogenesis of these infections in poultry is not clear but a feature of *B. pilosicoli* is its ability to attach by one cell end to enterocytes in the large intestine, forming a 'false brush border' of spirochaetes that can be seen on histological sections. This 'carpet-pile-like' form of colonization may occur throughout the large intestine, or be localized and focal, or not be observed at all – even though signs of disease are present. A spirochaetaemia caused by *B. pilosicoli* has been reported in debilitated and immunocompromised human patients, although whether this complication occurs in poultry and in other animal such as pigs remains to be determined.

B. intermedia does not specifically attach to enterocytes but may be found in large numbers in the mucus layer in an apparently loose association with the underlying enterocytes.

Clearly defined virulence determinants have not been described in either of these two pathogenic *Brachyspira* species. They are both highly motile in mucus and undergo chemotaxis, which is assumed to be important for colonization. *B. pilosicoli* is known to produce cell-surface-associated proteases but to date no specific toxins have been recognized.

Signs

The most consistent clinical sign of AIS is intermittent chronic diarrhoea, which typically may be seen in 5–20% of a flock. Faeces may be yellowish-brown, mucoid and/or foamy, with increases in both lipid and water ($\approx$15%) content. Eggs from infected hens become stained with faeces (preventing them from being sold as table eggs for direct consumption), and the feathers around the vent may be soiled ('pasty vents'). In flocks with widespread AIS, problems of 'wet litter' may be reported. This is manifest as faeces failing to 'cone' under cages, difficulties with mechanical cleaning and problems of increased odour emission and attraction of flies to the site. Furthermore, egg production may be delayed and/or reduced (by 5–10%), with eggs being smaller and lighter and having poorer shell quality. Broiler chicks hatched from infected broiler breeder hens also may be weak, with slow weight gain.

Gross lesions

There are no specific gross lesions seen in AIS. Affected caeca may be dilated with yellow-brown foamy or watery fluid. Histological examination may reveal a mild typhlitis and sometimes the obvious presence of spirochaetes.

DIAGNOSIS

Diagnosis is usually based on clinical signs, supported by the results of specific microbiological investigations.

The *Brachyspira* species involved in AIS typically can be grown on selective Trypticase Soy agar, containing 5% defibrinated ovine or bovine blood, 400 µg/mL spectinomycin and 25 µg/mL each of colistin and vancomycin. The plates are incubated in an anaerobic environment at 37–41°C for 3–10 days and any spirochaetal growth is observed under a phase-contrast or dark-field microscope. Typically, specific polymerase chain reaction (PCR) assays are then conducted on the primary growth to identify the species present. Differentiation by biochemical testing is possible but is not completely reliable. Isolates can be grown in specialized anaerobic broth media, and strain typing can be achieved using pulsed field gel electrophoresis.

CONTROL

Strict biosecurity should be maintained to prevent entry of infection, as well as spread between flocks on a site. This should include the presence of security fences around the site, minimization of movement of staff around the site, provision of footbaths outside sheds and the wearing of clean protective clothing and footwear. Measures should be taken to prevent hens from coming into contact with faeces from wild birds and animals. Treating infected laying flocks with antimicrobials is problematic because of the possibility of drug residues remaining in the eggs. If the eggs are to be consumed, then only registered antimicrobials that have no withdrawal periods should be used. Antimicrobials that have been used in the water to control AIS in some experimental studies include tiamulin (not to be used with ionophores: monensin, salinomycin and narasin), lincomycin, oxytetracycline and nitroimidazole derivatives. Where problems of AIS exist, the diet should be examined. If possible, wheat should be avoided, as well as cereal and legume sources rich in soluble nonstarch polysaccharides (which themselves can cause wet litter problems). No vaccines are currently available for AIS.

PUBLIC HEALTH CONSIDERATIONS

B. pilosicoli can colonize humans and may be invasive in immunocompromised individuals. The possibility that chickens could be a source of human infection should be considered.

FURTHER READING

Davelaar F G, Smits H F, Houvind-Hougan K et al 1986 Infectious typhlitis in chickens caused by spirochaetes. Avian Pathol 15: 247–258

Phillips N D, La T, Pluske J R, Hampson D J 2004 A wheat-based diet enhances colonisation with the intestinal spirochaete *Brachyspira intermedia* in experimentally-infected laying hens. Avian Pathol 33: 451–457

Phillips N D, La T, Hampson D J 2005 A cross-sectional study to investigate the occurrence and distribution of intestinal spirochaetes (*Brachyspira* spp.) in three flocks of laying hens. Vet Microbiol 105:
189–198

Stephens C P, Hampson D J 1999 Prevalence and disease association of intestinal spirochaetes in chickens
in eastern Australia. Avian Pathol 28: 447–454

Stephens C P, Hampson D J 2001 Intestinal spirochaete infections in chickens: a review of disease associations, epidemiology and control. Animal Health Res Rev 2: 101–110

Stephens C P, Hampson D J 2002 Experimental infection of broiler breeder hens with the intestinal spirochaete *Brachyspira* (*Serpulina*) *pilosicoli* causes reduced egg production. Avian Pathol 31: 169–175

Swayne D E, Bermudez A J, Sagartz J E et al 1992 Association of cecal spirochetes with pasty vents and
dirty eggshells in layers. Avian Dis 36: 776–781

BORRELIA ANSERINA SPIROCHAETOSIS (BLOOD SPIROCHAETES)

See Chapter 39 on parasitic diseases.

LISTERIA MONOCYTOGENES – LISTERIOSIS

This organism is widespread in nature and occasionally causes disease in humans and animals.

EPIDEMIOLOGY

Cause

Listeria monocytogenes is a small (0.4–0.5 μm × 0.5–2.0 μm) Gram-positive, nonsporing bacillus
or coccobacillus, which may be seen in groups of two or more and in a rough form it is filamentous. It is flagellate and, at 6–22°C, is motile with a tumbling motion. It can transform between
bacterial and L forms and there are 16 serotypes, all of which are considered to be potentially
pathogenic. It is ubiquitous and found in soil, silage, rotting vegetation and surface water, and
in poultry meat and in the intestine of apparently healthy and diseased animals and birds. It
can grow between 0°C and 43°C, with an optimal range of 30–37°C and a pH range of about
4.5–9.6. It can survive outside the body of the host, under moist conditions, for several years. It
is susceptible to pasteurization at 75°C for 10 s and, although varied in its susceptibility to antimicrobials, tetracyclines are commonly recommended in treatment.

Hosts

Many species of bird, fish and mammal may be infected with *L. monocytogenes* and the infection in poultry is of public health importance because it can be a source of infection for humans
through faeces and meat.

Spread

Among poultry, spread can occur through the faeces. However, with an organism as ubiquitous as this and able to survive for long periods outside the body, it may be difficult to determine the source and spread of infection. There is no evidence for egg transmission.

Influencing factors

The young are more susceptible than older birds and, apart from this, outbreaks of disease are associated with factors such as immunosuppression of the host and environmental cold and wet conditions.

DISEASE

Pathogenesis

Infection can follow ingestion, inhalation or wound contamination such as can occur after beak trimming.

Signs

In poultry enteric colonization with the organism may occur without the birds showing disease. Indeed, disease is rare in poultry although sporadic outbreaks do occur in chickens, turkeys, ducks, geese and pigeons, especially in temperate zones. Mortality can vary from very few to 40% of an affected flock.

The disease signs in birds occur either with progressive emaciation, nervous signs or sudden death and are associated with a septicaemic or encephalitic form or sometimes both. In neither are the signs pathognomonic. Depression is seen in both forms and in the former there may also be diarrhoea while in the less frequent encephalitic form the signs include incoordination, ataxia, torticollis and opisthotonos.

Lesions

The gross lesions associated with septicaemia are varied and include myocarditis with pale necrotic foci, hydropericardium, focal hepatic necrosis and, less frequently, splenomegaly with necrotic foci, nephritis, oedema of the lungs, thickening of the air sac walls, enteritis and conjunctivitis. In acute cases the only lesion may be congestion of the whole carcass with petechial haemorrhages on the serosa. In hens, salpingitis may occur following the acute disease. In the encephalitic form, small necrotic foci may be seen in the cerebellum, midbrain and medulla.

Microscopically, inflammatory cells and Gram-positive bacteria are seen in lesions.

DIAGNOSIS

Signs and lesions may be of some value but confirmation of disease can be made by isolation of the causal organism, demonstration of specific antigen in tissue or detection of DNA. Of these, culture of the bacterium is the most common method and, in attempting to grow the organism from uncontaminated sources such as myocardial lesions, unenriched medium is satisfactory. However, if there is contamination with other bacteria, a medium containing both enriching and selective agents is required or the prolonged 'cold enrichment technique' can be used. Isolation may also be achieved by culturing in the allantoic cavity of the developing chick embryo.

The organism may be identified by biochemical means, immunofluorescence or DNA analysis and an enzyme-linked immunosorbent assay (ELISA) has also been developed.

Since antibodies to *L. monocytogenes* are widespread in the blood of apparently normal animals, serological testing is not used for detecting infection.

For differential diagnosis, consideration should be given to conditions causing signs and gross and histological lesions of septicaemia or encephalitis, such as fowl cholera. fowl typhoid, Newcastle disease, avian influenza and *Pseudomonas aeruginosa* infection.

CONTROL

Control of disease in poultry is largely dependent on avoiding potential sources of infection and practising a high standard of management.

PUBLIC HEALTH CONSIDERATIONS

It is important to appreciate that this organism may be pathogenic to humans, particularly the very young and the immunologically compromised. Milk, vegetables, soft cheeses and meat, including poultry, may be sources of infection. It is important to realize also that the organism will continue to grow in some prepared foods kept at low temperatures and is of significance in human food-borne diseases.

FURTHER READING

Barnes J H 2003 *Listeria*. In: Saif Y M (ed) Diseases of poultry, 11th edn. Iowa State University Press, Ames, p 850

Gray M L, Killinger A H 1966 *Listeria monocytogenes* and listeric infections. Bacteriol Rev 30: 309–382

MEGABACTERIA

Although originally found to be associated with loss of condition in budgerigars, this organism has also been isolated from chickens and turkeys in poor condition and from fatalities in young ostriches. The causal organism is large, rod shaped and fungus-like. It is Gram-positive and periodic acid–Schiff-positive. However its classification awaits further study and in poultry it is uncertain whether it is a primary pathogen since, in some cases, other diseases have been found to coexist.

The disease associated with this organism particularly affects the proventriculus and occasionally the gizzard. There is an inflammatory response in the epithelium and considerable thickening of the wall. Diagnosis of the disease depends on thickening of the proventriculus and especially the epithelial surface from which numerous large organisms can be seen in smears or histological sections. Control is based on hygiene and the removal of infected stock.

FURTHER READING

Barnes H J 2003 Megabacteria. In: Saif Y M (ed) Diseases of poultry, 11th edn. Iowa State University Press, Ames, p 851

MORAXELLA OSLOENSIS – MORAXELLOSIS

This Gram-negative, short, plump, rod-shaped bacterium has been isolated from turkeys with a disease similar to fowl cholera, and from chickens with salpingitis. The organism differs from *Pasteurella multocida* by its growth on MacConkey medium and eosin–methylene blue medium.

FURTHER READING

Barnes H J 2003 *Moraxella*. In: Saif Y M (ed) Diseases of poultry, 11th edn. Iowa State University Press, Ames, p 851

Bisgaard M, Dam A 1981 Salpingitis in poultry. II. Prevalence, bacteriology and possible pathogenesis in egg-laying chickens. Nord Vet Med 33: 81–89

Emerson F G, Kolb G E, Van-Natta F A 1983 Chronic cholera-like lesions caused by *Moraxella osloensis*. Avian Dis 27: 836–838

MYCOBACTERIUM AVIUM – AVIAN TUBERCULOSIS

Avian tuberculosis occurs throughout the world in many avian and some mammalian species and in domestic poultry it is generally seen in mature stock kept in conditions of poor management. It usually runs a protracted course, causing reduction in condition, reduced egg production and eventually death. Although loss in a flock is intermittent it is invariably in adult fowls and this, together with the culling of unthrifty birds and the depression in egg production, can cause serious economic loss. The infection is of importance also because the disease occurs in wild birds, pigs, rabbits and mink.

EPIDEMIOLOGY

Cause

Mycobacterium avium is the name given to a complex group of mycobacterial organisms that, according to current taxonomy, consists of four subtypes:

- *M. avium* subsp. *avium* consists of three serotypes (1, 2 and 3) and several genotypes: this subtype is fully virulent for birds and small terrestrial mammals
- *M. avium* subsp. *hominissuis* consists of serotypes 4–6, 8–11 and 21, and several genotypes, and is found mainly in the external environment, dust, water, soil and invertebrates but some are virulent for birds
- *M. avium* subsp. *paratuberculosis* consists of a number of genotypes and affects ruminants and other animals
- *M. avium* subsp. *silvaticum* is isolated rarely and can be virulent for birds.

These mycobacteria are acid- and alcohol-fast when stained by the Ziehl–Neelsen method and the organisms often appear beaded. Of this large number of serotypes it is types 1, 2 and 3 that are most virulent and are mainly responsible for the disease in poultry. Even among these serotypes there is considerable variation in virulence. *M. avium*, compared with other mycobacteria, is relatively resistant to antimicrobials and relatively resistant to a number of disinfectants but is sensitive to ionic detergents. Outside the body it can survive for many years but the unprotected organism is killed by direct sunlight and within the carcass the organism survives for no more than a few weeks. It does not show tropism for any particular tissue but gross lesions of the liver, spleen, intestine and bone marrow are most commonly seen.

Hosts

It is probable that all species of bird can be infected but susceptibility among domestic species seems to be in the following order: chickens, ducks, geese and, least susceptible, turkeys, in which it is relatively uncommon. The disease is observed most commonly in older poultry because of the greater opportunity for infection with age and the generally long incubation period. However, occasionally, heavy losses may occur in pullets on multiage sites where the infection is endemic and the standards of hygiene poor. Game birds, particularly pheasants, are also susceptible. Some birds kept in zoological gardens seem to be prone to tuberculosis, perhaps because of the difficulty in adequately cleaning and disinfecting pens. Cage birds may also succumb to avian tuberculosis but tuberculosis in parrots and canaries may also be caused by *M. bovis* or *M. tuberculosis*. Surveys show that many species of wild bird become naturally infected and in some instances a predisposing factor is their close association with infection in domestic stock. Among mammals *M. avium* can cause progressive disease in swine, rabbits and mink and can cause sensitivity in cattle to the skin tuberculin test.

Spread

In the transmission of infection the most important source of the organism is the infected host, including domestic poultry, game birds and pet or wild birds. Next in importance, because of the prolonged survival of *M. avium* outside the body of the host, are items contaminated with the droppings and excrement of such birds. These commonly include litter, contaminated pens and pasture, equipment and implements that come into contact with infected hosts, and the hands, feet and clothing of attendants. 'Swill' containing offal or trimmings from tuberculous fowl or pigs can also be a source of infection. Eggs would seem to be only of minor importance in the spread of avian tuberculosis. Tubercular lesions have occasionally been noted in the reproductive tract (ovary and oviduct of the female and testes of the male) and tubercle bacilli have been reported, rarely, in the eggs laid by tuberculous hens. However, there is no evidence to suggest that chicks hatched from such eggs are likely to be infected or that disease is likely to be introduced into a flock by this means.

Influencing factors

The infections are worldwide but disease varies between and within countries. In domestic poultry lack of hygiene in management and the age of the birds influence the appearance of the disease since the organism is highly resistant in the environment and within the host is generally associated with a long incubation period.

DISEASE

Signs

Signs may be prolonged over a period of weeks or months before death. There is generally progressive but slow loss of condition and accompanying loss of energy and increasing lethargy. Although the appetite usually remains good, there is eventually gross emaciation with marked atrophy of the sternal muscles, with the 'keel' becoming prominent or even 'knife-edged'. The face and comb become pale and sometimes jaundiced and the comb is shrunken and often there is persistent diarrhoea with soiling of the tail feathers. Occasionally a bird will show a hopping, jerky type of locomotion, which is usually unilateral and is thought to be associated with tubercular lesions of the bone marrow of the leg bones or joints. Some may adopt a sitting position. Occasionally, birds may die suddenly in good bodily condition and yet show advanced lesions of tuberculosis. In such cases rupture of the affected liver or spleen with consequent internal haemorrhage is often the precipitating cause of death.

Lesions

Gross lesions, in the chicken, are most commonly seen in the intestines, liver, spleen and bone marrow but may be found in any organ or tissue. Irrespective of the organ involved, the lesions are typical tubercular granulomata. They are irregular, grey-white nodules, varying in size from pinpoint to large masses of coalescing tubercular material. When cut through, the nodules are firm and caseous and the centres may be a pale yellow colour, particularly those from the bone marrow. Those in the liver and intestine may show bile staining. The liver and spleen are often grossly enlarged and occasionally rupture, resulting in blood in the body cavity and sudden death. The smaller tubercles in these organs can be readily enucleated from the surrounding tissue, particularly when they protrude from the surface. Such protrusion of tubercles from the surface of the spleen gives the organ an irregular, 'knobbly' appearance. The wall of the intestine is invariably studded with similar lesions, varying in size from a millimetre to several centimetres in diameter. They usually involve the whole thickness of the intestinal wall and eventually ulcerate into the lumen of the intestine, with consequent discharge of bacilli and probably constituting the major source of infection within the droppings. The bone marrow of the long bones of the legs frequently contains tubercular nodules, which can best be seen macroscopically if the bones are split longitudinally, particularly in the region of the femoro-tibiotarsal and tibiotarsal–tarsometatarsal joints. They are pale yellow in colour and vary in size and number. This is one of the distinctive features of tuberculosis in the chicken. The lungs are less frequently affected in the domestic chicken but more commonly in waterfowl. Tubercle bacilli have been isolated from some cases of arthritis affecting the phalangeal joints ('bumble foot') in the fowl.

DIAGNOSIS

The clinical signs and gross lesions are strongly indicative of avian tuberculosis and the demonstration of acid/alcohol-fast tubercle bacilli in lesions or sections is supportive of this. There is seldom any difficulty in demonstrating the organisms, which are often present in very large numbers, particularly in young lesions and those from the bone marrow. Cultural examination, or even chick inoculation of suspect material, may be necessary when organisms are few or for isolation and identification of the causal agent. The agent can also be identified by DNA techniques.

Immunological tests are also of value in the recognition of infected birds during life. They include the tuberculin test, an agglutination test and ELISA. The tuberculin test in the fowl consists of injection of 0.05–0.1 mL of avian tuberculin into one wattle using a needle about 1 cm long and of 25 gauge. The other wattle remains uninjected as the control. When testing a flock it is usual to inject the tuberculin into the wattle on the same side for each bird. The needle is introduced at the lower edge of the wattle and is directed upwards into the centre. The test is read 48 h after the injection of tuberculin, although some positive reactions may be observed sooner than this. The test is read by palpating the two wattles simultaneously between the first finger and thumb of each hand. A positive reaction is recognized by a hot, soft, oedematous swelling of the injected wattle, which may be twice the size of the uninjected one or even larger. Most uninfected birds will show no reaction in the injected wattle and occasional small, firm, pea-like swellings can usually be ignored. The accuracy of the test, relative to gross lesions seen at necropsy, in detecting infected birds is about 80%. However, birds in an advanced stage of infection may give no reaction. It is possible, however, that such birds would be thin or emaciated on handling during the testing of a flock and thus arouse suspicion of tuberculosis.

Various modifications of the site of inoculation of tuberculin have been suggested for turkeys, ducks and other birds but this test has not yet proved to be reliable for these species. For these the whole-blood, stained antigen agglutination test may be preferable. In this test a drop of antigen (a suspension of avian tubercle bacilli) is mixed with a drop of blood from the bird under test. A positive reaction is indicated by agglutination within 1 min. The distinct advantage of this test is that birds have only to be handled once; however, its lack of specificity must be considered.

In differential diagnosis, at necropsy, most difficulty might be in differentiation from neoplasia but the simple enucleation of tubercular lesions from the surrounding tissues and the demonstration of typical acid fast organisms should be adequate.

CONTROL

In the control of this condition in poultry there are a number of basic features to be considered:

- The main sources of infection are infected hosts (live or dead) and anything that might be contaminated by their excretions or faeces. In this respect the resistance of the organism outside the body of the host must be appreciated. Other poultry, wild birds, pigs and other mammals may also be of significance as reservoirs of infection
- Infection can be monitored readily by clinical, necropsy, bacterial and serological means
- Neither drug therapy nor vaccination is economically feasible
- Greatest losses are experienced in stock older than about 18 months of age
- On some premises it may be impractical to attempt eradication of indigenous infection.

Control on infected premises may be by attempting eradication of infection, or by living with reduced infection. For eradication and the maintenance of freedom the requirements include (1) the removal of all infected material; (2) the introduction of stock that are free of infection (these could be day-old chicks or older stock considered to be free because of absence of clinical signs and lesions and negative serological tests); (3) the prevention of entry of the infection to the stock; and (4) monitoring, when appropriate, to determine freedom from infection.

Living with reduced infection can only be considered in circumstances in which it is not practical to attempt eradication. These include circumstances where the weight of infection, and thus the more adverse effects of the disease, may be reduced by such practices as (1) keeping stock no longer than the first laying season, (2) monitoring for infection and disposing of positive reactors and (3) practising all reasonable hygienic precautions to prevent entry of the infection and to remove it when the premises become empty. This is most difficult, if not impossible, under free-range management.

No vaccines are available for this infection.

PUBLIC HEALTH CONSIDERATIONS

Although the avian tubercle bacillus has been isolated in a few instances from humans, such cases are extremely rare and poultry would seem to be of little importance in the epidemiology of human tuberculosis. Nevertheless, carcasses of tuberculous poultry should be rejected for human consumption.

FURTHER READING

Boughton E 1969 Tuberculosis caused by *Mycobacterium avium*. Vet Bull 39: 457–465

Feldman W H 1983 Avian tuberculosis infections. Williams & Wilkins, Baltimore

Fulton R M, Thoen C O 2003 Tuberculosis. In: Saif Y M (ed) Diseases of poultry, 11th edn. Iowa State University Press, Ames, p 836–844

Keymer I F 1997 *Mycobacterium* infections of birds. Vet Rec 140: 292

Keymer I F, Jones D M, Pugsley S L, Wadsworth P F 1982 A survey of tuberculosis in the birds of Regent's Park Gardens of the Zoological Society of London. Avian Pathol 11: 563–569

Rozanska M 1965 Preparation of the whole blood rapid agglutination test and its specificity for diagnosis of avian tuberculosis. Bull Vet Inst Pulawy 20–25

Thorel M-F 2004 Avian tuberculosis. In: OIE Manual of diagnostic tests and vaccines for terrestrial animals, 5th edn. OIE, Paris, p 896–904

PSEUDOMONAS AERUGINOSA – PSEUDOMONIASIS

This organism causes disease in poultry as an opportunist pathogen.

EPIDEMIOLOGY

Cause

The genus *Pseudomonas* consists of many species but *Pseudomonas aeruginosa* is the one mainly involved in poultry disease and the infection is worldwide. The organism is a Gram-negative, motile, straight or slightly curved rod. It is a strict aerobe and will grow at 42°C but not at 4°C. Fluorescence can be demonstrated when the organism is grown in special media. The organism is ubiquitous in nature, being found in soil, water, sewage, lakes, on the surface of plants and in the intestinal contents of animals and birds. It is relatively resistant outside the body of the host, being able to survive on a very limited food supply. In general it is resistant to a number of antimicrobials but in this there is strain variation. It is an opportunist pathogen and its environmental and pathogenic promiscuity is due in part to its large and genetically diverse genome.

Hosts

Disease associated with pseudomonads has been recorded in a range of animals and plants and among poultry occurs in chickens, turkeys, ducks, geese, pheasants and ostriches; infection in eggs kills embryos.

Spread

P. aeruginosa is an opportunist pathogen and infection may occur through skin wounds, contaminated vaccines, contaminated antibiotic solutions, egg dipping or egg inocula or contamination of needles used for injection. These can result in high mortality in embryos or young chicks. Infection can also spread from infected to susceptible flocks on the same premises under conditions of inadequate hygiene.

Influencing factors

The adverse effect of the organism can be increased by concurrent infection with other pathogens and by stress and immunodeficiency of the host. All ages of poultry are susceptible but young birds are more susceptible than older stock.

DISEASE

The disease may be localized in such tissues as infraorbital sinuses, air sacs or integument (cellulitis) or it can be systemic, with septicaemic diseases of many organs and tissues. Morbidity and mortality varies from 2% to 100%. Greatest losses occur in very young birds.

Signs

Clinical signs are influenced by which organs and tissues are affected and may vary greatly. They can include one or more of the following: depression, incoordination, ataxia, torticollis, lameness, swelling of the head, wattles, sinuses and joints, especially of the leg, diarrhoea, conjunctivitis and respiratory signs. The period of incubation is very short – from a few hours to 2 days – and the duration of systemic disease is also of short duration.

Lesions

Lesions reflect the clinical disease and include: pericarditis, perihepatitis and air sacculitis; subcutaneous oedema, especially of the head and neck; cellulitis; exudate in affected joints; and necrotic focal lesions in the liver and spleen. In some cases they may be similar to those seen in colisepticaemia and the organism has been isolated occasionally from salpingo-peritonitis.

DIAGNOSIS

Differential diagnosis requires consideration of very many factors associated with systemic or localized lesions but it may be helpful to note the opportunistic nature of the organism and that infection frequently seems to be associated with poor hygiene or injury.

Diagnosis can be confirmed by the isolation and identification of the organism, which can be grown readily on common bacteriological media. Biochemical tests and the demonstration of specific pigments aid the identification. Genotypic methods are useful for epidemiological studies.

CONTROL

Prevention depends on responsible hygienic measures in all aspects of hatchery and bird management. Hygiene in hatcheries, especially in association with injection of eggs and vaccination of chicks, is of particular importance since infection of these can result in high mortality. The organism can also spread from infected flocks to susceptible ones on the same premises under conditions of inadequate hygiene.

Treatment may be of value if it can be applied early after infection. Although there is variation among isolates in their susceptibility to antimicrobials those found to be most effective include gentamicin, polymyxin B, neomycin and the fluoroquinolones or a combination of antibiotics.

FURTHER READING

Barnes H J 2003 *Pseudomonas*. In: Saif Y M (ed) Diseases of poultry, 11th edn. Iowa State University Press, Ames, p 852–854

Devriese L A, Viaene N J, DeMedts G 1975 *Pseudomonas aeruginosa* infection on a broiler farm. Avian Pathol 4: 233–237

Lusis P I, Soltys MA 1966 *Pseudomonas aeruginosa* Vet Bull 41: 169–177

STREPTOBACILLUS MONILIFORMIS – STREPTOBACILLOSIS

It is generally considered that this organism is a commensal of low pathogenicity for rats but is pathogenic for mice, guinea pigs, humans and turkeys.

Streptobacillus moniliformis is a Gram-negative filamentous bacterium that may be beaded.

The disease in turkeys particularly affects the legs, in which there is polyarthritis and synovitis. This is associated with infection of leg wounds with *S. moniliformis* following rat bites. Chickens seem to be resistant.

Diagnosis is by observation of wounds and the isolation and identification of the bacterium from lesions. Rodent control is required for prevention and a number of antimicrobials are useful for treatment, including penicillin.

Streptobacillus moniliformis can cause rat bite fever in humans.

FURTHER READING

Barnes H J 2003 *Streptobacillus*. In: Saif Y M (ed) Diseases of poultry, 11th edn. Iowa State University Press, Ames, p 854

Boyer C I Jr, Bruner D W, Brown J A 1952 A *Streptobacillus*, the cause of tendon sheath infection in turkeys. Avian Dis 2: 418–425

Mohamed Y S, Moorhead P D, Bohl E H 1983 Natural *Streptobacillus moniliformis* infection of turkeys, and attempts to infect turkeys, sheep and pigs. Avian Dis 13: 379–385

Yamamoto R and Clark G T 1967 *Streptobacillus moniliformis* infection in turkeys. Vet Rec 79: 95–100

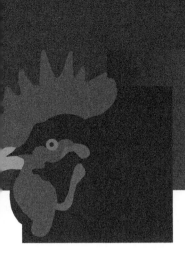

SECTION

3

Dennis J. Alexander

VIRAL DISEASES

Chapter **23**	*Herpesviridae*	**258**
Chapter **24**	*Retroviridae*	**276**
Chapter **25**	*Paramyxoviridae*	**294**
Chapter **26**	*Orthomyxoviridae* – avian influenza	**317**
Chapter **27**	*Poxviridae*	**333**
Chapter **28**	*Coronaviridae*	**340**
Chapter **29**	*Picornaviridae*	**350**
Chapter **30**	*Birnaviridae*	**359**
Chapter **31**	*Adenoviridae*	**367**
Chapter **32**	*Reoviridae*	**382**
Chapter **33**	*Astroviridae*	**392**
Chapter **34**	*Circoviridae*	**398**
Chapter **35**	*Parvoviridae*	**405**
Chapter **36**	*Caliciviridae* and hepeviruses	**410**
Chapter **37**	Arthropod-borne viruses	**415**

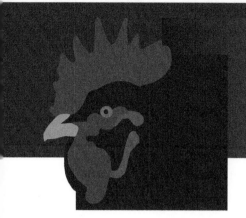

Venugopal Nair,
Richard C. Jones and
R. E. Gough

Herpesviridae

Members of the *Herpesviridae* are double-stranded, enveloped DNA viruses with roughly spherical morphology. Virus particles are usually 100–200 nm in diameter but sometimes larger. The capsid shows icosahedral symmetry. Members of the family show an enormous host range, particularly in avian species, but only three viruses appear to cause significant disease in poultry.

MAREK'S DISEASE VIRUS (VENUGOPAL NAIR)

Marek's disease, named after the Hungarian pathologist Jozsef Marek, is a lymphoproliferative and neuropathic disease of domestic chickens and, less commonly, turkeys, quails and geese caused by a highly contagious, cell-associated, oncogenic herpesvirus. Originally described in 1907 as a polyneuritis affecting the peripheral nerves, it was not until 1926 that the disease was recognized as a neoplastic disease producing tumours in several visceral organs. In the 1950s, the lymphomatous forms of the disease, referred to as 'visceral lymphomatosis' or 'acute leukosis', became widespread in the USA, particularly in broilers. The long-standing confusion between Marek's disease and other neoplastic diseases of chickens with regard to their aetiology was not resolved until 1967 when it was shown that Marek's disease was caused by a herpesvirus, in contrast to the retrovirus-induced leukoses and tumours.

Losses from the acute lymphomatous form of the disease reached their peak in the late 1960s in the USA and other countries. In 1970 the losses from carcass condemnation of broilers, mainly from Marek's disease, amounted to about US$200 million per annum, representing 1.6% condemnation of all broilers examined. With the widespread use of live Marek's disease vaccines, which became available in the early 1970s, there was a substantial reduction in losses worldwide. However with the increasing reports of vaccination breaks and emergence of more virulent pathotypes, Marek's disease still remains a significant avian disease of major economic importance. As it is not notifiable, the assessment of the true worldwide incidence and economic impact of Marek's disease is difficult. Nonetheless, a recent survey has indicated that it remains a major problem in many countries. The most recent estimates of economic impact of Marek's disease on the world poultry industry is in the range of US$1–2 billion annually.

EPIDEMIOLOGY

Cause

The causative agent of Marek's disease is a cell-associated lymphotropic herpesvirus, designated *Marek's disease virus* (MDV). Because of its lymphotropic nature, MDV was originally classified in the family *Herpesviridae* as a member of the subfamily *Gammaherpesvirinae* together with *Epstein–Barr virus* (EBV) and the oncogenic herpesviruses of nonhuman primates *Herpesvirus saimiri* and *Herpesvirus ateles*. However, on the basis of the genomic organization, MDV is currently placed in the genus *Mardivirus* together with alphaherpesviruses such as *Herpes simplex virus*. Within the genus *Mardivirus*, closely related but distinct species of viruses are grouped together. These include:

- Serotype 1 MDV (gallid herpesvirus type 2), which includes all the pathogenic strains of MDV as well as the attenuated strains such as CVI988
- Serotype 2 MDV (gallid herpesvirus type 3)
- Serotype 3 herpesvirus of turkey (HVT, meleagrid herpesvirus type 1).

Serotype 1 MDV consists of isolates that show wide variation in their pathogenicity and, on the basis of their pathogenic properties, can be grouped as mild (mMDV), virulent (vMDV), very virulent (vvMDV) and very virulent + (vv+MDV) pathotypes. The emergence of new pathotypes represents a continuous evolution of MDV towards greater virulence.

MDV DNA is a linear, double-stranded molecule of about 170 kb, consisting of a unique long region (U_L) flanked by a set of inverted repeat (TR_L and IR_L) regions and a unique short region (U_S) flanked by another set of inverted repeat (IR_S and TR_S) regions. Recently, the complete genome sequences of several MDV strains have been determined. The MDV genome has the capacity to encode more than 100 proteins, comprising both proteins homologous to those in other herpesviruses and proteins unique to MDV.

Hosts

MDV infection mainly occurs in domestic chickens and is ubiquitous among poultry populations throughout the world. The infection in other species is rare, but occasionally the disease occurs in turkeys and quails. Recently, Marek's disease has also been reported in migratory white-fronted geese in Japan. There is no conclusive evidence of human infection with MDV. In commercial chicken houses where the infection is rampant, virtually all birds become infected, commonly within the first few weeks of life, although on occasions this may be delayed. Because of the prevalence of serotype 1 viruses of varying pathogenicity and nonpathogenic serotype 2 in the poultry house environment, birds can be infected with more than one MDV strain. There is some evidence to suggest that, with increasing age of the birds, the frequency of isolation of nonpathogenic viruses becomes higher. Natural infection by nonpathogenic MDV can provide immunity to subsequent infection by a virulent strain.

Spread

The transmission of MDV occurs by direct or indirect contact, apparently by the airborne route. The epithelial cells in the keratinizing layer of the feather follicle replicate fully infectious virus and serve as a source of contamination of the environment. The shedding of the infected material occurs about 2–4 weeks after infection, prior to the appearance of the clinical disease, and can continue throughout the life of the bird. The virus associated with feather debris and dander in contaminated poultry house dust can remain infectious for many months. Although the inhalation of infected poultry house dust remains the commonest route of disease spread, other less common mechanisms of indirect transmission, such as those involving darkling beetles (*Alphitobius diaperinus*), may also play a minor role in transmission. There is no evidence for vertical transmission of MDV through the egg.

Because of the ubiquitous nature of the infection and the ability of MDV to survive for long periods outside the host, flock infections usually occur early in the life of the bird. In addition, hatched chicks in most flocks have maternally derived antibodies, which disappear in most chickens by 3–4 weeks of age. The rate of the spread of Marek's disease within a flock can vary greatly and depends on, among several factors, the level of initial exposure and the concentration of susceptible birds. A number of stress factors, including those from handling, change of housing and vaccination, are thought to increase disease incidence. There is also a sex influence on the disease, as females tend to develop more tumours.

DIAGNOSIS

Diagnostic procedures for Marek's disease include both pathological and virological methods. Pathological diagnosis identifies the nature of the tumour, whereas virological diagnosis identifies the aetiological agents present in a bird or flock.

Clinical signs

Although clinical signs associated with Marek's disease can occur in chickens from 4 weeks of age, signs are most frequently seen between 12 and 24 weeks of age and sometimes later. The incubation period can vary from a few to many weeks. In some of the virulent pathotypes that produce severe cytolytic disease, the incubation period can be shorter. The following are some of the characteristics of the different forms of the disease.

Classical form In this form of the disease, with mainly neural involvement, mortality rarely exceeds 10–15%, occurring over a few weeks or many months. The most common clinical sign is partial or complete paralysis of the legs and wings (Fig. 23.1). The signs can vary from bird to bird depending on the involvement of the different nerves. When the nerves controlling the neck muscles are affected, signs such as bending of the head or torticollis are seen. Similarly, the

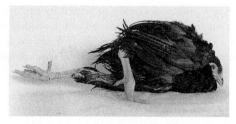

Fig. 23.1 Paralysis of the legs in a bird with Marek's disease.

involvement of the vagus nerve can result in the paralysis and dilation of the crop. Such birds may also show symptoms of gasping and respiratory distress.

Acute form In this form of the disease, where there is usually formation of lymphomas in the visceral organs, the incidence of the disease is frequently between 10–30% and in major outbreaks can go up to 70%. Apart from generalized manifestations such as depression, weight loss, anorexia and diarrhoea, the clinical signs are less marked. Mortality can increase rapidly over a few weeks, and then cease, or can continue at a steady or falling rate over several months.

Acute cytolytic disease In infections with some of the recently isolated vvMDV strains, an acute cytolytic disease with severe atrophy of the lymphoid organs is recognized. This form of the disease, also described as 'early mortality syndrome', results in very high mortality usually between 10 and 14 days of age.

Transient paralysis This is a rather uncommon manifestation of MDV infection that occurs between 5 and 18 weeks of age. Affected birds suddenly develop varying degrees of ataxia, paresis or paralysis of the legs, wings and neck. The disease is commonly observed 8–12 days after infection, usually lasts only for about 24–48 h and is associated with oedema of the brain. In some cases, the transient paralysis can be fatal.

Macroscopic lesions

In the classical form of Marek's disease, the characteristic finding is the enlargement of one or more peripheral nerves (Fig. 23.2). The most commonly affected nerves that are easily seen on post-mortem examination are the brachial and sciatic plexus and nerve trunks, coeliac plexus, abdominal vagus and intercostal nerves. The affected nerves are grossly enlarged and often two or three times their normal thickness. The normal cross-striated and glistening appearance of the nerves is lost: they have a greyish or yellowish appearance and are oedematous. Lymphomas are sometimes present in this form of the disease, most frequently as small, soft, grey tumours in the ovary, kidney, heart, liver and other tissues.

In the acute form, the typical lesion is the widespread, diffuse lymphomatous involvement of visceral organs such as the liver, spleen, ovary, kidney, heart and proventriculus. Sometimes lymphomas are also seen in the skin around the feather follicles and in the skeletal muscles. Affected birds may also show involvement of the peripheral nerves similar to that seen in the classical form. The liver enlargement in younger birds is usually moderate compared with that in adult birds, where the liver is greatly enlarged and the gross appearance is very similar to that seen in lymphoid leukosis. In the acute cytolytic form of the disease caused by some of the virulent isolates, extensive atrophic changes may result in the complete disappearance of the thymus and bursa of Fabricius.

Microscopic lesions

Although gross lesions can provide indications of the nature of the neoplasm, histopathological examination is essential for accurate diagnosis. For this, it is important that fresh tissues are collected into fixative from several cases from an affected flock. The most useful set of tissues to collect for the diagnosis of Marek's disease include the liver, spleen, bursa of Fabricius, thymus, heart, proventriculus, kidney, gonads, kidney, nerves, skin and other gross tumour tissues.

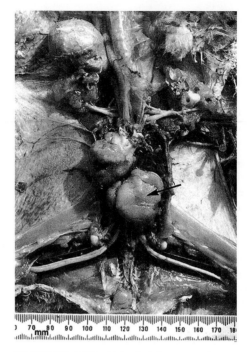

Fig. 23.2 Enlarged brachial and sciatic nerves and an ovarian lymphoma (arrow) in a chicken with Marek's disease.

The peripheral nerves in both classical and acute forms of the disease are affected by proliferative, inflammatory or minor infiltrative changes that are termed A-, B- and C-type lesions respectively. The A-type lesion consists of infiltration by proliferating lymphoblasts, large, medium and small lymphocytes and macrophages, and appears to be neoplastic in nature. Nerves with B-type lesions show oedema and infiltration by small lymphocytes and plasma cells with Schwann cell proliferation, and the lesion appears to be inflammatory. The C-type lesion consists of a mild scattering of small lymphocytes and plasma cells, often seen in birds that show no gross lesions or clinical signs, and is thought to be a regressive inflammatory lesion. Demyelination, which is frequently seen in nerves showing A- and B-type lesions, is responsible for the paralytic symptoms. Birds showing signs of acute transient paralysis have extensive vasculitis involving cerebellum, cerebrum and optic lobes.

Lymphomas seen in the visceral organs and other tissues are similar cytologically to the lymphoproliferations in the nerve A-type lesions. The lymphoid cells are usually of the mixed type, with a preponderance of small and medium lymphocytes. But sometimes, especially in adult birds, large lymphocytes and lymphoblasts may predominate. The polymorphic population of the lymphoid cells, as seen in impression smears or tissue sections of Marek's disease lymphomas, is an important feature in differentiating it from lymphoid leukosis (Table 23.1). The thymus and bursa of Fabricius in birds with acute cytolytic disease show severe atrophic changes replacing most of the lymphoid cells. Neoplastic lymphomatous lesions can also develop in these organs. Rarely, arterial lesions showing proliferative changes in the aortic, coronary, coeliac and mesenteric arteries are reported in cases of MDV-associated atherosclerosis.

Table 23.1 Important gross and microscopic features for the differential diagnosis of Marek's disease and lymphoid leukosis

FEATURE	MAREK'S DISEASE	LYMPHOID LEUKOSIS
Age	Few days to many weeks	Not less than 16 weeks
Clinical signs	Frequently paralysis	Nonspecific
Incidence	Usually more than 5% in unvaccinated flocks	Rarely more than 5% of infected flocks
Gross lesions		
Neural enlargement	Frequent	Absent
Bursa of Fabricius	Diffuse enlargement or atrophy	Nodular tumours
Proventriculus, skin and muscle tumours	May be present	Usually absent
Microscopic lesions		
Neural involvement	Frequent	Absent
Liver tumours	Mostly perivascular	Usually focal or diffuse
Spleen tumours	Usually diffuse	Mostly focal
Bursa of Fabricius	Interfollicular tumours and/or atrophy of lymphoid follicles	Intrafollicular tumours
Lymphoid proliferation in skin/feather follicles	Frequently present	Usually absent
Central nervous system	Lesions may be present	Usually absent
Cytology of tumours	Usually pleomorphic lymphoid cells consisting of lymphoblasts, small, medium and large lymphocytes and reticulum cells	Lymphoblasts of uniform morphology usually of clonal origin
Category of neoplastic lymphoid cell involved	T lymphocyte	B lymphocyte

Pathogenesis

The pathogenesis of Marek's disease is complex, with infection occurring through the respiratory route from the inhalation of poultry house dust contaminated with the virus (Fig. 23.3). After an early cytolytic infection mainly in the B lymphocytes in the bursa, spleen and thymus at 3–5 days post-infection, the virus infects the activated T lymphocytes, mainly of the CD4$^+$ phenotype. The infection in the T lymphocytes becomes latent at 6–7 days post-infection and the virus is spread throughout the body by the infected lymphocytes, which persist as a cell-associated viraemia. A secondary cytolytic infection occurs in the feather follicle epithelium from about 10 days after infection, from where infectious-cell-free virus is produced and shed into the environment in feather debris and dander. The latently infected T lymphocytes are subsequently transformed, leading to the development of lymphomatous lesions in the visceral organs. The main target cells for transformation in natural infections are the CD4$^+$ T cells, although the virus also has the potential to transform CD8$^+$ T cells.

Virus isolation

MDV infection in a flock can be detected by isolating the virus from the infected tissues. Materials commonly used for the isolation of the virus are buffy coat cells from heparinized blood samples, or suspensions of lymphoma and spleen cells. As MDV is highly cell-associated,

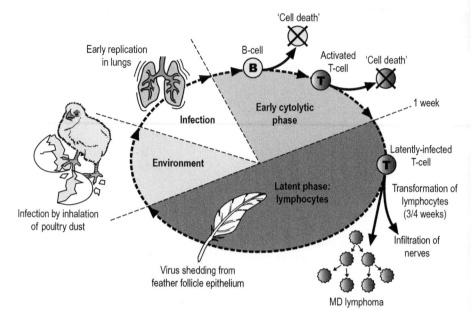

Fig. 23.3 Schematic diagram showing the different stages of the pathogenesis of Marek's disease.

it is essential that the suspensions contain viable cells. These cell suspensions are inoculated into monolayer cultures of chick kidney cells or duck and chicken embryo fibroblasts. Evidence of MDV replication in the culture can be seen as plaques, which appear in 3–4 days. Less commonly feather tips, from which cell-free MDV can be extracted, are also used for virus isolation.

Virus characterization

The MDV serotypes isolated in culture can be differentiated on the basis of the time of appearance, rate of development and morphology of the plaques and by using specific antibodies. Recently, molecular biological techniques such as polymerase chain reaction (PCR) tests have been used widely to differentiate between the oncogenic and vaccine strains. Quantitative PCR methods have also been used for accurate estimation of MDV genome copy numbers in various tissues. Such methods have shown that feather follicle epithelium is a rich source of MDV compared with the lymphoid cell targets. Diagnosis can also be made by detection of viral antigens or nucleic acids by immunofluorescence and immunohistochemical methods using polyclonal and monoclonal antibodies or by using in situ hybridization using MDV-specific nucleic acid probes or PCR.

Serology

The presence of antibodies to MDV in birds from about 4 weeks of age is an indication of infection. Antibodies detected in birds before that age are likely to represent maternally derived antibodies and are not considered evidence of active infection. Although there are no prescribed serological tests for detection of MDV-specific antibodies, the agar gel immunodiffusion (AGID) test is employed most commonly for this purpose. Disrupted MDV-infected tissue culture cells or the extracts of infected feather tips or feather tracts can be used as the antigen for this test.

CONTROL

Because of the highly contagious nature of MDV and its ability to survive for long periods, both within the host and in the environment, eradication of the disease is difficult. Control of the disease is based mainly on preventive vaccination, with improved management methods and use of genetically resistant birds.

Vaccination

The development of vaccines for the control of Marek's disease was a significant landmark both in avian medicine and basic cancer research, as this was the first example of a neoplastic disease controlled by the use of a vaccine. Vaccination represents, currently and at least for the foreseeable future, the main strategy for the prevention and control of Marek's disease. Live virus vaccines, used since 1970, are still the cornerstones of disease control programmes. These are usually administered to day-old chicks at hatching to provide protection against the natural challenge the chicks are exposed to early in life from the infected poultry house environment. With the introduction of in ovo immunization methods, an increasing number of birds are vaccinated by this route. Marek's disease vaccines are highly effective, often achieving over 90% protection under commercial conditions. Commercially available vaccines have been derived from all the three serotypes and are usually administered at the minimum recommended dose of 1000 plaque-forming units (pfu) per chick.

Serotype 1 vaccines Commercial vaccines developed from the members of this species include the attenuated HPRS-16 and the CVI988/Rispens strain of MDV vaccine. The CVI988/Rispens strain appears to be able to afford protection against the challenge from more recently isolated vvMDV and vv+MDV pathotypes.

Serotype 2 vaccines Naturally nonpathogenic strains of MDV belonging to serotype 2 are widespread among poultry flocks. Vaccines derived from these strains are protective against many virulent pathotypes but less so against very virulent strains. Cell-associated serotype 2 vaccines incorporating SB-1 and 301B/1 strains are available commercially.

Serotype 3 vaccines FC-126 strain of HVT is widely used commercially in many countries and is highly effective against virulent MDV strains but is less effective against some of the very virulent pathotypes. However, HVT continues to be widely used because of its low cost, availability as cell-free and cell-associated forms and effectiveness when field exposure is not severe.

Polyvalent vaccines The concept of polyvalent vaccine evolved from the demonstration of protective synergism, where the protection was greater with a combination of two vaccines than with individual components. HVT and SB-1 strains comprised the first commercial bivalent vaccine based on the protective synergism demonstrated between MDV-2 and HVT vaccines. Other bivalent vaccines that are available commercially include the combinations of HVT with either CVI988/Rispens or 301B/1 strains.

Recombinant vaccines Recombinant DNA technology potentially offers several advantages for the development of superior vaccines with very little residual pathogenicity. Experimentally, it has been demonstrated that fowl pox virus and HVT expressing the glycoprotein B (gB) gene of serotype 1 MDV offered significant levels of protection against MDV. Currently, two recombinant

HVT vaccines expressing *Newcastle disease virus* HN and F or MDV genes have been licensed for use in the USA.

Although Marek's disease vaccines were successful in controlling major losses from the disease, there have always been threats of vaccine failures. The causes of these failures include improper use of the vaccine, exposure to virulent viruses before the development of immunity, interference from maternally derived antibodies and emergence of virulent viruses that can break through the immunity.

Biosecurity

Since vertical transmission of infection does not occur in Marek's disease, chickens hatched and reared in isolation will be free of MDV. However, because of the highly infectious and ubiquitous nature of the virus, it is often difficult to maintain freedom from disease without vaccination programmes. Nevertheless, the use of vaccines should not be an alternative to good management or implementation of effective biosecurity measures. Management measures followed adequately should delay and lessen the seriousness of the disease. Young chicks should be reared in isolation from older flocks for the first 2–3 months, when the infection is most likely to have serious consequences. An 'all-in/all-out' policy should be the preferred option for the whole site. This would make it possible to break the infection cycle by disinfection when the houses are empty. Removal of used litter and disinfection of buildings are important aspects of disease control, especially in view of the possibility of selection for pathogens with increased virulence. Furthermore, placing the chicks in an environment heavily contaminated with virus before they have developed a solid immunity can lead to vaccination breaks. Strict biosecurity is also necessary to prevent the introduction of new MDV strains into a farm. Because insects could act as reservoirs of infection, treatment of premises with insecticides is desirable.

Selection for genetic resistance

Genetic resistance to Marek's disease is well documented and susceptible and resistant lines can be developed by progeny testing, selection from survivors of Marek's disease challenge, or blood typing. Two distinct genetic loci that play a major role in controlling resistance have been identified. The best characterized association is the one between the chicken major histocompatibility complex (MHC) and resistance to Marek's disease, the most notable being the association with the B^{21} allele. This association develops early in life and is accompanied by reduced numbers of infected T cells. A second type of resistance associated with non-MHC genes is provided by the observation that RPL line 6 and 7 chickens, which are both homozygous for the same MHC allele, differ markedly in Marek's disease susceptibility. Mapping of genes associated with resistance to Marek's disease is in progress and the recent availability of the chicken genome sequence and the panel of microsatellite and single nucleotide polymorphism (SNP) markers will assist in making major strides in this area in the future. As more such tools for selection for genetic resistance become available, poultry breeders will have the opportunity for genetic selection for resistance against Marek's disease.

ZOONOTIC POTENTIAL

The high prevalence of Marek's disease and the widespread use of live Marek's disease vaccines have raised some concerns about infection of humans. However, there is no conclusive evidence of human infection with MDV.

FURTHER READING

Davison T F, Venugopal Nair (eds) 2004 Marek's disease – an evolving problem. Elsevier Academic Press, London

Hirai K (ed) 2001 Marek's disease. Current topics in microbiology and immunology 255. Springer-Verlag, Berlin

Osterrieder N, Kamil J P, Schumacher D et al 2006 Marek's disease virus: from miasma to model. Nat Rev Microbiol 4: 283–294

Witter R L, Schat K A 2003 Marek's disease. In: Saif Y M (ed) Diseases of poultry, 11th edn. Iowa State University Press, Ames, p 407–465

INFECTIOUS LARYNGOTRACHEITIS (RICHARD C. JONES)

Infectious laryngotracheitis is a viral respiratory disease that affects chickens. It was first reported in the USA in 1924 and its earliest recorded occurrence in the UK was in 1935. It is recognized worldwide. The causal virus does not seem to be as invasive as other viral respiratory diseases and regions free of the infection seem to exist close to areas where the infection is indigenous. Serious disease outbreaks occur periodically when strains of infectious laryngotracheitis virus (ILTV) spread from persistently infected flocks to nonvaccinated birds. Both field strains and live attenuated vaccines have been shown to establish latent infections. The more severe forms of the disease are of considerable economic importance, since they may result in high mortality and greatly reduced production.

EPIDEMIOLOGY

Cause

The causal agent is a virus of the family *Herpesviridae* and the subfamily *Alphaherpesvirinae*, and is designated *Gallid herpesvirus* 1 (Iltovirus = ILT-like viruses). Antigenically, the virus strains appear to be homogeneous when examined by methods such as serum neutralization, immunofluorescence and enzyme-linked immunosorbent assay (ELISA). However, strains have been differentiated by restriction endonuclease analysis of DNA, PCR and restriction fragment length polymorphism and these techniques have allowed differentiation between field and vaccine strains. Field strains may show considerable variation in virulence.

ILTV can survive away from the host for several weeks under farm conditions and longer when the environment is very cold, especially in the presence of organic material such as mucus, blood and faeces.

The virus grows well on the chorioallantoic membrane of the chicken embryo, where it produces pocks, and it can be adapted to grow in the turkey and duck embryo. ILTV also grows readily in chick embryo liver, lung and kidney cell cultures where it causes syncytium-type cytopathic effects.

Hosts

The virus seems naturally to infect only domestic fowl and occasionally pheasants. All ages of fowl are susceptible and, although greatest susceptibility occurs in the very young, the disease is most commonly seen in the field in birds 3–9 months old. In endemic areas older birds are frequently immune. In general males are more susceptible than females and the heavier breeds more susceptible than light ones.

The disease may be exacerbated by concurrent infection with a variety of other pathogens such as Newcastle disease, infectious bronchitis and fowl pox viruses, and *Haemophilus paragallinarum* and *Mycoplasma gallisepticum*. Deficiency of vitamin A and excess ammonia in the atmosphere may also predispose birds to more severe disease.

Spread

Transmission of ILTV through the egg has never been reported and newly hatched chicks are free from infection. Virus enters the bird in infective droplets or mucus via the upper respiratory tract and conjunctiva and remains confined to the respiratory tract. It is shed mainly in exudates from the nares, oropharynx, trachea and conjunctiva and is transmitted in aerosol or expectorant form (blood and mucus). Among recovered birds and even birds given attenuated live vaccines, the virus can become latent and the birds become carriers. The virus remains in latent form in the trigeminal ganglia in the brain. Such birds, which usually show no signs of disease, may excrete the virus intermittently for long periods, perhaps for life, and a number of factors, such as the movement of stock, handling, social stress and the onset of lay, have been shown to precipitate re-excretion. These birds can act as an unsuspected source of infection.

The living infected bird is the most important source of infection and spread of disease, particularly in the early stages of infection. Movement of such birds, or even mildly affected stock or carriers, is a particularly potent method of spreading infection. Because of the survival of the virus outside the body of the host, fomites such as infected crates, receptacles, equipment and buildings and mechanical carriers such as personnel, wild birds, vermin and cats and dogs can be transmitters of the virus.

DIAGNOSIS

The history of ILT in individual birds and in a flock in a region where it has occurred before and the clinical signs and lesions in the more severe forms in which there is gasping respiration and tracheal haemorrhage, are virtually diagnostic of infectious laryngotracheitis. However, the mild form may be very difficult or impossible to distinguish clinically or at necropsy from other mild respiratory diseases. In these cases, for confirmation of infection, it is necessary to demonstrate the presence of the virus or an increase in antibody titre between acute and convalescent sera. Diagnostic methods available for infectious laryngotracheitis are: (i) histological examination of the trachea; (ii) virus detection and (iii) antibody detection.

Clinical signs

In the individual bird under commercial conditions, the period of incubation is about 6–12 days. Infection may result in peracute, acute or mild disease or asymptomatic infection. In the peracute form, birds may be found dead without prodromal signs or show sudden acute dyspnoea with severe coughing and expectoration of mucus, bloodstained exudate and blood clots, followed by death within 1–3 days. In acute infectious laryngotracheitis, dyspnoea is a feature but it is not as sudden in onset or as severe as in the peracute form. In some, increasing obstruction of the trachea with exudate causes the bird to breathe with long-drawn-out gasps, with a wide-open beak and often a high-pitched squawk, and invariably moist rales can be heard. There may be nasal discharge and conjunctivitis with frothy exudate at the anterior canthus of the eye. In most severely dyspnoeic birds there is cyanosis of the face and wattles and death usually occurs in 3–4 days. In others, the dyspnoea increases in severity over several days and then subsides and recovery occurs in 2–3 weeks.

In the mild form there may be one or more of the following signs: moist rales, slight coughing and head shaking, nasal exudate and conjunctivitis. Affected birds show depression commensurate with the severity of disease and the more severely affected birds are recumbent on their hocks. Egg production is also affected and may cease entirely for a time but, in those birds which recover, egg production in uncomplicated cases returns to the expected level. There is no loss of egg quality. The asymptomatic form occurs without clinical signs and its presence in a small flock may go undetected.

The nature of disease in flocks may mirror the condition in the individual birds. In some of the more severe outbreaks there is very high morbidity and as many as 70% of the affected birds may die. In some outbreaks, all forms of the disease may be seen throughout while in others only the milder form of the disease exists or as a sequel to a more severe form in the early part of an outbreak. In mild outbreaks most birds can appear clinically normal with perhaps a few showing conjunctivitis or tracheitis at necropsy.

Lesions

The gross lesions vary with the severity of the disease but in most cases are restricted to the upper respiratory tract. In the peracute form there is haemorrhagic tracheitis in which the trachea contains blood casts throughout the whole or part of its length or is filled with blood-stained mucus, and the primary bronchi may also be affected. This material is responsible for respiratory obstruction. In the acute form, caseous diphtheritic exudate, mucus and some haemorrhage occur in the trachea and frequently cause an obstructive or partially obstructive plug in the laryngeal and syrinx regions. The tracheas themselves are often very congested and cyanotic. In the mild forms there may be excess mucus with or without small amounts of diphtheritic exudate in the trachea. The nares may similarly show an inflammatory response but mainly with caseous exudates. Conjunctivitis is the most common ocular lesion. Occasionally there may be diphtheritic and caseous lesions in the oropharynx and larynx and this may be confused with the diphtheritic form of fowl pox or with avitaminosis A.

The lungs and air sacs are relatively rarely affected but there may be congestion of the lungs and some thickening of the interclavicular, thoracic and abdominal air sac walls and caseous exudate in the lumen.

Histologically the mucosa of the respiratory tract shows an inflammatory response and necrosis, with or without haemorrhage, which mirrors the severity of the clinical disease. A diagnostic feature is the presence of Cowdry type A intranuclear inclusion bodies in some epithelial cells. These are characterized by a condensed nucleus surrounded by a halo and margination of the chromatin. It is important to note that they are present only for a few days before desquamation of the epithelial cells and may be difficult to demonstrate.

Nonetheless, the development of these eosinophilic intranuclear inclusions in the respiratory and conjunctival epithelium is pathognomonic for infectious laryngotracheitis. Epithelial hyperplasia gives rise to multinucleated cells (syncytia), which include these inclusions with haemorrhage of the lamina propria. There is desquamation of the necrotic epithelium and loss of mucous glands. Regeneration occurs after about 6 days, after which it may no longer be possible to see the inclusions. Thus, their transient nature and the inability to see them does not exclude a diagnosis of infectious laryngotracheitis. Inclusion bodies may be observed after staining with Giemsa or haematoxylin and eosin after embedding the trachea in paraffin wax. Longitudinal sections of the trachea may provide a greater opportunity to observe the inclusions at different levels of the tissue.

Virus detection/isolation

The simplest method of virus identification in clinical material is by agar gel immunodiffusion (AGID) tests using a hyperimmune serum to ILTV. Virus is tested in macerated tracheal and laryngeal tissue from the affected bird but, although it is easy to perform, the test relies on a hyperimmune antiserum and is relatively insensitive. It is of value as a simple method of differentiating infectious laryngotracheitis from the diphtheritic form of fowl pox.

Isolation of ILTV may be conducted in embryonated eggs or cell cultures. Exudate and epithelial scrapings or tracheal swabs, taken as soon as possible after the onset of clinical signs, are emulsified in nutrient broth and the supernatants are inoculated on to the dropped chorioallantoic membrane of 10–12-day-old fertile chicken eggs or preformed monolayers of chick embryo liver cell cultures. Inoculation of eggs with ILTV results in the production of pocks on the chorioallantoic membrane. Inoculation of cell cultures causes syncytium formation after several days. In both instances, more than one passage may be required before the virus causes these effects. Then, the virus needs to be identified by some other means such as immunofluorescence, virus neutralization or electron microscopy. Identification by virus isolation is time-consuming and laborious but sensitive.

More rapid methods for detecting ILTV include immunofluorescence or immunoperoxidase staining of tracheal sections, an antigen capture ELISA, electron microscopy, DNA hybridization techniques and PCR. Immunofluorescence or immunoperoxidase testing is done on sections or epithelial scrapings from affected birds. The capture ELISA is claimed to be as accurate as but faster than virus isolation and more accurate than immunofluorescence. The use of direct electron microscopy for the examination of emulsified tracheal scrapings after negative staining provides potentially the most rapid method of detecting ILTV. From receipt of material, it is possible to observe herpesvirus particles in less than 1 h, although use of the electron microscope requires high titres of virus to be present in the samples, so it should not be relied upon as the only detection method.

Methods for identifying ILTV DNA in clinical samples are now used widely for diagnosis. Dot–blot hybridization assays and cloned virus DNA fragments have been shown to be highly sensitive for detecting virus when isolation and ELISA were negative. PCR has several advantages including being quick (1–2 days), more sensitive than virus isolation for clinical samples, especially when other contaminant viruses such as adenoviruses are present, and superior to isolation in the recovery phase. The use of PCR in conjunction with restriction fragment length polymorphism enables the differentiation between field strains and vaccine strains.

Serology

Techniques used for monitoring antibodies to ILTV in chicken serum, include AGID, virus neutralization, indirect immunofluorescence and ELISA. For AGID, antigen is provided by virus-infected chorioallantoic membranes or cell cultures. The test is very simple and can be performed in any laboratory but it is relatively insensitive. Virus neutralization tests are time-consuming and may be done using fertile chicken eggs inoculated by the chorioallantoic membrane route with enumeration of the pocks on the chorioallantoic membrane. Alternatively, they may be done more conveniently in cell cultures in microwell plates. Antibodies to ILTV can be demonstrated by indirect immunofluorescence by application of test sera to fixed, preinfected cell cultures. The method is sensitive but, since it relies on the intensity of fluorescence perceived by individuals, interpretation may be subjective.

ELISA offers ease of testing large numbers of sera, with semiautomation and commercial kits are available. It has been shown to be more sensitive than virus neutralization and of comparable sensitivity to indirect immunofluorescence. ELISAs are therefore the system of choice for flock testing.

CONTROL

In areas where the disease is indigenous it is extremely difficult to prevent the entry of the virus into susceptible flocks, especially on continuous production sites. In such circumstances vaccination is of value (see Ch. 4). For this purpose live vaccine is used. In high-risk areas it may be necessary to vaccinate at 1–3 days of age, although very young chicks are more likely to be adversely affected by vaccine than older stock. In other areas vaccination may be delayed to any age between 3 and 18 weeks. Birds may be vaccinated on more than one occasion with a period of 2–3 weeks between. The methods of vaccination include eye drop application, coarse spray, inclusion in the drinking water or (rarely) cloacal scarification. The protection produced seems variable but generally persists in a flock over several months. Because protection may be rapid following vaccination, it is worthwhile considering vaccination in the face of an outbreak, especially in the early stages.

A disadvantage of the use of live vaccine is the possible spread of the virus, particularly within a week or 10 days of vaccination, and the production of carriers, since the live virus can become latent. This may lead to infection becoming indigenous. For these reasons, in areas where the disease is not endemic but where an outbreak has occurred, it may well be economically sound to destock completely and thoroughly clean and disinfect before restocking with birds free of the infection.

Several features of infectious laryngotracheitis have led to the suggestion that the disease could be a candidate for eradication under certain circumstances. These include the relatively slow spread, the apparent lack of major hosts other than the chicken, no egg transmission and the single serotype. Such a strategy would depend on the provision of a genetically modified deletion vaccine and an appropriate ELISA to distinguish vaccinated birds from those infected naturally.

ZOONOSIS

There is no reported evidence that infectious laryngotracheitis is of zoonotic significance.

FURTHER READING

Bagust T J, Guy J S 2003 Laryngotracheitis. In: Saif Y M (ed) Diseases of poultry, 11th edn. Iowa State University Press, Ames, p 527–540

Bagust T J, Johnson M A 1995 Avian infectious laryngotracheitis: virus–host interactions in relation to prospects for eradication. Avian Pathol 24: 373–391

Bagust T J, Jones R C, Guy J J 2000 Avian infectious laryngotracheitis. Rev Sci Tech 19: 483–492

Hughes C S, Jones R C, Gaskell R M et al 1987 Demonstration in live chickens of the carrier state in infectious laryngotracheitis. Res Vet Sci 42: 407–410

DUCK VIRUS ENTERITIS (RICHARD E. GOUGH)

Duck virus enteritis (DVE), also called duck plague, is a contagious disease of waterfowl (Anseriformes) caused by a herpesvirus. The disease was first diagnosed in the Netherlands in 1949 and has since been reported in other European countries, North America and Asia. Outbreaks in commercial ducks and geese are usually associated with contact with wild waterfowl. As with many other herpesvirus infections there is evidence that birds that survive the disease may become carriers and intermittently excrete the virus for several years. A feature of DVE is the marked seasonality of the disease, with the majority of outbreaks in Europe and North America occurring between April and June.

EPIDEMIOLOGY

Cause

Duck enteritis herpesvirus (DEHV), anatid herpesvirus 1, is a member of the *Herpesviridae* family and is placed in the subfamily *Alphaherpesvirinae* but has not been assigned to either of the two genera currently specified. Enveloped virus particles have typical herpesvirus morphology but can range in size from 160–380 nm. The nucleocapsids are approximately 75–100 nm in diameter and the viral genome is dsDNA with a molecular weight of 119×10^6. DEHV is a heat-labile virus and similar to other herpesviruses in its sensitivity to chemicals, extremes of pH and disinfectants. Using plaque reduction, virus neutralization and cross protection tests no differences in antigenicity between isolates of DEHV had been demonstrated until a recent report from Vietnam suggested the presence of two subtypes of DEHV in that country.

Isolates of DEHV from North America, the UK and the Far East have been examined using restriction endonuclease and PCR analysis but significant differences were not detected, although minor differences in gel banding patterns were reported between vaccine and field strains of DEHV. Differences in virulence between isolates of DEHV have also been reported but as yet no molecular basis for these differences has been identified. Similar molecular studies have shown no relationship between DEHV and a selection of other avian herpesviruses.

A herpesvirus associated with high mortality in a flock of domestic geese in Australia has been shown to be antigenically and genomically distinct from DEHV.

Hosts

Outbreaks of DVE have occurred in a wide variety of domestic and feral ducks, geese and swans (Order Anseriformes). Some species are highly susceptible, such as domestic Muscovy ducks (*Cairina moschata*), while others, such as mallards (*Anas platyrhynchos*), appear more resistant to infection.

Anseriformes of all ages are susceptible to infection and frequently it is breeding birds that succumb. An outbreak in commercial Pekin ducks caused significantly higher mortality in breeders than in immature ducks.

Transmission studies in a variety of other nonwaterfowl species have failed to cause infection or an antibody response.

In captive or feral waterfowl several important factors will influence the course of disease including stress, concentration of birds, breeding condition, time of year, environment and species and interaction with other waterfowl. In North America and the UK over 80% of outbreaks occur during April to June, which coincides with the spring migration and the onset of breeding in wild and feral waterfowl. PCR testing for DEHV of cloacal swabs from captive and non-migratory waterfowl in the USA showed that shedding of virus peaked during the month of May and had significantly declined by September.

In commercial ducks introduction of the virus is usually due to transmission from wild water-fowl. Once the infection has been established many other factors related to commercial poultry production, including the environment, nutrition, management procedures and control measures, will influence the course of the disease.

There is no known public health significance associated with DEHV.

Spread

Water is particularly important for the transmission of DEHV in both commercial and feral waterfowl as virus is shed in large quantities via the cloaca, which is also the main portal of entry. An outbreak in commercial ducks and geese in the UK occurred when the fields on which the ducks were being fattened became flooded. Following contact with Mallard ducks that shared the flooded fields, the commercial ducks succumbed to DVE resulting in high mortality. It is most likely that natural infections of waterfowl may occur by either oral or cloacal routes.

In immunocytochemical studies the primary site of replication was found to be in the mucosa of the digestive tract, particularly the oesophagus and cloaca. Thereafter, spread to other organs occurs, principally the bursa of Fabricius, thymus, spleen and liver. Viral antigen can be detected in the nuclei and cytoplasm of epithelial, macrophage and lymphocyte cells.

Another important factor influencing the spread of infection is the ability of DEHV to remain latent in the immune host. Carrier birds may then shed virus and cause infection and disease among susceptible waterfowl. In North America it was shown that mallards, Canada geese and black ducks that had survived DVE were still shedding virus 4 years after infection. Outbreaks of DVE in collections of ornamental or domestic waterfowl in the UK are very often associated with contact with visiting mallards, particularly drakes.

Virus transmission through the egg has been reported in persistently infected Muscovy, Pekin and mallard ducks under experimental conditions.

DIAGNOSIS

Clinical signs

Because of the marked seasonality of the disease, unexplained deaths in waterfowl during April–June are suspicious of DVE. In commercial ducks and geese serious drops in egg production may also occur.

Ataxia is a common finding, with the birds using their wings to aid walking or swimming. Sick birds exhibit photophobia, pasted eyelids, nasal discharge, inappetence, extreme thirst with a watery, bloodstained diarrhoea. Adult male waterfowl may show prolapse of the phallus and in young birds congested beaks and bloodstained vents may be noted.

Birds that die from DVE are usually found to be in good bodily condition, although young growing ducks may show dehydration and loss of body weight.

Ducks that survive infection may excrete the virus for years. Persistently infected birds often have erosions near the orifices of the sublingual salivary glands that are in close proximity to the trigeminal nerve. It has been shown that DEHV in the trigeminal nerve of latently infected ducks can be reactivated following cocultivation with susceptible cells.

Lesions

Early lesions indicate the vascular damage that the disease causes. Multiple tissue haemorrhages are seen as well as free blood in body cavities and lumen of the gut. Petechial and larger haemorrhages may be seen on the heart, liver, pancreas, intestines, lungs and kidneys. In adult females the ovarian follicles may be deformed and discoloured. Haemorrhages are commonly seen on the mucosal surface of the alimentary tract. The oesophagus is typically involved, as is the caecum, large intestine and cloaca. Congestion or haemorrhage of the annular bands (lymphoid patches) of the small intestines is usually dramatic. In the later stages of the disease, lesions of the oesophagus and cloaca in particular develop into yellowish diphtheritic plaques. Whitish necrotic foci may be seen in the liver and other organs. The lesions of annular bands may also become necrotic. In young ducks, subcutaneous oedema of the neck and chest entrance may be seen, particularly during meat inspection following slaughter. Oedema of the thymus is also seen. Lesions in geese are often characterized by button-like haemorrhagic and necrotic lymphoid discs with raised rounded borders and depressed necrotic centres scattered along the length of the small intestine. Some species that die very rapidly, such as Muscovy ducks, may show only focal haemorrhages and necrosis of the cloaca.

Histologically, the disease is seen in its early stages to be one of vascular damage, and later areas of necrosis are seen. Intranuclear inclusion bodies can be seen in the cells surrounding necrotic foci and affected epithelia.

Although a presumptive diagnosis of DVE can be made on the basis of clinical and pathological findings, confirmation can only be made by virus isolation and identification. Duck embryo liver cell cultures are the most sensitive in vitro culture system, particularly those of Muscovy duck embryos. Several blind passages may be required before the virus causes a cytopathic effect, characterized by foci of rounded refractile cells. Confirmation of identity of the cytopathic agent can be obtained following electron microscopy examination of concentrated culture extracts for characteristic herpesvirus particles. Further identification can be obtained by virus neutralization in cell cultures using monospecific DEHV antiserum.

PCR assays have recently been developed to detect and identify DEHV in diagnostic samples. Both conventional and nested PCRs have been described to detect DEHV DNA in swabs or tissue samples from dead waterfowl and in carrier birds. The PCR primers are able to detect a conserved region of the virus genome. The method is reported to be highly sensitive, specific, rapid and easy to perform.

Antigen detection by immunofluorescence, immunoperoxidase, ELISA and dot immunobinding tests have also been described but are not routinely available.

CONTROL

In commercial duck flocks and game farms strict biosecurity is essential to prevent contact with wildfowl, particularly mallard ducks, some of which may be shedding virus. Contact with DEHV-infected carrier birds is much more difficult to control in collections of ornamental waterfowl, wildfowl sanctuaries and rescue centres, which frequently have contact with visiting wildfowl. Outbreaks in rescue centres are frequently attributed to the introduction of a sick bird that is incubating DVE. This has occurred on several occasions in swan rescue centres in the UK.

Attenuated live virus vaccines are available for prophylactic use in commercial ducks and geese and resident collections of waterfowl. Annual application of a live DVE vaccine to resident collections of waterfowl prior to the April–June 'DVE season' has been effective in reducing losses from the disease. However, it is not known whether live DVE vaccines can induce latency, particularly if transmission to wildfowl occurs, with subsequent reactivation of vaccinal virus. Inactivated vaccines for DVE have also been developed and evaluated under experimental conditions. The results showed that killed vaccines were as efficacious as modified live DVE vaccines in terms of protection in experimental challenge.

FURTHER READING

Friend M, Brand C J 1999 Duck plague. In: Friend M, Franson J C (eds) Field manual of wildlife diseases. Biological Resources Division, National Wildlife Health Center, Madison, p 141–151

Hansen W R, Gough R E 2007 Duck plague (duck virus enteritis). In: Thomas N J (ed) Infectious diseases of wild birds. Blackwell Publishing, Maldon, p 87–107

Hansen W R, Nashold S W, Docherty D E et al 2000 Diagnosis of Duck Plague in waterfowl by polymerase chain reaction. Avian Dis 44: 266–274

Woolcock P R 2004 Duck virus enteritis. In: OIE Manual of diagnostic tests and vaccines for terrestrial animals, vol. 2. Office International des Épizooties, Paris, p 913–920

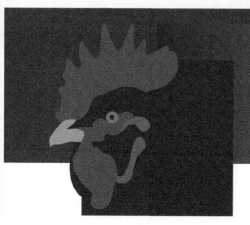

CHAPTER 24

Laurence N. Payne

Retroviridae

Three avian retrovirus species of the family *Retroviridae* are recognized to cause disease in poultry. Like all retroviruses, they are RNA viruses that replicate via a DNA proviral stage linearly present in the host genome, by virtue of the presence in the viral genome of a *pol* gene that encodes the enzyme reverse transcriptase necessary for the transcription of viral RNA to DNA. The three retroviruses are:

- **Avian leukosis/sarcoma group viruses (ALSV).** These include exogenous viruses that occur mainly in the domestic chicken and which cause a variety of leukotic disorders, sarcomas, and other tumours. Endogenous viruses with little or no pathogenicity belonging to this group occur in the domestic chicken and in various other species of bird
- **Reticuloendotheliosis viruses (REV).** These are exogenous viruses occurring in several species of domestic poultry and game bird that cause lymphomas and a runting disease syndrome
- **Lymphoproliferative disease virus of turkeys (LPDV).** This is an exogenous virus of turkeys that causes a lymphoproliferative disease.

Infections with these viruses have been responsible for significant but declining economic losses in the past. However, this situation was changed with the advent some 15 years ago of a new subgroup, designated J, of *Avian leukosis virus* (commonly termed ALV-J), which has caused serious losses worldwide in meat-type chickens. There are indications also that REV infections are becoming more prevalent. In contrast, LPDV infection now appears to be rare. An important feature of avian retroviruses is that they spread vertically as well as horizontally. Because of vertical transmission, vaccination does not offer an effective control method (although vaccination could limit horizontal spread) but in any case attempts to produce vaccines have been discouraging. Control of these diseases is in the hands of primary poultry breeding companies, who institute virus eradication programmes in order to produce virus-free breeding stock. However, disease problems can occur because of reinfection of birds on breeding and production farms.

Apart from their importance as causes of loss to the poultry industry, avian retroviruses are of importance and interest in biomedicine. Erythroid leukosis was the first leukaemic disease shown, by Ellermann and Bang in 1908, to be caused by a virus, and an avian sarcoma was the first solid tumour shown, by Rous in 1911, to be transmitted by a virus. Burmester and others provided proof of the viral aetiology of lymphoid leukosis in 1947. These diseases and their viruses have become widely used as model systems of viral oncogenesis. The viral enzyme reverse transcriptase, from which retroviruses get their name, was discovered in *Rous sarcoma virus* (RSV) and reported in 1970 by Temin and Mizutani, and the first cellular oncogene, *src*, was reported, in chickens, in 1976 by Stehelin, Varmus, Bishop and Vogt. Nobel prizes were awarded to Rous, Temin, Bishop and Varmus for their discoveries.

AVIAN LEUKOSIS/SARCOMA VIRUSES

The ALSVs cause erythroid, lymphoid and myeloid leukoses, a variety of other tumours, such as fibrosarcomas, haemangiomas and nephroblastomas, and the bone disorder osteopetrosis.

Of the neoplasms included in the leukosis/sarcoma group, lymphoid leukosis was until recently the commonest form, occurring mainly in layer-type birds. Over the past decade, myeloid leukosis and, to a lesser extent, erythroid leukosis have become common in meat-type broiler breeders and occasionally in broilers. Losses from these conditions have been of significant economic importance. The other conditions usually occur only sporadically. Subclinical infection by *Avian leukosis virus* (ALV), without the occurrence of neoplastic disease, has been found to depress egg production, egg weight, growth rate and other commercially important traits in both egg-type and meat-type stock and has provided an added incentive to prevention of infection.

EPIDEMIOLOGY

Cause

The ALSVs are placed in the *Alpharetrovirus* genus of the family *Retroviridae*. Members of the genus may be termed either ALV or *Avian sarcoma virus* (ASV). The viral RNA genome is diploid and in the prototypic virus has three genetic regions in the sequence 5′–*gag/pro–pol–env*–3′, which encode respectively the viral internal group-specific antigens and protease, RNA-dependent DNA polymerase (reverse transcriptase) and viral envelope glycoproteins. These structural genes are flanked by genomic sequences concerned with the regulation of viral replication, which in the DNA provirus form the viral long terminal repeats (LTRs). This genetic make-up is associated with slow neoplastic cell transformation and tumour development over several months. Other ALSVs cause rapid neoplastic transformation and tumour development within a few days or weeks. These acutely transforming viruses possess additional genes, termed viral oncogenes, responsible for oncogenic transformation, which originate by transduction of normal cellular genes, the proto-oncogenes. For example, RSV has the genetic structure 5′–*gag/pro–pol–env–src*–3′, the viral *src* gene being derived originally from a cellular *src* gene. Other acutely transforming ALSVs possess one (rarely two) of the dozen or so viral oncogenes that have been discovered. One of these oncogenes, *myc*, is present in a number of ALSVs that cause myelocytomas, and cellular *myc* (c-*myc*) is activated in bursal lymphoid cells during the induction of lymphoid leukosis. Most of the acutely transforming viruses have genetic deletions within the structural genes such that the oncogene-carrying virus is unable to replicate. It needs the presence of a nondefective ALV helper virus to complement the genetic defect. Most of the acutely transforming ALSVs that have been studied originated from field tumours but are now maintained as laboratory strains. Similar viruses are occasionally generated anew in ALV-infected flocks by transduction of cellular oncogenes. For example, acutely transforming variants of ALV-J occur that carry the c-*myc* oncogene and cause myelocytomas in chickens and turkeys.

The viral structural proteins include p27, the major group-specific (gs) antigen encoded by the *gag* gene, which is common to all viruses of the leukosis/sarcoma group and important in certain diagnostic tests. The envelope of the virion contains a glycoprotein, gp85, encoded by the *env* gene, which determines the subgroup specificity of the virus.

Virus infection of cells occurs through receptors on the cell membrane. Viral RNA is released in the cytoplasm and, under the influence of reverse transcriptase, a strand of viral DNA is synthesized on the template of viral RNA. A second strand of viral DNA is formed to produce linear double-stranded viral DNA, which migrates to the nucleus and becomes integrated in the DNA of the host. The proviral genes are integrated in the same order as their RNA copies in the virion and are flanked by the LTRs, which act as promoters and enhancers controlling transcription of proviral DNA to viral RNA. The transcribed viral RNA molecules serve either as genomic RNA in newly formed virions or as messenger RNAs, which are translated to produce the protein and enzymic products of the *gag/pro*, *pol* and *env* genes that form the virion. These products localize at the plasma membrane of the cell and form into spheroidal C-type virions, which are budded off from the cell.

Neoplastic transformation of the cell

Two types of mechanism are involved in tumour formation. Slowly transforming viruses, which do not carry a viral oncogene, transform cells by fortuitously integrating in the host genome adjacent to a normal cellular proto-oncogene, which is then abnormally expressed under the influence of the viral LTR promoter. This mechanism is termed 'promoter insertion'. In the induction of lymphoid leukosis, the c-*myc* oncogene in a B lymphocyte is activated. The acutely transforming viruses, which carry one or two of the various viral oncogenes, are oncogenic because of multiple viral insertions of the respective viral oncogene into the host genome, resulting in abnormal expression of the gene product. The particular oncogene present determines the type of neoplasm induced.

Virus subgroups

ALSVs in chickens are classified into six subgroups – A, B, C, D, E and J – on the basis of differences in their viral envelope gp85 glycoproteins, which determine virus-serum neutralization properties, viral infectivity interference patterns and host range in fowl of different genotypes. Subgroups F, G, H and I are allocated to endogenous ALVs occurring in pheasants, partridge and quail.

Sequence analyses of the gp85 encoding region of the *env* genes of viruses of the different subgroups have revealed hypervariable regions responsible for subgroup differences. The gp85 region of ALV-J *env* gene differs more greatly from the *env* genes of the other five subgroups, A to E, than the latter do amongst themselves (Fig. 24.1). Phylogenetic analyses of ALV-J isolates from various locations indicate marked *env* gene variability and continued viral mutation. The *env* gene of ALV-J shows very high homology to the avian endogenous retrovirus EAV-HP. It is believed that ALV-J arose de novo from a relatively recent genetic recombination between an unknown exogenous ALV and endogenous virus EAV-HP, and from which subsequent ALV-J isolates are derived.

Exogenous and endogenous avian leukosis viruses

According to how they are transmitted naturally, ALSVs can be classified as exogenous or endogenous. Exogenous leukosis viruses ('originating from the outside') spread as infectious virions, either vertically (congenitally) from dam to progeny through the egg or horizontally from bird

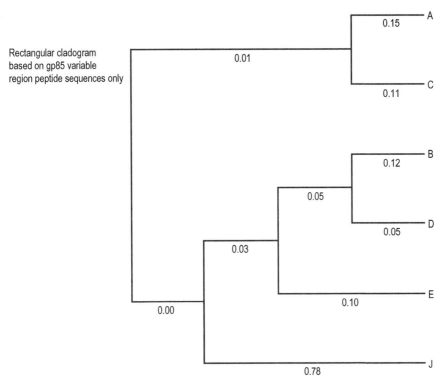

Rectangular cladogram
based on gp85 variable
region peptide sequences only

0.01

0.15 — A

0.11 — C

0.12 — B

0.05

0.05 — D

0.03

0.10

0.00

0.78 — J

E

Fig. 24.1 Phylogenetic tree of peptide sequences based on the variable regions of the envelope genes of avian leukosis viruses of subgroups A, B, C, D, E and J. The numbers represent the fraction of amino acid substitutions that define the branch; the larger the number the less similar the sequences. Relationships between subgroups A–E are closer than those between these subgroups and subgroup J. (Courtesy of Dr Peter Chesters.)

to bird by contact. Viruses of subgroups A, B, C, D and J spread in this way. Endogenous leukosis viruses ('originating from within'), including those of subgroup E, occur integrated as proviral DNA sequences in the genome of germ-line and somatic cells of normal chickens and are transmitted genetically in a Mendelian fashion by both sexes to their progeny. Several families of endogenous viruses are recognized: the endogenous viral (*ev*) loci, the moderately repetitive EAV and ART-CH families, and the highly repetitive CR1 family. The EAV family is of particular interest since it is apparently the origin of the *env* gene of ALV-J, as discussed above. These endogenous elements are examples of retroelements that are found in an extremely broad range of organisms and can make up 10% or more of the genome. Some retroelements are believed to be the evolutionary precursors of retroviruses while others, such as the *ev* loci, are believed to represent exogenous viruses that have become re-integrated on an evolutionary scale into the germ-line. Most endogenous viruses are genetically defective and lack the full complement of retroviral genes necessary for the production of infectious virus. The genes that are present may, however, be partially expressed as gene products such as gs antigen or reverse transcriptase. Some *ev* loci have a complete set of genes and may be expressed as subgroup E ALV, of which the virus strain RAV-0 is the prototype. The *ev*21 locus, which is genetically linked to the sex-linked slow feathering gene, *K*, on the Z chromosome, is expressed in chick embryos as the virus EV21. The EV21 virus may produce a tolerizing effect, weakening the immune response to exogenous ALV infection and increasing the incidence of, for example, lymphoid leukosis. Unlike the other sub-groups, subgroup E leukosis viruses have little or no oncogenicity for chickens, evidently because the LTR has weak gene promoter activity.

Oncogenic patterns of virus strains

Strains of ALSV often produce more than one type of neoplasm, although for each strain one particular neoplasm usually predominates. Some laboratory strains of virus consist of mixtures of viruses that contribute to the oncogenic variation, but studies with clone-purified strains indicate that these too can cause several types of neoplasm. The oncogenic spectrum is influenced by origin of the virus, virus dose, route of inoculation and the age and genotype of the host.

Spread

Exogenous ALVs are ubiquitous in commercial chickens on a worldwide basis. In the UK and USA ALV-A is commonly encountered and ALV-B is occasionally found. These subgroups cause mainly lymphoid leukosis. Subgroups C and D are very rare. *Ev* loci (including subgroup E viral loci) are present in virtually all chickens, as are the other endogenous virus families. ALV-J was first reported in the UK in 1991 in meat-type chickens and causes myeloid leukosis (myelocy-tomatosis) and other tumours. It has since spread in meat-type chickens throughout the world. In 2002, ALV-J was reported in commercial layer flocks for the first time, in China. Turkeys are susceptible to ALV-J but the infection has not been recognized in commercial stock. Dual infections by ALV-A and ALV-J have been observed in broiler breeder stock in Australia.

Most commercial chickens are exposed to and infected by exogenous ALV, and carry endog-enous leukosis viruses but usually only a few per cent develop leukosis or other tumours. Occasion-ally losses of 30% or more can occur. Economic losses in egg-laying stock arise principally from mortality from lymphoid leukosis occurring from 20 to 36 weeks of age and in meat-type stock from myeloid leukosis occurring mainly in adult birds from 25 to 55 weeks of age. The other neoplastic diseases occur more sporadically.

Exogenous ALV is transmitted both vertically (congenitally), from hen to progeny through the egg, and horizontally, between birds by direct or indirect contact. A small minority, usu-ally less than 10%, of chicks are infected vertically and the majority become infected by contact with vertically infected chicks during rearing. Vertical infection occurs from hens that shed ALV from the oviduct into the egg albumen, from whence it passes into the chick embryo. Chick embryos apparently do not become infected from the male. Congenitally infected chicks develop immunological tolerance to the ALV and fail to develop virus neutralizing antibodies but are permanently viraemic. Hens of this class have considerable amounts of virus in the oviduct and transmit this to most of their eggs and their embryos.

Chicks infected horizontally develop a transient viraemia and then usually develop virus-neutralizing antibodies without viraemia. Such birds become virus carriers. Lower proportions of hens of this type have an oviduct infection; they shed to their progeny intermittently. With subgroup J ALV infection of meat-type birds, early horizontal infection (up to 6 weeks of age) is more likely to produce permanent tolerant viraemic infection without antibody production.

Thus four classes occur in mature chickens: (1) tolerant viraemic, antibody-negative shedders ($V^+A^-S^+$); (2) nonviraemic, antibody-positive nonshedders ($V^-A^+S^-$); (3) nonviraemic, anti-body-positive shedders ($V^-A^+S^+$); and (4) nonviraemic, antibody-negative nonshedders ($V^-A^-S^-$), which are susceptible birds not yet infected or birds genetically resistant to infection. Infected birds with tolerant viraemia are more likely to develop leukosis than are immune birds with antibodies. The incidence of leukosis decreases if horizontal infection occurs after the first few weeks of life. Virus is present in the saliva, faeces and feather debris of infected birds but its survival outside the body is relatively short (a few hours) and consequently ALVs are not very contagious.

Virus-neutralizing antibodies in ALSV-infected hens are passed via the yolk to progeny chicks and provide a passive immunity to contact infection that lasts for 3–4 weeks. Actively acquired humoral and cell-mediated immune responses following infection similarly serve to reduce virus replication and hence neoplasia. Although some strains of ALSV have been shown to be immunosuppressive experimentally, there is no clear evidence that natural infections (including ALV-A and ALV-J) are significantly immunosuppressive.

Genetic resistance

Two types of genetic resistance to the ALSV group are recognized: resistance to virus infection and resistance to tumour development. Autosomal loci control responses to infection by ALSVs of subgroups A, B and C and are designated *tv-a* (tumour virus subgroup A), *tv-b* and *tv-c* respectively. The *tv-b* locus also controls responses to subgroup D and E viruses. Alleles for susceptibility and resistance occur at each locus, designated *tv-a^s*, *tv-a^r*, etc., and susceptibility is dominant over resistance. Susceptibility genes such as *a^s* encode the presence of subgroup-specific virus receptor sites through which the virus gains access to the cell; these receptors are decreased in number or are lacking in resistant cells. Receptors used by ALV have other normal physiological functions: thus the receptor for subgroup A ALV is a member of the low density lipoprotein receptor family and that for subgroup B, D and E is a member of the tumour necrosis factor receptor family. The ALV susceptibility phenotype is designated according to a convention that recognizes the species of the cell, e.g. chicken (C), and the subgroups of virus to which the cell is resistant (/). For example, the phenotype C/A denotes a cell or chicken resistant to subgroup A and susceptible to subgroups B, C, D, E and J; C/0 a cell or chicken susceptible to all six subgroups. Naturally occurring genetic resistance to cellular infection by subgroup J has not been recognized but a J-resistant cell line, DF-1/J, has been developed by genetic engineering for virus identification purposes.

Resistance to tumour development has been mainly studied with RSV-induced sarcomas, regression of which is influenced by genes within the major histocompatibility complex. Strains of chickens may vary in susceptibility to leukosis although they are all susceptible to infection. This is exemplified by the variable incidence of myeloid leukosis and other tumours following ALV-J infection of different chicken lines. The strength of the immune response to ALV-J also varies between lines.

PATHOGENESIS

Non-neoplastic conditions

ALV infection in the absence of neoplastic disease can adversely affect egg production traits in layers, including age at first egg, egg numbers, size, fertility and hatchability. Nonspecific mortality may increase. In meat-type birds, ALV infection (especially by ALV-J) can depress broiler growth rate.

Other non-neoplastic effects in ALV infection have been observed mainly in experimental infections. ALV infection has a tropism for myocardial cells, and a possible role of ALV-J in the causation of cardiomyopathy and ascites has been reported.

Lymphoid leukosis

Lymphoid leukosis is a common neoplasm caused by ALV of subgroups A and B (ALV-A and ALV-B). ALV-J has a weak ability to cause lymphoid leukosis, dependent on the strain of chicken. Lymphoid leukosis is characterized by enlargement of the liver (Fig. 24.2) by infiltrating lymphoblasts and the pattern of involvement is usually diffuse or miliary but can occasionally be nodular. Other organs are also tumorous. Nodular tumours can be found in the bursa of Fabricius in nearly all cases. Microscopically the lesions consist of diffuse areas or coalescing foci of extravascular immature lymphoid cells. In the bursa a follicular pattern of tumour growth can often be seen. The tumour cells in lymphoid leukosis invariably have the morphology of large lymphocytes or lymphoblasts; they have B-cell markers and carry surface IgM.

The incubation period from infection to the developed disease and death is 4 months or more. The target cells for neoplastic transformation in lymphoid leukosis reside in the bursa of Fabricius. At a variable time after infection of the bird, a proliferation of lymphoblasts can be observed in lymphoid follicles in the bursa, termed a focal preneoplastic hyperplasia. This process is the result of ALV proviral integration within the c-*myc* gene, leading to overexpression of Myc protein and blocked B-cell differentiation and migration. Many follicles are sometimes affected but the majority of these regress and only a few, due to activation of other cellular oncogenes, grow to give rise to nodular tumours in the bursa which are visible from about 14 weeks of age. Neoplastic lymphoid cells metastasize from the bursa to other organs such as the liver and spleen, causing death.

Spontaneous bursal lymphomas, independent of ALV infection, and enhanced by SB-1 serotype 2 Marek's disease vaccination, have been observed.

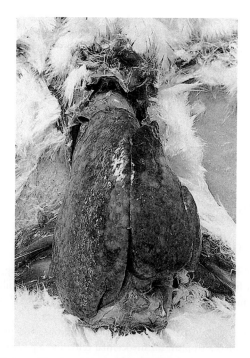

Fig. 24.2 Greatly enlarged tumorous liver in a chicken with lymphoid leukosis.

Erythroid leukosis (erythroblastosis)

This is a sporadic disease, affecting mainly adult chickens. It has become more common since the advent of subgroup J ALV, occurring also in young birds. Activation of the c-*erbB* gene in an erythroid cell by slowly transforming ALV gives rise to erythroid leukosis. Acutely transforming ALVs carrying the viral oncogene v-*erbB* exist and can cause erythroid leukosis. In cases of the disease, there is a variable anaemia, which is associated with the presence of a large number of immature red cells in the blood. The disease originates in the bone marrow and a leukaemia is present from the outset. It is a peculiarity of this condition that the malignant cells remain within the blood vessels throughout the course of the disease. This results in an erythrostasis in sinusoids in organs such as the liver, spleen and bone marrow, imparting to them a cherry-red colour that characterizes this condition post-mortem. The liver and spleen are moderately enlarged.

Myeloid leukosis (myeloblastosis and myelocytomatosis)

Myeloid leukosis involves an extravascular and intravascular proliferation of cells of the myeloid (granulocytic) series. It can occur as a sporadic disease mainly of adults but since the advent of ALV-J can also occur in higher incidence in adult birds and at times in broilers. It may occur as a myeloblastosis, originating in the bone marrow and involving immature myeloid cells, or as a myelocytomatosis in which more mature myelocytes are affected. Strains of subgroup J ALV that induce myeloid leukosis, such as strains HPRS-103 and ADOL-Hc1, lack a viral oncogene and are believed to induce the disease by activation of a cellular oncogene, apparently c-*myc*. Acutely transforming laboratory strains of ALV exist that can cause myeloblastosis or myelocytomatosis. The BAI-A strain of *Avian myeloblastosis virus* carried the oncogene v-*myb*; the MC29 strain of *Avian myelocytomatosis virus* carries v-*myc*. Similar acutely transforming viruses also occur naturally.

In diffuse myeloid leukosis (myeloblastosis) the liver and spleen are diffusely and greatly enlarged and the liver frequently has a granular, 'Morocco leather' appearance. Although the proliferative process is essentially extravascular, there is frequently an accompanying leukaemia.

The tumours of myelocytomatosis can be diffuse and/or discrete and nodular and have a creamy-white colour. The tumours may occur in a wide range of organs, including the liver, spleen and kidney, and have a predilection for the visceral surface of flat bones such as the ribs, skull, sternum and pelvis. Tumours may occur in the eye. Leukaemia may be present.

Other tumours and lesions

Solid tumours that can be caused by ALSVs include fibrosarcoma, chondroma, histiocytic sarcoma, endothelioma, haemangioma, nephroblastoma and hepatocarcinoma. They usually occur sporadically in young or older chickens and show features characteristic of their cellular origin. These other tumours are especially seen in flocks infected with ALV-J, accompanying myeloid leukosis and erythroid leukosis. Two recently described lesions of similar appearance occurring in broilers, termed multicentric histiocytosis by US workers and spindle-cell proliferative disease by Japanese workers, may also be associated with ALV-J infection. Also apparently associated with ALV-J infection are multiple mixed foci of myeloid and lymphoid cells in the liver of young birds. The lesion, termed lymphomyeloid hyperplasia, appears to be reactive rather than neoplastic. A new ALV-A has recently been implicated in causing fowl glioma and perineurioma.

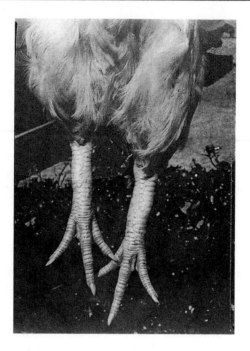

Fig. 24.3 Osteopetrosis.

Osteopetrosis

This is an uncommon bone disorder affecting mainly the long bones, notably of the legs and wings. Excessive osteoblast proliferation and bone formation results in gross thickening of the diaphyses of the long bones; occlusion of the marrow cavity may eventually give rise to anaemia (Fig. 24.3).

DIAGNOSIS

The signs in chickens affected by leukosis are nonspecific. The bird may be inappetent, weak and emaciated, diarrhoea may occur and the wattles may be pale. Osteopetrosis is readily apparent from thickening of the long bones.

Diagnosis involves pathological and virological examinations to determine the type of neoplasm responsible for mortality and which viruses are present in a flock. Because exogenous ALV is almost ubiquitous in commercial flocks, its isolation does not prove that it caused the tumour. Evidence that a virus isolate caused a particular type of tumour requires transmission experiments in which the tumour is reproduced. Virological testing is often also required to show that specific pathogen-free (SPF) flocks or live vaccines propagated in chicken cells are free of ALSV.

Signs and lesions

Identification of the type of neoplasm responsible for mortality is made by gross and histological examination of freshly killed or recently dying birds using the pathological criteria described above.

Cytological examination of May–Grünwald–Giemsa-stained impression smears of fresh tumour tissue is a useful aid to diagnosis. If possible, several birds should be examined. The main features for differentiating the leukoses are given in Table 24.1. The following set of tissues is recommended for the histological diagnosis of the leukoses and other neoplasms: liver, spleen, bursa of Fabricius, thymus, bone marrow, gonad, sciatic, brachial and coeliac nerves and any other tumour tissue. Differentiation of lymphoid leukosis from Marek's disease is important (see Ch. 23).

Virus isolation/detection

A variety of samples may be collected from a flock for detection of the presence of, or for isolation of, ALV or other tumour viruses. The presence of infection can be demonstrated most easily by detection of antibodies in serum. Viruses can be detected in and isolated from serum, plasma, buffy coat cells, tumour tissue, normal parenchymatous tissues (e.g. liver), feather pulp and tips, meconium, vaginal and cloacal swabs, egg albumen and embryos. Because the viruses are thermolabile at room temperature, samples should be collected from live or freshly killed birds, or from newly laid eggs, and stored and shipped at $-70°C$.

A variety of diagnostic tests are available for the detection of ALSV. The principles of the commonly used tests are outlined here; detailed procedures are available in laboratory manuals and technical articles.

Virus isolation is generally the ideal detection method, since the technique can detect all ALVs and is the starting point for several other investigative methods. Material (normally cell-free) to be tested for exogenous ALV is inoculated into specific-pathogen-free C/E chick embryo fibroblasts (CEFs) (susceptible to all ALV subgroups except E) growing in tissue culture plates or wells of microtitre plates, and the cultures are incubated for 7 days. Supernatants are collected and stored at $-70°C$ as virus isolates for other studies. The CEFs are sonicated and tested for the presence of ALV p27 gs antigen in an antigen enzyme-linked immunosorbent assay (ELISA) test (commercially available). A positive optical density (OD) reading for gs antigen compared with uninoculated CEF cultures (in which low levels of gs antigen of endogenous ALV origin may be detected) is indicative of the presence of exogenous ALV of subgroups A, B, C, D or J. Ideally, C/E CEFs from chickens free of endogenous gs antigen, such as line 0, should be used. If necessary, subgroup E ALV can be identified by inoculating test material on C/E CEF and quail embryo fibroblasts of phenotype Q/BJ. Subgroup E ALV will grow in the Q/BJ cultures but be excluded from the C/E cultures.

An antigen ELISA is available commercially for the detection of ALV p27 gs antigen in various materials such as egg albumen, meconium, vaginal and cloacal swabs, and feather pulp, as evidence of ALV infection. The test is used particularly to detect ALV shedder hens in ALV eradication programmes and is cheap, rapid and suitable for large-scale use. It is not subgroup specific for the different exogenous ALV subgroups (which is usually of no concern) but it has the disadvantage of also detecting gs antigen of endogenous ALV origin, although usually at a lower level. The testing of serum or plasma for gs antigen is not recommended because of the confusion between antigen of endogenous and exogenous origin. The antigen ELISA is also used to detect ALV growth in virus isolation tests in CEF as discussed above.

Virus characterization

The envelope subgroup of ALV isolates may be determined by several methods:

- **Viral interference assays**, which test the ability of an ALV isolate to prevent focus formation in C/E CEF cultures by RSV strains of known subgroup

Table 24.1 Main gross and microscopic features of importance in the differential diagnosis of the leukoses

FEATURE	LYMPHOID LEUKOSIS	ERYTHROID LEUKOSIS (ERYTHROBLASTOSIS)	MYELOID LEUKOSIS (MYELOBLASTOSIS)	MYELOID LEUKOSIS (MYELOCYTOMATOSIS)
Liver	Greatly enlarged; diffuse, miliary or nodular tumours; moderately firm	Moderately enlarged; diffuse infiltration; cherry red colour; soft	Greatly enlarged; diffuse infiltration; mottled; granular surface; firm	Often yellowish white nodular or diffuse tumours
Spleen	Usually enlarged; diffuse, miliary or nodular tumours; soft	Often enlarged; cherry-red; smooth; very soft	Often enlarged; diffuse tumour; mottled; smooth; soft	Often nodular or diffuse tumours
Bursa of Fabricius	Usually enlarged; nodular tumours	No changes	Sometimes tumorous	No changes
Bone marrow	Often tumorous; diffuse or focal	Semi-liquid; cherry-red	Diffuse, reddish-grey tumour infiltration	Usually diffuse yellowish-grey tumour infiltration
Blood	Occasionally lymphoblastic leukaemia	Erythroblastic leukaemia; immature erythrocytes; anaemia; thin buffy coat	Myeloblastic leukaemia; thick buffy coat	Myelocytic leukaemia; thick buffy coat
Cytology and histopathology	Lymphoblasts; mainly extravascular infiltrations	Erythroblasts; intravascular	Myeloblasts in intravascular and extravascular locations	Myelocytes in intravascular and extravascular locations
Other organs and tissues often grossly involved	Kidneys, ovary	Kidneys; may be haemorrhages in muscles	Kidneys, ovary	Kidneys, ovary, thymus, surface of bones (sternum, ribs, skull)

- **Virus neutralization assays**, in which the isolate, or the RSV pseudotype of the isolate, is exposed to antisera with known neutralization specificity to each subgroup, and examined for growth, or focus formation, respectively, in C/E CEF cultures (N.B. An RSV pseudotype is an RSV that can be created by coating a replication defective RSV with the viral envelope of an ALV, endowing the pseudotype with the subgroup characteristics of the ALV)
- **Host range assays**, in which the isolate, or the RSV pseudotype of the isolate, is placed in a subgroup depending on its ability to grow in, or transform, CEF cultures of varying ALV subgroup susceptibility phenotypes
- **Polymerase chain reaction (PCR) assays.** Primer pairs are available specific for the different ALV subgroups, including J. A problem with PCR methods is that the primer pairs used may not detect all variant viruses. Reverse-transcriptase PCR has also been developed for detection of viral RNA. PCR-induced sequences of various retroviral genes can be used to study viral relatedness and variability.

Serology

Detection of antibodies is used in flock surveillance to determine the presence or absence of infection by ALV of different subgroups, and to help to characterize the infective status of individual birds in epidemiological and eradication studies. Two types of test are mainly used:

- **Virus neutralization tests**, in which antibody is detected by ability to neutralize infectivity of ALVs, or RSV pseudotypes, of known subgroup; these tests are technically demanding and time-consuming
- **Antibody ELISA tests.** Tests for antibodies to subgroups A, B and J are available commercially and are rapid and suitable for large-scale testing.

A variety of other tests are available for testing for ALV and ALV antibodies. These include: the nonproducer (NP) cell activation tests for ALV; the phenotypic mixing test for ALV; the complement fixation test for ALV (COFAL); fluorescent antibody and other immunohistochemical tests for ALV and antibody; in situ hybridization for ALV; and chick and embryo inoculation tests for ALV pathogenicity. Highly sensitive tests for reverse transcriptase have been used to screen human vaccines produced in CEF for freedom from avian retroviruses. Details of these various tests can be found in laboratory manuals.

CONTROL

No treatment or vaccines are available and control must be based on obtaining birds from an ALV-free strain or from genetically resistant stock and on high standards of hygiene and flock management to prevent infection from the environment. Because the infection is egg-transmitted, it cannot be excluded by rearing in isolation unless the source is free of ALV.

Eradication of exogenous ALV from commercial flocks

Eradication of infection by exogenous ALV was formerly used only for the development of specific pathogen-free flocks for research or vaccine production but technical advances in methods for detecting ALV and infected birds have now extended control by virus eradication to commercial breeding layer and meat-type flocks. An ALV-free flock is developed by hatching and rearing in isolation a group of chicks free from congenitally infected birds. These chicks are obtained by selecting hatching eggs from hens that do not transmit exogenous ALV congenitally. ELISA testing of vaginal swabs or egg albumen (two eggs per hen) identifies birds that do or do not transmit ALV, as detected by presence of gs antigen. Chicks are hatched from non-shedder hens; meconium or cloacal swabs are taken at 1 day old and tested for gs antigen to eliminate any congenitally infected chicks that have been produced by transmitting hens that escaped detection. Thereafter, the ALV-free groups of birds are reared in isolation and monitored for freedom from infection by tests for antibody against ALV of subgroups A, B and J. Small-group hatching and rearing, with early testing and removal of infected groups, is considered to be a valuable adjunct to virus eradication programmes. Under some conditions, stock hatched free of ALV may later become exposed to horizontal infection but there are indications that this may not lead to disease or to vertical transmission.

Selection for genetic resistance

As discussed earlier, recessive genes that are present in varying frequency in commercial strains control resistance to infection. Commercial breeding companies can increase the frequency of the resistance genes and develop stock with resistance to ALV and thus to leukosis and other tumours. The genotypes of unknown parents can be determined by mating them to recessive tester birds, according to the segregation of susceptible and resistant progeny from a particular mating. The phenotypic classification of the progeny into susceptible and resistant classes is determined by inoculation of RSV of the appropriate subgroup (usually A and B) onto the chorio-allantoic membrane of chick embryos and embryos are classified based on the tumour pock count observed. Tests for the direct identification of the phenotype of adult birds are also available. Genes for resistance to infection by subgroup J have not been recognized. This approach to select genetically resistant stock has largely been replaced by commercial ALV eradication schemes.

PUBLIC HEALTH SIGNIFICANCE

There is no strong evidence to suggest that ALSVs present a health risk to humans. Certain strains of RSV can infect and transform human and other mammalian cells in culture and can cause sarcomas and other tumours in primates and other mammals. However, despite exposure of humans to ALV from live poultry, poultry meat and eggs, no conclusive epidemiological or other evidence exists of any risk of their causing human cancer. Also, exposure of humans to exogenous ALV present at one time (but not now) as a contaminant of live vaccines grown in embryonated eggs, such as those against yellow fever and measles, was not associated with any recognized hazard. Recently, low levels of reverse transcriptase and RNA of endogenous ALV and EAV retrovirus origin were detected in live human vaccines grown in SPF avian cells. There was however no evidence of these viruses, their provirus sequences or their antibodies in vaccine recipients and use of these vaccines was not considered to be harmful.

RETICULOENDOTHELIOSIS

The term reticuloendotheliosis includes several pathological syndromes caused by a group of retroviruses that are distinct from those causing the leukosis/sarcoma group of diseases of chickens. Natural infections by reticuloendotheliosis viruses (REVs) occur in chickens, ducks, geese, Hungarian partridge, pheasants, Japanese quail and turkeys. Resultant neoplastic disease has been observed sporadically in turkeys and, less commonly, in other species of bird.

EPIDEMIOLOGY

Cause

Viruses forming the REV group belong to the *Gammaretrovirus* genus of the family *Retroviridae* and are distinct from viruses of the leukosis/sarcoma group. The REV group includes antigenically closely related isolates from various sources, including strain T, *Chick syncytial virus, Spleen necrosis virus* and *Duck infectious anaemia virus*. Three antigenic subtypes of REV have been defined. A relationship between REV and certain mammalian retroviruses has been observed. Genetically nondefective strains of REV have *gag, pro, pol* and *env* genes and are slowly oncogenic, inducing B-cell lymphomas and T-cell lymphomas in chickens by promoter insertion adjacent to the cellular *myc* oncogene. Chronic lymphomas are also induced in turkeys and other species of birds but the mechanism has not been elucidated. The laboratory-propagated strain T REV consists of replication-defective virus that has acquired a viral oncogene, v-*rel*, derived from a cellular proto-oncogene, together with a nondefective REV helper virus needed for replication. Strain T is acutely oncogenic, inducing reticuloendotheliosis. Nondefective REV can be propagated in chickens, turkeys and quail fibroblast cultures. REV exhibits some cytopathic properties and plaques develop in duck embryo fibroblasts that can be used to assay the virus. A fluorescent focus assay for REV in fibroblasts grown under agar can also be used. Nondefective REV can serve as a helper virus for RSV and vesicular stomatitis virus; the resultant pseudotypes may be used to assay for virus neutralizing antibodies against REV.

Spread

Little is known about the epidemiology of REV infection in naturally infected turkey or chicken flocks. The infection has been reported in Australia, Egypt, Germany, Israel, Japan, the UK and the USA. In the USA, REV infection was found to be sporadic to frequent among commercial chickens and sporadic in turkeys. Data from experimental infections indicate that the infection can spread by contact with infected chickens and turkeys, and REV is present in faeces. Birds so infected develop a transient viraemia followed by the appearance of antibodies. Chickens and turkeys infected by embryo inoculation develop tolerant infections with persistent viraemia and absence of antibodies. Tolerantly infected chicken and turkey hens transmit the virus vertically to some of their progeny, and hens shed REV gs antigen and more rarely virus to egg albumen. Tolerantly infected turkey stags can transmit the infection to their progeny via semen. It is believed that mosquitoes and houseflies can transmit REV, and transmission has occurred with contaminated Marek's disease and fowlpox vaccines.

PATHOGENESIS

Acute reticulum cell neoplasia

Infection of newly hatched chickens and turkeys by replication-defective strain T virus results in high mortality from neoplastic disease 1–3 weeks later. Affected birds have enlarged livers and spleens, caused by focal or diffuse infiltration by proliferating reticulum cells and sometimes lymphocytes. Similar infiltrations occur in the gonads, heart, kidney and pancreas, giving rise to the original designation of the disease as a reticuloendotheliosis. The neoplastic target cells in reticuloendotheliosis are still unclear but appear to include immature B and T cells. It is uncertain whether this form of the disease occurs in the field.

Chronic lymphoid neoplasia

Nondefective strains of REV induce two types of more chronic lymphoid neoplasm in chickens. First, bursa-dependent B-cell lymphomas indistinguishable from lymphoid leukosis occur in chickens after a long latent period (4–10 months). Second, T-cell lymphomas have been induced experimentally that are comprised of large uniform lymphoreticular cells that arise in various visceral organs (but not the bursa) and peripheral nerves from 3 weeks after inoculation. Grossly, these tumours are somewhat similar to those of Marek's disease. Whether these T-cell tumours occur in chickens in the field is unclear. In turkeys, lymphoid tumours of uncertain nature have been found at 2–3 months after REV inoculation and T-cell lymphomas have been observed in commercial turkeys. In geese, inoculation of REV induces both very acute and chronic lymphomas. In ducks, experimental infection causes stunting, lymphoid tumours and sarcomas.

Birds infected with nondefective REV may develop a runting syndrome, with abnormal feathering and sometimes infiltration of peripheral nerves by lymphocytes and plasma cells, leading to nerve enlargement and sometimes paralysis. These nerve infiltrations may or may not be accompanied by lymphomas in other organs. Proventriculitis may also occur.

DIAGNOSIS

Clinical signs

No pathognomonic signs are observed during the development of acute or chronic neoplasia. Lymphomas in naturally infected turkeys have occurred between 15 and 20 weeks of age. A runting disease syndrome has occurred in flocks inoculated with vaccines accidentally contaminated with REV and some birds show a peculiar feathering abnormality (*nakanuke* in Japanese) in which wing feathers have adhesions of the barbule to part of the feather shaft. Some birds may show paralysis. REV infection can also cause immunosuppression.

REV-induced tumours in turkeys and chickens are morphologically varied and can be confused with Marek's disease, lymphoid leukosis caused by ALV, and lymphoproliferative disease of turkeys. Nerve lesions caused by REV infection are similar to those of Marek's disease. Serological diagnosis of the presence of REV is required to support a pathological diagnosis.

Virus detection

Viral antigen can be detected in serum from viraemic birds using the agar gel precipitin test and in cell extracts using a complement fixation test. ELISA tests for REV gs antigen and envelope antigen and PCR assays have been described.

Serology

The presence of infection in a flock can be determined by examination of sera for antibodies, using the ELISA test (commercially available), agar gel precipitin test, plaque reduction test, pseudotype-neutralization test or fluorescent antibody test.

CONTROL

Because REV infections are sporadic and often not associated with clinical disease, no control procedures have been developed. It is considered that procedures similar to those used for eradication of ALV in chickens could be applied if necessary. Freedom from REV is increasingly a requirement for exporting stock.

PUBLIC HEALTH SIGNIFICANCE

There is no direct evidence to associate REV with a human health hazard. But this question has received some attention because of the possible evolutionary relationship of REV to mammalian retroviruses, and its ability to infect and grow in cultured mammalian cells. Also, REV used as a vector virus can infect human cells, and plasmid REV DNA can transfect such cells, with integration and low-level replication. Continued vigilance is thus advisable.

LYMPHOPROLIFERATIVE DISEASE OF TURKEYS

Lymphoproliferative disease of turkeys was first reported from the UK in 1972 and has subsequently been recognized in other European countries and in Israel. It now appears to be rare in the UK but should be considered in the differential diagnosis of lymphoproliferative disorders of turkeys.

EPIDEMIOLOGY

Cause

Lymphoproliferative disease is caused by a retrovirus of the family *Retroviridae* that is distinct serologically and genetically from other avian retroviruses, although distantly related to ALSV. Characterization of LPDV has been hindered by the lack of any tissue culture system for propagating the virus. Nevertheless, some molecular characterization has been possible using virus prepared from plasma from viraemic turkeys.

The disease may be reproduced by inoculating turkey poults with tissue extracts and plasma from affected birds.

Spread

The infection can spread horizontally between turkeys and susceptibility to disease increases over the first few weeks of life. Vertical transmission has not been reported. Strains of turkey vary in their susceptibility to the disease. The incidence of infection is higher than that of the disease. Experimentally, ducks and geese were not susceptible to infection. Chickens were susceptible and gross and microscopic lymphoproliferative-disease-like lesions were observed.

PATHOGENESIS

Lymphoproliferative disease is characterized by marked enlargement of the spleen, which is usually pale pink in colour with a marbled appearance. The liver may be moderately enlarged, with miliary greyish-white foci. Miliary or diffuse tumour infiltration may also occur in kidney, gonad, intestinal wall, pancreas, lungs, myocardium and thymus. Peripheral nerves may be slightly enlarged and anaemia is often present. Leukocytosis or leukopenia has been observed.

The proliferative lesion is similar in all organs and tissues and consists of pleomorphic lymphoid cells, including lymphocytes, lymphoblasts, reticulum cells and plasma cells.

Following experimental infection of 4-week-old poults, early lymphoproliferative lesions are seen as early as 2 weeks in the spleen and thymus. By 3 weeks, splenic enlargement is present and foci of lymphoproliferative lesions are seen in many organs. Small focal lesions consisting of lymphocytes, with germinal centres, may also occur and increase in frequency with time; these may be regressing lesions.

Viraemia occurs by 5 days after infection and persists for several weeks. An antibody response has not been detected but markedly elevated serum IgG levels are reported. Immunosuppression is observed in experimental infections.

DIAGNOSIS

The disease is seen mainly in growing turkeys between 7 and 18 weeks of age and occasionally in adults. Affected birds die suddenly, sometimes after preceding depression. Up to 20% of the flock may be affected.

Diagnosis of lymphoproliferative disease is based on gross and microscopic lesions in affected birds, detection of reverse transcriptase activity in plasma, which is higher with magnesium ions than with manganese ions, detection of LPDV in tissues by immunofluorescence or in plasma by an ELISA test and PCR assay. Differentiation of lymphoproliferative disease from reticuloendotheliosis is important, employing especially the virological and serological tests for REV.

CONTROL

No specific control measures for the disease have been developed. Control has been by elimination of infected turkey strains.

PUBLIC HEALTH SIGNIFICANCE

There is no evidence that LPDV represents any hazard to humans.

FURTHER READING

Biggs P M 1997 Lymphoproliferative disease of turkeys. In: Calnek B W et al eds. Diseases of poultry, 10th edn. Iowa State University Press, Ames, p 485–489

Coffin J M, Hughes S H, Varmus H E (eds) 1997 Retroviruses. Cold Spring Harbor Laboratory Press, Woodbury

De Boer G F (ed) 1987 Avian leukosis. Martinus Nijhoff, Boston

Fadly A M 2000 Isolation and identification of avian leukosis viruses. Avian Pathol 29: 529–535

Fadly A M, Payne L N 2003 Leukosis/sarcoma group. In: Saif Y M (ed) Diseases of poultry, 11th edn. Iowa State University Press, Ames, p 465–516

Fadly A M, Witter R L 1998 Oncornaviruses: leukosis/sarcoma and reticuloendotheliosis. In: Glisson J R et al, eds. A laboratory manual for the isolation and identification of avian pathogens, 4th edn. American Association of Avian Pathologists, Kennett Square, p 185–196

Kaleta E F, Payne L N, Heffels-Redmann U (eds) 2000 Proceedings of the international symposium on ALV-J and other avian retroviruses. Institut für Geflugelkrankheiten, Giessen

Payne L N, Venugopal K 2000 Neoplastic diseases: Marek's disease, avian leukosis and reticuloendotheliosis. Rev Sci Tech 19: 544–564

Venugopal K 1999 Avian leukosis virus subgroup J: a rapidly evolving group of oncogenic retroviruses. Res Vet Sci 67: 113–119

Witter R L, Fadly A M 2003 Reticuloendotheliosis. In: Y M Saif (ed) Diseases of poultry, 11th edn. Iowa State University Press, Ames, p 517–536

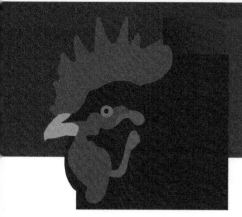

CHAPTER 25

Dennis J. Alexander and
Richard C. Jones

Paramyxoviridae

The family *Paramyxoviridae* is placed in the order *Mononegavirales* with two other families *Rhabdoviridae* and *Filoviridae*. Members of the family *Paramyxoviridae* are enveloped RNA viruses that possess nonsegmented, single-stranded genomes of negative sense. The RNA undergoes capsid assembly in the cytoplasm and envelopment at the surface of infected cells. By negative contrast electron microscopy, particles appear pleomorphic, usually 100–500 nm in diameter if roughly spherical, or about 100 nm across if filamentous.

The family has been divided into two subfamilies: *Paramyxovirinae* and *Pneumovirinae*.

PARAMYXOVIRINAE (NEWCASTLE DISEASE AND OTHER PARAMYXOVIRUSES) (DENNIS J. ALEXANDER)

The subfamily *Paramyxovirinae* is divided into five genera:

- ***Morbillivirus***. The type species is measles virus, the genus includes canine distemper and rinderpest viruses
- ***Respirovirus***. The type species is *Human parainfluenza virus* 1; the genus includes bovine and human parainfluenza 3 and *Sendai virus*
- ***Henipavirus***. Formed from *Nipah virus* and *Hendra virus*
- ***Rubulavirus***. The type species is mumps virus, the genus includes some other mammalian parainfluenza viruses
- ***Avulavirus***. *Newcastle disease virus* (NDV or APMV-1), the type species, and the other avian paramyxoviruses (APMV-2 to APMV-9) are placed in this genus. The name is derived from 'avian *Rubulavirus*' as at one time the avian paramyxoviruses were placed in the same genus as mumps virus.

The members of the *Avulavirus* genus show all the typical properties of their family. They have a herringbone nucleocapsid of about 18 nm in diameter and a pitch of 5 nm. The virus particles have typical projections covering the surface, which are inserted into the envelope. There are two sizes of surface projection, or spike; the longest (about 8 nm) consists of a single glycoprotein

Table 25.1 The avian paramyxoviruses (APMV)

PROTOTYPE VIRUS STRAIN	USUAL NATURAL HOSTS	DISEASE PRODUCED IN POULTRY
APMV-1 (*Newcastle disease virus*)	Numerous	Varies from extremely pathogenic to inapparent, depending on strain and host infected
APMV-2/chicken/California/Yucaipa/56	Turkeys, chickens, passerines	Mild respiratory disease or egg production problems; severe if exacerbation occurs
1. APMV-3*/turkey/Wisconsin/68	Turkeys	Mild respiratory disease but severe egg production problems worsened by exacerbating organisms or environment
2. APMV-3*/parakeet/ Netherlands/449/75	Psittacines, passerines	None known
APMV-4/duck/Hong Kong/D3/75	Ducks, geese	None known
APMV-5/budgerigar/Japan/ Kunitachi/74	Budgerigars and related birds	No infections of poultry reported
APMV-6/duck/Hong Kong/199/77	Ducks, geese, turkeys	Mild respiratory disease and slightly elevated mortality in turkeys; none in ducks or geese
APMV-7/dove/Tennessee/4/75	Pigeons and doves	Mild respiratory disease in turkeys, infection of ostriches reported
APMV-8/goose/Delaware/1053/76	Ducks and geese	No infection of poultry reported
APMV-9/domestic duck/ New York/22/78	Ducks	None known

* Serological tests may distinguish between turkey and psittacine isolates.

(HN) with which both haemagglutination and neuraminidase activities are associated. The smaller spikes are formed by the F glycoprotein, which is associated with the ability of the virus envelope to fuse with cell membranes, allowing insertion of virus genetic material into the host cell, and to cause fusion of infected cells, resulting in the characteristic cytopathic effect of syncytial formation.

NDV was first isolated in 1926 from chickens in Newcastle-upon-Tyne, from which the name was derived, and for 30 years remained the only known avian paramyxovirus. However, since the early 1970s innumerable isolations have been made from avian species of paramyxoviruses serologically distinct from NDV. To date, haemagglutination inhibition (HI), immunodouble diffusion, serum neutralization (SN), neuraminidase inhibition, other serological tests and structural and genetic properties have been used to show nine distinct groups of avian paramyxoviruses. The serotypes have been termed APMV-1 to APMV-9 (APMV-1 being NDV). The method of nomenclature used for influenza A isolates has been adopted for avian paramyxoviruses so that an isolate is named by: (1) serotype, (2) species or type of bird from which it was isolated, (3) geographical location of isolation, (4) reference number or name and (5) year of isolation.

In Table 25.1 the prototype strains of each serotype are listed with the usual natural host and the disease signs seen in affected poultry. With the exception of APMV-6 viruses, which have occasionally been isolated from turkeys, and APMV-7 viruses, which have been isolated from turkeys and ostriches in the USA, disease in poultry has been associated only with viruses of APMV-1, APMV-2 and APMV-3 serotypes and these will be considered in more detail.

NEWCASTLE DISEASE (APMV-1)

EPIDEMIOLOGY

Cause

Newcastle disease is caused by a group of closely related viruses that form the *Avian paramyxovirus* type 1 (APMV-1) serotype. Some serological relationships have been demonstrated between NDV and other paramyxovirus serotypes, the most significant being that with viruses of APMV-3 serotype. For many years NDV strains and isolates were considered to form a serologically homogeneous group and this has been the basis of the vaccination procedures employed prophylactically in most countries. However, more exact serological techniques, most notably the use of mouse monoclonal antibodies, have shown that considerable antigenic variation exists between different strains of NDV. Such differentiation of isolates has been extremely helpful in understanding the epizootiology of NDV. More recently, detailed phylogenetic studies have shown that NDV isolates form at least six and possibly seven or eight distinct genetic lineages; generally these lineages correlate with antigenic groups detected by monoclonal antibodies.

A striking feature of NDV strains and isolates is their ability to cause quite distinct signs and severity of disease, even in the same host species. Based on the disease produced in chickens under laboratory conditions NDVs have been placed in five pathotypes:

- **Viscerotropic velogenic NDVs** cause a highly virulent form of disease in which haemorrhagic lesions are characteristically present in the intestinal tract
- **Neurotropic velogenic NDVs** cause high mortality following respiratory and nervous signs
- **Mesogenic NDVs** cause respiratory and sometimes nervous signs with low mortality
- **Lentogenic respiratory NDVs** cause mild or inapparent respiratory infection
- **Asymptomatic enteric NDVs** cause inapparent enteric infection.

However, such groups should be regarded only as a guide as there is always some degree of overlap and some viruses are not easily placed in a specific pathotype.

Hosts

Over 250 species of bird have been reported to be susceptible to natural or experimental infections of NDV and it seems probable that many more if not all species are susceptible to infection. NDV strains have been shown to infect all the major and minor species of domestic poultry, although some species (e.g. ducks) tend to show few signs of disease even when infected with the strains of NDV most virulent for chickens.

Panzootics

The history of Newcastle disease is marked by at least three panzootics in domestic birds. The first began with the emergence of the disease in fowl in the mid-1920s and spread slowly from the Far East throughout the world, with extremely rapid spread within some countries. The second panzootic appeared to emerge in domestic fowl in the Middle East in the late 1960s and spread much faster than the first, reaching all continents and most countries by 1973. Several authors associated this rapid spread with the movement of infected psittacine birds as a consequence of the international pet bird market. A third panzootic was associated with a mainly neurotropic and enteric disease in pigeons. It too appeared to emerge in the Middle East and between the late 1970s and the mid-1980s spread throughout the world in racing, show, meat and feral pigeons; in some countries spread to other birds and poultry occurred. The viruses responsible for this panzootic could be distinguished from other NDVs by monoclonal antibodies and formed a distinct genetic lineage. For pragmatic purposes this strain of NDV has become known as *Pigeon paramyxovirus* type 1 (PPMV-1).

Spread

The mode of transmission from bird to bird is clearly dependent on the organs in which the virus multiplies. Birds showing respiratory disease presumably shed virus in droplets and aerosols of mucus, which may be inhaled by susceptible birds. Viruses that are mainly restricted to intestinal replication may be transferred by ingestion of contaminated faeces, either directly or in contaminated food or water, or by inhalation of small infective particles produced from dried faeces. Such considerations may drastically affect the rate of spread. Viruses transmitted by the respiratory route in a community of closely situated birds (i.e. in an intensive broiler house) may spread with alarming rapidity. Viruses excreted in the faeces and transmitted chiefly by the oral/faecal route may spread only slowly, especially if birds are not in direct contact (i.e. caged layers).

Assessments of airborne spread of NDV over large distances have produced varied results. During the panzootic of 1970–1973 this type of spread was considered to be of major importance in some countries but of much less significance in others. If airborne spread occurs at all over more than quite short distances it probably requires very specific conditions.

Humans seem to play the central role in the spread of NDV, usually by the movement of live birds, fomites, personnel and poultry products (including dead birds and faeces for fertilizer) from affected premises to susceptible birds.

Feral birds and other wildlife have undoubtedly contributed to the spread of disease during epizootics, either by infection or by mechanical transfer, but their exact role has not been fully evaluated. Virulent NDV does seem to be endemic in cormorants in North/Central America and there has been some suggestion that such birds have been involved in recent outbreaks in Europe.

A carefully documented epizootic in fowl occurring in the UK in 1984 demonstrates the interactions between the methods of spread that may occur. The form of NDV that has been termed PPMV-1 was introduced into the country, probably by stray racing pigeons. The virus proceeded to spread rapidly among UK racing pigeons and from these to feral pigeons. This resulted in the infection of a flock of pigeons living on food stored at a dockyard. Food contaminated with pigeon faeces from these stores was fed untreated to fowls, who subsequently developed disease. There was relatively little secondary spread but where it was seen it was inevitably related to the agency of humans in the movement of personnel, contaminated vehicles and unfumigated eggs.

A key to the successful spread of NDV is the ability of the virus to survive in the dead host or excretions. In infected carcasses NDV may survive for several weeks at cool ambient temperatures or several years if held frozen. Faeces, in which virus may be present in high titres, also represents an excellent medium for the survival of NDV, and even at 37°C infectivity has been reported to be retained for over a month. NDVs are usually regarded as heat labile and readily destroyed by cooking. In one study using meat infected artificially with strain Herts 33, the time required to reduce the virus titre by $1 \log_{10}$ was calculated as 120 s at 65°C, 82 s at 70°C, 40 s at 74°C and 29 s at 80°C, so depending on the starting titre of the virus heating at fairly high temperatures for a number of minutes may be required to reduce the probability of virus survival to an acceptable level.

DIAGNOSIS

Clinical signs

As indicated above in defining pathotypes, the disease produced following infection with NDV may vary considerably with the infecting virus. In addition, the species of bird, the immune status, age and conditions under which they are reared may also greatly affect the disease signs seen, while the presence of other organisms may greatly exacerbate even the mildest forms of disease. As a consequence, no disease signs may be regarded as pathognomonic.

The highly virulent viruses may produce peracute infections of fully susceptible chickens where the first indication of disease is sudden death. Typically, disease signs such as depression, prostration, diarrhoea, oedema of the head and nervous signs may occur, with flock mortality reaching 100%. The appearance of shell-less or soft-shelled eggs, often laid outside the nest boxes, followed by complete cessation of egg laying, may be an early sign in adult fowl.

The moderately virulent, or mesogenic, viruses usually cause severe respiratory disease, followed by nervous signs, with flock mortality up to 50% or more. The variant virus associated with the pigeon panzootic in the 1980s produced no respiratory signs in infected fowl. In these infections diarrhoea and nervous signs were the main presentation of the disease, preceded by catastrophic drops in egg production in laying hens.

The viruses of low virulence may cause no disease, or mild respiratory distress for a short time in chickens and turkeys. However, the presence of other organisms or poor husbandry may cause disease comparable to that seen with more virulent virus. Respiratory disease in broilers at the end of the rearing period, often with significant mortality, has been associated with multiple infections of the respiratory tract with various combinations of avian pneumovirus, infectious bronchitis and vaccine strains of NDV. Even inapparent infections may result in loss of weight gain in broiler chickens and small reductions in egg production.

Lesions

No gross lesions are pathognomonic for any form of Newcastle disease. Viruses producing clinically inapparent infections cause no gross lesions, while the organs affected by other pathotypes relate directly to the disease signs seen.

Viruses causing respiratory disease may induce inflammation of the trachea, often with haemorrhages. The air sacs may also be inflamed and appear cloudy and congested. The virulent viscerotropic viruses usually cause haemorrhagic lesions of the intestinal tract, particularly the proventriculus. These lesions may vary greatly in size and severity.

Microscopic lesions vary considerably and also have little value in the diagnosis of Newcastle disease. The highly virulent viruses cause necrotic lesions, frequently with haemorrhages, in a range of organs of infected chickens. When the respiratory tract is involved, inflammation, cellular infiltration and haemorrhage of the trachea may be seen, sometimes with proliferative and exudative lung lesions. In milder forms lymphocyte infiltration in the air sac walls, lungs and trachea may be seen as clinical signs in the flock diminish. Where nervous signs have been dominant, examinations of the CNS have resulted in reports of neuronal degeneration, perivascular cuffing of lymphocyte cells and proliferation of the endothelial cells.

Virus isolation

Sampling from live birds of any species for virus isolation should consist of both cloacal swabs (or faeces) and tracheal swabs, regardless of the clinical signs. From dead birds, intestines, intestinal contents and tracheas should be sampled, together with organs and tissues obviously affected or associated with the clinical signs (e.g. the brain if nervous signs are present).

Samples should be placed in phosphate-buffered isotonic saline containing antibiotics at pH 7.0–7.4 (checked after the addition of antibiotics), faeces and minced tissues as 10–20% (w/v) suspensions. The exact mixture of antibiotics does not appear to be critical and may be varied to meet local conditions. However, high concentrations are usually necessary, especially for faeces and cloacal swabs. An example is: penicillin 10 000 units/mL, streptomycin 10 mg/mL, gentamicin 250 µg/mL, nystatin 5000 units/mL with 50 µg/mL oxytetracycline when *Chlamydia* infection may be a possibility. Samples should be left at room temperature for 2 h in the antibiotic solution or up to 3 days at 4°C.

NDVs will grow in a large range of cell culture systems, although viruses of low virulence may require the addition of 5 µg/mL trypsin and no serum in the media to facilitate growth. These may be chosen for virus isolation where local conditions preclude the use of specific pathogen-free embryonated fowls' eggs. However, the latter, at 9–10 days of age, are the preferred method for the isolation of NDV. Supernatant obtained after light centrifugation of the samples in antibiotic solution should be inoculated into the allantoic cavity of a minimum of five eggs and held at 37°C until dead or dying, or for 5–7 days. Eggs should be chilled at 4°C and the amnio-allantoic fluid harvested and tested for haemagglutination of chicken red blood cells. Negative fluids should receive at least one more passage through eggs.

Haemagglutination activity in bacteria-free fluids may be due to any of the avian paramyxoviruses or avian influenza viruses. NDV may be confirmed by HI test using specific NDV antiserum. Some isolates of the other avian paramyxovirus serotypes may give low titres with NDV polyclonal antiserum. This is most likely with viruses of APMV-3 serotypes, which are often isolated from birds held in quarantine and occasionally from turkeys. Confusion between these groups of virus can usually be avoided by the use of adequate control sera, especially specific monoclonal antibodies.

Virus characterization

Because of the wide range of pathotypes, the almost universal use of live Newcastle disease vaccines and the effect of exacerbative organisms or environmental conditions on the clinical signs produced by lentogenic viruses, mere isolation and identification of NDV are inadequate for diagnosis and disease control purposes. Further characterization in the laboratory, especially of the virulence for chickens, is therefore necessary.

The molecular basis that controls the virulence of NDV strains is now largely understood and it is possible, using nucleotide sequencing techniques, to assess whether or not an isolate has the genetic make-up to be highly pathogenic in poultry. As discussed above the viral F protein brings about fusion between the virus membrane and the cell membrane so that the virus genome enters the cell and replication can begin. The F protein is therefore essential for replication, but during replication NDV particles are produced with a precursor glycoprotein, F0, which has to be cleaved to F1 and F2 polypeptides that remain bound by disulphide bonds for the virus particles to be infectious. This post-translation cleavage is mediated by host cell proteases.

The cleavability of the F0 molecule has been shown to be related directly to the virulence of viruses in vivo. Studies of the deduced amino acid sequences of the F0 precursor showed that viruses virulent for chickens had the sequence ^{113}R–Q–K/R–R^{116} at the *C*-terminus of the F2 protein and F (phenylalanine) at residue 117, the *N*-terminus of the F1 protein. In contrast the viruses of low virulence had sequences in the same region of ^{113}K/R–Q–G/E–R^{116} and L (leucine) at residue 117. Thus there appeared to be the requirement of a basic amino acid at residue 113, a pair of basic amino acids at 115 and 116 plus a phenylalanine at residue 117 if the virus was to be virulent for chickens. The presence of these basic amino acids at these positions means that cleavage can be effected by a protease or proteases present in a wide range of host tissues and organs but, for lentogenic viruses, cleavage can occur only with proteases recognizing a single arginine (i.e. trypsin-like enzymes). Lentogenic viruses are therefore restricted in the sites where they are able to replicate to areas with trypsin-like enzymes, such as the respiratory and intestinal tracts, whereas virulent viruses can replicate and cause damage in a range of tissues and organs, resulting in a fatal systemic infection.

That the virulence of NDV strains is governed by the F0 cleavage site is sufficiently established that it has been incorporated into the most recent definition of Newcastle disease adopted by the World Organization for Animal Health (OIE):

'Newcastle disease is defined as an infection of birds caused by a virus of avian paramyxovirus serotype 1 (APMV-1) that meets one of the following criteria for virulence:

(a)   The virus has an intracerebral pathogenicity index (ICPI) in day-old chicks (*Gallus gallus*) of 0.7 or greater.

or

(b)   Multiple basic amino acids have been demonstrated in the virus (either directly or by deduction) at the C-terminus of the F2 protein and phenyl-alanine at residue 117, which is the N-terminus of the F1 protein. The term 'multiple basic amino acids' refers to at least three arginine or lysine residues between residues 113 to 116. Failure to demonstrate the characteristic pattern of amino acid residues as described above would require characterization of the isolated virus by an ICPI test.

    In this definition, amino acid residues are numbered from the N-terminus of the amino acid sequence deduced from the nucleotide sequence of the F0 gene, 113–116 corresponds to residues –4 to –1 from the cleavage site.'

It should be noted that an in vivo test has been retained and is necessary to confirm a low-virulence virus. This is to overcome the problems that may be experienced with the sequencing technology if mixtures of virulent and avirulent are isolated. The definition allows confirmation of the presence of virulent virus by sequencing, but an in vivo test is required to give a negative result. The recommended in vivo test is the intracerebral pathogenicity index test in day-old chicks. This involves the inoculation of virus derived from fresh infective allantoic fluid into the brain of 10 1-day-old chicks from specific-pathogen-free parents. Each bird is examined at 24 h intervals for 8 days and scored 0 if normal, 1 if sick and 2 if dead; sick birds that are too ill to eat or drink must be killed humanely and scored as dead at the next observation. The index is the mean score per bird per observation over the 8-day period. The most virulent viruses give ICPI values approaching the maximum score of 2.0, while lentogenic viruses give values of or close to 0.0.

Molecular techniques in diagnosis

There has been increasing use of reverse-transcription polymerase chain reaction (RT-PCR) and other similar techniques to detect NDV in clinical specimens, the advantage being the extremely rapid demonstration of the presence of virus. Oropharyngeal swabs are often used as the specimens of choice because they are easy to process and usually contain little extraneous organic material that can interfere with RNA recovery and amplification by PCR. However, tissue, organ and faeces samples have been used with some success.

Usually, RT-PCR systems have been used to amplify a specific portion of the genome that will recognize all NDV strains and one that will give added value; e.g. amplifying part of the F gene that contains the F0 cleavage site so that the product can be used for assessing virulence. Perhaps the most serious problem in the use of RT-PCR in diagnosis is the necessity for post amplification processing because of the high potential for contamination of the laboratory and cross-contamination of samples. Extreme precautions and strict regimens for handling samples are necessary to prevent this.

More recently, real-time RT-PCR (rRT-PCR) techniques have come into prominence in the diagnosis of Newcastle disease. The rRT-PCR assays are based on fluorogenic hydrolysis probes or fluorescent dyes and eliminate the postamplification processing step that can lead to con-tamination problems with conventional RT-PCR. In addition, results may be obtained rapidly, sometimes in less than 3 h. The most successful application of a rRT-PCR test was in the USA during the Newcastle disease outbreaks of 2002–2003, when the rRT-PCR assay employed showed a sensitivity of 95% compared with virus isolation for more than 1400 specimens. The test used in the USA has three sets of primers and probes that are used in separate reactions: a matrix primer/probe set that is designed to detect most strains of NDV, a fusion primer/probe set that can identify virulent strains of NDV and a primer/probe set designed to detect low viru-lence strains of the virus. Samples are first screened with the matrix primers/probe then positive specimens are tested with the low-virulence and fusion and primers/probe sets to confirm pres-ence of low-virulence or highly virulent virus respectively. In the future it may be possible to carry out all three reactions simultaneously in a single tube.

Phylogenetic studies

Development of improved techniques for nucleotide sequencing and the demonstration that even relatively short sequence lengths could give meaningful results in phylogenetic analyses have led to a considerable increase is such studies in recent years. Considerable genetic diver-sity has been detected but viruses sharing temporal, geographical, antigenic or epidemiological parameters tend to fall into specific lineages or clades and this has proved valuable in assessing both the global epidemiology and local spread of Newcastle disease.

Although in the past phylogenetic studies have been impracticable as a routine tool, the greater availability and increased speed of production of results obtained using sophisticated, commer-cially available kits for RT-PCR and automatic sequencers now means such studies are within the capabilities of many more diagnostic laboratories and can give meaningful results that are con-temporaneous rather that retrospective. It has been proposed that genotyping of NDV isolates should become part of diagnostic virus characterization for reference laboratories by producing a 375-nucleotide sequence of the F gene, which includes the F0 cleavage site, routinely for all viruses and comparing the sequences obtained with other recent isolates and viruses representa-tive of the recognized lineages and sub-lineages. Such analysis should allow rapid epidemiological assessment of the origins and spread of the viruses responsible for Newcastle disease outbreaks.

Serology

A wide range of tests may be used to detect antibodies to NDV in poultry sera and tests based on neutralization or enzyme-linked immunosorbent assay (ELISA) reactions have been used in support of the diagnosis of Newcastle disease. Currently, the HI test is most widely used.

The value of any serological method in the diagnosis of disease is clearly dependent on the expected immune status of the birds involved and is therefore complicated in the case of Newcastle disease by the worldwide use of vaccines.

For most avian sera a positive HI titre may be regarded as 1/16 if 4 haemagglutinin units (HAU) of antigen are used and 1/8 if 8 HAU are used (titres are more usually expressed as the reciprocal of the end-point dilution in several forms of notation, i.e. 8, 2^3, $\log_2 3$). In unvaccinated birds, positive serology and clinical signs may be considered as strong diagnostic evidence of the disease.

HI and other tests may be used to measure the immune status of vaccinated birds. Mean levels expected following vaccination range from 2^4–2^6 after a single live vaccine to 2^9–2^{11} with multi-dose programmes, including oil-emulsion inactivated vaccines. Some authors have attempted to correlate HI titres to NDV with protection against a fall in egg production or disease when stock are challenged with virulent virus. These estimates have been based on laboratory experiments and at best are an oversimplification, as it is impossible to allow for the multifarious exacerbating conditions that may be encountered in the field.

CONTROL

Legislation

Most countries free of Newcastle disease have legislation aimed at preventing the introduction of disease by infected birds or contaminated produce. Such legislation may be extremely complicated and variable as it depends on the disease situation, internal control policies and vaccination status in both the importing and the exporting country.

In view of the association of the spread of the 1970–1973 panzootic in the western hemisphere with the transportation of exotic birds, many countries impose quarantine on such birds on importation, which is aimed specifically at the detection and elimination of birds infected with NDV. Generally the requirement is for isolation for a period of at least 35 days, with close veterinary supervision and virus isolation monitoring for NDV.

The spread of NDV by pigeons during the 1980s resulted in several countries imposing restrictions on such birds, including bans on races from specific areas or compulsory vaccination. Measures enforced in European Union (EU) countries restrict races to pigeons that have been vaccinated.

Legislative powers may also be applied to control disease within a country. Many countries have a slaughter policy for birds with Newcastle disease, with compulsory disposal of all birds and produce on site. Restrictions may also be imposed by law on the movement of poultry and produce within a defined affected area. In some countries 'ring vaccination' may be obligatory following an outbreak, while in other countries prophylactic vaccination of all poultry is required by law.

In recent years the control of Newcastle disease in EU countries has been tackled by a series of legislative directives defining disease, the measures to prevent introduction and spread, and the method of stamping out disease if outbreaks occur. All legislative control measures require careful definition and are inevitably dependent on nationally effective diagnosis, monitoring and enforcement.

Vaccination

Basically, there are three types of commercially available vaccine for Newcastle disease: live lentogenic, live mesogenic and inactivated. Live lentogenic vaccines are usually derived from field viruses that have been shown to have low pathogenicity for poultry but produce an adequate mmune response. Typical vaccine strains are Hitchner B_1 and La Sota – possibly the two most widely used animal vaccines – and F strain and V4. However, these viruses have frequently been subjected to selection pressures by manufacturers in order to improve their immunogenicity or to enable their use by a particular method of application.

Live lentogenic vaccines may be given to birds individually by eye drop or beak dipping but it is usually more practical to use methods of mass application such as in the drinking water or by machines generating sprays or aerosols. Aerosols have particular use during epizootics in the face of quickly spreading disease, as administration of lentogenic vaccine strains in this way may enable rapid vaccination of large numbers of birds and generally the immune response is particularly fast. However, sprays and aerosols, particularly aerosols with small particle size that may penetrate deeply into the respiratory tract, result in reactions that will be most severe in fully susceptible birds. Use of aerosols of La Sota vaccine on such birds may result in heavy mortality.

Mesogenic vaccines such as Roakin, Mukteswar, Komarov and H have usually been derived in the laboratory from fully virulent strains. Their use is generally restricted to countries where there is a problem due to enzootic virulent viruses. Methods of application vary with strain. Some may be given in drinking water while others require intradermal inoculation via the wing web. Mesogenic vaccine viruses are capable of causing severe disease and must only be administered following primary vaccination with lentogenic viruses. Mesogenic vaccines are capable of producing a high secondary immune response and are frequently used in countries in the Middle and Far East; in most Western countries their use is prohibited. Birds infected with mesogenic vaccine viruses would fall within the OIE definition of Newcastle disease.

Inactivated vaccines are usually prepared from egg-grown virus that is killed by treatment with formalin or β-propiolactone. Aqueous inactivated vaccines have been used but in recent years these have been superseded by those based on oil. The immunogenicity of such vaccines may vary considerably with the type and ratios of the components of the vaccine. Both virulent and avirulent viruses have been used as a source of antigen for inactivated vaccines. From a safety aspect, viruses of low virulence would seem the most sensible source of antigen and have the added advantage of usually growing to higher titres in eggs.

Inactivated vaccines must be given individually to birds by intramuscular or subcutaneous injection. Thus, in addition to their higher production costs, they are also much more expensive to administer than live vaccines.

The timing of application and the type of vaccine is extremely important in the efficacy of Newcastle disease vaccination. Many different parameters must be considered in devising vaccination programmes and these include: the disease situation, disease control policies, availability of vaccine, maternal immunity, use of other vaccines, presence of other organisms, size of flock, expected life of the flock, available labour, climatic conditions, economics of vaccination or type of vaccine and past performance of vaccination programmes.

Maternal immunity represents a particular problem in vaccination against Newcastle disease as it may prevent the effectiveness of primary vaccination. To overcome its effect, birds are either left until 3–4 weeks of age before primary vaccination or vaccinated with live virus at 1-day-old by eye drop or coarse spray, to establish infection in some birds that will spread to others as they become susceptible, followed by revaccination at 3–4 weeks of age. Oil-emulsion inactivated vaccines have also been used successfully in 1-day-old, maternally immune chicks.

Except during epizootics of Newcastle disease, vaccination past 3 weeks of age is usually only practised in egg-laying birds. In order to maintain antibody levels, either slightly more virulent live vaccines than the primary vaccines are given at regular intervals or inactivated vaccines are used; the latter may be followed by mild live vaccines at intervals to maintain the immune response.

In many countries, where outbreaks of Newcastle disease are rare, vaccination of broiler chickens is not practised as birds are kept such a short time after protection due to maternal immunity has waned.

In some countries, particularly developing countries, many chickens are reared as scavenging village chickens, which frequently act as reservoirs for NDV. Satisfactory vaccination of such birds represents a considerable challenge. Over recent years the use of a thermostable lentogenic virus that can be presented by coating food has been evaluated. Under field conditions this has met with variable success.

Hygiene and disease security

Under field conditions vaccination alone is insufficient to bring about effective control of Newcastle disease and must be accompanied by good hygiene. In poorly managed, overcrowded, badly ventilated conditions with inevitable underlying bacterial infections even the mildest live vaccine strains may produce disease sufficiently severe to mimic Newcastle disease of high pathogenicity. Good hygiene complemented by good management is therefore of critical importance at all times and not merely during an epizootic of disease.

Hygiene measures should involve both maintaining the birds in a healthy environment and imposing some degree of biosecurity. Ideally, this should begin at the planning stage of developing a commercial poultry farm. Poultry farms and flocks are best sited well away from each other and not in the typical clusters seen in most highly developed countries. Houses and food stores should be bird-proofed to prevent potential spread from feral birds. Some form of security should be imposed on all farms and houses to prevent easy access of humans and fomites. Ideally, vehicles should be thoroughly disinfected on entering and leaving premises. Any movement directly between premises, such as food deliveries, egg collection, dead carcass collection, etc., should be particularly avoided. On some farms, involving highly valuable genetic stock, owners have installed change of clothes and showering facilities for staff entering and leaving the site. Such procedures are highly desirable and should be more widely applied.

When outbreaks of disease do occur, further problems of hygiene arise at a farm level. Where there is no slaughter policy, depopulation should nevertheless be contemplated, especially on sites involving birds of different ages where the continual presence of susceptible birds may result in the perpetuation of the virus despite the use of vaccines.

After depopulation all poultry and products, including faeces, should be disposed of correctly. For countries with a slaughter policy this may involve burial or incineration on site. However, in more and more countries alternatives to these methods of disposal have to be sought to comply with antipollution laws. Trials have shown that carefully regulated and monitored composting of materials, including carcasses, results in the removal of infectious virus provided that sufficiently high temperatures are reached, and in some recent outbreaks in Europe carcasses have been removed to rendering plants for destruction. The latter method has some risks since it involves the movement of infective carcasses off the infected site.

ZOONOSIS

NDV is a human pathogen. Reported infections have been non-life-threatening and usually not debilitating for more than a day or two. The most frequently reported and best substantiated clinical signs in human infections have been eye infections, usually consisting of unilateral or bilateral reddening, excessive lacrimation, oedema of the eyelids, conjunctivitis and subconjunctival haemorrhage. Although the effect on the eye may be quite severe, infections are usually transient and the cornea is not affected.

Reports of other clinical symptoms in humans infected with NDV are less well substantiated but suggest that a more generalized infection may sometimes occur resulting in chills, headaches and fever, with or without conjunctivitis.

There is evidence that both live vaccine and virulent (for poultry) strains of NDV may infect and cause clinical signs in humans.

Human infections with NDV have usually resulted from direct contact with the virus, infected birds or carcasses of diseased birds. There have been no reports of human to human spread, although spread by contagion is theoretically possible. The types of person known to have been infected with NDV include: laboratory workers (usually as a result of accidental splashing of infective material into the eye), veterinarians in diagnostic laboratories (presumably as a result of contact with infective material during post-mortem examinations), workers in broiler processing plants and vaccination crews – especially when live vaccines are given as aerosols or fine dust.

AVIAN PARAMYXOVIRUS TYPE 2 (APMV-2)

EPIDEMIOLOGY

Cause

Viruses of the APMV-2 serotype are also termed 'Yucaipa-like', indicating their close serological relationship with the prototype strain (Table 25.1). These viruses may show wide serological variation in HI tests, and marked lability of the haemagglutination activity of some strains and isolates has been recorded.

Hosts

APMV-2 viruses have been reported to infect both chickens and turkeys. Isolates have also been obtained from a wide variety of feral birds but are most frequently associated with birds of the order Passeriformes. Isolations of APMV-2 viruses are often obtained from exotic birds held in quarantine, where their association with disease is uncertain. The incidence of isolations is much higher from quarantined passerines than psittacines, suggesting that the virus is introduced by these species and spreads to psittacines.

APMV-2 viruses are not known to infect humans, although there has been one report of infected primates.

Geographical distribution

APMV-2 viruses have been reported to infect both chickens and turkeys in the USA, Canada and Israel (although in these countries they show greater prevalence in turkeys), chickens in the former USSR and Japan and turkeys in Italy and France. Recently APMV-2 infections of chickens in the UK have been reported.

Isolations from feral or quarantine birds have been made in countries representing North and South America, Asia, Europe and Africa. The wide distribution of viruses of this serotype is probably related to the migratory nature of some of the species shown to be frequently infected.

Spread

Little is known of the transmission of APMV-2 viruses from bird to bird but the ease of isolation from the respiratory and intestinal tracts of infected birds suggests very similar mechanisms to NDV. However, reports indicate relatively slow spread through a flock and that closely situated flocks do not always become infected.

The prevalence of viruses of this serotype in small birds, which may invade poultry houses, suggests mechanisms by which the virus may be introduced to poultry populations. Introduction as a result of the importation of infected turkeys has been reported.

There is little evidence indicating the mode of secondary spread of APMV-2 viruses but it may be assumed that all the mechanisms by which NDV is disseminated from farm to farm may be similarly involved in the transfer of APMV-2 viruses.

DIAGNOSIS

Clinical signs

In uncomplicated infections, APMV-2 viruses may cause mild respiratory disease and reduced egg production in chickens and turkeys. However, in the presence of exacerbative organisms or environmental stress, the disease signs may be far more serious, with severe respiratory disease, cessation of egg production and even high mortality.

No signs or post-mortem lesions are specific for APMV-2 virus infections.

Virus isolation and identification

Recommended virus isolation procedures in embryonated fowls' eggs are identical to those for NDV. Virus identification requires monospecific antiserum to APMV-2 virus for use in HI tests. It is preferable to use antisera to more than one APMV-2 strain because of occasional marked antigenic variation. APMV-2 viruses show extremely low pathogenicity indices in day-old chicks or 6-week-old chickens.

Serology

Antibodies to APMV-2 viruses may be detected by HI tests. Serological surveys in some countries have indicated the presence of APMV-2 antibodies in flocks which have shown no overt disease.

CONTROL

Many aspects of the introduction and spread of APMV-2 viruses will be controlled by legislation and procedures aimed at the prevention of Newcastle disease. However, the frequent isolation of the virus from small birds indicates the importance of keeping poultry in bird-proofed buildings. When clinical disease has been associated with the presence of APMV-2 virus, control has usually involved antibiotic treatment or medication aimed at the probable exacerbating organisms. On some occasions depopulation has been necessary.

Applications of the hygiene, biosecurity and management procedures outlined for NDV will help in the prevention of secondary spread of APMV-2 viruses.

AVIAN PARAMYXOVIRUS TYPE 3 (APMV-3)

EPIDEMIOLOGY

Cause

Viruses of the APMV-3 serotype have been differentiated into two serological groups that, at present, appear to coincide with the isolation of virus from either psittacines and passerines or turkeys. This distinction is indicated by conventional serology in HI tests but has been more clearly confirmed by the use of mouse monoclonal antibodies. APMV-3 viruses may show serological relationships with NDV (APMV-1) isolates.

Hosts

APMV-3 viruses have been obtained from two sources: domestic turkeys and exotic pet birds held in quarantine. Despite the high prevalence of APMV-3 viruses in turkeys in some countries, there have been no reports of APMV-3 viruses infecting chickens, although their susceptibility has been demonstrated in the laboratory. Occasionally, HI antibodies to APMV-3 viruses have been reported in chickens, but it seems most likely that these are the result of the cross-relationships with NDV in well-vaccinated birds.

In birds held in quarantine the incidence of APMV-3 virus isolations is much higher in psittacine species than passerine species, suggesting the introduction with psittacines with subsequent spread to passerines. In contrast to viruses of APMV-2 serotype there have been no confirmed reports of APMV-3 isolates from feral birds. The assumption is that APMV-3 viruses are enzootic in feral psittacines but there is no evidence to verify this.

APMV-3 viruses have not been reported to infect humans.

Geographical distribution

APMV-3 viruses have been isolated from exotic pet or zoo birds in the Netherlands, the UK, the USA, Belgium, France, Germany and Japan. Isolations from turkeys have been made in the USA, Canada, the UK, France and Germany.

Spread

It has been suggested that the introduction of APMV-3 viruses into the turkey populations of different countries may be due to the importation of infected birds. At present the evidence for this is purely circumstantial.

Little is known of the methods of secondary spread of APMV-3 viruses among the turkey population, although humans and fomites are strongly implicated. Spread from house to house on a single site appears to occur only slowly. Outbreaks of disease in turkeys often recur at an affected premises, despite precautionary measures such as cleaning, disinfecting and delay in restocking.

DIAGNOSIS

Clinical signs

Although APMV-3 viruses have been associated with nervous disease with high mortality in captive psittacines in aviaries, their presence is not always marked by specific disease outbreaks in birds held in quarantine.

In turkeys, viruses of this serotype appear to be responsible for mild respiratory disease and reduction in number and quality of eggs laid. The effect on egg production in turkeys may show considerable variation in severity, depending on the presence of other organisms, environmental factors and the time at which infection occurs. Generally, there is a rapid fall in the number of eggs produced, with a high level of white-shelled eggs. Recovery to normal egg production levels may occur within a few weeks if there is little secondary involvement.

Virus isolation and identification

Procedures for the isolation of APMV-3 viruses in embryonated fowls' eggs are identical to those used for NDV. Although frequently isolated from exotic birds dying in quarantine, attempted isolations from affected turkeys have not always resulted in a high success rate.

Virus identification is by using monospecific antiserum in HI tests. The cross-relationship with NDV (APMV-1) may occasionally cause problems in typing isolates. However, using conventional sera, adequate controls usually resolve any doubts, while monoclonal antibodies may confirm specific typing.

APMV-3 viruses from either turkeys or exotic birds usually have very low pathogenicity indices in day-old chicks or 6-week-old chickens. Some psittacine isolates have shown ICPI values comparable to those reported for mesogenic NDV isolates.

Serology

Antibodies to APMV-3 viruses can be detected in HI tests. High antibody titres may be obtained following the use of inactivated vaccines in turkeys. HI titres to APMV-3 viruses in turkeys vaccinated against NDV have been reported as absent or very low but the possibility of positive APMV-3 titres due to cross-relationship with NDV should not be ignored in the serological diagnosis of APMV-3 infection.

CONTROL

Quarantine measures aimed at the control of NDV are applied in many countries and have resulted in the awareness of APMV-3 viruses in exotic birds. However, little further action is taken in isolation of APMV-3 viruses in any of the countries imposing quarantine and it is not known what actual or potential effect these viruses may have on the health of the pet bird or poultry populations of the countries to which they are introduced.

In turkeys, strict hygiene has been implemented to combat the effects and spread of APMV-3 viruses. In addition, commercially available, oil-emulsion-inactivated vaccines have been used successfully to control egg production problems associated with APMV-3 infections.

FURTHER READING

Aldous E W, Alexander D J 2001 Technical review: detection and differentiation of Newcastle disease virus (avian paramyxovirus type 1). Avian Pathol 30: 117–128

Alexander D J 2001 Newcastle disease – the Gordon Memorial Lecture. Br Poult Sci 42: 5–22

Alexander D J 2003 Newcastle disease, other avian paramyxoviruses and pneumovirus infections: Newcastle disease, other avian paramyxoviruses. In: Saif Y M (ed) Diseases of Poultry, 7th edn. Iowa State University Press, Ames, p 63–92

Alexander D J 2004 Newcastle disease. OIE Manual of standards for diagnostic tests and vaccines, 5th edn. Office International des Épizooties: Paris, p 270–282

Alexander D J, Bell J G, Alders R G 2004 A technology review: Newcastle disease – with special emphasis on its effects on village chickens. FAO Animal Production and Health Paper 161. Food and Agriculture Organization, Rome, p 63. Available on line at: www.fao.org/documents/show_cdr.asp?url_file=/docrep/006/y5162e/y5162e00.htm

Council Directive 92/66/EEC of 14 July 1992 Introducing community measures for the control of Newcastle disease. Offic J Eur Commun 1992; L260: 1–20

PNEUMOVIRINAE (Richard C. JONES)

The subfamily *Pneumovirinae* consists of two genera: *Pneumovirus* – in which the pneumoviruses responsible for infections of mammals are placed, the type species being human respiratory syncytial virus and *Metapneumovirus* – the pneumoviruses infecting avian species, the type species being *Turkey rhinotracheitis virus* (TRTV). The genomic organization of APVs resembles that of mammalian pneumoviruses, including *Bovine respiratory syncytial virus* and *Human respiratory syncytial virus*, but with some distinct differences. In the USA, avian pneumoviruses are referred to as 'avian metapneumoviruses' and disease in the turkey is called 'avian metapneumovirus infection of turkeys'.

Avian pneumoviruses are the cause of turkey rhinotracheitis, a highly contagious respiratory disease of turkeys, which may involve high morbidity and variable mortality. Turkey rhinotracheitis results in significant falls in egg production in breeder turkeys. Avian pneumoviruses also cause respiratory infection in chickens and are reported to cause loss of egg production in breeders and layers. This has frequently been referred to as turkey rhinotracheitis in chickens but is more correctly described as *Avian pneumovirus* (APV) infection of chickens. Often the term avian rhinotracheitis is used for infection in both species. The precise role of APV as a primary pathogen in the chicken is less clear than in the turkey, since experimental infection of chicks with the virus usually produces very mild or asymptomatic disease. However, APV infection has been associated with loss of egg production in layers and breeders and APV vaccines are effective in preventing such losses. Swollen head syndrome is sometimes a consequence of infection of chickens with APV.

Turkey rhinotracheitis was first described in South Africa in the late 1970s and soon appeared in Europe and the Middle East. APV infections in turkeys and chickens are now virtually worldwide in distribution and of considerable economic significance, particularly in the turkey, where it has arguably been the most important disease for more than 20 years. Until 1997, there was no evidence of APV infection in North America, when a virus isolated from outbreaks of respiratory disease among turkeys in Colorado, which later appeared in Minnesota, was shown to be a pneumovirus that had some differences from the strains seen elsewhere. The disease is no longer in Colorado but continues to be a problem in the turkey industry in Minnesota.

EPIDEMIOLOGY

Cause

APV is a pleomorphic, enveloped, RNA virus with an outer envelope bearing fusion (F) and glycoprotein (G) spikes (Fig. 25.1). Originally, it was thought that there was only one type of APV but work in the early 1990s, using monoclonal antibodies and nucleotide sequences of the G protein, showed that there were at least two subtypes, identified as A and B. Originally, type A was found in South Africa and the UK and type B in the rest of Europe. However, it is now recognized that both subtypes are present in the UK, in continental Europe and in most other parts of the world where chickens and turkeys are kept, except for the USA, Canada and Australia. These viruses grow in tracheal organ cultures (TOC), where they cause ciliostasis; they also grow in fertile fowls' eggs inoculated via the yolk sac. They can be adapted to grow in avian cell cultures and cell lines such as Vero cells. Both subtypes have been isolated from and can infect chickens and turkeys. Commercial live and killed vaccines have been produced to both types A and B and while, under experimental conditions, cross-protection offered by each vaccine against the other is generally good, the existence of two types does lead to difficulties in interpretation of ELISA tests, depending on the antigen used (see below).

In 1997, a pneumovirus was confirmed as the cause of respiratory disease of turkeys in the USA, a country believed until then to be free of infection with APV. First encountered in Colorado and then in Minnesota, molecular studies have shown this virus to differ from types A and B, to a similar extent that A and B differ from each other. Initial comparisons of the nucleotide (nt) and predicted amino acid (aa) sequences of the fusion and matrix genes from the Colorado APV showed that it shares 60% nt and 78% aa sequence identity, while the F gene shares 71% nt and 67% aa sequence identity with subtypes A and B respectively. In contrast, subtypes A and B had predicted aa sequence identities of 83–89% for M and F genes. Thus, the US virus, possessing significant genetic identity, was called subtype C (Colorado). It has been suggested that it may be a different serotype. It was originally isolated in Vero cells or chick embryo fibroblasts, is not neutralized by antisera to types A or B, does not induce ciliostasis in TOC, and its antibodies are only detected by ELISAs with homologous antigen.

More recently, French viruses originally isolated from turkeys in the mid-1980s have been shown to be non-A, non-B and not subtype C. These viruses were assigned to subtype D. Another APV isolated from Muscovy ducks in France was shown to be subtype C but of a different genetic lineage from the American subtype. Whether the French C or D subtypes are

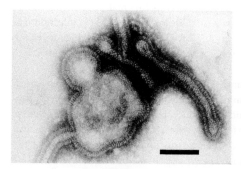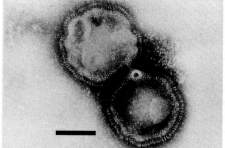

Fig. 25.1 Electron micrograph of negatively stained particles of avian pneumovirus. The virions are pleomorphic and covered with a regular fringe of spikes. Bar = 100nm.

important in disease in Europe has not been reported. However, it seems possible that more subtypes of APV may be detected in due course.

In 2000, the first report of a human metapneumovirus was published and several others followed from other parts of the world. They were isolated from young children suffering from mild to severe respiratory illnesses. Serological studies have shown that these viruses have been circulating in human populations for more than 40 years. Nucleotide and amino acid sequences indicate that the human metapneumovirus is more closely related to APV subtype C than A, B or D.

Most of the descriptions to follow refer to what is known about APV subtypes A and B.

Hosts

APVs have been demonstrated in turkeys, chickens, pheasants, guinea fowl, Pekin ducks and Muscovy ducks and antibodies have been detected in ostriches in Zimbabwe and herring gulls in Germany. In countries with large populations of guinea fowl, they may be important in the epidemiology of respiratory diseases. It is suspected that wild birds may be important in the transmission of APV over large distances. In the USA, several studies have detected APV subtype C infection in wild migratory birds. APV RNA has been detected in the nasal turbinates of wild sparrows, geese, swallows and starlings captured in the north central region and molecular studies have shown them to be very closely related to isolates from turkeys. While these results may suggest that APV can replicate in wild avian species, the precise role of migratory birds in APV epidemiology is unclear. For example, the states surrounding Minnesota and Canada to the immediate north have not reported serious APV outbreaks. Furthermore, while subtypes A and B are present in South and Central America and migratory flight paths extend to the north, neither of these variants has been reported in the USA.

Spread

Following infection of chickens or turkeys, APV is shed from the respiratory tract, primarily the nares and trachea. In experimental infections, virus has sometimes been shown to be shed in the faeces but the importance of this in the field is uncertain. The virus can spread rapidly within a flock, suggesting the importance of droplet and aerosol transmission, although mechanical means are likely to be significant between flocks. While experimental evidence suggests that infected birds shed virus for only a relatively short time (6–8 days) postinfection, following its introduction into a susceptible turkey population, APV infection spreads rapidly and frequently occurs as an explosive epizootic. This was well documented in the UK when, between July and December 1985, almost every turkey flock in England and Wales (but not Scotland) became infected. During the primary wave of infection, turkey flocks of all ages are affected; subsequently, the disease becomes enzootic. Thereafter, successive waves of infection occur, affecting only those farms that have been depleted and restocked with susceptible poults. The frequency of these secondary waves appears to be, at least in part, dependent upon the density of the turkey populations. In high-density areas, most flocks will experience disease between 3 and 10 weeks of age. Conversely, in low-density areas secondary waves may be only rarely encountered.

The somewhat uneven global spread of APV infection remains an enigma. Turkey rhinotracheitis first appeared in South Africa in the late 1970s and then Israel and Europe. It was subsequently reported in many other parts of the world, but not the USA until the first report of a pneumovirus in 1997, which proved to be a different subtype (C) from the familiar subtypes A and B. Whether wild birds can transmit virus between continents in addition to local flocks and whether this is done mechanically or because they are infected is unknown. Australia remains free of infection.

No evidence of prolonged virus persistence could be demonstrated in chickens or turkeys after chemical T-cell immunosuppression, nor using sentinel birds. Although APV has been isolated from very young poults and experiments have shown that there are abundant amounts of virus in the oviduct epithelium of the infected turkey hens, there are no confirmed reports of egg transmission in either turkeys or chickens.

Little work has been done on the survival of APV strains away from the host, although American work with the subtype C virus suggests that it may survive many days in litter. However, these viruses are easily killed by common disinfectants.

Other factors

Exacerbating factors for APV infection are the common ones for respiratory diseases and include high ammonia and dust levels in the atmosphere, overcrowding and intercurrent infections. Infectious agents that have been shown to have a synergistic effect include *Escherichia coli*, *Ornithobacterium rhinotracheale*, *Mycoplasma gallisepticum* and *Chlamydophila*. *Mycoplasma synoviae* does not appear to have an exacerbating effect. In contrast to synergism, when chicks are infected with both APV and *Infectious bronchitis virus* (IBV), IBV limits the replication of APV but still allows a protective response and this has a bearing on vaccine programmes for young chicks (see below). Simultaneous dual vaccination of chicks with live APV and NDV vaccines does not have the adverse effect that IBV vaccines do. Dual infections with immunosuppressive viruses have not been investigated.

E. coli infection is invariably present in swollen head syndrome in broiler chickens, which sometimes follows APV infection. However, APV is not the only virus associated with the condition and reports indicate the involvement of IBV in some outbreaks.

PATHOGENESIS

Susceptible turkeys and chickens become infected via the respiratory tract and virus replication can be demonstrated by immunostaining of the epithelium of the turbinates and the trachea by 2 days postinfection. Infectious virus usually cannot be isolated from these sites for more than 6–8 days and the lungs and air sacs do not usually contain virus. However, intercurrent infection with *E. coli*, *O. rhinotracheale* and other agents may exacerbate and prolong the respiratory disease and permit greater penetration of virus into the lower respiratory tract. Intercurrent infection with *M. gallisepticum* may increase the overall morbidity within a flock.

In mature female turkeys without antibodies, virus has been demonstrated in the epithelium of the oviduct in all regions on days 7–9 postinfection. It is thought that infection here causes a sequence of events leading to loss of egg production and sometimes egg quality (white, thin shells) although without the permanent effects IBV can have on the reproductive tract of the chicken. It is likely that virus reaches the oviduct from the respiratory tract after a viraemic phase. In the chicken, a direct effect of virus on the oviduct has been harder to establish and, although infection adversely affects egg production, it may be mainly due to the stress of infection. Experimentally, loss of production in hens has only been induced after intravenous inoculation of virus. Natural infections have been reported to cause loss of pigment in normally brown eggs.

Infection with APV results in the development of virus-neutralizing and ELISA antibodies in the serum, but these antibodies appear to have little importance in controlling the respiratory disease. When poults were B-cell immunosuppressed by cyclophosphamide and vaccinated at

1 day old, despite their inability to produce circulating antibodies, they were immune to challenge with virulent APV given at 21 days of age, suggesting that cell-mediated immunity is important. Indeed, more recent work has confirmed that cell-mediated immunity helps birds recover from respiratory infection. Circulating antibodies however, play an important role in protecting the oviduct after infection of laying birds and this is the rationale behind the use of killed vaccines following priming with live vaccines.

Maternal antibodies have been shown to be ineffective in the face of early challenge of poults and chicks and they have little adverse influence on early vaccination with live vaccines. Locally produced antibodies appear to be actively involved in protection. Virus-specific IgA and IgG can be detected in the tears of both chicks and poults after infection with virulent APV and the tears have virus-neutralizing activity. However, following infection with an attenuated APV, the turkey reacts much more vigorously than the chicken in terms of lachrymal antibodies, so the local immune responses of the turkey and chicken appear to differ in terms of degree. This may be of importance in relation to vaccine strategies for the two species.

DIAGNOSIS

Signs and lesions

Turkeys

APV infection results in an acute disease of the upper respiratory tract in turkeys from an early age. The condition most commonly affects turkey flocks aged between 3 and 10 weeks and is characterized by rapid onset, with high flock morbidity that frequently approaches 100%. Clinical signs may include depression, change of voice, gasping, moist tracheal rales, snicking, coughing, submandibular oedema, swollen infraorbital sinuses, foamy ocular discharge and excess mucus detectable at the nostrils. In uncomplicated cases recovery is rapid and may be complete in 7–14 days with low or no mortality. However, high mortality rates, often exceeding 50%, have been reported and these are associated with secondary bacterial invasion, particularly by *E. coli*. Mortality rates may also be increased by poor hygiene or ventilation, overstocking and cold, damp weather.

There appears to be wide variation in the severity of clinical signs between birds in a flock and between flocks, and in the morbidity rate. The signs are similar to those outlined for turkey coryza. Rarely, flocks may exhibit no overt signs, yet seroconversion can be detected. Generally, the clinical signs are reduced in flocks older than 10 weeks of age and those housed in open-sided sheds or on free range.

In breeding flocks clinical signs may be less severe and are closely followed by a drop in egg production. Typically the loss is about 50%, but this may vary considerably. Egg production usually returns to normal in 2–4 weeks and the recovery phase is commonly associated with increased numbers of white and thin-shelled eggs. Reduction in hatchability may occur. The effects on egg production are more severe if the flock has rhinotracheitis in the first 2–3 weeks of lay. Prolapse of the oviduct may occur in turkey hens affected in lay as a result of violent coughing.

At necropsy, excess respiratory mucus is found in the nares and trachea, which at first is clear but may become mucopurulent with time, especially where bacteria are involved. In complicated outbreaks typical lesions of colisepticaemia are found in several organs. In affected breeders, the oviducts may contain masses of inspissated albumen and occasionally solid yolk. Oviduct regression may be accompanied by egg peritonitis.

Microscopic changes occur in the mucosa of the nares and trachea between 4 and 10 days after infection. The first abnormality seen is focal loss of the surface ciliary layer at 2 days. By day 4 the loss of cilia is most extensive and the mucosal surface is irregular as a result of extrusion of epithelial cells. Within the epithelium there is vacuolation and occasional cell debris. Subepithelial hyperaemia is also present with intraepithelial heterophils and lymphocytes. Copious inflammatory exudate is observed. These degenerative and inflammatory changes become most marked between days 4 and 10. In the later stages, subepithelial lymphocyte accumulations become conspicuous. Beyond 10 days after infection, recovery occurs and the tracheal epithelium returns to normal. The changes are not pathognomonic.

Chickens

The role of APV as a primary pathogen of the chicken is poorly understood. Strains of virus that cause overt clinical disease in turkeys induce an antibody response in chickens but only mild disease, with a clear nasal exudate, or subclinical infection. In broilers, APV may be one of several agents involved in respiratory disease of multiple aetiology. Experimentally, concurrent infection of chicks with APV and other agents such as *E. coli* or *M. gallisepticum* has been shown to exacerbate and prolong respiratory signs and lesions. In uncomplicated APV infection, microscopic lesions in the respiratory tract are usually less marked than in the turkey. In breeders or commercial layers, APV infection is associated with reduced egg production and loss of shell colour.

Swollen head syndrome, consisting of swelling of the periorbital and infraorbital sinuses with associated torticollis and cerebral disorientation, usually in less than 4% of chickens in a flock, has been associated with earlier APV infection. Swollen head syndrome is not exclusively the result of APV infections and appears to be the consequence of secondary bacterial infection and *E. coli* is invariably involved. It has never been produced experimentally with APV alone and the mechanism of development of swollen head syndrome has never been elucidated. Nonetheless, APV vaccines are effective against the condition. Pneumovirus infections are regarded as a common predisposing factor to secondary adventitious bacterial infections in mammals, most notably respiratory syncytial virus leading to otitis media in children.

Virus isolation/detection

Clinical signs due to APV infection in the turkey and the chicken may resemble those caused by other respiratory agents, so laboratory methods are needed for confirming a diagnosis. The diagnosis of APV infection depends on the demonstration of the virus, by isolation or by RT-PCR or specific serum antibodies by ELISA.

If virus isolation is attempted from clinical specimens, it is essential to obtain fresh material from affected birds in the early stages of the disease. Difficulty may be encountered in isolation since, by the time clinical signs are evident, infectious virus may be very difficult to isolate. Upper respiratory tract material is preferred to that from the trachea. Ocular, nasal or tracheal exudate or swabs bearing this material are agitated with antibiotic broth and inoculated into TOC which are examined for up to 11 days for evidence of ciliostasis. A further one or two passages may be necessary if the samples are negative on first passage. Virus identity needs to be confirmed by immunofluorescence staining of infected TOC, by an SN test in TOC using an anti-APV serum or by RT-PCR. An alternative to TOC is to use fertile eggs after 6 days of incubation, inoculated via the yolk sac. APV infection causes haemorrhages on the embryos with some mortalities, usually after two or three passages. Egg-passaged material will then induce syncytial-type cytopathic effect in tissue culture of chick embryo origin. However, for primary isolation of types A and B virus, tissue cultures of turkey or chick origin or mammalian cell lines are usually considered to be of little value, although cell cultures were used successfully for isolation of the US subtype C virus which is not ciliostatic in TOC. Virus isolation is expensive and time-consuming. An alternative to isolation is the use of sentinel birds, which also has these disadvantages. Immunofluorescence (fluorescent antibody) staining of tracheal epithelial smears or frozen sections is a rapid way of detecting virus but only of value in the early stages after infection.

Molecular methods have been developed for detecting APV in clinical material. RT-PCR with appropriate primers is capable of distinguishing between subtypes A, B and C. This methodology has the advantages of high specificity and speed and can detect vestiges of viral nucleic acid in clinical samples when complete infectious virus can no longer be isolated. Because of these features, RT-PCR is now widely used in most diagnostic laboratories. The recommended protocol is to take dry swabs from the oropharynx and choanal cleft, usually at least 10 from each flock. These swabs can be transported at ambient temperature without significant loss of ability to detect viral nucleic acid by RT-PCR. However, it is worth remembering that the molecular method does not provide the live virus, so, if it is needed for further studies, then isolation will need to be done as well.

Serology

Serum antibodies may be detected by indirect immunofluorescence, serum neutralization tests or ELISA. The latter is the method of choice for large-scale flock testing. Several commercial ELISAs are available for subtypes A and B viruses but discrepancies have arisen because of apparent false negatives, since ELISAs using plates coated with heterologous antigen subtype may be less sensitive for detecting antibodies to the homologous subtype. When birds have been vaccinated with one type and challenged with the other, or perhaps both, interpretation of tests may be difficult. In order to obviate this problem, new approaches to expressing the viral proteins essential for ELISA testing are being developed to provide subtype specific or bi- or trivalent tests. Normally, antibodies to the US type C virus can only be detected with an ELISA using the homologous antigen.

While detection of antibodies to APV is valuable in indicating the presence of field infection in a flock and assessing vaccinal 'takes', it must be remembered that failure to detect antibodies after vaccination does not necessarily indicate lack of immunity.

CONTROL

There is no treatment for APV infection. Application of antimicrobials to treat secondary bacterial infections may have some success, especially on multiage sites. However, the main approach to control has been through the use of vaccines.

Live attenuated and inactivated oil-adjuvanted vaccines are available and generally give good protection, provided that they are given carefully, so that each bird receives the appropriate dose. The live vaccines are used to protect against disease in growing turkeys and broilers and are effective in the face of maternal antibodies. Turkeys are usually vaccinated at 1 day old by spray, but broiler vaccination may be delayed by about 1 week, since there is evidence that simultaneous vaccination with live IBV vaccine at 1 day old impairs the response to APV vaccines. This is unlikely to occur with NDV vaccines. Sometimes turkeys are revaccinated during rearing by spray or in the drinking water, although the latter method is less effective. Although it has been shown that live vaccines developed from subtypes A and B protect against challenge with the heterologous virus, vaccines of both types are frequently used for the same flock and are sometimes given alternately or simultaneously with half or full doses of each.

Live vaccines also act in priming future layers and breeders before application of inactivated vaccines. Both chickens and turkeys can be protected against loss of egg production and quality by the use of live priming and killed vaccines before laying begins. Killed vaccines may be given alone or in combination with other killed preparations.

Immunity to APV infection of the respiratory tract is not dependent on circulating antibodies and birds that are negative by ELISA may still be protected.

From time to time, flocks may experience apparent vaccine failure after APV vaccines. It has been shown experimentally that multiple bird-to-bird passage of attenuated APV virus in nonimmune birds can result in exaltation to a virulent form. For this reason, it is important to ensure that all birds receive a full dose of vaccine so that they all have the chance to develop full immunity. In order to eliminate the adverse effects of reversion, several novel approaches to APV vaccines are being investigated, such as vector vaccines and infectious clone 'reverse genetics' vaccines.

ZOONOTIC IMPLICATIONS

Although the human pneumovirus is more closely related to APV subtype C than to subtypes A, B or D, they are different viruses and there is no evidence that the avian viruses can infect humans.

FURTHER READING

Cook J KA 2000 Avian rhinotracheitis. In: Beard C W, McNulty M S (eds) Disease of poultry: world trade and public health implications. Rev Sci Tech19: 602–613

Cook J K A, Huggins M B, Orbell S J et al 1999 Preliminary antigenic characterisation of an avian pneumovirus isolated from commercial turkeys in Colorado, USA. Avian Pathol 28: 607–618

Gough R E 2003 Newcastle disease, other avian paramyxoviruses and pneumovirus infections: avian pneumoviruses. In: Saif Y M (ed) Diseases of Poultry, 7th edn. Iowa State University Press, Ames, p 92–101

Jones R C 1996 Avian pneumovirus infections: questions still unanswered. Avian Pathol 25: 639–648

Njenga M K, Lwamba H M, Seal B S 2003 Metapneumoviruses in birds and humans. Virus Res 91: 163–169

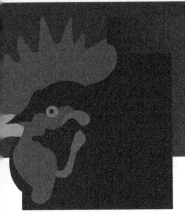

CHAPTER 26

Dennis J. Alexander

Orthomyxoviridae – avian influenza

Viruses forming the family *Orthomyxoviridae* are enveloped RNA viruses with single-stranded genomes of negative sense (i.e. the virus RNA is complementary to the messenger RNA) that are divided into eight segments. Proteins are associated with the RNA genome to form the nucleoprotein–RNA–polymerase complex. The matrix protein surrounding the genome complex is enveloped in a lipid membrane covered by two different surface projection glycoproteins with which haemagglutination and neuraminidase activities are associated separately. The haemagglutinin is responsible for attachment of the virus to cell receptors and eventually for the fusion of the virus and cell membranes, allowing the virus genome to enter the cell and replication to take place. Six of the segments of the virus genome are single genes coding for a single structural protein or precursor protein. The two matrix protein genes are on one segment, as are the two nonstructural proteins. This segmentation is an important property of these viruses as it allows reassortment of genes to occur if two viruses infect and replicate in the same cell.

By negative contrast electron microscopy, orthomyxoviruses appear as roughly spherical or filamentous particles 80–120 nm in diameter or cross-section.

At present the *Orthomyxoviridae* family consists of five genera: *Influenzavirus A*, *Influenzavirus B*, *Influenzavirus C*, *Thogotovirus*, tickborne viruses that occasionally infect mammals, and *Isavirus,* the virus responsible for infectious salmon anaemia. Only viruses of the *Influenzavirus A* genus are known to infect poultry.

EPIDEMIOLOGY

Cause

A disease capable of causing extremely high mortality among infected fowl was first differentiated from other diseases in 1878 and became known as 'fowl plague'. The causative organism of this disease was shown to be a virus as early as 1901 but it was not until 1955 that the relationship with mammalian influenza A viruses (first isolated in the 1930s) was demonstrated. This finding led to the recognition that other isolates from birds, which were serologically distinguishable from the 'fowl plague' viruses and usually caused only mild disease, were also influenza A viruses. Furthermore, it was shown that influenza A viruses capable of causing the virulent form of the disease in chickens could be of at least two subtypes of influenza A and that viruses of low virulence could be antigenically indistinguishable from those of high virulence. This resulted in some problems of definition, since 'fowl plague' viruses had been considered to be of a specific serological subtype. As a result, the term 'highly pathogenic avian influenza' (HPAI) was adopted to apply to viruses capable of causing the severe disease (i.e. fowl-plague-like disease) in poultry regardless of their subtype and the term low pathogenic avian influenza (LPAI) to other viruses.

To date, only influenza A viruses have been isolated from birds. Viruses are placed in genera or types A, B or C on the basis of the nucleocapsid or matrix antigens, which are common for all viruses of the same type/genus. Influenza A viruses are subtyped on the basis of the haemagglutinin (H) or neuraminidase (N) antigens; it is these antigens that are important in protective immunity and show the greatest variation. At present there are 16 recognized H subtypes and nine N subtypes. Each virus possesses one H and one N subtype and most of the possible combinations have been isolated from avian species.

There are strict rules for naming influenza isolates. The name should show: (1) antigenic type; (2) host of origin; (3) geographical location; (4) strain reference number; (5) year of isolation; and (6) for type A viruses the H and N subtypes, e.g. A/turkey/England/199/79 (H7N7).

Because of the marked difference of the disease in susceptible poultry caused by avian influenza (AI) viruses depending on the virulence of the virus strain (see Clinical signs, below) it is necessary to make clear definitions of the different viruses for trade and control purposes. This is further complicated by the fact that the virulent viruses appear to arise by mutation of LPAI viruses of H5 and H7 subtype and that this occurs in poultry. In some instances the mutation from LPAI to HPAI appears to have occurred very quickly after introduction into poultry but on other occasions the low virulence virus of H5 or H7 subtype has circulated for some time before the mutation has taken place. In recent years the consensus among those concerned with the control of avian influenza and international trade in poultry products has been that to avoid the emergence of HPAI there should be control measures aimed at LPAI viruses of H5 and H7 subtypes. The World Organization for Animal Health (OIE) has addressed this in the 2005 Terrestrial Animal Health Code with the following definitions:

> For the purposes of this Terrestrial Code, avian influenza in its notifiable form (NAI) is defined as an infection of poultry caused by any influenza A virus of the H5 or H7 subtypes or by any AI virus with an intravenous pathogenicity index (IVPI) greater than 1.2 (or as an alternative at least 75% mortality) as described below. NAI viruses can be divided into highly pathogenic notifiable avian influenza (HPNAI) and low pathogenicity notifiable avian influenza (LPNAI):
>
> (a) HPNAI viruses have an IVPI in 6-week-old chickens greater than 1.2 or, as an alternative, cause at least 75% mortality in 4- to 8-week-old chickens infected intravenously. H5 and H7 viruses which do not have an IVPI of greater than 1.2 or cause less than 75% mortality in an intravenous lethality test should be sequenced to determine whether multiple basic amino acids are present at the cleavage site of the precursor haemagglutinin molecule (HA0); if the amino acid motif is similar to that observed for other HPNAI isolates, the isolate being tested should be considered as HPNAI.
>
> (b) LPNAI are all influenza A viruses of H5 and H7 subtype that are not HPNAI viruses.

The term LPAI is then used to define all infections caused by AI viruses that are not NAI viruses. The revision of the definition of avian influenza has resulted in modified trade requirements, as these now also apply for LPAI of H5 and H7 subtypes, i.e. LPNAI viruses.

Hosts

Not until the 1970s was it realized that vast pools of influenza A viruses exist in the feral bird population; since then this aspect of the ecology of influenza viruses has received considerable attention. Surveys of wild birds have resulted in the isolation of viruses from species representing all the major avian families throughout the world. However, the frequency and number of isolations from other species has been overshadowed by the presence of these viruses in waterfowl, especially ducks. Analysis of the various published reports of surveillance studies indicates an overall isolation rate of about 11% from sampled birds. However, that isolation rate fell to about 2% if ducks and geese were excluded, and within the Order Anseriformes the large majority of viruses were isolated from birds of the genus *Anas*, particularly mallard ducks (*Anas platyrhynchos*). Isolation rates for ducks congregating on lakes prior to migration have been very high, usually in the range of 20–60%, although somewhat lower further along migratory routes. Nevertheless, this indicates the potential for the spread of influenza viruses throughout the world by migratory birds. Despite the predominance of AI viruses in waterfowl, studies suggest that waterfowl do not act as a reservoir for all avian influenza viruses. It seems likely that part of the influenza gene pool is maintained in shorebirds and gulls, from which the predominant number of isolated influenza viruses are of different subtypes from those isolated from ducks.

In domestic poultry there is good evidence that the highly pathogenic disease was widespread in Europe at the end of the 19th and beginning of the 20th centuries. During the 1920s disease was also reported in the USA, Africa and the Far East. By 1959 reports of the disease were extremely rare but in that year chickens in Scotland showed classical signs of 'fowl plague' and were shown to be infected with a virus of H5 subtype; until that time all HPAI viruses had been of H7 subtype. The viruses responsible for the reported outbreaks of HPAI in domestic poultry since 1959 are listed in Table 26.1. It should be noted that, so far, all have been of H5 or H7 subtype.

Prior to 1955, infections of poultry with influenza viruses of low pathogenicity appear to have gone largely unreported or unrecognized, although a few isolates, such as A/chicken/Germany/N/49 (H10N7), were available and were identified as influenza viruses some years after isolation. In more recent years, such viruses have been reported from most countries with developed poultry industries as occasionally infecting chickens and turkeys. Commercial ducks have also frequently been shown to be infected with influenza viruses but this has rarely been associated with disease because of the marked clinical resistance these birds show, even to strains that are highly virulent for chickens and turkeys. Most of the minor poultry species have been shown to be susceptible to infection with influenza virus and isolations of virus have been reported from Muscovy ducks, geese, quail, guinea fowl, chukars, partridges, pheasants, ostriches and other ratites. The susceptibility of pigeons (*Columba livia*) remains unclear. Historically, pigeons have been considered to be resistant to all types of AI virus and, in experiments, attempted infections of pigeons have usually failed even with HPAI viruses. However, there have been several reports of Asian HPAI H5N1 isolates obtained from pigeons.

Spread

Influenza viruses replicate in the respiratory and intestinal tracts of infected birds and bird-to-bird transmission would appear to occur through virus in droplets or aerosols from the respiratory

Table 26.1 Reported highly pathogenic avian influenza (HPAI) isolates obtained from primary outbreaks in poultry* since 1959

	HPAI VIRUS	SUBTYPE	APPROXIMATE NUMBERS OF POULTRY INVOLVED	AMINO ACIDS AT THE HA0 CLEAVAGE SITE (/ = POINT OF CLEAVAGE)
1	A/chicken/Scotland/59	(H5N1)	One small farm	PQRKKR/GLF
2	A/turkey/England/63	(H7N3)	29 000	PETPKRRRR/GLF
3	A/turkey/Ontario/7732/66	(H5N9)	8000	PQRRKKR/GLF
4	A/chicken/Victoria/76	(H7N7)	58 000	PEIPKKREKR/GLF
5	A/chicken/Germany/79	(H7N7)	1 200 000 chickens	PEIPKKKGR/GLF
6	A/turkey/England/199/79	(H7N7)	80 geese	PEIPKRKGR/GLF§
7	A/chicken/Pennsylvania/1370/83	(H5N2)	9000	PEIPKKKRKR/GLF§
8	A/turkey/Ireland/1378/83	(H5N8)	17 000 000	PQKKKR/GLF
9	A/chicken/Victoria/85	(H7N7)	307 000, mostly ducks	PQRRKKR/GLF
10	A/turkey/England/50–92/91	(H5N1)	240 000	PEIPKKREKR/GLF
11	A/chicken/Victoria/1/92	(H7N3)	8000	PQRKRKTR/GLF
12	A/chicken/Queensland/667–6/94	(H7N3)	18 000	PEIPKKKKR/GLF
13	A/chicken/Mexico/8623–607/94	(H5N2)	22 000	PEIPRKRKR/GLF
14	A/chicken/Pakistan/447/94	(H7N3)	Unknown – millions?	PQRKRKTR/GLF§
15	A/chicken/NSW/97	(H7N4)	>6 000 000	PETPKRRKR/GLF
16	A/chicken/Hong Kong/97†	(H5N1)	160 000	PEIPKRRKR/GLF
17	A/chicken/Italy/330/97	(H5N2)	3 000 000	PQRRRRKKR/GLF
18	A/turkey/Italy/99	(H7N1)	8000	PQRRKKR/GLF
19	A/chicken/Chile/2002	(H7N3)	14 000 000	PEIPKGSRVRR/GLF
20	A/chicken/Netherlands/2003	(H7N7)	≈700 000	PEKPKTCSPLSRCRETR/GLF§
21	A/chicken/Eurasia&Africa†/2003–6	(H5N1)	>25 000 000	PEIPKRRR/GLF
22	A/chicken/Texas/2004	(H5N2)	Unknown – 100s of millions	PQRERRRKKR/GLF§
23	A/chicken/Canada-BC/2004	(H7N3)	6600	PQRKKR/GLF
24	A/ostrich/S. Africa/2004	(H5N2)	16 000 000	PENPKQAYRKRMTR/GLF
25	A/chicken/S. Korea/2005	(H5N2)	30 000	PQREKRKKR/GLF
		(H7N7)	219 000	PEIPKGRHRRPKR/GLF

tract or through faeces, either directly or in contaminated water or food. In view of the relatively slow and inefficient spread observed in both natural and experimental infections when individual birds are not in very close contact, especially with HPAI viruses, the faecal–oral route may be the main route of spread. There is little evidence that airborne spread occurs over long distances.

Until recently it appeared that the epidemiology of AI consisted of the perpetuation of LPAI viruses of all H subtypes in wild birds, where they caused little or no disease, with spread from time to time to poultry. Very occasionally introductions of LPAI viruses of H5 or H7 subtype into poultry resulted in the mutation of these viruses to virulent viruses that caused HPAI. In the large majority of HPAI outbreaks (i.e. excluding the Asian H5N1 HPAI virus) HPAI viruses had rarely been isolated from free-living birds and when they had been isolated it was usually in the vicinity of outbreaks of HPAI in poultry or geographically and chronologically close to known outbreaks in poultry. The one exception, prior to the Asian H5N1 virus, was an outbreak in terns in South Africa in 1961 caused by H5N3 HPAI virus with no apparent poultry connection.

The degree to which LPAI or HPAI viruses spread in poultry appeared to be considerably variable and depended on the levels of biosecurity and concentration of poultry in the vicinity of the initial outbreaks or the emergence of HPAI virus. However, events during the late 1990s and especially after 2003 have completely changed our concepts of AI epidemiology and the spread of LPAI virus of H9N2 subtype and HPAI virus of H5N1 subtype need separate consideration from the general situation.

General situation

All available evidence suggests that normally the primary introduction of LPAI viruses into a poultry population is a result of wild bird activity, usually waterfowl but gulls and shorebirds have also been implicated. This may not necessarily involve direct contact, as infected waterfowl may take the viruses to an area and these may then be introduced to poultry by humans, other types of birds or other animals, which do not need to be infected but may transfer the virus mechanically in infective faeces from the waterfowl. Surface water used for drinking water may also be contaminated with influenza viruses and a source of infection. There is much evidence implicating waterfowl in the vast majority of primary LPAI outbreaks and in summary this is as follows:

- There is a much higher prevalence of infection of poultry on migratory waterfowl routes
- There is a higher prevalence of infection of poultry kept in exposed conditions (e.g. turkeys on range, ducks on fattening fields) and, conversely, where there have been regular LPAI infections and change to a policy of confinement has been pursued LPAI problems largely disappear
- Surveillance studies in areas with LPAI problems in poultry have shown the same variation in virus subtypes in sampled waterfowl and turkey outbreaks
- Influenza outbreaks show a seasonal occurrence in high-risk areas, which coincides with migratory activity
- In most documented specific outbreaks evidence has been obtained of probable waterfowl contact at the initial site.

Although waterfowl and other wild birds appear to be responsible, albeit indirectly, for most influenza introductions to domestic poultry, other possibilities should not be ruled out. For example, it seems highly likely that H1N1 viruses may pass readily between pigs, humans and turkeys and the introduction of viruses of this subtype to turkey flocks from infected pigs has been well documented.

In most recorded outbreaks of influenza virus infections of poultry, secondary spread has been considered to be primarily by the agency of humans, generally by the transference of live birds or infective faeces from infected to uninfected flocks. In many developed poultry industries most collections and deliveries are done on a contractor basis, resulting in considerable numbers of different people and equipment travelling from one farm to another. Obviously, such traffic particularly lends itself to the efficient spread of the virus.

Until the 1990s infections with LPAI viruses, even where outbreaks in poultry occurred regularly, were usually thought to have usually occurred as fresh introductions, sometimes remaining present in the poultry in some areas for some time causing extended outbreaks, but were not considered to be endemic in any poultry compartment throughout the world. Since such viruses have not been the subject of notification and control aimed at eradication it was not clear why they had not become more ubiquitous and endemic in poultry across large geographical areas as had other viruses such as avian pneumoviruses or avian infectious bronchitis viruses. However, since the mid-90s it has become clear that this situation has changed. In addition to the problems seen with viruses of H9N2 and H5N1 subtypes described in the next two sections, there have been other areas where virus appears to have become established in poultry. In the USA, for example, LPAI of H7N2 subtype appears to have been maintained in live bird markets and a number of outbreaks in conventional commercial poultry have been traced to these markets. In Mexico LPAI viruses of H5N2 have continued to be isolated from poultry since their emergence in 1994 and despite the widespread use of vaccines.

It also appears that when HPAI viruses have emerged secondary spread has been far more significant in recent years than in the past. In the first 12 outbreaks since 1959 there was relatively little spread from the farm where the virus was first detected, except in Pennsylvania in 1983/84 when there were 448 outbreaks and 17 000 000 birds died or were slaughtered. In contrast, since 1994 there has been significant spread to numerous sites, resulting in huge economic losses in Mexico in 1994, Pakistan in 1994, Hong Kong in 1997, Italy in 1999/2000, the Netherlands in 2003 and Canada in 2004 (Table 26.1). Even these massive outbreaks have been dwarfed by the Asian HPAI H5N1 outbreaks discussed below.

LPAI H9N2 virus

Infections of poultry, mainly chickens, with LPAI viruses of H9N2 seem to have become geographically widespread and in some areas endemic. In the mid-1990s outbreaks in poultry due to H9N2 AI viruses occurred in Germany, Italy, Ireland, South Africa, USA, Korea and China. Since 2000, H9N2 infections of poultry have been reported in countries across from the Middle East to east Asia (Israel, United Arab Emirates, Saudi Arabia, Jordan, Kuwait, Lebanon, Libya, Iraq, Iran, Pakistan, China and Korea), often causing widespread and persistent outbreaks in commercial poultry. Several of these countries have implemented wide-scale vaccination programmes against the H9N2 virus.

Asian HPAI H5N1 virus

The emergence of HPAI H5N1 virus in south-east Asia and its spread across Asia and into Europe has also presented wholly new concepts in the epidemiology of AI. The apparent progenitor virus for the subsequent outbreaks of HPNAI of H5N1 subtype was obtained from an infection of geese in Guandong province PR China in 1996. In some reports it has been considered that the virus continued to circulate in southern China, primarily in domestic ducks and showing some genetic variation. This apparently low-level, but probably endemic, situation changed dramatically in December 2003 to February 2004 when suddenly eight countries in E and SE Asia reported outbreaks of HPNAI due to H5N1 virus. Although there seemed to be some success in controlling the outbreaks in some countries, it appeared to re-emerge in a second wave in July 2004 onwards. Malaysia reported an outbreak in poultry in August 2004 and became the ninth country in the region to be affected. The virus appeared to affect all sectors of the poultry populations in most of these countries, but its presence in free-range commercial ducks, village poultry and fighting cocks seemed especially significant in the spread of the virus.

If HPAI virus becomes widespread in poultry, especially in domestic ducks that are reared on free range, spillover into wild bird populations is inevitable. In the past such infections have been restricted to wild birds found dead in the vicinity of infected poultry, but there has always been concern that infections of wild birds in which HPAI virus caused minimal or no clinical signs (e.g. ducks) could result in spread of the virus over large areas and long distances. Outbreaks affecting many wild bird species at two waterfowl parks in Hong Kong were recorded in 2002 and further, possibly more significant, outbreaks in wild migratory birds were reported in China and Mongolia in 2005. In particular it was suggested that presence of virus in migratory birds at Lake Qinghai in Western China could be the means by which the H5N1 virus could spread west and south.

There is no good evidence that wild birds were responsible for the introduction into Russia but HPAI H5N1 virus genetically closely related to isolates obtained at Lake Qinghai reached poultry there in the summer of 2005. Whether spread from there to other western Asian and some eastern European countries occurred or whether virus was introduced independently is not clear; neither is it clear whether spread was associated with movements of poultry or wild birds – possibly both were involved – but during 2005 and the beginning of 2006 genetically closely related H5N1 viruses appeared in a number of countries in the region.

Reports of HPAI H5N1 virus infections continued in the first 3 months of 2006 and by early April 2006 31 countries from Asia, Europe and Africa had reported HPNAI caused by H5N1 virus to the World Organization for Animal Health (OIE) since the end of 2003 (Table 26.1).

Two isolated incursions of HPAI H5N1 virus into Europe occurred in 2004 and 2005 and are good examples of the influence of humans in the potential spread of AI viruses. The first was detected when eagles smuggled from Thailand and confiscated at Brussels Airport, Belgium were shown to be infected with H5N1 virus genetically similar to those isolated in Thailand. The second was when investigations of deaths in captive caged birds held in quarantine in England, ostensibly from Taiwan, showed them to have resulted from HPAI H5N1 infection. In this case the virus was genetically closest to viruses isolated in China.

Isolates from dead swans were obtained in Croatia in October 2005. These infected swans were a forerunner of the apparent importance of these birds in the spread of HPAI H5N1 and during January to April 2006 wild mute swans or other wild birds were shown to be infected in Azerbaijan, Iran, Kazakhstan, Georgia and 20 European countries. What appears to have occurred was that mute swans, or other birds, overwintering on the Black Sea became infected at a time when adverse weather conditions made the Black Sea inhospitable and the birds dispersed to other areas. However, this would not explain the appearance of ostensibly the same H5N1 strain in swans and wild birds on the Baltic Coast at the same time.

The spillover and circulation of H5N1 in wild birds represents the first occurrence in recorded history of such an event. The virus has infected over 50 wild bird species that represent a broad taxonomic and genetic spectrum and in which HPAI infections are likely to have quite different consequences and epidemiology. At the time of writing it is impossible to make any forecasts or speculations on the impact of such occurrence on AI ecology and epidemiology.

DIAGNOSIS

Clinical signs

The clinical signs of avian influenza are influenced by the following factors: the strain of virus, the species and age of host; the immune status of the host against the virus, the presence of other exacerbating infections, deficiency conditions and environmental factors (such as excess ammonia and dust). The disease caused by different viruses varies in severity from high mortality, with sudden deaths preceded by few or no clinical signs, to a very mild form or even inapparent infection.

Often the first sign of HPAI in chickens or turkeys is the sudden onset of high flock mortality, which may approach 100% within a few days. Clinical signs, which may be associated with high mortality, are cessation of egg laying, respiratory signs, rales, excessive lacrimation, sinusitis, oedema of the head and face, subcutaneous haemorrhage with cyanosis of the skin, particularly of the head and wattles, diarrhoea and occasionally nervous signs. Usually these signs are most marked in birds that take some time to die.

The less virulent viruses may also cause considerable disease. In uncomplicated infections these influenza viruses may cause drops in egg production, respiratory disease, anorexia, depression, sinusitis and low but elevated mortality. When other organisms such as pneumoviruses, *Newcastle disease virus* (NDV) or other avian paramyxoviruses, *Escherichia coli*, *Pasteurella* sp. or *Mycoplasma* are also present and exert an exacerbative effect, or the birds are under stress due to adverse environmental conditions, mortality may rise to as high as 60–70% of the flock, even higher in young turkey poults, and clinical signs show a marked increase in severity.

Ducks tend to be refractory, even to the viruses that are highly pathogenic for chickens, although they may be carriers. In complicated infections, sinusitis, blepharitis, respiratory distress and increased mortality may be seen. There have been varying reports of the virulence of the Asian HPAI H5N1 virus for commercial ducks. It appears that some strains of this virus, but not others, may cause severe disease and mortality in ducks.

Influenza viruses of both low and high virulence for chickens have produced disease problems in ostriches. There appears to be a big variation in the seriousness of disease with the age of the ostriches and it seems likely that they are not fully susceptible to HPAI.

Clinical signs may arouse considerable suspicion but are not reliable in diagnosis, for which demonstration of virus or specific antibody is required.

Lesions

The gross lesions observed generally reflect the clinical signs and are therefore equally varied and unhelpful in diagnosis. In the most severe cases, birds show various congestive and haemorrhagic lesions on the skin, liver, spleen, heart, kidneys and lungs. However, in birds that died suddenly these are usually absent. Infections with influenza viruses of low virulence are usually associated with lesions of the respiratory tract, most notably sinusitis, sometimes with mucopurulent to caseous exudates. Gross kidney lesions have also been associated with infections of chickens with influenza viruses of low virulence. Pancreatitis has been reported in birds infected with influenza viruses of both high and low virulence.

Detailed histological studies with HPAI virus infections have failed to demonstrate any pathognomonic lesions and different results, particularly of the organs involved, have been obtained with viruses of different virulence. In general, highly pathogenic infections result in oedema, hyperaemia, haemorrhage and degenerative necrotic foci in the visceral organs.

Myocardial necrosis and myocarditis are often noticeable features of some virulent virus infections. Some viruses have shown marked central nervous involvement and, with these infections, widespread perivascular cuffing and necrosis of the neuronal cells are often seen; less frequently, oedema and haemorrhage in the nervous tissue may be evident.

Virus isolation

Samples taken from dead birds for virus isolation should include faeces or intestinal contents and trachea. In addition, organs such as lungs, air sacs, intestine, spleen, brain, liver and heart may be processed separately or as an organ pool. From live birds, oropharyngeal and cloacal swabs (the latter should show evidence of sampling faeces with as much as 1 g of faeces being optimal) should be taken. Some small, fragile birds may be harmed by swabbing and fresh faeces from these should be substituted. The preferred method of virus isolation is by inoculation of embryonated fowls' eggs and the techniques described for NDV (see Ch. 25) should be followed.

Haemagglutination activity in bacteria-free allantoic fluid may be due to an influenza virus or any of the avian paramyxoviruses. In view of the widespread use of live Newcastle disease vaccines it is probably simplest to exclude the isolation of NDV by HI test with specific NDV antiserum at this stage. The recommended method for the demonstration of the presence of an influenza A virus is by immunodiffusion, using specific antiserum positive for one or both of the type antigens, the matrix and the nucleocapsid proteins, and concentrated virus. Virus may be concentrated by high-speed centrifugation, or precipitation by adding 1 M hydrochloric acid to the infective allantoic fluid until the pH is approximately 4.9, chilling the mixture for 1 h at 0°C, followed by light centrifugation to clarify, then discarding the supernatant. The concentrated virus is then solubilized by resuspension in 1% sodium lauroyl sarcosinate buffered to pH 9.0 with 0.5 M glycine.

Virus characterization

Further virus characterization involves subtype identification and an estimate of virus pathogenicity. The methods recommended for the identification of influenza A subtypes by the World Health Organization Expert Committee involved the use of specific antisera prepared against the isolated antigen. Such sera are not generally available and this approach is therefore not practicable for most diagnostic laboratories. An alternative is to use a series of polyclonal antisera prepared against whole viruses. This requires at least two sera with different combinations for each H and N subtype to avoid interference; more may be necessary for conclusive typing because of the occurrence of antigenic variation within a subtype. It is usually necessary for non-specializing laboratories to refer samples to reference centres for full antigenic characterization.

Once an influenza virus is isolated it is also necessary to make some estimation of the virulence for chickens to comply with the OIE definition of notifiable AI.

The OIE definition has both in vivo and molecular tests for virus virulence. HPNAI viruses give either 75% mortality of eight 4- to 8-week-old susceptible chickens within 10 days following intravenous inoculation with 0.2 ml of a 1:10 dilution of a bacteria-free, infective allantoic fluid or viruses that have an intravenous pathogenicity index (IVPI) greater than 1.2. The IVPI test in chickens involves the intravenous inoculation of virus derived from fresh infective allantoic fluid into 10 6-week-old specific pathogen-free chickens. Each bird is examined at 24-h intervals for 10 days and scored 0 if normal, 1 if sick, 2 if very sick or paralysed and 3 if dead. Birds that are so sick they are unable to eat or drink should be killed humanely and scored as dead at the next observation. The index is the mean score per bird per observation over the

10-day period. The HPAI viruses give IVPI values approaching 3.0, while viruses of low virulence give values of 0.0.

The second part of the definition:

> For all H5 and H7 viruses of low pathogenicity in chickens, the amino acid sequence of the connecting peptide of the haemagglutinin must be determined. If the sequence is similar to that observed for other highly pathogenic AI isolates, the isolate being tested will be considered to be highly pathogenic

takes into account the current knowledge of the molecular basis of pathogenicity and that to date only viruses of H5 and H7 subtype have been shown to cause HPAI in susceptible species.

For all influenza A viruses the important haemagglutinin glycoprotein is produced as a precursor, HA0, which requires post-translational cleavage by host proteases before it is functional and virus particles are infectious. The HA0 precursor proteins of avian influenza viruses of low virulence for poultry have a single arginine at the cleavage site and another at either position -3 or -4 from the cleavage site. These viruses are limited to cleavage by extracellular host proteases such as trypsin-like enzymes and thus restricted to replication at sites in the host where such enzymes are found (i.e. the respiratory and intestinal tracts). HPAI viruses possess multiple basic amino acids (arginine – R and lysine – K) at their HA0 cleavage sites, either as a result of apparent insertion or apparent substitution, and appear to be cleavable by an intracellular ubiquitous protease(s), probably one or more proprotein-processing subtilisin-related endoproteases of which furin is the leading candidate. These viruses are able to replicate throughout the bird, damaging vital organs and tissues which results in disease and death. Demonstration of multiple basic amino acids at the cleavage site of HA0 confirms the actual or potential pathogenicity of the virus. The HA0 cleavage sites of some typical LPAI and HPAI viruses are shown in Table 26.1. The Chile 2002 and the Canada 2004 H7N3 HPAI viruses show distinct and unusual cleavage site amino acid sequences. These viruses appear to have arisen as a result of recombination with other genes (nucleoprotein gene and matrix gene respectively) resulting in an insertion at the cleavage site of 11 amino acids for the Chile virus and 7 amino acids for the Canadian virus.

As with Newcastle disease (see Ch. 25) the definition allows confirmation of the presence of virulent virus by sequencing, but an in vivo test is required to give a negative result as the possibility of dual infections or virus cultures containing mixed populations of viruses of high and low virulence cannot be ruled out.

Molecular techniques in diagnosis

There has been increasing use of reverse-transcription polymerase chain reaction (RT-PCR) and other similar techniques to detect AI viruses in clinical specimens, the advantage being the extremely rapid demonstration of the presence of virus. Oropharyngeal swabs are often used as the specimens of choice because they are easy to process and usually contain little extraneous organic material that can interfere with RNA recovery and amplification by PCR. However, tissue, organ and faeces samples have been used with some success.

Usually RT-PCR systems have been used initially to amplify a specific portion of the genome that will recognize all AI viruses, i.e. a conserved part of the matrix or nucleoprotein gene to identify the presence of AI virus. Further RT-PCR on positive samples have been aimed at detecting H5 and H7 subtypes, often amplifying a portion of the HA gene coding for the HA0 cleavage site so that the product can be used for assessing virulence. Perhaps the most serious problem n the use of RT-PCR in diagnosis is the necessity for postamplification processing because of the high potential for contamination of the laboratory and cross-contamination of samples. Extreme precautions and strict regimens for handling samples are necessary to prevent this.

The post 2003 spread of Asian H5N1 has resulted in a huge increase in diagnosis and surveillance for AI in many countries throughout the world, with a desire for obtaining results as rapidly as possible. Many laboratories have turned to real time RT-PCR (rRT-PCR) techniques to handle the large number of samples as efficiently as possible; especially as results may be obtained rapidly sometimes in less than 3h. In addition, rRT-PCR assays are based on fluorogenic hydrolysis probes or fluorescent dyes and eliminate the postamplification processing step that can lead to contamination problems in conventional RT-PCR. The strategy for rRT-PCR in the diagnosis of AI viruses has been similar to conventional RT-PCR with different sets of primers and probes used in separate reactions: a matrix or nucleoprotein gene primer/probe set that is designed to detect most strains of AI, a HA gene primer/probe set that can identify the presence of H5 subtype and another for H7 subtypes. Samples are first screened with the matrix/nucleoprotein gene primers/probe, then positive specimens are tested with the H5 and H7 primers/probe sets to confirm presence of these subtypes.

Antigen detection

Commercially available kits for the direct detection of virus antigens in samples, which are usually based on an antigen-capture enzyme immunoassay system, have been used for detecting the presence of influenza A viruses in poultry. In particular the Directigen® Flu A kit (Becton Dickinson Microbiology Systems) has been used widely in several countries. It uses a monoclonal antibody against the nucleoprotein and should therefore be able to detect any influenza A virus. Although it was developed to detect virus in mammalian infections, it has been successfully applied to poultry and other birds. There may be some variation in the sensitivity for different specimens; oropharyngeal or tracheal samples provide the best sensitivity. The main advantage of antigen detection tests are that they can demonstrate the presence of influenza A virus within 15 minutes. The disadvantages are that they may lack sensitivity, have not been validated for different species of birds and types of specimens (e.g. cloacal swabs), subtype identification is not achieved and the kits are expensive. These tests should be used as a flock test, i.e. taking multiple samples, and not as an individual bird test.

Serology

The diversity of influenza A virus surface antigens imposes severe limitations on the use of conventional serology in the diagnosis of infection. The numerous subtypes and variations within subtypes mean that the HI test is of value only when the H subtype of the infecting virus is already known, and is therefore usually limited to monitoring outbreaks. A more practicable approach to general influenza diagnosis is to use immunodiffusion tests to detect one of the type antigens, the nucleocapsid and matrix proteins. Immunodiffusion, using a nucleoprotein-rich extract from infected chorioallantoic membranes, has been usefully employed to monitor poultry flocks at risk from influenza infections, on a routine basis, with considerable success in detecting infected flocks. One drawback to the use of this test is that some birds, particularly waterfowl, rarely produce precipitating antibodies following influenza A infection. A suitably validated enzyme-linked immunosorbent assay (ELISA) test for detecting antibodies either to specific H subtypes or matrix or nucleoprotein may be used, although the problem with this is that, unless a competitive test is used, the test is host-specific, since it is dependent on the detection of host immunoglobulins.

CONTROL

Control and eradication of AI is unlikely to be achieved by pursuing a single strategy and the latter goal will only be reached and/or maintained if there are policies and practices in place that ensure: awareness and knowledge of AI, good biosecurity, rapid diagnosis, surveillance and prompt, safe depopulation of birds on infected establishments.

Control policies

Control policies adopted at national or international level require legislative enforcement to be effective and the extent to which these will be forthcoming for avian influenza will be influenced by the perceived threat to the poultry industry, the size of the industry and its importance to the country's economy. Since the turn of the century this perception has been high and there have been considerable changes made in international control policies and the AI viruses that should be the subject of such controls. As indicated in the definition above, the OIE has extended viruses that fall into the category of notifiable for trade purposes to include viruses of H5 and H7 subtypes that are not HPAI. Similarly, many countries, including all European Union members, have extended control legislation to include H5 and H7 virus infections. In practice, such legislation, which does not necessarily involve stamping out for LPNAI, has made formal the control strategies for LPNAI virus, often involving stamping out, that had been practised in countries where outbreaks had occurred in recent years.

In addition to the changes in which viruses should be considered notifiable, the OIE has also introduced the concept of 'compartmentalization' for avian influenza. In general terms this allows that, if a given country cannot provide sufficient evidence of freedom from NAI, an enterprise within that country, in collaboration with the official veterinary service, may generate a compartmentalization programme demonstrating that it is free from infection. In addition, an enterprise that has one exporting production line (e.g. layers) and other production lines that are not destined for export may certify only the layer compartment as free, provided that the management practices comply with those required for a separate compartment within the enterprise. This would mean that were NAI identified in, for example, fattening ducks in a country, it should not necessarily result in international trade restrictions in a different compartment, for example, chicken meat, provided that the broiler sector can demonstrate that it is free of NAI.

A feature of HPAI outbreaks over the last 10 years has been the occurrence of several outbreaks in geographical areas with extreme concentrations of poultry farms usually referred to as 'densely populated poultry areas' (DPPA). In such areas eradication by conventional stamping out alone has proved difficult, because of the speed of spread of the disease and in at least three of these episodes – Hong Kong 1997, the Netherlands 2003 and Canada 2004 – the authorities have resorted to pre-emptive culling of large numbers of birds to bring about control and eradication.

Management

Considerable success in the control of influenza infections of domestic poultry by prevention of introduction and secondary spread may be achieved by good management, and biosecurity (encompassing bioexclusion and biocontainment) represents the first and most important means of prevention. In countries with developing poultry industries, such management should begin at the planning stage, ensuring that farms are situated away from migratory waterfowl routes and not developed in the clusters frequently seen in countries with established industries.

Where possible, birds should be reared in confinement in wild-bird-proofed houses. Surface water should not be used untreated for drinking water.

Prevention of secondary spread after an initial outbreak will also depend on good biosecurity procedures, especially control of movements of personnel and equipment to and from the premises. Measures such as: minimizing movements on and off the farm; ensuring that all equipment, especially vehicles, is disinfected before access to the site is permitted; and ensuring that movements between different farms (e.g. egg collection, carcass collection, food delivery) are to and from specified collection and delivery points away from the poultry flocks need to be enforced. Possibly the most important consideration is who has actual contact with the flock. Access to the birds should be kept to a minimum. If it is unavoidable, then visits by personnel who may have visited other poultry farms, such as food deliveries, bleeding, thinning or vaccination crews, inseminators and veterinarians, must be considered the most likely method of introduction of avian influenza and regimens of clothing change, equipment disinfection and other basic hygiene controls should be enforced before access to the birds is allowed. In areas of high risk the most stringent methods of biosecurity must be imposed and these should include changing of clothes and, ideally, showering for staff working with poultry.

When outbreaks do occur, depopulation should be considered even for the less virulent and non-notifiable virus infections in the absence of any statutory requirement. After depopulation all poultry and products, including faeces, should be buried or incinerated on site, and restocking should not take place until at least 2 weeks after thorough cleansing and disinfection.

Vaccination

For many years vaccination against HPAI viruses and therefore LPAI of H5 or H7 subtypes was actively discouraged or banned in some countries because it was considered that it would interfere with the diagnosis of HPAI. Vaccination with autogenous inactivated vaccines was carried out in a few areas where LPAI viruses of other subtypes were a problem, mainly in turkeys, in the USA and Italy. However, the marked increase in outbreaks of HPAI since the 1990s and the spread of H9N2 infections across Asia has led to considerable pressure to use vaccination as part of control policies, either as an emergency measure or prophylactically for both HPAI and LPAI.

Current AI vaccines when selected properly and administered correctly will protect against clinical signs and mortality, reduce the levels and duration of virus excretion and increase the resistance of the host to infection by raising the minimum infectious virus dose needed to infect the bird. However, AI viruses (especially HPAI) may still infect and replicate in vaccinated birds without the presentation of clinical signs. Infection with HPAI virus without clinical signs may lead to delays in notification and diagnosis resulting in spread of infection and could result in an endemic situation. Additionally, notifiable AI, as defined by OIE, would still be confirmed in healthy, infected, vaccinated birds.

Even if vaccination is employed the goal should be to eradicate the virus and vaccination alone should not be considered the solution for the control of NAI or even LPAI subtypes. Without the application of monitoring systems, strict biosecurity and depopulation in the face of infection, there is the possibility that these viruses could become endemic in vaccinated poultry populations. Long-term circulation of the virus in a vaccinated population may result in both antigenic and genetic changes in the virus.

Inactivated vaccines

Conventionally, AI vaccines have been prepared from infective allantoic fluid inactivated by β-propiolactone or formalin and emulsified with mineral oil. Some vaccination strategies against

LPAI viruses have been to produce autogenous vaccines (i.e. prepared from isolates specifically involved in an epizootic); others have been to use vaccines prepared from LPAI viruses possessing the same haemagglutinin subtype that yield high concentrations of antigen. LPAI H5 and H7 subtypes are used so that high biosecurity facilities are not required. Inactivated vaccines aimed at H5, H7 and H9 subtypes are now commercially available and have been licensed for use in a number of countries. In China a so-called 'genetically modified vaccine' has been used. This is essentially a conventional inactivated vaccine but the vaccine virus was produced by reverse genetics using the six internal genes from a human influenza vaccine strain (PR8) and the H5 and N1 genes from A/goose/Guangdong/3/96, the progenitor virus of the Asian H5N1 HPAI viruses. Further, the H gene was modified to give a LPAI HA0 cleavage site. The logic of the PR8 genes is that this results in a virus that grows to high titres in eggs.

Recombinant vaccines

Recombinant vaccines for AI viruses have been produced by inserting the gene coding for the influenza virus haemagglutinin into a live virus vector and using this recombinant virus to immunize poultry against AI. These vaccines have certain advantages in that they are live vaccines, stimulating both humoral and cellular immunity, can be easily administered and allow easy distinction between vaccinated and infected birds. But there may be problems if birds have immunity to the vector vaccine, e.g. *Fowlpox virus* or infectious laryngotracheitis viruses for recombinant vaccines available currently, and the vector virus may also have limited host range.

Detection of infection in vaccinated flocks and vaccinated birds

Many countries and international agencies are insisting that any use of vaccination must involve a strategy that allows 'differentiation of infected from vaccinated animals' (DIVA). A DIVA strategy is necessary because, while in poultry vaccination will protect challenged birds from disease, increase the amount of virus needed to infect the vaccinated bird and decrease the amount of virus excreted, vaccinated birds will not show clinical signs if challenged with AI and therefore HPAI or LPAI of H5 or H7 subtypes could infect a flock and circulate for some time in that flock unnoticed. There is therefore a need to be able to identify vaccinated birds that have subsequently become infected with field virus so that other control measures, e.g. stamping out, can be implemented.

At the flock level, a simple method is to regularly monitor sentinel birds left unvaccinated in each vaccinated flock but this approach may have some management problems. As an alternative, or in addition, testing for field exposure may be performed on the vaccinated birds. Several systems have been developed in recent years that would allow the detection of field challenge of vaccinated birds.

One method is to use a vaccine containing a virus of the same haemagglutinin (H) subtype but a different neuraminidase (N) from the prevailing field virus. Antibodies to the N of the field virus act as natural markers of infection. This system has been used in Italy following both emergency and prophylactic vaccination strategies. Problems with this system would arise if a field virus emerges that has a different N antigen to the existing field virus or if subtypes with different N antigens are already circulating in the field. The use of vaccines containing only HA, e.g. recombinant vaccines, allows classical AGID tests or ELISA tests based on nucleoprotein or matrix protein to be used to detect infection in vaccinated birds. For inactivated vaccines, a test that detects antibodies to the nonstructural virus protein, which are only produced during natural infection, has been described but has yet to be validated in the field.

The development of rapid and sensitive virus-detection methods, especially those that can be automated, such as rRT-PCR, means that these could be used for simple widespread and regular testing of vaccinated birds for the presence of field virus.

ZOONOSIS

Early experimental work suggested that AI viruses were unlikely to cause any significant infections of humans directly. This was reinforced by the lack of reports of AI infections. Up to 1995 there had been only three recorded instances of AI viruses infecting humans: in 1959 virus was isolated from a patient in the USA suffering from hepatitis, and in 1977 and 1981 laboratory accidents had resulted in eye infections of laboratory staff presenting as conjunctivitis; interestingly all three of these were due to H7N7 subtype viruses (Table 26.2). However, since 1996 there have been regular reports of natural infections of humans with avian influenza viruses. Infections with the Asian H5N1 have received the greatest attention because, at the time of writing, of the 223 people infected since May 1997 123 (55%) have died, but human infections with other viruses have occurred in a number of countries (Table 26.2). These infections, of mainly H7 subtype AI viruses, but also H9N2, have usually caused conjunctivitis or mild flu-like illness but in the Netherlands there was one fatality. Transmission between humans appears to have occurred only on very rare, exceptional occasions and in nearly all reported cases of human infections with AI viruses there has been close association with infected birds or infective carcasses.

Table 26.2	Human infections with avian influenza viruses to May 2006				
YEAR	**SUBTYPE**	**HPAI/LPAI***	**COUNTRY**	**NO. INFECTED**	**SYMPTOMS**
1959	H7N7	HPAI	USA	1	Hepatitis?
1977	H7N7	HPAI	Australia	1*	Conjunctivitis
1981	H7N7	LPAI	USA	1*	Conjunctivitis
1996	H7N7	LPAI	England	1	Conjunctivitis
1997–April 2006	H5N1	HPAI	Hong Kong, China, Vietnam, Thailand, Cambodia, Indonesia, Azerbaijan, Djibouti, Egypt, Iraq, Turkey	223	Influenza-like illness, **123 deaths**
1998/9	H9N2	LPAI	Hong Kong/China	2 (+5?)	Influenza-like illness
2002	H7N2	LPAI	USA (VA)	1	None
2003	H7N2	LPAI	USA (NYC)	1	Influenza-like illness
2003	H7N7	HPAI	Netherlands	83 (>1000?)	Conjunctivitis, influenza-like illness, **1 death**
2004	H7N3	HPAI	Canada (BC)	2	Conjunctivitis
2006	H7N3	LPAI	UK (England)	1	Conjunctivitis

* Highly pathogenic avian influenza (HPAI), or low pathogenic avian influenza (LPAI).

However, there is an even more alarming aspect to the human infections with AI viruses, which relates to the emergence of influenza pandemics. Influenza A infections in humans have been marked throughout history by serious pandemics every 10–50 years. In the 20th century the sudden emergence of antigenically different strains in humans, termed antigenic shift, resulted in pandemics occurring on four occasions, 1918 (H1N1), 1957 (H2N2), 1968 (H3N2) and 1977 (H1N1). By far the worst influenza pandemic for which there are accurate records was the one beginning in 1918. It has been estimated that during the pandemic more than 40 million people died. Because the viral RNA of influenza viruses is segmented, genetic reassortment can occur in mixed infections with different strains of influenza A virus. This means that, when two viruses infect the same cell, progeny viruses may inherit sets of RNA segments made up of combinations of segments identical to those of either of the parent viruses. Both the H2N2 1957 and the H3N2 1968 pandemic viruses differed from the prevailing viruses in the human population as a result of reassortment with avian influenza viruses. These reassortments brought about antigenic shift resulting in viruses with both surface glycoprotein genes from the avian virus for the 1957 virus and the important HA gene from the avian virus for the 1968 virus, but retained internal protein genes that allowed these viruses to be readily transmissible in the human population. The current concern is that human infections with the Asian H5N1 virus (or any other AI virus) could lead to reassortment, antigenic shift and the emergence of a pandemic virus if the person was also infected with an influenza virus currently circulating in the population. The potential of these human infections with AI virus to result in a pandemic virus emerging has been added to by the determination of the entire genome of the 1918 pandemic virus and the suggestion that this virus emerged by a complete avian virus adapting to humans without reassortment.

FURTHER READING

Alexander D J 2005 Avian influenza. In: OIE Manual for diagnostic tests and vaccines for terrestrial animals, 5th edn. OIE, Paris, ch 2.07.12. Available on line at: http://www.oie.int/eng/normes/ MMANUAL/A_00037.htm

Capua I, Alexander D J 2004 Avian influenza – recent developments. Avian Pathol 33: 393–404

EFSA Scientific Panel on Animal Health and Animal Welfare 2005 Animal health and welfare aspects of avian influenza. EFSA J 266(Annex): 1–21

European Commission 2006 Council Directive 2005/94/EC of 20 December 2005 on Community measures for the control of avian influenza and repealing Directive 92/40/EEC. Offic J Eur Commun L10: 16–65

Sims L D, Domench J, Benigno C et al 2005 Origin and evolution of highly pathogenic H5N1 avian influenza in Asia. Vet Rec 157: 159–164

Swayne D E, Halvorson D A 2003 Influenza. In: Saif Y M (ed) Diseases of poultry, 7th edn. Iowa State University Press, Ames, p 135–160

World Organization for Animal Health 2003 Terrestrial animal health code, 14th edn, chapter 2.7.12.1 Avian influenza. OIE, Paris. Available on line at: www.oie.int/eng/normes/mcode/en_chapter_2.7.12. htm

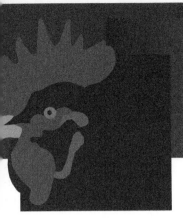

Michael A. Skinner

Poxviridae

Poxvirus infections of birds are caused by viruses currently defined by the International Committee on Taxonomy of Viruses as members of a single genus. The *Avipoxvirus* genus is one of the eight genera of the subfamily *Chordopoxvirinae*, all of which infect vertebrates. Viruses of the other seven genera all infect mammals. The avipoxviruses appear incapable of causing disease in mammals; therefore there appears to be no zoonotic potential. Like other poxviruses they contain a double-stranded DNA genome, ranging up to more than 300 kbp, and replicate within the cytoplasm of the cells they infect.

Fowlpox virus (FWPV) is the best studied and prototypic species of the avipoxviruses. There are currently nine other recognized species, yet avipoxvirus infections have been observed in more than 230 of the known 9000 species of bird, spanning 23 orders. Very little is currently known about the genome diversity, host-range and host-specificity of the causative agent(s).

EPIDEMIOLOGY

Cause

Because of its characteristic lesions and physical nature, FWPV was one of the earliest viruses identified. It also played important roles in the development of modern virology during the middle decades of the 20th century. Fowlpox was one of the first diseases of livestock and poultry for which effective vaccines were developed, as early as the late 1920s. These vaccines led to effective control of the disease and its virtual eradication from commercial poultry production in the temperate regions; consequently the research effort was scaled back.

Like other poxviruses, the brick-shaped avipoxviruses are large enough (at 300 × 250 × 100 nm) to be resolved by light microscopy. Indeed, the particles were originally observed following staining with basic dyes (such as basic fuchsin in Gimenez stain) and were termed elementary particles or Borrel bodies. Their size means that poxviruses are, unlike the majority of smaller viruses, not truly filterable – being substantially excluded by 200 nm pore-size filters.

The avipoxviruses also appear to have some of the largest known genomes of viruses of vertebrates, more than 300 kbp for *Canarypox virus* (CNPV), encoding about 300 proteins (by way of comparison, this is 100 times the size of the smallest poultry virus genome, that of *Chicken anaemia virus*, and half the size of the genome of the smallest free-living bacterium).

Hosts

Although evidence of poxvirus infection has been observed in many avian species, little is known about the natural host range of the causative agents, because of the lack of robust techniques for the identification and differentiation of isolates. Initially, viruses were distinguished by their ability to cause disease in a range of test species, such as chickens, pigeons, turkeys and quail. Such infectivity studies probably overestimate the degree of similarity between the viruses, as many seem able to cause disease in the test species, although this may be due to high doses used in the artificial inoculation. More meaningful data were obtained from the in vivo studies by analysing antigenic cross-reactivity, grouping or distinguishing viruses by their ability or inability to induce protective immunity against each other. Thus *Psittacinepox virus* offered no protection against FWPV or *Pigeonpox virus*, or vice versa; neither did *Quailpox virus*. Similarly, *Mynahpox virus* showed no cross-protection with fowl, pigeon, psittacine, quail or turkey poxviruses and a condor poxvirus induced no protection against FWPV. The development of in vitro serological techniques allowed such serological comparison in the laboratory. Such techniques were applied to only a small proportion of the observed isolates, often because initial propagation in chick embryos or chick embryo fibroblast cells failed. Possibly as a consequence of the limited characterization of isolates, there are only ten recognized species of *Avipoxvirus*: *Canarypox virus*, *Fowlpox virus*, *Juncopox virus*, *Mynahpox virus*, *Pigeonpox virus*, *Psittacinepox virus*, *Quailpox virus*, *Sparrowpox virus*, *Starlingpox virus* and *Turkeypox virus*.

Taxonomy and epidemiology

Taxonomy and classification of avipoxviruses may appear to be of solely academic interest. However, both are important to the study of epidemiology and hence to our future ability to control the diseases. Recent molecular studies confirm earlier impressions that avipoxviruses can jump species to cause disease. Thus isolation of a virus from a turkey, for instance, is not sufficient to demonstrate that *Turkeypox virus* is the cause and, more importantly, that the outbreak can be controlled by a *Turkeypox virus* vaccine. When new disease challenges emerge, it is therefore important that we can quickly and accurately identify the nature of the causative agent.

Recent molecular studies (see below) have demonstrated that avipoxviruses fall into three major groups: the FWPV-like viruses, the CNPV-like viruses and the psittacinepox viruses. As the name suggests, the psittacinepox viruses have so far only been isolated from psittacines. In contrast, viruses of the FWPV-like and CNPV-like groups either appear inherently capable of infecting a wider range of birds or have evolved and adapted to be able to infect different birds. FWPV-like viruses have been isolated from turkeys, pigeons, ospreys, albatrosses, doves and falcons. Viruses closely related to, and even barely distinguishable from, CNPV can cause disease in great tits, sparrows, stone curlews and houbaras. CNPV-like viruses have been isolated from pigeons and starlings. A recent report from Virginia in the USA indicates that one particular CNPV-like virus has caused disease in a wide range of birds (robins, crows, herons, finches, doves, hawks, gnatcatchers, mockingbirds and cardinals). It is not yet known whether the virus that caused this epornitic has a wider geographical distribution throughout the USA.

It is therefore apparent that pigeon pox can be caused by two distinct types of virus, one FWPV-like and one CNPV-like. The FWPV-like virus is very closely related to viruses from turkeys and osprey, and a little less closely related to those from an albatross, a falcon and a dove. The CNPV-like virus is closely related to one from a starling.

We are only just beginning to glimpse the complexity of avipoxvirus host range and epidemiology. A clear understanding will require more sampling from healthy wild birds, as well as from diseased birds (both accompanied by more detailed record keeping of host species, clinical history and presentation) and more extensive genome sequence data from a wider range of distinct viruses.

Infection of birds outside the normal host range of the avipoxvirus may result in reduced or enhanced pathogenesis. The former is exemplified by a virus that had caused an aggressive, diphtheritic form of the disease in the Andean condor (*Vultur gryphus*) from which it was isolated but which produced only small, localized cutaneous lesions in inoculated chickens. Enhanced pathogenesis is less well documented, because we know little about mild diseases in their natural hosts. It is, however, suspected that canaries, in which poxviruses cause devastating disease, may not be the natural reservoir for CNPV. More surveys of wild birds, such as that in the Canary Islands, which found mild poxvirus lesions in 50% of short-toed larks (*Calandrella rufescens*) and 28% of Berthelot's pipits (*Anthus berthelotti*), will clarify this situation, especially if they are coupled with studies of phylogeny based on molecular techniques.

Reintroduction programmes in the Middle East for the houbara bustard have suffered losses due to *Avipoxvirus* infections from unknown sources. Reintroduction programmes such as that for the closely related great bustard on Salisbury Plain, Wiltshire in the UK may face similar threats. There are also concerns that avipoxviruses might threaten marginal species such as the flightless, nocturnal New Zealand owl parrot or kakapo.

Spread

Poxviruses produce two infectious forms: the intracellular form shed into the environment, in a stable form resistant to desiccation, by desquamation of skin lesions and the extracellular form released into the blood to spread to secondary sites of infection. The primary route of infection, particularly in the wild, is mechanical transmission of blood-borne, extracellular virus by biting insects. This explains the preferential localization of lesions to the unfeathered areas (around the eyes and nares, on the comb, wattle or legs). It also explains why fowlpox remains a problem essentially in situations where control of biting insects becomes more problematic. Therefore fowlpox is generally not a problem for intensive production systems in the temperate areas of northern Europe and the northern USA, even in the absence of vaccination, although problems have been observed with free-range flocks, which are obviously more exposed to biting insects. Under subtropical and tropical climates, fowlpox affects even intensive, commercial production. After Newcastle disease, fowlpox is the most important viral pathogen of backyard flocks in Africa. Pecking by infected birds may provide an alternative route of mechanical transmission. Infection via both these routes leads primarily to the cutaneous forms of the diseases.

Inhalation or ingestion of virus (or virus-infected cells shed from cutaneous lesions), leads to the diphtheritic forms of disease, with lesions on the mucous membranes of the mouth, pharynx, larynx and sometimes trachea. This route of infection is more likely to occur at high population density, such as is found with commercial poultry flocks or collections of captive or domesticated birds (including quarantine facilities). Such lesions may also form as a consequence of secondary viraemia following primary cutaneous lesions. *Avipoxvirus* infections of canaries and finches can cause significantly higher rates of mortality than those of chickens or turkeys.

DIAGNOSIS

Clinical signs

Fowlpox in chickens, spread mechanically by biting insects, is relatively mild in its cutaneous form but causes higher mortality in its diphtheritic form, by occlusion of the oropharynx. It is primarily a disease of mature birds. A third, pneumonia-like form of poxvirus disease has been described in canaries, in which mortality is high. The reasons for these differences cannot be elucidated without more knowledge of the molecular phylogeny and epidemiology of these viruses.

Cutaneous lesions are difficult to detect in their early stages, particularly when few birds are infected. They start as small, hard nodules or papules, which increase in size and vesiculate, then pustulate and finally form a crusty scab. The scab is dark and obvious. Individual lesions may be dismissed as trauma wounds (perhaps from pecking) but multiple lesions are frequently present, they may even coalesce, rendering diagnosis common at this stage. After a couple of weeks, the scabs (which contain infectious virus) will drop off, leaving resolved lesions. Coalesced lesions can show considerable thickening; on the eyelids this can result in closure of the eye. The thickening is attributed to epithelial cell hyperplasia, which may be caused by virus-encoded, cellular growth factors (resembling nerve growth factor in the avipoxviruses; epidermal growth factor in the mammalian poxviruses). Large lesions may take several weeks to resolve. Lesions near the nostrils or eyes may (via the conjunctiva) precipitate the diphtheritic (or wetpox) form, in which the initial nodules coalesce to form raised caseous lesions on the mucous membranes of the mouth, oesophagus, pharynx, larynx or trachea. These lesions can thicken sufficiently to interfere with feeding or breathing, explaining the higher mortality of this form of the disease. Such lesions can be discriminated from those of infectious laryngotracheitis (caused by a herpesvirus) by histological examination. The *Avipoxvirus* infections seen in canaries and finches often present as systemic infections with the development of pneumonia, leading to cyanosis and high mortality (up to 100%).

Smears of material scraped from cutaneous lesions, or post-mortem sections from diphtheritic lesions (or airway epithelium in the case of pneumonia), can be stained with haematoxylin/eosin or Gimenez. The presence of eosinophilic inclusions (A-type inclusions, Bollinger bodies) in the cytoplasm is diagnostic of poxviruses. Basophilic (or B-type) inclusion bodies may also be seen in the cytoplasm (these represent the sites of virus replication, the so-called 'viral factories'), as may Borrel bodies (the virions themselves).

Virus isolation/detection

Virus may be passaged and amplified in vivo through specific-pathogen-free chickens via wing web scarification or through embryonated eggs via chorioallantoic membrane infection. The method of choice for virus propagation, however, is in vitro on chick embryo fibroblast cell cultures (CEFs) for amplification through liquid culture or for plaque purification under semisolid overlay. Not all *Avipoxvirus* isolates will form plaques, or even propagate, on CEFs. Primary cultures of other poultry species (duck, turkey or quail) may also be used.

Avipoxvirus replication is limited to avian cells. Relatively few avian cells lines are available and suitable for propagation of viruses (as many permanent cell lines were transformed by avian retroviruses or *Marek's disease virus* and may be producers of the transforming viruses). Quail cell lines (QT6 and QT35) can be used for propagation of FWPV (and possibly other avipoxviruses) but it has been shown that these cells naturally carry latent *Marek's disease virus*. Unfortunately, FWPV fails to plaque and replicates poorly in the recently derived chicken fibroblast cell line DF-1.

Serology

Evidence for prior infection, or for ongoing infection in the flock, can be determined by serological methods. The older technique of gel precipitation has essentially been superseded by enzyme-linked immunosorbent assay (ELISA), as used in commercial flock monitoring kits. Virus neutralization tests are more specific but are technically more demanding.

Monoclonal antibodies

Monoclonal antibodies against the three major immunodominant structural antigens of FWPV have been isolated and characterized. One target is the 39K immunodominant core protein equivalent to the vaccinia virus A4 protein. Variability is observed in the size of this protein between different isolates and strains, because of diagnostic differences in the number of repeats of a 12-amino-acid motif. Another target is the 35K protein, equivalent to VACV H3, found on the surface of the infectious, intracellular form of the virus, as is the third target, the 63K p4c protein, responsible for virion entry into A-type inclusion bodies. None of these monoclonal antibodies appears to be neutralizing.

Molecular diagnostics

Restriction enzyme digestion and Southern blotting

Before the acquisition of genome sequence data, Southern blotting had been used as a molecular diagnostic to prepare restriction enzyme digest fingerprints of the different avipoxviruses. The method is relatively insensitive, both in the amount of viral DNA required for the assay and in its ability to discriminate between closely related strains.

Polymerase chain reaction – restriction fragment length polymerization and sequence analysis

Since DNA sequence data became available for FWPV, amplification by polymerase chain reaction (PCR) has become a useful way to identify the presence of an avipoxvirus. Normally this has been based on the sequence of the gene encoding the p4b protein, with primers for a 578 bp fragment. However, all avipoxviruses produce fragments of the same length so the specific nature of the avipoxvirus could only be identified either by sequencing the PCR product or by restriction enzyme fragment polymorphism (RFLP) profiling. Analysis of the sequence at the p4b locus has been extremely useful in gaining a preliminary picture of the molecular phylogenetic relationships of the avipoxviruses. The FWPV and CNPV proteins share only 64.2% amino acid identity, representing a substantial level of divergence.

A new PCR locus has recently been identified, the H3 locus, which works with most (but not all) avipoxviruses. However, this locus has the advantage that viruses of the two major groups (CNPV-like and FWPV-like) can be discriminated purely on the basis of the size of the PCR product, a sensitive and fairly straight-forward procedure, without recourse to RFLP or sequence analysis (though the latter provides further detail on the identity of the isolate).

The genome sequences of the standard USDA challenge strain of FWPV, an extensively culture-passaged, attenuated, plaque-purified FWPV (FP9) and a pathogenic CNPV have been determined. The sequences have confirmed the extensive divergence and considerable differences between the avipoxviruses and the mammalian poxviruses, typified by *Vaccinia virus*. In fact, phylogenetic analysis shows that avipoxviruses are most closely related to molluscum contagiosum virus of humans, a relationship confirmed by other specific aspects of their molecular biology.

Despite having sequence information for the prototypic members of the two major groups of avipoxviruses, it has still proved extremely difficult to identify conserved primer sequences that will work in PCR reactions against all other members of the genus, further illustrating the extent of sequence divergence and diversity within this group of viruses.

Intraspecies and interstrain differentiation

The high level of conservation within species of avipoxviruses makes it difficult to differentiate between different strains or isolates. This becomes particularly relevant where there is a need to differentiate between vaccines and pathogenic strains. We have surveyed numerous loci within FWPV and, apart from the heterogeneous terminal repeat region (which presents considerable technical difficulties), only one locus has been found that allows clear differentiation. Termed the H9 locus, it appears to be an unstable region, resulting in deletions of different lengths in various FWPV strains, isolates and vaccines (and probably in CNPV too). For example, three commercial fowlpox vaccines appear to have the parental sequence as found in two clinical isolates, while two other different commercial fowlpox vaccines appear to share an identical deletion at this locus.

CONTROL

Vaccines

Vaccination against fowlpox was introduced in the 1920s, using live FWPV or pigeonpox virus, some strains of which we now know to be antigenically closely related to FWPV. Vaccine strains are currently available commercially from various companies. Most originate from early isolates, with a minority derived from field isolates collected in the mid-1960s.

Depending on the nature of the particular vaccine strain, vaccination with commercial products may be undertaken from 10 days or 4 weeks of age into the wing web using a bifurcated needle or by scarification of the thigh. A good take is indicated by the presence of a small lesion at the site of vaccination 6–8 days later, with immunity developing in 8–15 days. Birds to be vaccinated should always be healthy; spread of vaccine to nonvaccinated birds should be avoided by thorough infection control measures.

Treatment

There are no demonstrated effective treatments for avipoxvirus infections. Topical treatments are often used to treat lesions on backyard poultry. The effectiveness of these is not clear but they may help prevent or treat secondary bacterial infections. Studies are underway in South Africa on the effectiveness of oral plant-derived extracts based on folk medicine remedies.

Variant fowlpox viruses

There have been reports of outbreaks of fowlpox within flocks previously vaccinated with FWPV or pigeonpox virus vaccines. Assuming vaccination had been effective, this suggests that antigenic variation had occurred within the isolates. Little is known about protective epitopes for humoral or cellular immune responses in FWPV and there has only been preliminary characterization of the 'variant' isolates. In Brazil, FWPV has also been associated with cases of dermal squamous cell carcinoma. Whether FWPV is a causative agent and whether a variant is involved is not clear.

The role of integrated *Reticuloendotheliosis virus* sequences

A vaccine strain of FWPV, FPV-S, known to be contaminated with *Reticuloendotheliosis virus* (REV) was found to carry a near full length, infectious progenome of the retrovirus inserted within its poxviral genome. The provirus has been found in most, if not all, pathogenic isolates of FWPV but the majority of vaccine strains of FWPV carry only noninfectious, long terminal repeat (LTR) sequences of REV. When examined, the provirus and the LTR sequences have only ever been found at the same single locus, although differences exist between the retained REV sequences found in different isolates. It appears likely that a single, ancestral event inserted the provirus into the FWPV genome between FPV201 and FPV203, in contrast to the multiple REV insertions that have been observed in *Marek's disease virus*. There are no REV sequences in the completely sequenced genome of CNPV but they have been detected in a commercial CNPV vaccine as well as in some commercial pigeonpox virus vaccines. Full-length REV sequences have recently been detected in an isolate from a turkey.

Recombinant FWPV vaccines

Systems for isolating recombinant vaccinia virus were developed in the early 1980s, bringing the prospect of developing whole new generations of vaccines based on recombinant viruses. Shortly thereafter, considerable interest emerged in developing FWPV as an equivalent recombinant vector for use in poultry. Several of the commercial vaccine and laboratory attenuated strains were used as the basis for the development of recombinant FWPV (rFWPV) against a number of important poultry pathogens, notably *Avian influenza virus*, *Newcastle disease virus*, *Infectious bronchitis virus*, *Avian haemorrhagic enteritis virus*, *Marek's disease virus* and *Infectious bursal disease virus* as well as *Mycoplasma gallisepticum*. Commercial rFWPV for *Newcastle disease virus* and for avian influenza virus were produced early and have been licensed for commercial use in the USA. rFWPV against avian influenza have also been licensed for use in Mexico; indeed between 1997 and 2003, approximately 708 million doses of a killed H5N2 vaccine and an additional 459 million doses of a recombinant fowlpox-H5 vaccine were used in Mexico to control H5N2. It, and similar viruses developed in China, are being used in south-east Asia to counter the highly virulent avian influenza H5N1 strain. rFWPV effective against *Marek's disease virus*, *Turkey rhinotracheitis virus* and REV have also been developed. Attempts to derive effective vaccines against *Infectious bronchitis virus* have been less successful. Recombinant avipoxvirus vaccines have yet to be licensed for agricultural use in Europe.

FURTHER READING

OIE 2004 Fowlpox diagnostic tests and vaccines. In: Manual of diagnostic tests and vaccines for terrestrial animals, 5th edn. OIE, Paris. Available on line at www.oie.int/eng/normes/mmanual/A_00113.htm

Skinner M A, Laidlaw S M, Eldaghayes I et al 2005 Fowlpox virus as a recombinant vaccine vector for use in mammals and poultry. Expert Rev Vaccines 4: 63–76

Tripathy D K, Reed W M 2003 Pox. In: Saif Y M (ed) Diseases of poultry, 11th edn. Iowa State University Press, Ames, p 253–269

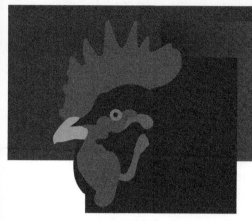

CHAPTER 28

Jane K. A. Cook

Coronaviridae

The family *Coronaviridae* is a member of the order *Nidovirales*, the only other family in the order being the *Arteriviridae*. These are linear, single-stranded RNA viruses of positive sense. The *Coronaviridae* family is divided into two genera, *Coronavirus* and *Torovirus*, but only viruses of the *Coronavirus* genus have been reported to infect birds. Coronaviruses are enveloped, pleomorphic but usually spherical virus particles of 120–140 nm in diameter. The important antigenic and functional proteins are present as distinct, club-shaped projections (known as spikes), spaced widely apart and dispersed evenly over the surface of the virion. In addition to avian species, coronaviruses have been reported to infect cattle, dogs, cats, pigs, rodents and humans. Coronaviruses are divided into three groups, based on antigenic relationships and gene sequencing data. All known avian coronaviruses are placed in group 3, although there is some experimental evidence to suggest that a group 2 coronavirus, *Bovine coronavirus*, can infect turkeys and cause enteric disease in them. The possibility exists, therefore, that birds may be infected with coronaviruses belonging to other groups.

The best-known avian coronavirus and the most important economically and from a welfare point of view, is avian *Infectious bronchitis virus* (IBV; Fig. 28.1), the type species of the *Coronavirus* genus and a major pathogen in chickens. However, coronaviruses of turkeys, pheasants and other avian species are now recognized.

INFECTIOUS BRONCHITIS

Infectious bronchitis was first reported in North Dakota, USA, in 1931 as an acute, highly infectious respiratory disease of chickens. It now has worldwide distribution. The primary target organ is the respiratory tract, where initial infection and disease occurs. IBV also affects egg-laying performance, and renal damage associated with infectious bronchitis has become increasingly important, particularly in broilers. Economically, the most important aspects are the effects on egg production and quality in laying hens and production performance in broilers, where the initial respiratory infection is frequently exacerbated by secondary infections.

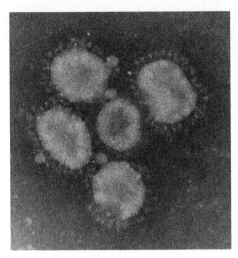

Fig. 28.1 *Infectious bronchitis virus* negatively stained. Electron micrograph courtesy of the Institute for Animal Health, UK.

EPIDEMIOLOGY

Cause

The IBV contains four structural proteins: a surface projection, known as the spike, a nucleoprotein, a membrane protein and a small membrane protein. The spike (S) glycoprotein is responsible for attachment to and fusion of the virus membrane with the host cell membrane, as well as for inducing protective immune responses. Molecular studies have shown that the *S* gene of IBV is also responsible for determining the serotype or genotype of an IB virus or variant. It is now known that only a small number of amino acid changes in the S1 part of the spike can result in what is defined by laboratory tests as a new variant. Since it is possible for concurrent infection with more than one type of IBV to occur, new variants may emerge as a result of both recombination between two different IBVs, as well as by mutations of the genome. Many different IBV variants are recognized both on the basis of antigenic variation, determined by virus neutralization (VN) tests, and increasingly by molecular analysis of the genome (genotyping). Variants of economic importance include: Massachusetts, which is the serotype most commonly found worldwide; Connecticut, Arkansas and Delaware 072 from the USA; T from Australia; D274; D1466; 793B (4/91); B1648; Italian 02 from Europe, and so on. IBVs in Australia have evolved in their own distinct lineages and other areas, for example parts of south-east Asia, have their own unique IBV variants, as well as ones found in other parts of the world. The number of new IBV variants continues to increase as simpler methods for their detection become available. While these different variants are important epidemiologically, their significance in terms of control of infection is less clear. This is because new variants are defined by a very small number of amino acid changes, so that the majority of the genome is conserved.

In addition to antigenic variation within IBVs, variations in virulence are now reported. There have been reports from the USA and Europe of IBV strains with increased virulence compared with previous isolates of the same serotype. There may also be variations in pathogenesis. One such example of this is the 793B (4/91) variant, which has been associated with both muscle myopathy and scouring in broilers, as well as with mortality in adult breeding hens. More recently a variant IBV isolated in Europe, designated D388 (QX), has been associated with 'false layers'.

Hosts

Although domestic fowl have usually been regarded as the exclusive host of IBV, there are reports of IBV isolations from other avian species. In turkeys, coronaviruses (TCoV, also called *Bluecomb disease virus* and *Turkey enteric coronavirus*) are known to be associated with enteric disease, mortality and underperformance and to affect egg-laying performance in older birds. In pheasants, coronaviruses have been associated with respiratory disease and renal problems. Sequence data for coronaviruses from turkeys and pheasants show them to be at least as closely related to IBV as different IBV strains may be to each other and it is clear that the host range of IBV itself extends beyond the chicken.

In the last few years, possibly as a result of renewed interest in coronaviruses with the emergence of the severe acute respiratory syndrome (SARS) virus, coronaviruses have been reported in other gallinaceous birds, including partridge, guinea fowl and peafowl, as well as in nongallinaceous birds such as teal (in this case, the virus was possibly an IBV that had spread from nearby chickens). In some cases, analysis of the genome of these coronaviruses has shown them to be IBV, and examples exist to indicate both reisolation of a vaccine strain and isolation of a virulent field strain. However, some recent coronavirus isolates from gallinaceous birds, for example mallard duck and a pigeon, have two small extra genes near the 3' end of the genome, indicating that they cannot be classified as IBV and may represent new species. This is a new area of investigation and, while the coronaviruses detected in some gallinaceous and nongallinaceous birds have not so far been associated with disease, these species are potential carriers of IBV and other coronaviruses and could therefore play a role in global transmission of infection.

Avian coronaviruses are not known to pose any human health risk.

Spread

IBV is highly infectious and only a few virus particles may initiate an infection. After a short incubation period of 1–3 days, bird-to-bird transmission occurs rapidly and signs are seen in most birds in a susceptible flock. Virus is shed via both the respiratory tract and the faeces and a high standard of biosecurity is essential to minimize both entry of infection to a flock and spread between flocks. The virus may be shed for several weeks after clinical recovery and can persist in the intestinal tract for several months. The virus is rapidly killed by common disinfectants but its survival in the environment has not been adequately studied. Direct airborne transmission of virus from the respiratory tract to susceptible birds is probably the most common method of spread, particularly when respiratory signs are present. However, transmission through infected faeces is also important and spread by fomites certainly occurs. The greatest source of infection is birds in which virus is rapidly replicating. While true egg transmission is not believed to be significant, surface contamination of eggs is likely to occur. Because the virus may persist in the bird for many weeks, carrier birds may exist. There is no evidence for the involvement of vectors in IBV transmission.

DIAGNOSIS

Clinical signs

Respiratory signs are the first and most common clinical manifestation in birds of all ages and include tracheal rales, gasping, sneezing, watery nasal discharge, sometimes accompanied by

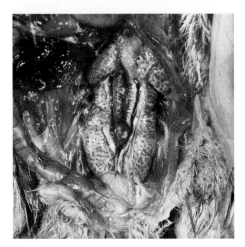

Fig. 28.2 Kidneys of a chicken experimentally infected with an *Infectious bronchitis virus* isolate capable of causing nephritis.

lacrimation, and facial swelling. Generally birds appear huddled and depressed; food conversion and weight gain are usually affected. Mortality is generally negligible in the uncomplicated disease, except in very young chicks and in the absence of maternal antibody. However, significant morbidity and mortality may occur as a result of secondary bacterial infection. The uncomplicated disease may last 10–14 days but secondary infection may increase the duration.

Renal problems caused by IBV often follow an initial respiratory infection in broilers. Affected birds, commonly at 3–6 weeks of age, show depression, scouring and wet litter, associated with increased water intake. In the mild form there may be little or no mortality, but mortality can reach 30%. The kidneys are often pale, swollen and blotchy and the distended tubules are white, because of the presence of urates (Fig. 28.2).

In IBV infection of commercial layers or broiler breeders, respiratory signs may or may not be observed and the most common manifestation is the effect on egg production and egg quality. Flocks infected prior to or during lay are affected. In unprotected flocks, the drop in egg production may exceed 50%. However, in birds that have received a complete vaccination programme but are challenged with field strains against which those vaccines do not provide complete protection, the disease may present as failure to lay at the full potential or production falls of up to approximately 10% (Fig. 28.3). Production may take 4–6 weeks to return to normal, or this may never be achieved.

As production begins to increase, deterioration in external and internal egg quality is seen. Eggs may be smaller than normal; they may be misshapen or show ridging. The shells may be depigmented, some becoming almost completely white (Fig. 28.4), or have calcareous deposits. Eggs are often very thin-shelled or completely shell-less. Internally, the albumen loses its viscosity ('watery whites') and the chalazae are often broken so that the yolk floats free. Small haemorrhages may be seen in the albumen or yolk. Some birds in an infected flock may lay normally, despite showing respiratory signs.

It has been known for many years that infection of very young, susceptible chicks with a particularly virulent IBV strain may be followed by aberrant oviduct development. There may be partial, or almost complete absence of the duct, or vestiges that are nonpatent or cystic. At maturity affected birds may ovulate normally, with the ova then being shed into the body cavity. Such birds go through the motions of oviposition but fail to lay ('blind or false layers'). Sometimes

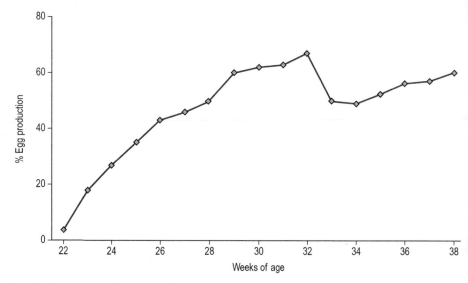

Fig. 28.3 Egg production (%) of a flock of laying hens vaccinated against infectious bronchitis from which a variant *Infectious bronchitis virus* was isolated at 32 weeks of age. (Redrawn with permission of Taylor & Francis from Cook J K A 1984 The classification of new serotypes of infectious bronchitis virus isolated from poultry flocks in Britain between 1981–1983. Avian Pathol 13: 733–741; www.tandf.co.uk/journals)

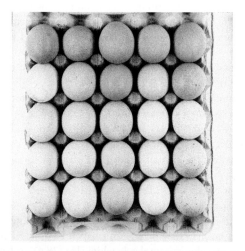

Fig. 28.4 Eggs laid by different hens (columns) prior to inoculation with a variant *Infectious bronchitis virus* (top row) and between 2 and 7 days later (rows 2 to 5). (Reproduced with permission of Taylor & Francis from Cook J K A, Huggins M B 1986 Newly isolated serotypes of infectious bronchitis virus: their role in disease. Avian Pathol 15: 129–138; www.tandf.co.uk/journals)

ova pass along a patent but abnormal oviduct, giving eggs of reduced shell and albumen quality. Until recently, there was little evidence to suggest that this phenomenon was a significant problem under normal commercial conditions. However, since 2004, there have been reports from parts of Europe of poor egg production in otherwise apparently healthy flocks, but in which some hens may present with a pendulous abdomen. In such cases, ovaries may appear to be normal and functional, whereas the oviduct is thin-walled and frequently contains large, watery cysts. A novel IBV variant (designated D388 or QX) has been detected in a number of such cases; however, experimental reproduction of the condition with this isolate has yet to be reported.

Lesions

Gross lesions

These include excess mucus in the trachea, nasal cavity and sinuses, accompanied by inflammation and catarrhal exudate that may become caseous. This may lead to formation of mucoid plugs of pus in the primary or secondary bronchi, frequently causing asphyxia. Lungs may be congested and air sac walls may be cloudy and thickened, often with yellow, caseous exudate.

In infected layers, the oviduct may appear normal. However, deposits of yolk may accumulate in the abdomen: so called 'egg peritonitis'.

Histological lesions

Within about 18 h of infection, the trachea and bronchi show loss of cilia with epithelial hyperplasia and metaplasia, often with sloughing of the surface cells. Subepithelial thickening is marked, with oedema and massive monocyte and lymphocyte infiltration of the lamina propria and loss of mucous glands.

Disease of the mature oviduct results in regression in size with metaplasia of the epithelium, glandular dilatation, infiltration of subepithelial tissues with monocytes and proliferation of lymphoid follicles and later fibroplasia. When aberrant oviduct development follows infection with a highly virulent strain at a very young age, there is hypoplasia of the epithelium and tubular glands and the lumen may be obliterated.

In renal infections, interstitial lymphocytic infiltration occurs, with granular degeneration, vacuolation and necrosis of the tubular epithelium, together with accumulation of urates and necrotic material in the lumen. In the ureters there is metaplasia and necrosis of the epithelium with sloughing into the lumen. Visceral gout is sometimes seen.

Host factors

Some innate increase in resistance to infectious bronchitis infection occurs with increasing age. The immune status of the host influences protection, and both maternal immunity and active immunity, resulting from natural infection or vaccination, may prevent or reduce disease and limit virus excretion. Experimental data suggest that there are differences between inbred lines of chicken in their susceptibility to IBV infection, but there are no data to suggest that this extends to commercial breeds. There is evidence that onset of lay (probably associated with hormonal changes) can cause re-excretion of virus that has been latent in the host following an earlier infection.

Factors influencing disease

In young chickens, particularly broilers where stocking density is highest, infection with other pathogens may result in more severe and prolonged respiratory disease. Such pathogens include *Newcastle disease virus*, *Infectious laryngotracheitis virus*, avian pneumoviruses, bacteria such as *Haemophilus paragallinarum* or *Escherichia coli*, and *Mycoplasma gallisepticum* or *Mycoplasma synoviae*. Chilling in brooding chicks can exacerbate the disease, as can poor ventilation and build-up of ammonia levels in the shed. Immunosuppressive agents, such as *Infectious bursal disease virus*, may reduce the protective immune response to vaccination or field challenge. In the nephritic form of the disease, some breeds appear to be more severely affected and a high-protein diet is an exacerbating factor.

Clinical diagnosis

The clinical features and gross and histological lesions are not diagnostic. The respiratory infection may resemble diseases caused by other pathogens, either alone or as part of a multifactorial disease syndrome. Poor egg production and quality may be caused by many infectious and noninfectious factors, including poor management. There are also other causes of abnormal oviduct development, and kidney disease may be associated with nutritional deficiencies or be of unknown cause. Therefore, proof of IBV infection depends on detecting either the virus itself or an increase in specific antibody levels in serum.

Virus isolation/detection

The detection of IBV in respiratory tract tissues is easiest in the early stages of infection, when virus is replicating most rapidly. Beyond about 7–10 days after infection virus is difficult to isolate. At later stages, or when cases of aberrant egg production are being investigated, faeces, intestinal tract tissue (possibly caecal tonsil) or kidney are the material of choice for virus isolation attempts. Oviduct is not a rewarding site from which to attempt IBV isolation. Sentinel birds have been used successfully to aid the isolation of IBV. Specific-pathogen-free (SPF) chickens, possibly vaccinated against the IBV serotypes common to the area, are introduced into a flock and sampled at weekly intervals thereafter.

For attempted virus isolation from field material, the most successful systems are embryonated chicken eggs inoculated via the allantoic route or chick embryo tracheal organ cultures (TOCs). Material is homogenized with broth containing antibiotics and centrifuged or filtered to remove debris and contaminants. The material is then inoculated into the allantoic cavity of 9–11-day embryonated chicken eggs or into TOCs. Following embryo inoculation, IBV if present, will cause characteristic embryo dwarfing and curling by the 18th day of incubation, but several 'blind' passages, to allow embryo adaptation of the virus, may be required. Three or four passages are therefore usually given before a sample is discarded as negative, making it an expensive and time-consuming procedure. In TOCs, IBV causes ciliostasis within 2–3 days of inoculation. This is easily observed by low-power microscopy. As with embryo inoculation, two or three passages at 1–2-day intervals may be necessary. The identity of the virus isolated in either system should be confirmed. This may be achieved by examining centrifuged allantoic fluid or TOC supernatant by electron microscopy, immunochemical assays, antigen-detecting enzyme-linked immunosorbent assays (ELISAs) or increasingly by using molecular methods. By incorporating serotype-specific monoclonal antibodies into an assay it is possible to identify the IBV serotype involved.

In situations where it is not essential to actually obtain an isolate of the virus, IBV may be detected by immunochemical assays (immunofluorescence or immunoperoxidase using an anti-IBV serum) and increasingly by molecular methods. These involve the reverse-transcription polymerase chain reaction (RT-PCR) together with restriction enzyme fragment length polymorphism (RFLP) analysis, DNA probes or nucleic acid sequencing. They are increasingly used for the detection of IBVs generally, as well as for the differentiation of specific variants. These techniques have also facilitated molecular epidemiological studies to monitor the distribution of specific variants. While direct sequencing of the genome is the most accurate method for identifying new variants, RFLP, which identifies sites unique to a particular serotype, is acceptable and has provided a rapid method for variant identification. The RNA required for these techniques can be extracted directly from either swab material or appropriate tissues of infected birds, or from allantoic fluid or TOC supernatant of samples from which virus isolation is being attempted. Since viral nucleic acid is what is being detected, it is not necessary for live virus to be present and RT-PCR probably detects the presence of IBV for longer than is possible by virus isolation methods. While, for many purposes, the lack of a live virus is not a problem, for epidemiological studies and for further research, the availability of an isolate could be necessary.

For use in genome analysis, universal oligonucleotide primer sets, designed to detect all known IBVs, as well as ones designed to detect only specific serotypes, have been developed. Initially these were based on sequence data from parts of the spike protein gene. However, as this is the part of the genome showing the most variation, sequence data from parts of the membrane and nucleoprotein genes have also been used. More recently, effort has concentrated on the use of the 3' end of the genome, an area known to be conserved in coronaviruses. By so doing, it is hoped to develop assays that will detect and differentiate not only IBV strains but also novel coronaviruses of other avian species.

Molecular techniques give results more quickly than virus isolation methods. However, their sensitivity means that great care is needed to avoid contamination of reagents and the tests should be performed only in a dedicated laboratory where a high level of technical expertise is available.

Serology

The methods available to detect IBV antibodies include agar gel precipitation (AGP), haemagglutination inhibition (HI), immunofluorescence, ELISA and VN. The VN test is the most reliable test for identifying and differentiating IBV variants but is time-consuming and expensive and is only performed when it is important to identify the particular serotype involved in an outbreak, or for epidemiological studies. It can be performed in indicator systems such as chicken embryos, TOCs, or avian cell culture using a cell-culture-adapted virus. The HI test is a simple and reliable test but the virus must first be treated with an appropriate enzyme. When performed carefully with appropriate controls, the HI test can differentiate between responses to particular serotypes. However, following exposure to more than one IBV serotype, differentiation by HI becomes unreliable. The other assays all detect group-specific antibodies. The AGP test is simple to perform but relatively insensitive. Some birds never develop precipitins while in others they are present for only a few weeks. For this reason, the only advantage of this test is that a positive result indicates recent exposure to the virus. The ELISA detects all known IBV serotypes and therefore cannot be used to identify particular variants. It is the most commonly used test for monitoring responses to vaccination and to indicate possible field challenge. Because of the availability of reliable commercial kits, it is widely used for flock screening.

CONTROL

Attention to management factors, such as temperature and ventilation, are essential, particularly in controlling the effects of secondary bacterial infection. The use of antimicrobials may also be beneficial against secondary infections. However, drug therapy is of no value in controlling the virus. While strict biosecurity is an important part of disease control, because IBV is ubiquitous and spreads rapidly it is impossible to exclude it completely by hygienic means. Thus control depends on increasing the resistance of the bird by vaccination.

Live attenuated and inactivated (oil-adjuvanted) vaccines are highly effective and widely used. The live attenuated vaccines are used to prevent and control infection in young birds and to 'prime' future breeders and layers prior to administration of inactivated vaccines. It is important to remember that, for inactivated vaccines to be effective, chickens must have been 'primed' with a live vaccine. To achieve optimal benefit from the inactivated vaccine, at least 4–6 weeks should elapse between the last application of live vaccine and administration of the inactivated vaccine. Ideally the live vaccine should contain IBV serotypes that will stimulate protection against the variants existing in a particular area. The Massachusetts serotype is the one most commonly included but, depending on local circumstances, other serotypes, where this is permitted by the regulatory authorities, may be included in order to optimize protection. Frequently, two or more applications of live attenuated vaccine are given, often varying the serotype of IBV in the later vaccinations.

Despite the apparent protective effect of maternally derived immunity in very young chicks, live vaccines can be administered successfully from 1 day of age by coarse spray, beak dipping or nasal or eye drop. Older birds may be vaccinated via the drinking water, by eye drop or coarse spray. Different vaccination protocols are available, designed for different types of bird (see Ch. 5) but the most important point is to ensure that the vaccine is carefully and correctly administered so that each bird receives the required dose. Whatever protocol is followed, a highly attenuated live virus vaccine is given initially. For broilers this is likely to be given in the hatchery by coarse spray. Revaccination of broilers, possibly at 2–3 weeks of age, is now common practice in some areas. In order that protection against both infectious bronchitis and Newcastle disease may be achieved by one application of vaccine, the two vaccines may be combined. Because of the risk that, if it is present in excess, the infectious bronchitis vaccine may interfere with the response to the Newcastle disease vaccine, the use of a combined product is preferable to the use of two separate vaccines given together. For future breeders or layers, the first vaccination is usually given at about 3 weeks of age, in the drinking water or by spray, and may be followed by one or more further applications of live attenuated vaccine. Before onset of lay an inactivated vaccine is given intramuscularly or subcutaneously. Increasingly, the inactivated vaccine is likely to be a multivalent one containing possibly two different IBV antigens, as well as antigens to other important poultry pathogens.

Excellent protection against homologous challenge is obtained, provided that vaccination is carried out carefully. However, there is now increasing evidence that licensed vaccines provide heterologous protection against challenge with some different IBV serotypes or variants, although it is not currently possible to predict when this might occur based on either serotyping or genotyping. Recent data suggest that, if two antigenically distinct live-attenuated IBV vaccines are applied, preferably separated by at least 2 weeks, good protection may be achieved against challenge with a range of heterologous IBV serotypes. This is probably because of the very small number of amino acid differences between different serotypes or variants in the immunity-inducing part of the virus.

Although a high antibody titre following vaccination or natural infection is indicative of protection, particularly against the homologous strain of IBV, a low titre, even against homologous strains, may not indicate poor protection. This is because local and cell-mediated immunity are very important in protecting against IBV challenge but are difficult to measure by currently available methods. Locally produced antibody in the upper respiratory tract is the important first line of defence against IBV challenges. It is therefore very important that the live attenuated infectious bronchitis vaccines are applied very carefully to ensure good, even stimulation of local antibody in every bird.

FURTHER READING

Bijlenga G, Cook J K A, Gelb J Jr, de Wit J J 2004 Development and use of the H strain of avian infectious bronchitis virus from the Netherlands as a vaccine. A review. Avian Pathol 33: 550–557

Cavanagh D 2005 Coronaviruses in poultry and other birds. Avian Pathol 34: 439–448

Cavanagh D, Naqi SA 2003 Infectious bronchitis. In: Saif Y M (ed) Diseases of poultry, 7th edn. Iowa State University Press, Ames, p 1101–1119

Cook J K A, Mockett A P A 1995 Epidemiology of infectious bronchitis virus. In: Siddell S G (ed) The Coronaviridae. Plenum Press, New York, p 317–335

De Wit J J 2000 Detection of infectious bronchitis. Technical review. Avian Pathol 29: 71–93

Guy J S Turkey coronavirus enteritis. In: Saif Y M (ed) Diseases of poultry, 7th edn. Iowa State University Press, Ames, p 300–307

Ignjatovic J, Sapats S 2000 Avian infectious bronchitis virus. Rev Sci Tech 19: 493–508

Kaleta E, Heffels-Redmann U (eds) 2006 Proceedings of the international symposium on avain corona- and pneumoviruses and complicating pathogens, Rauischholzhausen, Germany

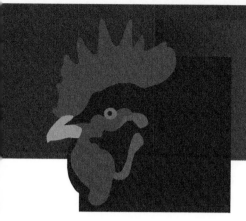

CHAPTER 29

Richard E. Gough and
M. Stewart McNulty

Picornaviridae

The family *Picornaviridae* contains small, 22–30 nm, non-enveloped, icosahedral, single-stranded RNA viruses and is divided into nine genera. No virus isolated from avian species has been assigned to these genera, although avian encephalomyelitis has tentatively been placed in the *Hepatovirus* genus. A number of viruses that are pathogenic for chickens, turkeys and ducks have been provisionally identified as picornaviruses and, on the basis of their biological characteristics, are considered to be most like viruses of the *Enterovirus* genus. However, these viruses are poorly characterized and their true taxonomic status has not been determined. They include the causal viruses of duck virus hepatitis type 1, turkey viral hepatitis and others.

AVIAN ENCEPHALOMYELITIS (EPIDEMIC TREMOR) VIRUS

The first record of avian encephalomyelitis was published in 1932 and concerned an outbreak in baby chicks in the USA 2 years earlier. The disease in chickens is now worldwide and was recognized in turkey poults in 1968. The natural disease has also been recognized in pheasants, Japanese quail and pigeons. Its economic significance stems from disease in chicks (paralysis, ataxia and muscular dystrophy), reduced egg production of a temporary nature in laying hens and an accompanying lowered hatchability of fertile eggs.

EPIDEMIOLOGY

Cause

Avian encephalomyelitis virus (AEV) has physical and chemical properties consistent with those of enteroviruses of the family *Picornaviridae*. However, recent characterization of its genome indicates that it is more closely related to *Hepatitis A virus* than to enteroviruses, and it has now been provisionally classified as a tentative species in the genus *Hepatovirus* in the family *Picornaviridae*. All strains seem to be antigenically uniform but there are variations in neurotropism and irulence. Field strains are mainly enterotropic while fowl-embryo-adapted strains such as the Van Roekel (VR) strain are mainly neurotropic and are much more likely to kill embryos. The virus s relatively resistant to physical and chemical agents but there is little published information on ts susceptibility to disinfectants.

Hosts

The natural host range is limited to chickens, turkeys, Japanese quail, pheasants and pigeons. In addition, ducklings and guinea fowl are susceptible to experimental infection, while mice, guinea pigs, rabbits and monkeys are refractory. It seems to be of no significance to public health although other species of virus belonging to the *Hepatovirus* genus cause disease in mammals.

Spread

The humoral immune status of the host appears to be the main factor influencing the outcome of infection. Maternal antibody can protect young birds against systemic infection and it generally becomes increasingly difficult to produce disease in chicks as they become older. This is attributed to increasing immunocompetence with age and the development of a protective humoral response. However, recent field observations have shown that chickens vaccinated by the oral route at 14 weeks of age may develop typical central nervous system lesions and clinical signs within 2–5 weeks of vaccination. It is considered that immunosuppression may have predisposed the birds to the clinical signs of disease in this instance. In birds infected or vaccinated during the rearing period, the immune response to natural infection or vaccination prevents subsequent egg transmission of the virus and provides protective maternal immunity that lasts through the highly susceptible period of the life of the young bird. When susceptible birds are infected after they come into lay, transmission of the virus occurs through the egg, and spreads horizontally from vertically infected to susceptible stock housed together and through fomites. Egg transmission occurs during the period from the infection of susceptible laying hens to the development of flock immunity: a period of 3–4 weeks. Transmission of infection from vertically infected to susceptible chicks can occur in the hatchery and during brooding and in older stock. It has been suggested that some infected birds become enteric carriers of the virus and excrete virus in their droppings for extended periods. The comparative resistance of the virus to physical inactivation also supports indirect spread through fomites.

In the pathogenesis of the condition the virus enters the tissues from the infected egg in vertically infected chicks, while the oral route is most probable after hatching. In very young chicks the virus may be disseminated over a variety of tissues, including the brain, viscera and muscles. A proportion of infected embryos may be killed during the last few days of incubation; most of those that hatch show signs at 1–7 days of age. For those infected after hatching, the incubation period is at least 11 days. Thus the disease pattern may involve a reduction in hatchability, clinical signs in vertically infected chicks, which appear during the first 10 days of life, and signs in those infected after hatching, which are seen at 2–5 weeks. Although infection may be generalized following entry of the virus at any age, disease of the nervous system is normally seen only in the first few weeks of life.

DIAGNOSIS

The clinical signs in young birds, the absence of gross lesions and the histological lesions in the brain, spinal cord and viscera, together with the absence of other virus infections and nutritional deficiencies affecting the nervous system, are strongly suggestive of avian encephalomyelitis and are frequently used for routine presumptive diagnosis.

In differential diagnosis it is necessary to consider other causes of neurological disorders, such as nutritional encephalomalacia and virus infections such as Newcastle disease, Marek's disease, and equine encephalomyelitis and infectious meningoencephalomyelitis of turkeys, both of which are restricted geographically.

A definitive diagnosis of avian encephalomyelitis requires demonstration of the virus by isolation or by other means.

Signs

Clinical signs include depression, ataxia and tremors in chicks and some depression in egg production in layers, with reduced hatchability. Opacity of the lens, either unilateral or bilateral, occurs in relatively few survivors of a diseased flock and is thought to be caused by the virus. The nervous signs may be seen at or soon after hatching but are more commonly first seen at 1 week of age. The ataxia varies from slight incoordination to sitting on the hocks and lateral recumbency, when death results from inanition or trampling by other members of the flock. Very mildly affected birds may recover completely. Tremors may be absent from some outbreaks or may occur in only a few birds in an affected flock. They usually follow the initial stages of incoordination and may be confined to the head and neck, or be observed over the whole body. Some affected birds emit a plaintive cheep. Morbidity may be as high as 60% but is more commonly 15% of the flock, but mortality in affected birds is high. Fresh cases rarely occur after 5–6 weeks of age but avian encephalomyelitis has been reported in birds of more than 17 weeks. They showed paralysis of the legs and increased flock mortality of 0.2–1% per week.

In layers the fall in egg production is about 5–10% and lasts for 5–14 days, with return to full potential production at the end of this time. The fall in hatchability accompanying the depression in production is about 5% of fertile eggs. In turkey poults and turkey hens the corresponding clinical signs are usually less severe. Clinical signs associated with natural infection of pigeons include paralysis of the wings, opisthotonos, torticollis and head tremor, particularly in birds up to 3 months of age. In adult birds diarrhoea also features.

Lesions

There are no gross lesions in the young or older bird apart from rare pale areas in the gizzard muscle of chicks and opacity and fixation of the lens in a small proportion of survivors. Histologically there are lesions in the brain, spinal cord (but not the peripheral nerves) and viscera. Gliosis occurs in the molecular layer of the cerebellum as nodular aggregates. More diffuse gliosis is seen in the brainstem and midbrain and these changes, together with central chromatolysis of neurones in these areas, are considered by some to be almost pathognomonic. Neuronal degeneration is seen in Purkinje cells and neurones throughout the brain and spinal cord, especially in the pons, medulla oblongata and ventral horn cells of the cord. Perivascular cuffing with small lymphocytes is seen throughout the central nervous system and foci of infiltrating lymphocytes are seen in the dorsal root ganglia and in the proventriculus, gizzard, pancreas and other viscera. Similar lesions have been described in pigeons naturally infected with AEV.

Virus isolation/detection

For virus isolation a suspension of brain, pancreas or duodenum from affected chicks is inoculated into the yolk sac of 5–6-day-old susceptible chick embryos. Eggs are candled daily and

12 days after inoculation some of the embryos are examined for gross signs of AEV infection, consisting of inertia, muscular dystrophy and occasional mortality. Virus neutralization tests in embryonated eggs, using extracts of brain suspension from affected embryos and AEV mono-specific antiserum, have been used to confirm the identity of the virus. The remaining embryos are hatched and during the first 10 days of life the chicks are observed for typical clinical signs of avian encephalomyelitis.

Examination of smears from the brain or cryostat sections stained by direct immunofluorescence may also be used to demonstrate virus; positive results are confirmatory but negative results are often unreliable. Increased sensitivity and specificity have been obtained by including an AEV monoclonal antibody in the assay.

A nested polymerase chain reaction (PCR) has been described for the detection of AEV RNA in chicken embryos and in vaccinated chickens. However, the PCR is not yet routinely used in the diagnosis of AEV infection.

Serology

A number of serological tests are available for determining the presence of infection. A virus neutralization (VN) test involves the inoculation of dilutions of an egg-adapted strain of virus alone and virus together with serum into susceptible chick embryos. By this means the neutralizing index of the serum can be determined and an index of $\log_{10}$ 1.1 or greater is considered positive. The test may be made on acute and convalescent paired sera from birds showing a fall in egg production. A rise in titre indicates recent infection. Another method of demonstrating specific antibody is the embryo susceptibility test: 36–48 eggs from a flock are incubated for 6 days and then each live embryo is inoculated into the yolk sac with 100 EID_{50} (infective dose for 50%) of VR virus. The embryos are incubated for a further 12 days and examined. If fewer than 50% of them show muscular dystrophy the flock is considered to be immune. An indirect immunofluorescence test, immunodiffusion and an enzyme-linked immunosorbent assay (ELISA) have also been developed and compare favourably with the VN test. Because of its specificity and sensitivity, rapidity of performance and amenability to large-scale screening, the ELISA has replaced other tests for antibody, including the assessment of efficiency of vaccination.

CONTROL

Drug therapy is of no value and under commercial conditions it is impracticable to attempt the elimination of infection by high standards of hygiene. Thus control is dependent on the vaccination of stock. Live and inactivated vaccines are available. Live vaccines are more commonly used; these can be given by mass administration, usually in the drinking water, and stimulate a durable and adequate degree of protection.

Vaccination is undertaken to protect primarily against egg transmission of the virus and consequent disease in the progeny, and against a fall in egg production and hatchability. Commercial layers are often unvaccinated, since the total fall in egg production is small. The age at which birds are vaccinated with live vaccine should be chosen so that the virus will not produce adverse effects or fail to stimulate immunity. During the first 6 weeks of life live vaccine may produce disease, and during the first 8 weeks maternal antibody may interfere with the immune response. Live vaccine given to birds in lay may cause egg transmission and disease in the progeny. Thus, such vaccines are usually given between 8 and 16 weeks of age. A period of at least 2 weeks on either side of vaccination is allowed between this and the administration of other vaccines.

Vaccines similar to those used for chickens can be used for turkeys. In an outbreak in chicks or poults, affected birds are best destroyed, since most will succumb.

Inactivated vaccines may be used for protecting susceptible laying flocks that are close to or currently in lay without causing a fall in egg production as might occur with live vaccines. Although certain features of the spread of this infection are not understood, hygienic precautions such as cleaning and disinfection between flocks and disposal of carcasses and litter must be practised in order to limit, at least, the build-up and spread of virus.

FURTHER READING

Calnek B W 1993 Picornaviridae. In: McFerran J B, McNulty M S (eds) Virus infections of vertebrates, vol 4. Virus infections of birds. Elsevier, Amsterdam, p 465–478

Calnek B W 2003 Avian encephalomyelitis. In: Saif Y M (ed) Diseases of poultry, 11th edn. Iowa State Press, Ames, p 271–278

Calnek B W, Fabricant J 1981 Immunity to infectious avian encephalomyelitis. In: Rose M E et al (eds) Avian immunology. Poultry Science Symposium No. 16. British Poultry Science, Edinburgh, p 235–254

Marvil P, Knowles N J, Mockett A P A et al 1999 Avian encephalomyelitis virus is a picornavirus and is most closely related to hepatitis virus. J Virol 80: 653–662

Tannock G A, Shafren D R 1994 Avian encephalomyelitis virus: a review. Avian Pathol 23: 603–620

Todd D, Weston J H, Mawhinney K A et al 1999 Characterisation of the genome of avian encephalomyelitis virus with cloned cDNA fragments. Avian Dis 43: 219–226

DUCK VIRUS HEPATITIS

Duck virus hepatitis was first described in 1950, causing severe losses in ducklings in Long Island, New York, then the major duck-growing area of the USA. It has since been described in most important duck-growing areas of the world. The disease has usually become endemic in these regions.

Duck virus hepatitis is an acute, highly infectious viral disease of ducklings aged from 2 days to 3 weeks. Older ducklings may be diseased, particularly if affected by toxic substances or suboptimal nutrition, but adult stock are resistant. Age resistance to disease is essentially complete from 7 weeks of age.

EPIDEMIOLOGY

Cause

Three antigenically distinct viruses have been described that cause clinical signs and lesions sufficiently similar that they have been called *Duck hepatitis virus* (DVHV) type I, type II and type III.

The originally described classic duck hepatitis (type I) agent is probably a picornavirus, while type II virus is an astrovirus (see Chapter 33). Type III virus, described in the USA, is also probably a picornavirus but it has not been fully characterized. The type I virus is more widespread and more virulent than the type II and III viruses. The viruses belonging to types I and III do not cross-protect. DVHV type I is highly resistant to physical and chemical conditions and the virus can remain viable in the environment for long periods of time. Variant strains of the virus have been reported from several countries.

Hosts

While experimental infection has been described in other poultry species, natural infections with type I virus have been reported only in ducks.

Spread

Type I and type III viruses remain viable for many weeks in faeces, etc., and it is therefore probable that infection follows the ingestion by susceptible ducklings of virus from the environment. Spread between sites is probably by means of contaminated equipment, vehicles and personnel. Egg transmission is not thought to occur.

Within a flock the disease spreads rapidly to all susceptible ducklings.

DIAGNOSIS

Signs

Signs of type I infection are peracute and death usually follows within an hour of their onset. Affected birds are often in good condition but start to lose contact with the main flock. Soon they fall over on their sides and, after a short struggle, with paddling movements of the legs, the birds die. The head is usually stretched upwards and backwards (opisthotonos; Fig. 29.1). The mortality rate may be over 90% of the flock, although in the endemic situation a 5–10% loss is more common. The highest losses occur in ducklings less than 7 days of age. Signs of type III virus infection are similar, but less severe, with mortality usually below 30%.

Any disease causing sudden death in young ducklings must be considered for differential diagnosis, the main ones being duck virus enteritis, bacterial septicaemia, coccidiosis and mycotoxicosis.

Lesions

The main lesions are in the liver (Fig. 29.2), which is enlarged and has a number of petechial and ecchymotic haemorrhages. In older birds, a bacterial septicaemia may be superimposed,

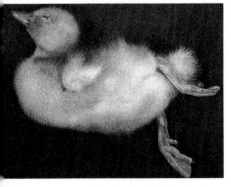

Fig. 29.1 A young duckling that has died from duck virus hepatitis. Note the typical position of opisthotonos and the cleanliness of the down and feet.

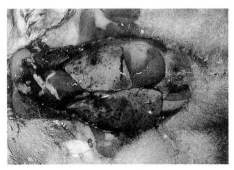

Fig. 29.2 Young duckling showing typical liver lesions of duck virus hepatitis.

although the liver haemorrhages should still be evident. In addition, fatty kidneys described as duck fatty kidney syndrome may be caused by DVHV.

Virus isolation

The sudden onset of a disease causing high mortality in young ducklings, the opisthotonos of the dead bird and the characteristic liver haemorrhages are together sufficient to justify the diagnosis of duck virus hepatitis. Laboratory diagnosis of type I virus infection is based on virus isolation following the inoculation of blood or organ suspension from affected ducklings into the allantoic sac of 9-day-old embryonating chicken eggs or 10- to 14-day-old duck embryos. Most embryos die within 6 days of infection. Rapid diagnosis using direct immunofluorescence may be made on the livers of affected ducklings. Type III virus can be isolated following inoculation of liver suspensions on to the chorioallantoic membrane (CAM) of duck embryos. Susceptible 1-day-old ducklings and duck cell cultures have also been used for virus isolation. Molecular techniques have not been described for the detection of DVHV type 1 in clinical material.

Serology

Serological tests have not proved useful in diagnosis of type I DVHV. Neutralization tests in embryonated chicken eggs can be used to detect antibodies in convalescent serum samples and to determine the response to vaccination.

CONTROL

Immunization of breeders with live attenuated vaccines provides maternally derived antibodies that prevent high mortality in young ducklings due to DVHV types I and III. Multiple vaccinations of breeders with attenuated type I virus are often required, both during the rearing period and continuing throughout lay. In some cases, breeder vaccination is augmented by passive immunization of their progeny using convalescent duck sera or egg antibodies derived from hyperimmunized fowl; this procedure has also been used to control outbreaks in the progeny of unvaccinated breeders.

Experimental inactivated, adjuvanted type I vaccines for breeders have also been used successfully; priming with live vaccines gave best results.

Vaccination of newly hatched ducklings with a single dose of live attenuated type I vaccine has also been used. These vaccines have been administered by a variety of routes, including foot web stab, subcutaneous, intramuscular, aerosol spray and drinking water. This strategy is dependent on the ducklings being fully susceptible (i.e. free from maternal antibodies) and on their being exposed to fairly low doses of virus following development of active immunity. Live vaccines readily revert to virulence following passage in susceptible ducklings.

In theory, the disease can be prevented by rearing ducklings in strict isolation; in practice this is very difficult to achieve.

FURTHER READING

Crighton G W, Woolcock P R 1978 Active immunization of ducklings against duck virus hepatitis. Vet Rec 102: 358–361

Woolcock P R 2003 Duck virus hepatitis. In: Saif Y M (ed) Diseases of poultry, 11th edn. Iowa State Press, Ames, p 343–354

OTHER AVIAN ENTEROVIRUS-LIKE VIRUSES

A number of other enterovirus-like viruses have been detected in samples from several avian species, including chickens, turkeys, guinea fowl, pheasants, partridge, ostriches and psittacine species. In most cases virus particles have been observed by electron microscopic examination of intestinal contents or faeces and attempted propagation of the viruses has not generally been successful. However, several enterovirus-like viruses from chickens and turkeys have been isolated and propagated in the yolk sac and CAM of embryonated chicken and turkey eggs and partially characterized. They include isolates from the faeces of a broiler chicken, designated 84-700, from the meconium of dead-in-shell chicks from flocks with runting stunting syndrome, designated FP3, and from broilers with respiratory disease, designated 612. These isolates are antigenically unrelated to each other by cross-immunofluorescence or to AEV and duck hepatitis viruses.

Antibodies to 612 and FP3 viruses are widely distributed in chickens in the UK. However, although 84-700 was isolated from chicken faeces, serological studies have shown that antibodies to 84-700 are widespread in turkeys.

Turkey enterovirus-like viruses have been isolated from turkey poults with enteric problems in the USA and France. The US viruses are the best characterized and some of these are now known to be astroviruses.

Enterovirus-like viruses from chickens and turkeys have been associated with a variety of conditions, including transmissible enteritis, runting and stunting syndrome and baby chick nephropathy. Experimental transmission studies with some of these isolates resulted in histopathological lesions of varying severity in the small intestine and the kidneys.

Horizontal spread occurs readily, probably through ingestion of faecally contaminated material and vertical transmission through the egg probably occurs with most of these viruses.

With the development and availability of molecular techniques it is probable that more enterovirus-like viruses will be detected and fully characterized in the future. Recent molecular investigations have already resulted in several viruses, formerly referred to as 'enterovirus-like viruses' (*Avian nephritis virus*, turkey small round viruses and entero-like viruses), being classified as species of *Astrovirus*. Indeed, it may transpire that more of the enterovirus-like viruses detected by electron microscopy in the past are in fact astroviruses.

There is no evidence suggesting that these viruses are transmissible from avian species to humans or other mammals. Their transmissibility between avian species is also unknown.

Vaccines and other specific control measures are not available.

TURKEY VIRAL HEPATITIS

Turkey viral hepatitis is an acute, highly contagious disease of turkeys. It has been recognized in the USA, Canada, Italy and the UK. Outbreaks are usually seen in turkeys under 6 weeks of age. The condition is usually diagnosed only at post-mortem examination, when lesions are seen in the liver and sometimes the pancreas. Liver lesions are macroscopic pale foci 1–2 mm in diameter, occurring on the surface and in the parenchyma of the liver. Foci represent focal necrosis of hepatocytes and infiltration with mononuclear cells. Electron microscopic examination of degenerating hepatocytes has revealed the presence of intracytoplasmic aggregates of enterovirus-like viruses. The causal virus is currently classified as an unassigned virus in the family *Picornaviridae*. Turkey viral hepatitis is often subclinical but disease may be precipitated by stress. Depression, anorexia and increased mortality are the main signs. Morbidity can be very high but mortality is normally low and occurs for only 1–2 weeks. Infection of laying turkeys may impair reproductive performance but deaths are not seen in birds over 6 weeks of age. Vertical transmission probably occurs.

The causal virus can be grown in the yolk sac of chicken and turkey embryos, but has not yet been grown in cell cultures. Infected embryos die, with subcutaneous oedema and congestion, and may be stunted. As these signs are nonspecific, confirmation that turkey viral hepatitis is present requires intraperitoneal inoculation of day-old turkey poults with yolk sac material harvested from dead embryos. If the virus is present, necropsy of the inoculated poults 6–9 days later should reveal typical liver lesions.

There are no effective treatments or control measures.

FURTHER READING

Guy J S 1998 Virus infections of the gastrointestinal tract of poultry. Poult Sci 77: 1166–1175

Guy J S 2003 Turkey viral hepatitis. In: Saif Y M (ed) Diseases of poultry, 11th edn. Iowa State Press, Ames, p 399–403

Macdonald J W, Randall C J, Dagless M D 1982 Picorna-like virus causing hepatitis and pancreatitis in turkeys. Vet Rec 111: 323

McFerran J B 1993 Avian enterovirus infections. In: McFerran J S, McNulty M S (eds) Virus infections of vertebrates, vol 4: Virus infections of birds. Elsevier Science, London, p 497–503

McNeilly F, Connor T J, Calvert V M et al 1994 Studies on a new enterovirus-like virus isolated from chickens. Avian Pathol 23: 313–327

McNulty M S, Guy J S 2003 Avian enterovirus-like viruses. In: Saif Y M (ed) Diseases of poultry, 11th edn. Iowa State Press, Ames, p 326–332

McNulty M S, Connor T J, McNeilly F et al 1990 Biological characterization of avian enteroviruses and enterovirus-like viruses. Avian Pathol 19: 75–87

Thierry van den Berg*

Birnaviridae

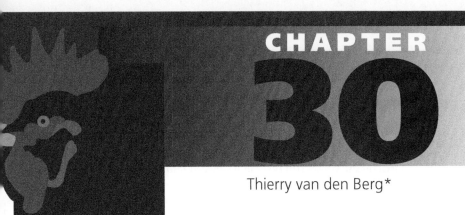

The virus responsible for infectious bursal disease (IBD) is a member of the *Avibirnavirus* genus, within the family Birnaviridae. It is non-enveloped with a single-shelled icosahedral capsid and has a diameter between 55 and 60 nm (Fig. 30.1). This relatively simple structure confers on the virus a high resistance in the outside environment, which represents a key issue in the control of the disease. The genome of the virus consists of two segments, A and B, of double-stranded RNA. Segment A encodes the viral structural proteins VP2 and VP3 as well as VP4, the viral protease, and VP5, a protein of regulatory function. As an external capsid protein, VP2 elicits the neutralizing antibody response and represents the molecular basis for antigenic variation whereas the internal capsid protein VP3 is more stable and induces group-specific antigens. Segment B

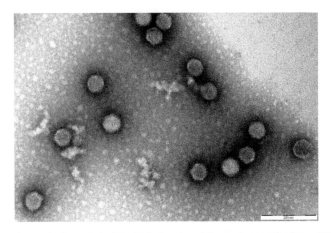

Fig. 30.1 Electron micrograph of negatively stained *Infectious bursal disease virus* particles (bar = 200 nm). (Courtesy of Dr J. Mast, VAR.)

* The author wishes to acknowledge the contribution of W. Baxendale, author of this chapter in the 5th edition.

encodes VP1, the viral polymerase, involved in replication and transcription of the virus and thus playing some role in the virulence of the virus.

EPIDEMIOLOGY

Cause

Infectious bursal disease viruses (IBDVs) can be divided into two main serotypes by neutralization tests. Within the serotype 1 group, there is considerable variation in virulence, from apathogenic to very virulent strains that may cause up to 50% mortality in a flock. These viruses, in contrast to serotype 2 viruses, have a tropism for precursor B lymphocytes of the bursa and cause depletion of this organ. No disease has been attributed to serotype 2 infections of chickens. Both serotype 1 and 2 viruses infect turkeys and ducks but cause no disease in these species.

The high mutation rate of the RNA-polymerase of RNA viruses generates a genetic diversification that could lead to the emergence in the field of viruses with new properties allowing them to persist in immune populations. In the case of IBDV, these mutations can lead to antigenic variation and/or modification of virulence, and the evolution of the virus since 1984 has been marked by two major events. The first was the discovery of an antigenic drift in serotype 1 viruses. Starting in 1984, several viral strains of this serotype were isolated in the USA in flocks of broilers that had been properly vaccinated. The new viruses did not cause the characteristic clinical signs of the infection but had a major immunosuppressive potential. They were called 'variant' since they were capable of infecting subjects with an antibody titre considered protective in normal circumstances. The second major epidemiological event was the emergence, starting in 1987, of European very virulent viruses (vvIBDVs), particularly in farms that were perfectly well managed and in which all hygiene and sanitary control measures had been implemented. Significantly more pathogenic than the classical viral strains, these viruses are also capable of infecting birds with normally protective antibody titres. As no antigenic mutation allowing for characterization of the vvIBDVs was discovered, these viruses are generally considered to be pathotypical variants.

Hosts

Only chickens (*Gallus gallus*) develop an infectious and highly contagious disease after infection with pathogenic serotype 1 virus, the severity of which varies according to the dose and virulence of the strain, age and breed of the birds and the presence or absence of passive immunity. Indeed, young chicks with maternally derived antibody (MDA) are immune to infection while antibody levels are high but become susceptible when titres drop. vvIBDVs appear to be capable of breaking through MDA at an earlier age. There is evidence that light breeds, such as Leghorns, are more susceptible to disease than others. No carrier state or vertical transmission has been demonstrated.

IBDV is highly host-specific. Experimental inoculation of other bird species (e.g. quails, partridges, pheasants, guinea fowl, turkeys and ducks) with serotype 1 viruses failed to induce any clinical sign or disease, even when a vvIBDV strain was used for challenge. In this case, only quails showed some replication without clinical signs.

Spread

Following infection of susceptible chicks, the virus is excreted in the faeces as early as 2 days post-infection (thus shortly before the first clinical signs) and for at least 10–14 days.

Transmission in a flock occurs mainly via the faecal–oral route but infection through aerosol is also likely to occur in highly infected areas. In infected flocks, morbidity is high, with up to 100% positive serology after the passage of the virus, while mortality is variable and typically occurs in successive waves, with a peak 3–5 days post-infection. Initial infection in a given farm is generally very acute, with very high mortality rates if a very virulent strain is involved. If the virus persists in the farm and is transmitted to successive flocks, the clinical forms of the disease appear earlier and are then gradually replaced by subclinical forms. Nonetheless, acute episodes may still occur. Moreover, a primary infection may also be inapparent when the viral strain is of low pathogenicity or if maternal antibodies are present.

IBDV is very stable and remains infective in the poultry environment for many months. The virus is transmitted by direct contact with excreting subjects, or by indirect contact with inanimate or animate (farm staff, material, animals) contaminated vectors. The virus can survive for months in contaminated premises and mealworms as well as litter mites have been shown to be infective for up to 8 weeks.

PATHOGENESIS

The target organ of IBDV is the bursa of Fabricius at its maximum development, where B lymphocytes mature in avian species. Bursectomy can prevent illness in chicks infected with virulent virus. Actively dividing, surface-immunoglobulin-M-bearing B cells are lysed by infection but cells of the macrophage lineage can be infected in a persistent and productive manner and play a crucial role in the dissemination of the virus. The severity of the disease is directly related to the number of susceptible cells present in the bursa of Fabricius; therefore, the highest age susceptibility is between 3 and 6 weeks, when the bursa is at its maximum development. This age susceptibility is extended in the case of vvIBDV infection. Necropsies performed on birds that die during the acute phase (2–4 days following infection) reveal hypertrophied, hyperaemic and oedematous bursas. After oral infection or inhalation, the virus replicates primarily in the lymphocytes and macrophages of the gut-associated tissues. Then virus reaches the bursa via the blood stream where replication will occur. By 13 h post-infection most follicles are positive for virus and by 16 h a second and pronounced viraemia will start, with secondary replication in other organs. This second wave coincides with an important inflammatory response in the bursa of Fabricius and is associated with clinical disease and death. Similar kinetics is observed for vvIBDVs but multiplication at each step is amplified and the acute phase might start earlier. Repopulation of the bursa with B lymphocytes is variable; in some cases starting by 8 days and in others after 3 weeks post-infection, depending on the severity of the disease.

There is a growing evidence for a role of proinflammatory cytokines in the pathogenesis of IBD. Indeed, during the acute phase of IBD, there is a dramatic infiltration of T cells around the site of virus replication, including the bursa of Fabricius, spleen and caecal tonsils. T lymphocytes do not support viral replication but are activated and exhibit upregulation of cytokine genes that has an effect on macrophage function with an exacerbated production of promediators such as interferon (IFN)1, tumour necrosis factor (TNF) α, interleukin (IL) 6 or IL8. This cytokine storm induces a shock in the bird, which becomes prostrated and reluctant to move (Fig. 30.2). A direct activation of bursal macrophages by virulent IBDV has also been demonstrated recently.

Recovery from disease or subclinical infection is followed by immunosuppression with more serious consequences if the strain is very virulent and infection occurs early in life. In field conditions, chickens tend to become infected toward the age of 2–3 weeks, when MDA declines and there is considerable evidence that the virus can have an immunosuppressive effect up to

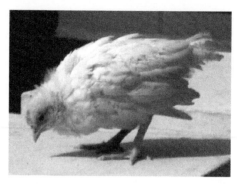

Fig. 30.2 Clinical signs during the acute phase of infectious bursal disease: depression, prostration, soiled vents, anorexia, ruffled feathers and reluctance to move.

the age of 6 weeks at least. Although the immunosuppression caused by IBDV is principally directed towards B lymphocytes, an effect on cell-mediated immunity has also been demonstrated, thus increasing the impact of IBDV on the immunocompetence of the chicken. In addition to its zootechnical impact and its role in the development of secondary infections, IBD may thus also affect the immune response of the chicken to subsequent vaccinations, essential in all types of intensive farming.

DIAGNOSIS

Clinical signs

As indicated above, the severity of the clinical signs is dependent upon the age, breed and MDA level of the chick, as well as upon the virulence of the virus. Therefore, the clinical picture may vary considerably from one farm, region, country or even continent to another.

The acute form is characterized by sudden onset, short course and state of apparent health after recovery. After a short incubation period of 2–3 days, affected chicks show depression, white, watery diarrhoea, soiled vents, anorexia, ruffled feathers, prostration, closed eyes and sudden death (Fig. 30.2). With vvIBDV, mortality rate ranges from 10–20% in heavy breeds and 40–50% in light breeds, occasionally reaching 30% in broilers and 60% in layers at initial infection. With classical and variant strains, mortality rarely exceeds 2–3%.

The milder form of disease may result in the absence of apparent acute phase of disease, with little or no signs other than suboptimal growth and sometimes an increase in other diseases, affected flocks showing increased susceptibility to infection with opportunistic pathogens, often leading to chronic disease situations and also suboptimal vaccine responses. This subclinical infection results in lower than expected economic outputs and downgrading of carcasses, with antibiotic therapy frequently used as the means of control.

Lesions

The carcasses of birds dying from IBDV are dehydrated; there are petechial haemorrhages in the leg and thigh muscles, and occasionally on the mucosa of the proventriculus, and increased mucus in the intestine. The liver may be swollen and show peripheral infarcts; in some cases

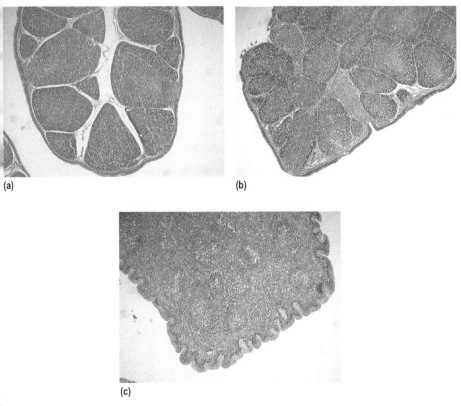

Fig. 30.3 Bursal lesions. Bursa of noninfected chicken (a), of chicken infected with a moderately pathogenic strain (b) and of chicken challenged with the Faragher strain 52/70 (c) was sliced and sections were prepared following standard procedures and haematoxylin/eosin stained. (With permission from COST Action 839 Ring Trial, organized and prepared by Drs E. Mundt and J. P. Teifke.)

splenomegaly occurs. Although macroscopic lesions are observed mainly in the bursa of Fabricius, which presents all stages of inflammation following an acute infection, in some birds the kidneys appear swollen and may contain urate deposits and cell debris, which is probably the result of blockage of the ureters by a severely swollen bursa. Also, disseminated petechiae, muscle haemorrhage and impairment of clotting are often observed and must be related to excessive inflammatory response consecutive to the cytokine storm.

The histological changes in the bursa of Fabricius reflect the initial inflammatory response with hyperaemia, oedema and infiltration of heterophils and T lymphocytes accompanied by B-cell necrosis. There is hyperplasia of reticuloendothelial cells and interfollicular tissue. With decline of the acute inflammatory response, the corticomedullary epithelium proliferates and cystic cavities develop in the medullary areas of the follicles (Fig. 30.3). In the spleen and caecal tonsils there is some necrosis of lymphoid cells and there may be plasma cell depletion in the harderian gland.

In most cases, the history, clinical signs and gross lesions are adequate for recognition of acute disease. In the case of subclinical IBD, differential diagnosis may be necessary and will include avian coccidiosis, Newcastle disease in some viscerotropic forms, malabsorption syndrome, water deprivation, mycotoxicoses or infectious bronchitis in its nephropathogenic form.

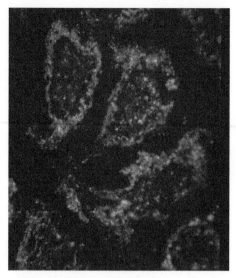

Fig. 30.4 Immunofluorescence staining on bursa of Fabricius of birds dying of infectious bursal disease: medullary areas of the follicles are depleted whereas cortical areas are stained.

Virus detection/isolation

Confirmation of clinical diagnosis may be made by detection of viral antigen in a gel diffusion test against a known positive antiserum or by immunofluorescence (Fig. 30.4) or immunostaining in frozen bursal sections or smears. Several antigen-capture enzyme-linked immunosorbent assays (ELISAs) using specific monoclonal antibodies for capture or detection have been developed for antigenic typing of IBDV strains.

Although virus isolation is rarely used for diagnosis as it is time-consuming. IBDV can be grown on the chorioallantoic membrane of 10–11-day-old embryonated eggs. Some strains grow on primary isolation in chick embryo cells, Vero cells or certain lymphoblastoid cell cultures.

Molecular tests are now more and more widely used in avian laboratories. Several reverse-transcription polymerase chain reaction (RT-PCR) tests allowing the detection of viral RNA have been developed, either using highly conserved regions of the virus for general diagnosis or using the variable region of VP2 for typing of the IBDV strain.

No virulence marker has been identified so far and determination of the pathogenicity of an IBDV isolate requires experimental inoculation in susceptible chickens, compared with reference strains.

Serology

Current serological tests cannot distinguish between antibodies induced by pathogenic IBDV and those induced by vaccine viruses, and thus serological diagnosis is of little interest in endemic zones. Nonetheless, the quantification of IBDV-induced antibodies is important for the medical prophylaxis of the infection in young animals, in order to measure the titre of passive antibodies and determine the date of vaccination or in laying hens in order to verify proper vaccine intake.

Antibodies can be detected by seroneutralization, which is the most sensitive but also the most laborious test, or by ELISA or precipitation tests, which can be used for serological surveys. The seroneutralization test is considered to be the gold standard in IBDV serology, notably for the detection of low levels of residual maternal antibody, which can interfere with vaccine administration. Nonetheless, ELISA can be used instead of seroneutralization, provided that the correlation has been well established between tests and preferably supported by proficiency testing.

CONTROL

Because of the very high resistance of IBDV in the outside environment and its wide distribution, hygienic measures alone, while essential, are often insufficient to prevent infection. There is evidence, however, that thorough cleaning and disinfection of houses between flocks and good management can reduce or even suppress the challenge virus, but these practices are poorly cost-efficient. Eradication in affected countries thus seems unrealistic and prevention of IBD necessitates both hygienic measures and medical prophylaxis. Indeed, no vaccine can solve the problem if major sanitary precautions are not taken. These include 'all-in/all-out' farming methods, cleaning and disinfection of premises and observance of a 'down time' period. Formaldehyde and iodophors are effective disinfectants.

In practice, the economic impact of clinical and subclinical IBD warrants the use of efficient vaccines. While a role for cell-mediated immunity in protection has been demonstrated, good protection correlates with the induction of neutralizing antibodies, as demonstrated by the passive protection of young chicks by MDA. A satisfactory level of protection can be induced either passively by immunizing parent flocks with inactivated vaccines or actively by immunizing the chick with live vaccines given in the drinking water. The ideal vaccine must not cause disease or bursal lesions, must not be immunosuppressive and must confer long-lasting immunity even in birds with a high level of maternal immunity. Such a vaccine does not exist and a proper balance between efficacy (immunogenicity) and safety (residual pathogenicity) has to be found.

Inactivated vaccines are safe but costly and are, therefore, essentially used to produce high, uniform and long-lasting antibody titres prior to lay in hens that have been vaccinated with a live virus. These vaccines are administered by the subcutaneous or intramuscular route at the age of 16–20 weeks in order to transmit high levels of MDA to the progeny. Until the 1980s, this practice could protect broilers until the end of their growing period, since challenge strains were less pathogenic. But with the emergence of vvIBDV, it was no longer possible to protect the progeny passively during the whole fattening period and a live vaccination became necessary. Therefore, the interference of MDA with vaccination has become the key issue in the establishment of a successful vaccination schedule, and serological monitoring is usually necessary to determine the optimal timing for vaccination.

Live IBD vaccines achieve broad, efficient, long-lasting protection and are widely used. They are made from viral strains that have been attenuated by serial passages on embryonated eggs and/or cell culture. Depending on their degree of attenuation, the vaccine strains cause histological lesions of varying severity to the bursa of Fabricius of specific-pathogen-free chickens and are classified as mild, intermediate or hot strains. The hot strains induce, in specific-pathogen-free chickens, histological lesions comparable to those caused by pathogenic strains, the only difference being that they do not cause mortality.

In the field, there is often strong competition between the vaccine and the challenge strain. Mild vaccine strains that cause no bursal lesions cannot be used effectively in chicks with MDA until about 4 weeks of age as they are neutralized and cannot compete with pathogenic strains.

Intermediate vaccine strains that are less affected by MDA can be given with some success as early as 2–3 weeks, depending upon MDA titres. In regions where a too strong challenge with vvIBDV occurs, hot strains are used to break through MDA as early as possible. This approach however is risky and must be used in a very timely and limited manner as these vaccines induce immunosuppression and carry the risk of reversion to virulence.

In countries where antigenic variants exist (e.g. the USA), inactivated vaccines for use in parent stock to provide MDA may therefore contain both classical and variant strains to ensure broad-spectrum antibodies. Vaccines used for active immunization, however, need not contain variant strains as the antibody titres induced are sufficiently high to provide adequate cross-protection against current variants in the field.

New strategies have been developed to overcome the interference of MDA. The first approach is the in ovo inoculation of the vaccine at an embryonic age (18 days) when the absorption of passive antibody into the embryo is not yet completed. To reduce the residual pathogenicity of the vaccine for the embryo, a new concept, consisting of the preparation of a virus–antibody complex, has been developed using a specific hyperimmune serum (or 'virus neutralizing factor', VNF) mixed with the vaccine virus. The second approach uses recombinant vaccines expressing the VP2 protein that are, by definition, insensitive to IBDV MDA as the IBDV antigen is only expressed during replication of the vector. So far, only a HVT-VP2 recombinant has been commercialized, that presents the further advantage of being applicable in ovo.

FURTHER READING

De Wit J J 1999 Gumboro disease: optimizing vaccination. Int Poult Prod 7: 19–21

Kaleta E (ed) 1994 Proceedings of the First International Symposium on Infectious Bursal Disease and Chicken Infectious Anaemia, Rauischolzhausen, Germany

Kaleta E (ed) 2001 Proceedings of the Second International Symposium on Infectious Bursal Disease and Chicken Infectious Anaemia, Rauischolzhausen, Germany

Lukert P D, Saif Y M 2003 Infectious bursal disease. In: Saif Y M (ed) Diseases of poultry, 11th edn. Iowa State University Press, Ames, p 161–179

Müller H, Schnitzler D, Bernstein F et al 1992 Infectious bursal disease of poultry: antigenic structure of the virus and control. Vet Microbiol 33: 175–183

Sharma J M, Kim I, Rautenschlein S, Yeh H 2000 Infectious bursal disease virus of chickens: pathogenesis and immunosuppression. Dev Comp Immunol 24: 223–235

Van den Berg T (ed) 1999, 2000, 2001, 2002 Proceedings of the EU COST Action 839 on Immunosuppressive Viral Disease of Poultry. European Commission, Office SDME, Brussels

Van den Berg T P 2000 Acute infectious bursal disease of chicken. A review. Avian Pathol 29: 175–194

Van den Berg T P, Eterradossi N, Toquin D, Meulemans G 2000 Infectious bursal disease (Gumboro disease) in diseases of poultry: world trade and public health implications. Rev Sci Tech 19(special edn): 509–543

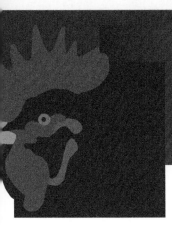

CHAPTER 31

Joan A. Smyth and
M. Stewart McNulty

Adenoviridae

The adenoviruses are members of the family *Adenoviridae*, which currently comprises four genera: *Mastadenovirus*, *Aviadenovirus*, *Siadenovirus* and *Atadenovirus*. The adenovirus species found in birds to date are members of the latter three genera (Table 31.1).

Adenoviruses are icosahedral, non-enveloped double-stranded DNA viruses that range in size from 74–90 nm and have a characteristic morphology (Fig. 31.1). They have 252 structural units or capsomeres, which surround a core 60–65 nm in diameter and are arranged into 20 triangular faces with 12 vertices. The capsomeres found at the vertices are called pentons, while the nonvertex capsomeres are called hexons. Each triangular face has six capsomeres along each edge. One pin-shaped projection, called a fibre, projects from each vertex of members of the *Mastadenovirus*, *Siadenovirus* and *Atadenovirus* genera, while members of the *Aviadenovirus* genus have two fibres at each vertex. Adenoviruses replicate in the nucleus (Fig. 31.2), producing characteristic inclusions; these can be demonstrated histologically, by ultrastructural examination or by immunofluorescence in infected cells, both in vitro and in vivo (Figs 31.2–31.5).

Classification of adenoviruses has undergone major revision in the last 5 years. Adenoviruses that infect mammals belong to the genera *Mastadenovirus* and *Atadenovirus*, while those that infect birds belong to one of three genera: *Aviadenovirus*, *Siadenovirus* and *Atadenovirus*. The genus *Aviadenovirus* contains the so-called conventional group I avian adenoviruses (Table 31.1), with *Fowl adenovirus* A (CELO/Phelps) as the type species. *Duck adenovirus* B, *Pigeon adenovirus* and *Turkey adenovirus* B are tentative species in the *Aviadenovirus* genus. The genus *Siadenovirus* contains the so-called group II avian adenoviruses (turkey haemorrhagic enteritis (THE) virus, marble spleen disease (MSD) virus of pheasants and the avian adenovirus splenomegaly (AAS) virus of chickens), which are now considered to be strains of one virus species, *Turkey adenovirus* A. The other virus species in this genus, *Frog adenovirus*, is the type species of the genus. The genus *Atadenovirus* includes the haemagglutinating viruses associated with egg drop syndrome (EDS) 1976 in domestic fowl. These viruses are now

Table 31.1 | Classification of adenoviruses from birds (2005).

GENUS	SPECIES	SEROTYPES	REPRESENTATIVE STRAIN
Aviadenovirus	*Fowl adenovirus* A	*Fowl adenovirus* 1	Celo (Phelps)
	Fowl adenovirus B	*Fowl adenovirus* 5	340
	Fowl adenovirus C	*Fowl adenovirus* 4	KR95
		Fowl adenovirus 10	CFA20
	Fowl adenovirus D	*Fowl adenovirus* 2	GAL-1
		Fowl adenovirus 3	75
		Fowl adenovirus 9	A2-A
		Fowl adenovirus 11	380
	Fowl adenovirus E	*Fowl adenovirus* 6	CR-119
		Fowl adenovirus 7	YR-36
		Fowl adenovirus 8a	TR-59
		Fowl adenovirus 8b	764
	Goose adenovirus	*Goose adenovirus* 1	
		Goose adenovirus 2	
		Goose adenovirus 3	
	(*Duck adenovirus* B)	*Duck adenovirus* 2	
	(*Pigeon adenovirus*)	*Pigeon adenovirus* 1	
	(*Turkey adenovirus* B)	*Turkey adenovirus* 1	
		Turkey adenovirus 2	
Siadenovirus	*Turkey adenovirus* A	*Turkey adenovirus* 3	
Atadenovirus	*Duck adenovirus* A	*Duck adenovirus* 1	127, BC-14, JPA-1, 126

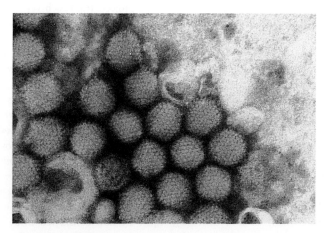

Fig. 31.1 Negatively stained fowl *Aviadenovirus* particles.

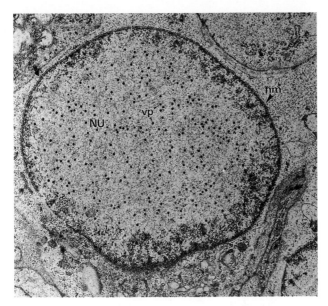

Fig. 31.2 Electron micrograph of turkey spleen infected with *Turkey haemorrhagic enteritis virus*. Virus particles (vp) are seen in the nucleus (NU), which is separated from the cytoplasm by the well-defined nuclear membrane (nm).

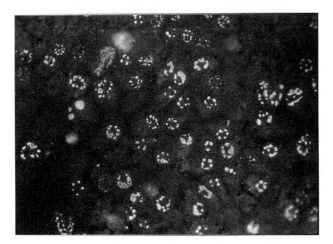

Fig. 31.3 Immunofluorescent staining of chick embryo liver cells infected with a type 9 fowl *Aviadenovirus* using a type 1 conjugated antiserum.

classified as strains of the species *Duck adenovirus* A. *Ovine adenovirus* D is the type species of this genus.

PUBLIC HEALTH SIGNIFICANCE

There have been no reports of the adenoviruses of birds infecting mammals, including humans.

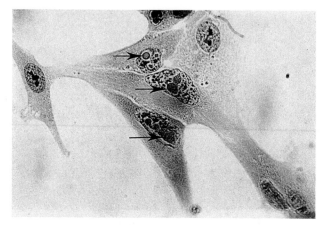

Fig. 31.4 Inclusion bodies (arrowed) in chick embryo liver cells infected with fowl *Aviadenovirus* type 7. Haematoxylin/eosin stain.

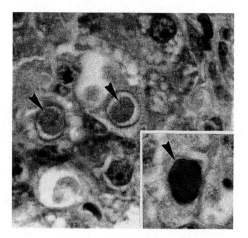

Fig. 31.5 Liver from a natural case of inclusion body hepatitis. The eosinophilic intranuclear inclusions are arrowed. The inset shows liver from an experimental type 5 *Aviadenovirus* infection. Note the dark basophilic inclusion. Haematoxylin/eosin stain.

AVIADENOVIRUSES IN DOMESTIC FOWL

EPIDEMIOLOGY

Cause

At least 12 serotypes of fowl *Aviadenovirus* (Table 31.1) have been recognized on the basis of virus neutralization tests. These serotypes and the other aviadenoviruses share a common group antigen, demonstrable by immunodiffusion or immunofluorescence tests. This group antigen is distinct from that shared by the human and the majority of animal adenoviruses, and these viruses were previously referred to as conventional or group I fowl adenoviruses. The occurrence of prime strains and strains of broad antigenicity (i.e. showing partial cross neutralization) complicates virus classification by serotyping. Under the new classification scheme, which considers additional criteria, such as calculated phylogenetic distance and restriction fragment length polymorphism (RFLP) analysis of the genome, the former group I viruses remain members of the genus *Aviadenovirus*, with the 12 serotypes assigned to one of five virus species, i.e. *Fowl adenovirus* A–E (Table 31.1). Only serotype 1 (*Fowl adenovirus* A) has haemagglutination activity, but it agglutinates only rat red blood cells.

Pathogenesis

Following experimental infection of specific-pathogen-free (SPF) chicks in the first few days of life, using natural routes of exposure, initial growth of fowl aviadenoviruses occurs mainly in the epithelium of both the large and the small intestine. A viraemia then occurs, so that virus can be subsequently detected in many organs, including liver, kidney, respiratory tract, bursa of Fabricius, spleen and bone marrow. However, in the field, infections with aviadenovirus are not normally detected during the first few days of life but isolations from 3 weeks onwards are common. In these cases, virus can be readily isolated from faeces, ocular and nasal mucosa, and bursa of Fabricius. In naturally occurring infections, *Aviadenovirus* is excreted in the faeces for about 3 weeks, with the peak excretion between 4 and 7 days after infection.

Aviadenoviruses can establish latent infections and chickens that have been infected with *Aviadenovirus* are potential lifelong carriers. Carriers probably excrete the virus at intervals throughout their life. Reactivation of latent virus causes a recall of serum antibody to the common group antigen and, if the birds are in lay, virus may be transmitted through the egg. Aviadenoviruses are commonly isolated from hens around the time of peak egg production.

Spread

Following primary infection or reactivation of latent virus, fowl aviadenoviruses can be transmitted vertically through the embryonated egg; this is the main method of spread from one generation of intensively reared poultry to the next. Subsequently, horizontal spread, primarily by contact with infected faeces, occurs. Airborne spread is not considered to be important. Spread by fomites or personnel is possible because aviadenoviruses are relatively resistant to inactivation. They resist treatment with lipid solvents, trypsin, 2% phenol and 50% alcohol. Similarly, exposure to pH 3 or pH 9 does not inactivate adenoviruses but 1:1000 formalin does. Aviadenoviruses are relatively resistant to thermal inactivation: some strains survive heating at 60°C for 30 min.

Chicks hatching from infected eggs may excrete the virus in faeces from hatching but more usually virus excretion is detected in the flock at 2–4 weeks of age. In-contact chicks will become infected and, as most commercial flocks are made up of the progeny of several parent flocks, there is often considerable exchange of serotypes. It is not uncommon to isolate two serotypes from the same bird and a broiler flock may well have four or more serotypes present. By the time a bird reaches sexual maturity it may well have been infected with the majority of the 12 recognized serotypes.

DIAGNOSIS

Clinical signs

Aviadenoviruses have been isolated from virtually every clinical condition. However, they have been most commonly associated with inclusion body hepatitis (IBH), hydropericardium syndrome, respiratory disease, falls in egg production, diarrhoea, tenosynovitis, poor growth and reduced feed conversion. An isolate causing pancreatitis, anaemia and severe lymphoid depletion of the bursa of Fabricius and spleen has been described. Cholecystitis, cholangitis and gizzard erosions have also been found associated with aviadenoviral replication in these organs in broiler chickens, and the disease was experimentally reproduced in broiler and SPF chickens infected by both oral and ocular routes with the virus.

However, it must be stressed that infections with aviadenoviruses occur frequently in healthy birds and aviadenoviruses may be commonly isolated from them under all systems of management. This does not mean that they do not cause disease, but it does mean that isolation of aviadenoviruses from diseased birds forms no basis for assuming that they are the cause of the disease. There is no relationship between *Aviadenovirus* antigenicity and pathogenicity; viruses belonging to the same serotype may differ in pathogenicity.

Inclusion body hepatitis

This condition is usually seen in meat-producing chickens aged 3–7 weeks. However, it has also been recorded in younger and older birds, and in replacement pullets. It is a rare disease in turkeys. It is characterized by a sudden increase in mortality. This is normally between 2 and 10% of the flock but up to 30% has been described. Significant mortality persists for only a few days. The other birds in the flock often appear normal or they may be depressed for a few days. Overall feed conversion and weight gain are usually depressed. The liver in diseased birds is pale and swollen, and frequently has haemorrhages. Microscopically there is a diffuse and generalized hepatitis, with intranuclear inclusion bodies which are often eosinophilic in the hepatocytes (Fig. 31.5). Necrotizing pancreatitis and intranuclear inclusions have also been reported in some outbreaks. Anaemia, icterus of the skin and subcutaneous fat, haemorrhages in various organs, especially the muscles, and bone marrow degeneration are usually present, but vary in severity. It is likely that some of these changes are due to simultaneous infection with chicken anaemia virus.

The aetiology of this disease has not been properly established. It is incorrect to talk of an IBH virus. Virtually every serotype of fowl *Aviadenovirus* has been isolated from naturally occurring cases of IBH. Furthermore, all the known *Aviadenovirus* serotypes will produce hepatitis when young SPF chicks are inoculated parenterally. However, using natural routes of inoculation, most attempts to reproduce a disease similar to the naturally occurring disease in the age group usually affected have been unsuccessful.

Furthermore, most experimental *Aviadenovirus* infections produce basophilic inclusion bodies in the hepatocytes, with many viral particles demonstrable by electron microscopy in the nucleus. However, the inclusion bodies that predominated in many of the early described field cases of IBH in birds over 2 weeks old were eosinophilic and adenovirus particles were not present. If aviadenoviruses are involved, they appear to act with some other factor. It has been suggested that a combined infection with infectious bursal disease (IBD) virus and aviadenoviruses will produce IBH. However, very many flocks undergoing combined infections with these viruses have remained healthy. Furthermore, outbreaks of IBH occurred in both Northern Ireland and New Zealand before IBD virus was introduced into those countries. Some outbreaks of disease described as IBH closely resemble haemorrhagic syndrome/infectious anaemia caused by *Chicken anaemia virus*.

Outbreaks of IBH described in Australia in the early 1990s differ significantly from the above. They occurred in much younger chicks (i.e. under 3 weeks of age), have caused higher mortality and predominantly basophilic inclusion bodies were present in hepatocytes. Aviadenoviruses belonging to serotypes 6, 7 and 8 have been isolated from field cases and have reproduced the disease in experimentally infected chicks using natural routes of exposure. Interestingly, while the fowl aviadenoviruses capable of reproducing the disease under experimental conditions belonged mostly to serotype 8, restriction endonuclease analysis of the DNA of 16 of these isolates, including some from serotypes 6 and 7, showed that they comprised a single distinct group, designated group E, which did not include antigenically related nonvirulent or mildly virulent aviadenoviruses isolated from other conditions. Similarly, isolates belonging to serotypes 1, 8 and 12 associated with severe outbreaks of IBH in New Zealand were also assigned to group E but were distinct from Australian group E viruses. Group E viruses belonging to serotypes 6 and 8 have also been isolated from peracute IBH outbreaks in the USA.

Hydropericardium syndrome

This condition, also known as Angara disease, was first recognized in 1987 in Pakistan. It has subsequently been reported in many other parts of the world. The disease is similar to IBH but the mortality is higher, ranging from 20–80% in broilers, and is characterized by the accumulation of up to 10 mL of clear fluid in the pericardium. Aviadenoviruses belonging mostly to serotype 4 have been implicated in the aetiology but other factors may also be involved, e.g. immunosuppression and/or coinfection with chicken anaemia virus.

Respiratory disease

Aviadenoviruses are frequently isolated from air sacs, lungs and trachea of chickens with respiratory disease. Varying success has been reported in attempts to reproduce respiratory disease experimentally. With the exception of *Quail bronchitis virus* (an FAdV-1 strain) in young bobwhite quail (see below), it is unlikely that most aviadenoviruses are significant respiratory pathogens. However, they may become more important, particularly if birds are immunosuppressed.

Falls in egg production

These viruses are not regarded as an important cause of egg production problems. Under most management systems, birds will reach sexual maturity having been infected by a large number of *Aviadenovirus* serotypes. Aviadenoviruses have been isolated from laying hens, both from normal flocks and flocks with egg-production problems. This emphasizes the point made earlier that isolation of *Aviadenovirus* does not always imply aetiological involvement.

Viral arthritis/tenosynovitis

A number of workers have reported that aviadenoviruses are isolated as frequently as reoviruses from the joints or tendons of birds with this condition. However, poor success has been achieved in experimental reproduction of this disease using aviadenoviruses.

Virus isolation/detection

Virus detection is usually achieved by virus isolation. DNA detection methods for aviadenoviruses are still mainly used as research tools at present.

Virus isolation is best achieved by inoculating both a 10% suspension of the affected organ and a faeces suspension into cell cultures. Chick embryo liver or lung cells, or chick kidney cells, are all sensitive but chick embryo fibroblasts are relatively insensitive. At least two passages, each of 6 days duration, are required. While most strains grow in embryonated eggs, only serotypes 1 (Celo) and 5 (Tipton) will consistently kill the embryos.

Virus growth in cell cultures can first be detected by rounding of the cells or demonstration in stained cells of large basophilic intranuclear inclusions. This can be confirmed by immuno-fluorescent staining or by direct electron microscopy.

Virus characterization

If desired, the serotype can be determined using the neutralization test. Similarly, digestion of the whole viral DNA with restriction endonucleases has been used in classifying isolates. Polymerase chain reaction (PCR) combined with restriction endonuclease analysis has also been used in classifying isolates and, for some of the virus strains, the results suggest different group-ings from those of the current classification. As discussed above, because aviadenoviruses are widely distributed in healthy birds, their isolation from birds with disease is not proof that they have caused the disease.

Serology

The double immunodiffusion test has been commonly used to detect antibody to the *Aviadeno-virus* group antigen. While this is quick, cheap and technically easy to carry out, it is relatively insensitive. Furthermore, because of the ubiquitous nature of aviadenoviruses it is difficult to interpret the results. If a test for detecting group antibodies is required, for example in monitor-ing SPF flocks, then more sensitive tests such as indirect immunofluorescence or enzyme-linked immunosorbent assay (ELISA) should be used.

Type antibodies can be detected by the serum neutralization test but this test is expensive even when the microtitre technique is used.

CONTROL

With the exception of the recent outbreaks of IBH in Australia, and hydropericardium syndrome in Pakistan and Mexico, there has been little need for the development of vaccines to control fowl *Aviadenovirus* infections, because of the lack of a well-established case for their pathogenicity. In Pakistan, vaccines based on formalin-inactivated liver suspensions pro-tected broilers under field conditions; similar results were obtained in Mexico. Other inac-tivated vaccines were also reportedly effective in preventing hydropericardium syndrome in India.

AVIADENOVIRUSES OF OTHER BIRDS

The genus *Aviadenovirus* also contains goose adenoviruses 1, 2 and 3; these belong to the species goose adenovirus. Two serotypes of aviadenovirus from turkeys (TAdV-1 and TAdV-2), a pigeon isolate and one serotype from Muscovy ducks are currently classified as strains of tentative spe-cies in the genus *Aviadenovirus* (Table 31.1).

The turkey isolates grow only in cells of turkey origin. Antibody studies demonstrate that these viruses are widely distributed in turkeys. In addition, at least some fowl adenoviruses can infect turkeys; these viruses can be isolated in cells of fowl and turkey origin. The turkey viruses have mostly been isolated from outbreaks of respiratory and enteric disease and falls in egg production, but there is no convincing evidence that these viruses cause serious disease.

BH in 1-day-old and 4-week-old turkeys associated with *Turkey adenovirus* serotype 2 and an untyped *Aviadenovirus* respectively has been described in the USA. Basophilic intranuclear inclusions were present in hepatocytes in both cases. An adenovirus-associated tracheitis in young goslings with up to 12% mortality between 4 and 11 days of life has been described in Canada. No information is available on the virus type (see also Atadenoviruses, Respiratory disease in geese). Aviadenoviruses belonging to serotypes isolated from fowl have also been isolated from ducks, guinea fowl, pheasants, pigeons, quail and budgerigars. Outbreaks of adenovirus-associated IBH in pigeons and pancreatitis in guinea fowl have been described in several countries.

Quail bronchitis virus, which is antigenically indistinguishable from FAdV-1, causes respiratory disease in young (usually less than 3 weeks old) bobwhite quail. Morbidity and mortality may exceed 50%. At necropsy, necrotizing tracheitis, bronchitis and pneumonia are present. There is no specific treatment or preventative.

FURTHER READING

Balamurugan V, Kataria J M 2004 The hydropericardium syndrome in poultry: a current scenario. Vet Res Commun 28: 127–148

Benko M, Harrach B, Both G W et al 2005 Adenoviridae. In: Fauquet C M et al (eds) Virus taxonomy, classification and nomenclature of viruses. Eighth report of the International Committee on the Taxonomy of Viruses. Elsevier, San Diego, p 213–218

Erny K M, Barr D A, Fahey K J 1991 Molecular characterization of highly virulent fowl adenoviruses associated with outbreaks of inclusion body hepatitis. Avian Pathol 20: 597–606

Hess M 2000 Detection and differentiation of avian adenoviruses: a review. Avian Pathol 29: 195–206

McFerran J B, Adair B M 1977 Avian adenoviruses – a review. Avian Pathol 6: 189–217

McFerran J B, Smyth J A 2000 Avian adenoviruses. Rev Sci Tech 19: 589–601

Meulemans G, Couvreur B, Decaesstecker M et al 2004 Phylogenetic analysis of fowl adenoviruses. Avian Pathol 33: 164–170

SIADENOVIRUSES OF BIRDS

Adenoviruses differing from those in the genus *Aviadenovirus* have been isolated from turkeys, pheasants and chickens throughout the world. These have become commonly known as turkey haemorrhagic enteritis (THE) virus, marble spleen disease (MSD) virus and avian adenovirus splenomegaly virus respectively. They have not been grown in the commonly available cell cultures or chicken embryos, but one of them, THE virus, has been grown in vitro in turkey leukocyte cell cultures. Growth also occurs in a turkey lymphoblastoid B-cell line (MDTC-RP19) derived from a tumour induced by *Marek's disease virus*. These viruses were previously called group II avian adenoviruses because they share a common group antigen which is, however, distinct from that of aviadenoviruses. Only one serotype of avian siadenoviruses has been recognized, i.e. TAdV-3. These viruses are now grouped as one species, *Turkey adenovirus* A, within the genus *Siadenovirus*. Common features of this genus are relatively small genome size (26 kb) and a putative sialidase gene. Infections by these viruses produce different manifestations in each of the three bird species affected, and thus the disease in each species has previously been assigned its own name. For simplicity, each disease is described separately.

TURKEY HAEMORRHAGIC ENTERITIS

EPIDEMIOLOGY

Cause

Variation in virulence occurs among isolates of TAdV-3 virus made from turkeys. Antibody to TAdV-3, also known as THE virus, is widely distributed in turkeys in the UK; most flocks develop antibody between 8 and 19 weeks of age without showing signs of disease. Outbreaks of disease may be precipitated by overcrowding, chilling or a low plane of nutrition, when mortalities up to 60% have been recorded, although lower levels are more usual. Younger turkeys, under 4 weeks of age, protected by maternal antibodies, appear to be resistant.

TAdV-3 virus is spread in the faeces. There is no evidence of egg transmission.

DIAGNOSIS

The history of sudden deaths and the post-mortem findings of the acute disease are often taken as diagnostic. Diagnosis may be confirmed by recognition of the characteristic nuclear inclusions by histology, or demonstration of antigen or virus.

Clinical signs

These vary considerably from flock to flock because of the varying virulence of the agent and influencing factors.

In acute cases, sudden deaths may occur in a flock over a 5–10-day period. The tail feathers are often stained with blood and the whole carcass may appear pale. In less acute outbreaks, the birds may be depressed and have wet droppings.

In more chronic cases, the birds are depressed, often sitting back on their hocks, disinclined to move, and have dark, tarry droppings that make white birds look dirty. In these less acute cases, there is very little mortality.

THE virus is immunosuppressive and may predispose to outbreaks of colibacillosis.

Lesions

The carcasses of the birds that die of the condition are pale because of blood loss and the intestine is full of blood and mucosal debris, invariably involving the duodenum but extending as far as the caecum in severe cases. The intestinal mucosa of the duodenum has a velvety appearance and may show occasional necrotic areas. The spleen is enlarged and mottled, with intranuclear inclusion bodies in lymphoreticular cells. Survivors sometimes show a thickening of the duodenal wall and mild catarrhal enteritis and have enlarged mottled spleens for several weeks. These are often found on the processing line at slaughter. The demonstration of intranuclear inclusion bodies in the lymphoreticular cells of the spleen and the lamina propria of the intestine and other organs confirms the diagnosis.

Virus detection/isolation

The agar gel immunoprecipitation test can be used to demonstrate the presence of either the agent or antibodies. Virus isolation can be attempted using the MDTC-RP19 cell line. More sensitive tests such as ELISA and PCR have also been used.

CONTROL

There is no specific treatment: concentrate on removing any predisposing cause and providing a warm, dry and well-ventilated environment. Electrolyte and vitamin therapy may be useful. Recovery and resistance develop in about 2 weeks.

Various vaccines based on avirulent strains and administered in the drinking water between 4 and 6 weeks of age are available in some parts of the world. A tissue culture attenuated vaccine has been used extensively but such vaccines have been reported to be immunosuppressive. In a recent study, a prototype subunit vaccine was protective experimentally when given by injection at 3 weeks of age. Good management practices, ensuring optimal nutrition and the avoidance of overcrowding and chilling, and the practice of biosecurity measures designed to minimize transfer of virus from flock to flock, all help to reduce the occurrence and severity of disease.

AVIAN ADENOVIRUS SPLENOMEGALY VIRUS INFECTION OF DOMESTIC FOWL

A virus antigenically related to, if not identical with, THE virus and designated avian adenovirus splenomegaly (AAS) virus of chickens has been isolated from domestic fowl. If fowl are inoculated with THE virus, they develop enlarged, mottled spleens. The significance of AAS virus infection of fowl has not yet been fully established, although the enlarged spleens have resulted in condemnation of broilers at meat plants.

MARBLE SPLEEN DISEASE OF PHEASANTS

This disease is characterized by sudden mortality of 2–20% of the flock, which may extend over 10–14 days. Flock mortality can approach 100%. It is most commonly seen in birds 3–8 months old. The birds apparently die from asphyxia as a result of acute pulmonary oedema. The spleens are also enlarged, with grey necrotic foci. Laboratory diagnostic methods are similar to those used for THE except that intestine is not a good site to look for antigen in pheasants. Vaccines administered via the drinking water and based on naturally occurring avirulent viral isolates have been used in the USA.

FURTHER READING

Arbuckle J B R, Parsons D, Luff P R 1979 Haemorrhagic enteritis syndrome of turkeys. Vet Rec 104: 435–436

Benko M, Harrach B, Both G W et al 2005 Adenoviridae. In: Fauquet C M et al (eds) Virus taxonomy, classification and nomenclature of viruses. Eighth report of the International Committee on the Taxonomy of Viruses. Elsevier, San Diego, p 213–218

Bygrave A C, Pattison M 1973 Marble spleen disease in pheasants. Vet Rec 92: 534

Carlson H C, Al-Shiekly F, Petit J R et al 1974 Virus particles in spleens and intestines of turkeys with haemorrhagic enteritis. Avian Dis 18: 67–73

Domermuth C H, Gross W B, Douglass C S et al 1977 Vaccination for haemorrhagic enteritis of turkeys. Avian Dis 21: 557–565

Domermuth C H, Gross W B 1975 Haemorrhagic enteritis of turkeys antiserum – efficacy, preparation and use. Avian Dis 19: 657–775

McFerran J B, Smyth, J A 2000 Avian adenoviruses. Rev Sci Tech 19: 589–601

ATADENOVIRUSES OF BIRDS

EGG DROP SYNDROME 1976

EPIDEMIOLOGY

Cause

The cause of EDS is an adenovirus that differs from aviadenoviruses and siadenoviruses in that it agglutinates avian but not mammalian red blood cells to high titres, has a relatively high adenine–thymine content and has a gene for a novel structural protein p32K. Although EDS virus apparently shares the *Aviadenovirus* group antigen, this can be detected only by indirect means. It is now classified as a species, *duck Adenovirus* A, in the genus *Atadenovirus*.

EDS virus is a naturally occurring adenovirus of ducks, geese and other waterfowl that has infected domestic fowl. It grows best in duck and geese cell cultures but also grows well in chick embryo liver and chick kidney cells. It grows to very high titres in embryonated duck eggs but poorly in chicken embryos. All virus isolates belong to one serotype (DAdV-1) but a collection of isolates has been divided into three genotypes using restriction endonuclease analysis. Recent studies in Japan suggest that the virus circulating in chickens has not changed in over 20 years since it was introduced to chickens. However, a study of isolates from India showed major differences (4.6%) in the hexon gene of one isolate.

Pathogenesis

Following experimental infection of laying hens, the virus grows to a limited extent in the nasal mucosa. This is followed by a transient viraemia, with virus growth in lymphoid tissue. At 8 days after infection there is a massive growth in the pouch shell gland region of the oviduct, coincident with the occurrence of eggshell changes. Both eggs with normal and affected shells contain virus, both externally and internally, for the next 2–3 weeks.

Chicks hatching from these infected eggs often do not develop antibody but they may be latently infected. At around peak egg production, the virus is reactivated and horizontal spread occurs. In a minority of cases there is horizontal spread of the virus between birds during the growing period but, as the amount of virus excreted is small, this spread is limited.

The pathogenesis of EDS virus differs from that of aviadenoviruses in that growth in the surface epithelial cells of the intestine has not been detected.

Spread

Three patterns of EDS have become evident over time. Classical EDS followed the introduction of EDS virus into primary broiler breeder stock, most probably through a vaccine grown in duck cells. Vertical transmission with reactivation of the virus around the time of peak egg production gave an apparent breed and age susceptibility. The virus was subsequently eradicated from primary breeding stock. The second pattern (the endemic form) has resulted from lateral spread between flocks. Spread is primarily associated with contaminated eggs or Keyes trays and is usually seen in commercial egg layers. Any age of laying flock may be affected and there is often an association between affected flocks and an egg packing station. The third (sporadic) form is also seen in any age or breed of chicken. It results from introduction of infection from ducks, geese or any infected wild bird, either through direct contact or indirectly through contaminated drinking water.

The main source of virus in the droppings is secretions from the oviduct. Lateral spread between flocks via contaminated personnel or fomites, other than Keyes trays, can occur, but does not appear to be a major hazard. Other methods of spread could be via contaminated needles and, possibly, biting insects.

DIAGNOSIS

Clinical signs

The first sign is usually a loss of shell pigmentation. This is quickly followed by production of thin-shelled, soft-shelled and shell-less eggs (Fig. 31.6). Eggshells may have focal thickenings; however, ridging and misshapen eggs are not a feature. In experimental studies, there was no depression in egg numbers (i.e. the fall in production is apparently due to affected eggs being eaten or lost in the litter). Fertility and hatchability are unaffected if obviously affected eggs are discarded. The birds are normally healthy but sometimes appear slightly depressed for 48 h or so. Diarrhoea has been described but this is probably due to excess oviduct secretions in the droppings.

Classical EDS is manifested either by a sudden apparent fall in production around peak egg production or by a failure to achieve or hold predicted production. In the first case the flock

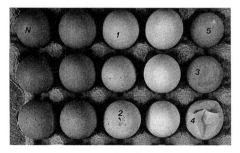

Fig. 31.6 Eggs from birds infected with egg drop syndrome virus. These changes range from the normal brown eggs (N), through loss of shell pigment (1), thinning of the normal eggshell (2) and cracks where the eggs roll on to the wire of the cages (3) to soft-shelled (4) and shell-less (5) eggs.

will have been devoid of detectable antibody before the drop in production. In the second case, a small percentage of the flock will have developed antibody during the growing period. It takes 4–10 weeks for usable egg production to recover. There may be compensation later in lay. Overall, the loss has been estimated at 10–16 eggs per bird.

The vast majority of outbreaks of EDS have occurred in domestic fowl but infection with EDS virus has been associated with a similar disease in quails. Drops in egg production and appearance of soft-shelled eggs have been associated with seroconversion to EDS virus. Turkeys and pigeons are susceptible to experimental infection but show no apparent signs.

The combination of a sudden fall in egg production, associated with production of thin-shelled, soft-shelled and shell-less eggs in a flock of apparently healthy birds, is highly suggestive of EDS. However, in cage units spread may occur over a period of many weeks and the main signs may be only a small depression in egg numbers. A careful examination will show that typically affected eggs are present in some cages.

Virus isolation/detection

Although virus has been isolated from cloacal swabs, virus recovery can be a problem because excretion is transient and it is often difficult to identify the correct bird to sample. The easiest method is to feed affected eggs to individually caged susceptible hens. Once they produce affected eggs, the pouch shell gland is harvested and samples are inoculated into either duck kidney or fibroblast cell cultures or embryonated duck eggs. Chick embryo liver or lung, or chick kidney cells, can also be used but are less sensitive. Virus growth is detected by testing for haemagglutinin activity. At least two 7-day passages are required.

EDS viral antigen can be detected in pouch shell gland epithelium by immunofluorescent or immunocytochemical staining but its presence is transient and examination of randomly selected birds has usually been negative.

Antigen-capture ELISA methods have been reported but have the same diagnostic limitations as the above methods. PCR detection methods have been described but their usefulness for diagnosis in field cases is not yet reported.

Serology

Detection of antibodies to EDS virus by the haemagglutination inhibition test using fowl red blood cells is sensitive and easy, and is the diagnostic method of choice in unvaccinated flocks. ELISA is now also used. As spread can be slow, especially in cage units, it is imperative to select the correct birds for sampling. By the time birds produce affected eggs they have already seroconverted and blood should therefore be taken from cages in which affected eggs occur.

CONTROL

The classical form has apparently been eliminated from all primary breeders.

Endemic EDS can be controlled by vaccination and effective inactivated oil-adjuvanted vaccines are available. These are given intramuscularly between 14 and 18 weeks of age and are often combined with other antigens, such as *Newcastle disease virus* or IBD virus. As the main method of horizontal spread is by the infected egg and Keyes tray, plastic Keyes trays that are washed and sterilized before returning to the farm should be provided where possible. Other methods of spread, such as contaminated transport, personnel and needles, seem to be less important. Aerial spread is not important.

Sporadic EDS can be controlled by segregation of fowl from ducks, geese and other waterfowl. If lake, dam or other surface water is given to birds, this water should be chlorinated or replaced by borehole-derived water.

RESPIRATORY DISEASE IN GEESE

A severe outbreak of tracheitis and bronchitis due to EDS virus infection has been reported in Hungary. Nuclear inclusions were present in the superficial epithelial cells of the trachea and bronchi. The disease was reproduced experimentally.

FURTHER READING

Benko M, Harrach B, Both G W et al 2005 Adenoviridae. In: Fauquet C M et al (eds) Virus taxonomy, classification and nomenclature of viruses. Eighth report of the International Committee on the Taxonomy of Viruses. Elsevier, San Diego, p 213–218

Smyth J A, McFerran J B 1989 Egg drop syndrome. Prog Vet Microbiol Immunol 5: 83–108

UNCLASSIFIED ADENOVIRUSES

A novel adenoviral enteritis of goslings has been described in China. The virus has not been classified. It produces a severe necrotizing enteritis.

Adenoviruses that were not neutralized by antisera to known adenoviruses have been recovered from diseased long-tailed ducks (Alaska) and common eider ducks (Baltic Sea). It is not known if these viruses are related to each other. The former produced IBH and enteritis in orally inoculated long-tailed ducks.

Adenovirus-like viruses that appear to be distinct from the currently known types of adenovirus of birds have been demonstrated in a transmissible proventriculitis of chickens.

Adenoviral inclusions have been reported as an incidental finding in the kidney of Japanese quail on toxicity studies.

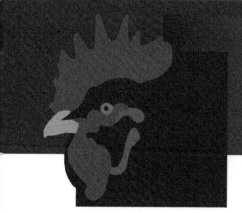

M. Stewart McNulty,
Richard C. Jones and
Richard E. Gough

Reoviridae

The family *Reoviridae* contains three genera, *Orthoreovirus* (reoviruses), *Orbivirus* and *Rotavirus*, with members that infect birds. Current knowledge indicates that orbiviruses do not cause disease in domestic poultry; therefore this chapter is restricted to reoviruses and rotaviruses.

REOVIRUSES (M. STEWART MCNULTY AND RICHARD C. JONES)

EPIDEMIOLOGY

Cause

The reovirus virion is a double-shelled structure 75–76 nm in diameter and composed of 92 hollow capsomeres (Fig. 32.1). The genome consists of 10 segments of double-stranded RNA. Replication is in the cytoplasm. There is no envelope and the virus is resistant to chloroform, pH 3, sodium deoxycholate and trypsin, although some strains are now known to be sensitive to this enzyme. Reoviruses are relatively resistant to inactivation by heat and disinfectants. Unlike the mammalian reoviruses, the avian strains do not agglutinate red blood cells.

Reoviruses grow well in chick kidney and embryo chick liver and lung cell cultures. They grow less well in chick embryo fibroblasts. They form syncytia with prominent cytoplasmic inclusions. They also grow well in embryonated eggs when inoculated into the yolk sac or on to the chorioallantoic membrane.

The fowl reoviruses have a common group antigen, as detected by immunofluorescence, complement fixation and gel diffusion, but the cross-reaction between strains is by no means complete. These viruses are not antigenically related to the mammalian reoviruses. On the basis of the serum neutralization (SN) test five serotypes have been recognized in Japan and four in the USA. A study comparing strains from many areas has suggested that there are at least 11 serotypes. However, there is considerable antigenic overlap between serotypes. Work in Australia showed

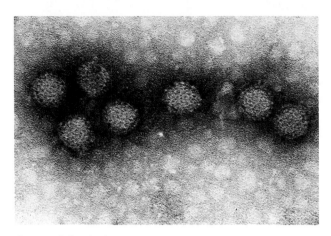

Fig. 32.1 Avian reovirus, negatively stained.

that reassortment of genes can occur when a cell is infected by more than one reovirus, so it is likely that new antigenic variants appear from time to time.

More recently, restriction fragment profiles obtained from two cDNA fragments of the σC-encoding and σNS-encoding genes were used to differentiate and classify avian reovirus isolates. A small group of Taiwanese isolates were classified into four distinct groups, which were consistent with serological characterization using the SN test. Furthermore, isolates within groups could be distinguished, indicating that this technology could be useful in following the spread and evolution of particular isolates.

There is wide variation in virulence between antigenically similar isolates. While reovirus infections are ubiquitous in domestic fowl, the vast majority of reoviruses isolated appear to be nonpathogenic. Despite many molecular studies comparing avian reoviruses from normal and diseased chickens, the factors responsible for pathogenicity have not been elucidated.

Hosts

Although primarily of disease concern in domestic fowl, principally because of viral arthritis or tenosynovitis, reoviruses have been isolated from a range of other avian species. Of the farmed avian species, infections have also been described in turkeys, ducks and geese.

Reoviruses have also been isolated from domestic pigeons with diarrhoea, and from African grey parrots with subcutaneous haemorrhages, necrotic lesions in liver, spleen, bone marrow and intestinal lamina propria, air sacculitis and epicarditis.

Reoviruses have been isolated from other psittacine species, including budgerigars, black-tailed gulls, common eiders, pheasants, bobwhite quail and mallard ducks. It is not clear whether and to what extent reoviruses infecting a particular avian species are distinct. It is known that cross-infection between some avian species occurs. There is some evidence that reoviruses from wild birds can cause joint lesions in chickens experimentally, but whether they represent a real threat to poultry is unknown.

No public health problems are known to exist with avian reoviruses.

Spread

Horizontal spread occurs readily from bird to bird, mainly by ingestion of contaminated faeces but infection via the respiratory tract may also occur. Vertical transmission through the embryonated egg also occurs, not only during the acute phase but also at intervals through life. Although, as with most viruses, the rate of vertical transmission of avian reoviruses is low, egg transmission is important in the epidemiology of avian reovirus infections and a small group of vertically infected chicks can easily become a nucleus of infection for hatchmates.

The virus is widely disseminated in intensive poultry flocks. Reoviruses are commonly isolated from normal healthy chickens from the first week of life onwards.

DIAGNOSIS

Clinical signs

Shortly after infection there is a viraemia. Virus grows in virtually all organs. The highest titres are found in the alimentary tract, spleen, tendons and respiratory tract. There is some dispute about the time during which virus can be recovered from these organs. Some workers could constantly recover virus only for about 2 weeks, whereas others have recovered virus for up to 4 months, especially in tendon sheaths.

In domestic fowl, reoviruses have been associated with enteric conditions such as cloacal pasting and ulcerative enteritis, acute and chronic respiratory disease, pericarditis and hydropericardium, anaemia, inclusion body hepatitis and death. Although some of these conditions have apparently been reproduced experimentally, there is little evidence to suggest that reoviruses are significant causes of these conditions in the field. An exception to this is the strain that consistently caused acute hepatitis and deaths in broilers under 10 days of age. Work from the Netherlands, Australia and the USA has suggested that reoviruses may be involved in the malabsorption syndrome in broilers characterized by runting, abnormal feather development, proventriculitis, diarrhoea and skeletal changes. However, this remains to be confirmed and other agents have been implicated in studies carried out elsewhere.

It is generally accepted that reoviruses cause tenosynovitis or viral arthritis. This is a condition normally seen in meat-producing birds between 4 and 8 weeks but has been recorded in younger birds, in broiler breeders at peak of lay and in 9-month-old white Leghorns. It is characterized by swelling of one or both of the hock joints and of the associated tendons. This produces lameness and the birds are reluctant to move. Chronic tendonitis may result and this may lead to rupture of the gastrocnemius tendon (Fig. 32.2). In severe cases erosion of the articular cartilage may also occur. While morbidity is very variable, it is usually below 10%; similarly, mortality is usually under 1% but can reach 10%. However, condemnations due to synovitis are usually 1–2%, although in some outbreaks much higher figures have been found. Tenosynovitis

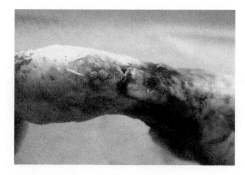

Fig. 32.2 Tendon rupture associated with reoviral arthritis.

associated with reovirus infection has also been recorded in young turkeys, but the aetiological role of the virus has not been proved.

Tenosynovitis may be reproduced by infecting young specific-pathogen-free (SPF) chickens with reoviruses and they can be reisolated from or detected by fluorescent antibody techniques in the damaged joint tissue. However, it has also been observed that the virus may be readily isolated from many internal organs of birds 1–2 weeks old and that these flocks do not develop tenosynovitis. This can be explained by the observation that the ability of reoviruses to cause joint and tendon lesions is highly variable and differs between virus strains.

The signs and lesions of reovirus arthritis/tenosynovitis are not pathognomonic and resemble those caused by *Staphylococcus aureus* and *Mycoplasma synoviae*, both of which can sometimes be detected, with reovirus, in affected joints.

In turkeys, a reovirus has been isolated from cases of poult enteritis and mortality syndrome (PEMS) in the USA. PEMS is characterized by diarrhoea, dehydration, weight loss, anorexia, growth depression and high mortality. Experimental infections showed that the isolate produced only some of the signs and lesions; it is unlikely to be the cause of PEMS. Reoviruses have been isolated from turkeys with tenosynovitis and with a variety of enteric conditions. However, as with PEMS, reoviruses are unlikely to be the cause.

A disease of young Muscovy ducks caused by a reovirus has been described in South Africa, France and Israel. It was characterized by debility, diarrhoea, serofibrinous pericarditis, spleno- and hepatomegaly with necrotic foci, and tenosynovitis in some chronic cases. Morbidity in Israel was 30% and mortality was 20%. A similar condition, also caused by a reovirus, has been present in geese in Hungary for more than three decades.

Virus isolation/detection

Detection of reoviruses is usually achieved by isolation of the virus in cell culture or in embryonated eggs. Alternative methods such as polymerase chain reaction (PCR) and in situ hybridization for detection of viral nucleic acid are being used in some diagnostic laboratories.

Faeces and spleen are probably the best sources of virus. However, if arthritis is present, the preferred samples are the hypotarsal sesamoid and the tendons that pass through it, hock articular cartilage and synovial membrane. The chances of virus recovery are improved if these samples are macerated rather than simply swabbed.

Reoviruses are best isolated in chick embryo lung or liver cells or chick kidney cells. Chick embryo fibroblasts are not very sensitive. Virus growth is recognized by syncytial formation with cytoplasmic inclusion bodies. Virus identity can be confirmed by immunofluorescent staining (Fig. 32.3) or by direct negative contrast electron microscopy. Care must be taken in examination of infected cultures, because the syncytia may detach from the glass, leaving holes in the monolayer, giving the impression of an old, degenerating culture. Adenoviruses may also be isolated from affected joints but are unlikely to be of any significance. Where arthritis is present, isolation of reoviruses from affected joints may be considered diagnostic but, because reovirus infections are common in apparently healthy birds, their isolation from other systems and tissues should be interpreted with caution.

An alternative method of isolation of reoviruses is to use embryonated eggs and these are probably as sensitive as cell culture. Eggs and cell cultures should be derived from an SPF source. The yolk sac is the route of choice. High virus concentrations cause embryo death within 5–6 days, with congestion and haemorrhages of the skin and necrotic lesions in the liver. At lower viral concentrations the embryos live longer, become dwarfed and have necrotic foci on the spleen, liver and heart. Inoculation on to the chorioallantoic membrane causes pocks.

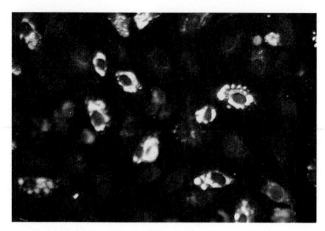

Fig 32.3 Immunofluorescence of fowl reovirus in infected cell culture.

Serology

Antibody to the avian reovirus group antigen can be detected by the immunodiffusion test, indirect immunofluorescence and enzyme-linked immunosorbent assay (ELISA). The antigen for immunodiffusion is usually prepared from the chorioallantoic membranes of infected embryos. Infected cell cultures can also be used. However, as reovirus antibody is so widespread in healthy birds, interpretation of serology is very difficult. ELISA is frequently used to monitor reovirus antibodies in breeding stock, particularly when they have been vaccinated.

Type-specific antibody can be detected using the SN test but is not done routinely. Chick embryo liver cells are the best system and either a plaque reduction or a tube test can be used.

CONTROL

Inactivated oil-adjuvanted vaccines, frequently based on the S1133 strain, have been used in chicken breeding stock to reduce egg transmission of the virus and to stimulate good levels of maternal antibody in the chicks. This is based on the observation that chicks are most susceptible to pathogenic reoviruses at 1 day of age but develop an age-associated resistance from 2 weeks of age. Live vaccines, using attenuated reoviruses, have also been used. Reoviruses can replicate in the gut even when high levels of homologous maternally derived antibody are present. It is not clear how much cross-protection there is between the reovirus serotypes; neither has it been determined which serotypes are the most important in the aetiology of viral arthritis or indeed whether serotype identity is relevant. It is not surprising, therefore, that reports on the effectiveness of the vaccines have been varied. Commercial reovirus vaccines are available in some countries for protection against malabsorption syndrome even though their role in this condition appears uncertain.

Where outbreaks of viral arthritis have caused problems, particular attention should be given to cleansing and disinfection of the house and equipment after clear-out to prevent problems in the next crop of broilers. Reoviruses are very robust away from the host and can survive for many days on materials associated with the poultry house.

FURTHER READING

Kibenge F S B, Wilcox G E 1983 Tenosynovitis in chickens. Vet Bull 53: 431–444

McNulty M S 1993 Reovirus. In: McFerran J B, McNulty M S, eds. Viral infections of vertebrates, vol 4. Virus infections of birds. Elsevier, Amsterdam, p 181–193

Rosenberger J K, Jones R C 2003 Reovirus infections. In: Saif Y (ed) Diseases of poultry, 11th edn. Iowa State University Press, Ames, p 283–298

ROTAVIRUSES (RICHARD E. GOUGH AND M. STEWART MCNULTY)

Rotaviruses are a widespread cause of enteritis and diarrhoea in a variety of mammalian and avian species. Their aetiological role as a cause of diarrhoea in young calves was first established in 1969. Since that time they have been associated with enteric disease in the newborn of many mammalian species, including humans, in which they cause acute gastroenteritis in young children. Avian rotaviruses were first described in the USA in 1977 in turkey poults with diarrhoea. Subsequently they were detected in commercial poultry, including game birds, in Europe, South America, Asia and Africa. It is probable that *Rotavirus* infection occurs commonly worldwide in domestic poultry and other avian species, in which their significance has yet to be determined.

EPIDEMIOLOGY

Cause

Rotaviruses are classified as a genus in the family *Reoviridae*. Intact virions have a double-shelled icosahedral capsid and are approximately 70 nm in diameter. Particles with only the inner capsid layer are approximately 60 nm in diameter. Rotaviruses possess a double-stranded RNA genome, which can be separated into 11 segments following electrophoresis in polyacrylamide gels. The overall pattern of the migration of the RNA segments has allowed avian rotaviruses to be classified into electropherogroups. These groups can be further divided into electropherotypes, which show differences based on the migration of one or more individual segments. To date, five distinct electropherogroups have been recognized in turkeys and chickens. Rotaviruses belonging to electropherogroups 1, 2 and 3 have been detected in chickens and turkeys; electropherogroup 4 has been found only in chickens and 5 only in turkeys. Rotaviruses have also been subdivided into at least five serogroups (A–E) based on antigens that are common within a serogroup but distinctive outside that serogroup. Antigenic characterization of isolates representing different electropherogroups has shown that these viruses also belong to different serogroups. One serogroup of avian rotaviruses, designated group A, is antigenically related to group A mammalian rotaviruses. So far, group D rotaviruses have been recognized only in avian species. Antigenic heterogeneity in the form of different serotypes also occurs within the serogroups. In the literature, the non-group-A rotaviruses are frequently described as atypical rotaviruses or rotavirus-like viruses. The molecular biology of mammalian rotaviruses has been extensively studied, but similar investigations with avian rotaviruses have been much more limited.

Hosts

Rotaviruses have been detected in a variety of avian species, including chickens, turkeys, pheasants, partridges, ducks, guinea fowl, ratites, pigeons and parrots. During the first few weeks of life *Rotavirus* infection may lead to significant morbidity and mortality, particularly in turkeys and game birds. However, there is no age resistance to infection and rotavirus-associated diarrhoea has been recorded in commercial laying hens and other adult birds.

Rotaviral enteritis is a significant problem in pheasant chicks under 2 weeks of age, causing up to 70% mortality in some instances. Most outbreaks result in 10–15% losses in susceptible pheasant chicks that become infected during the first few days of life. In older pheasants, outbreaks of diarrhoea have been reported following periods of stress. Although the mortality is usually low in these situations the morbidity may be high and infection may predispose the birds to secondary enteric infections.

Rotavirus infections are commonly subclinical, particularly in chickens and turkeys.

Several factors will influence the course and severity of the disease. These include putative differences in virulence between rotavirus strains, the level of maternally derived antibody in exposed chicks, stocking densities, the interaction with other infectious agents, managemental factors and environmental stress. The widespread practice of custom hatching pheasant eggs from different suppliers has been identified as an important factor in outbreaks of rotavirus-associated disease in pheasant chicks.

There is no known public health significance associated with avian rotaviruses.

Spread

Rotaviruses are excreted in the faeces in very large numbers. It has been shown that experimentally infected turkey poults shed virus for up to 24 days. As rotaviruses are generally considered to be moderately resistant to physical and chemical inactivation, this leads to heavy and persistent contamination of the environment. Infection will obviously accumulate and persist in poultry houses where litter is reused. Transmission of virus in or on the egg has been suggested to explain infection in 3–4-day-old turkey and pheasant chicks. However, there is no evidence that vertical transmission via the egg occurs even under laboratory conditions. On a number of large game farms the scrupulous cleaning of pheasant eggs prior to setting has led to a reduction in *Rotavirus* outbreaks in chicks under 1 week of age. This suggests that virus can be transmitted from contaminated eggs to susceptible chicks in the hatchery.

Horizontal transmission occurs readily between birds in direct and indirect contact probably by the faecal/oral route. There is no evidence of a carrier state in birds or of the existence of biological vectors.

DIAGNOSIS

Clinical signs

Following ingestion the principal site of virus replication is the mature villous epithelial cells of the small intestine, resulting in villous atrophy.

Occasionally, replication has been reported to occur in the epithelial cells of the large intestine. The mechanism by which rotaviruses cause diarrhoea in birds has not been fully investigated, although it is probably similar to the situation in mammals. Following destruction of the epithelial cells, compensatory crypt hypertrophy occurs, resulting in replacement of mature epithelial cells by immature cells that are deficient in digestive enzymes and in the ability to transport water and electrolytes. This will result in diarrhoea due to malabsorption and increased water secretion. Following experimental infection of SPF chickens and turkeys, maximum virus excretion in the faeces occurred from 2 to 5 days post-inoculation. Similar results were obtained in transmission studies in susceptible pheasant chicks.

The principal clinical sign associated with rotavirus infection in young birds is diarrhoea, with associated dehydration, poor feed conversion and weight gains, and increased mortality. Infection in turkey poults may result in 'wet litter' problems accompanied by litter eating, inflammation of the vent with associated pecking and general restlessness. Clinical signs may vary in severity depending on the age of the bird and its immune status. In pheasant and partridge chicks typical signs in chicks under 2 weeks of age are depression, drooping wings, yellowish watery diarrhoea and increased mortality. Chicks surviving *Rotavirus* infection may be severely stunted and succumb to secondary enteric pathogens.

The clinical signs associated with *Rotavirus* are not pathognomonic and other enteric viruses, such as turkey astrovirus, may produce similar signs, either alone or in combination with rotaviruses. *Rotavirus* infections in chickens, turkeys and other avian species are commonly subclinical. It is therefore often difficult to evaluate the significance of rotavirus infections in diseased birds.

Lesions

The most consistent post-mortem finding is the presence of abnormal amounts of fluid and gas in the distended caeca and intestinal tract. Other features include signs of dehydration, inflamed vents and anaemia due to vent pecking.

The most obvious histopathological lesions in experimentally infected turkeys are villous atrophy and crypt hypertrophy in the small intestine, with leukocytic infiltration of the lamina propria, basal vacuolation of the epithelial cells and surface scalloping of the villous tips. Loss of microvilli from the surfaces of the enterocytes has also been reported. Surprisingly, the overall lesions in older turkeys (12–16 weeks) were considered to be more severe than those observed in younger birds (<17 days) following experimental infection with a group A *Turkey rotavirus*. There are few detailed reports on the histopathological findings following natural rotavirus infection. Degeneration and inflammation of the duodenum and jejunum has been reported in poults with rotaviral enteritis.

Virus detection/isolation

At present the diagnosis of avian *Rotavirus* infection in clinical samples is based on the demonstration of the virus by electron microscopy or by detection of its antigens and/or RNA (Fig. 32.4).

Negative contrast electron microscopic examination of intestinal contents or faeces is routinely used in diagnostic laboratories for the detection of rotaviruses. The technique is sensitive, can reveal the presence of other viruses and can give rapid results. Disadvantages are that visualization of the virions gives no indication of the serogroup to which the *Rotavirus* belongs. Immune electron microscopy using *Rotavirus* group-specific antisera prepared in SPF chickens or turkeys can also be used. This technique has been used to distinguish group A from group D turkey rotaviruses in clinical specimens.

Rotavirus RNA can be demonstrated directly in faecal or intestinal content samples after extraction and analysis by polyacrylamide gel electrophoresis. Following staining, *Rotavirus* RNA can be identified by the characteristic migration pattern of the 11 genome segments. The technique provides a convenient means of distinguishing between different electropherogroups and electropherotypes and also detecting unusual isolates.

Attempts to isolate and propagate rotaviruses in vitro are generally unreliable and are not used in routine diagnostic laboratories. Group A avian rotaviruses have been isolated in primary

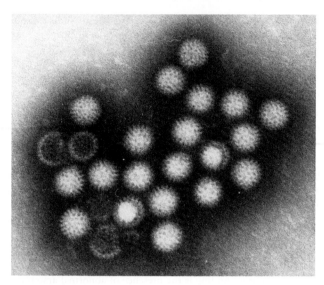

Fig. 32.4 Group of avian *Rotavirus* particles.

chicken embryo liver and kidney cells and the MA104 mammalian cell line. The incubation of the sample with a proteolytic enzyme, such as trypsin, facilitates activation of the virus and the growth of avian group A rotaviruses in cell cultures. Non-group-A rotaviruses have proved extremely difficult to isolate and propagate in cell cultures.

Commercial ELISA kits that have been developed to detect group A mammalian rotaviruses have been used to detect avian group A rotavirus antigens in faeces samples. However, as most rotaviruses associated with disease in poultry are non-group-A, these ELISAs cannot be recommended for routine diagnosis.

Molecular methods such as PCR have not been developed for routine detection of avian rotaviruses.

Serology

Antibodies to rotaviruses are widespread in domestic avian species. In view of this, coupled with the multiplicity of serogroups and the difficulty in growing non-group-A rotaviruses in cell cultures, serology is not used routinely for diagnostic purposes. Indirect immunofluorescence using infected cell cultures and virus neutralization tests have been used to screen SPF chicken and pheasant flocks for antibodies to group A rotaviruses.

CONTROL

Given the widespread occurrence of *Rotavirus* infection in poultry, it is not feasible to attempt to maintain commercial flocks free of infection. In flocks where rotaviral enteritis is a problem, improved hygienic measures have prevented build-ups of infection between successive crops of birds. Management factors, such as reducing stocking densities, increasing turnaround times and using fresh litter for successive crops of birds will reduce the impact of *Rotavirus* infection. Outbreaks of *Rotavirus*-associated enteritis in pheasant chicks have been significantly reduced on game farms where good hatchery and breeder hygiene is practised. Reducing stocking densities in the rearing sheds and adopting a 'closed flock' breeding programme have also reduced losses from rotavirus infection. The effect of diarrhoea on the litter, the so-called 'wet litter' syndrome, can be minimized by increasing temperature and ventilation and by the addition of fresh litter.

In pheasant chicks under a week old, oral rehydration therapy with electrolyte solutions has been used to ameliorate the effects of rotavirus infection.

At present there are no avian *Rotavirus* vaccines available. Obvious problems in vaccine development include the diversity of serogroups and the difficulty in propagating the non-group-A rotaviruses in cell cultures. However, an experimental group A *Rotavirus* vaccine has been evaluated in pheasants. A good serological response was produced in the breeding pheasants following one inoculation of inactivated vaccine. When the progeny of the vaccinated hens were challenged at 2–3 days of age a significant reduction in mortality was recorded compared with chicks from unvaccinated parents.

FURTHER READING

McNulty M S 1993 Rotavirus infections. In: McFerran J B, McNulty M S (eds) Virus infections of birds. Elsevier Science, Amsterdam

McNulty M S 2003 Rotavirus infections. In: Saif Y M (ed) Diseases of poultry, 11th edn. Iowa State University Press, Ames, p 308–320

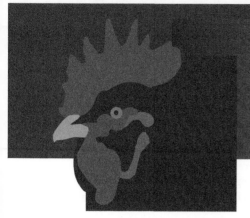

CHAPTER
33

Richard E. Gough and
M. Stewart McNulty

Astroviridae

The family *Astroviridae* comprises two genera, *Mamastrovirus* and *Avastrovirus*, which infect mammalian and avian species respectively. Astroviruses are spherical, non-enveloped, positive-sense, single-stranded RNA viruses typically 28–30 nm in diameter. In contrast to picornaviruses, which are similar in size but have no obvious surface structure, negative staining of astroviruses may reveal the presence of five- or six-pointed star-shaped profiles, which occupy most of the presenting surface of about 10% of the virus particles (Fig. 33.1). Astrovirus infection has been associated with outbreaks of diarrhoea in a variety of mammalian species, including humans, pigs, lambs, calves, dogs, cats, deer and mice; astroviruses appear to be host-restricted. At least eight serotypes of human astrovirus and two serotypes of bovine astrovirus have been

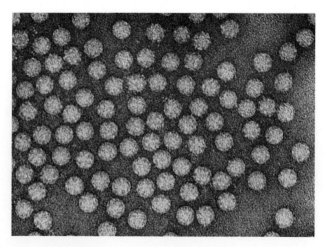

Fig. 33.1 *Turkey astrovirus*, negatively stained.

recognized. Astrovirus infection has been identified as the cause of duck virus hepatitis (DVH) type II and of nephritis in chickens and has also been associated with enteric disease in turkey poults, including the so-called 'poult enteritis and mortality syndrome' (PEMS). Characterization studies have shown that there are at least two genetically distinct serotypes of turkey astrovirus.

It is likely that astrovirus infections occur in many species of domestic poultry. There are reports of their occurrence in chickens in the UK and in guinea fowl with enteritis in Italy. As the star-shaped profiles on the virions may not be present or may be difficult to recognize, it is possible that some of the small, round viruses described in the faeces of a number of different avian species may be astroviruses. Amplification and analysis of viral nucleic acid sequences is a much more reliable way of identifying putative astroviruses than negative-contrast electron microscopy.

TURKEY ASTROVIRUS

EPIDEMIOLOGY

Cause

Astrovirus infection of turkeys has been described in the UK, Italy and the USA. It is likely that these infections occur worldwide. Infection in turkeys occurs very commonly in the first 4 weeks of life. In a flock survey in the USA, astrovirus was detected in 79% of diseased flocks, as opposed to 29% of normal flocks. In the USA, mixed infections of astrovirus and group D *Rotavirus* occurred frequently in diseased flocks. More recently, astroviruses have been detected in the USA in association with PEMS (turkey astrovirus type 2) and have been shown to be antigenically and genetically distinct from previously described turkey astroviruses (*Turkey astrovirus* type 1). There is no evidence for vertical transmission of astroviruses in turkeys or in other species. Spread probably occurs horizontally by ingestion of infected faecal material. Turkey astroviruses are extremely resistant to inactivation by a variety of physical and chemical agents. It has been reported that treatment with a peroxymonosulphate disinfectant, 0.3% formaldehyde or 90% methanol inactivates astrovirus in turkey embryo intestinal homogenates.

DIAGNOSIS

Clinical signs

In the USA, astrovirus infection in commercial turkey poults has been associated with a syndrome, usually occurring between 1 and 3 weeks of age and characterized by diarrhoea, nervousness, litter eating, stunting and slightly increased mortality. The main economic impact of this syndrome stems from the stunting.

The precise role of astrovirus in this syndrome is still to be defined. However, oral inoculation of specific-pathogen-free (SPF) poults with astrovirus resulted in the production of watery droppings and frothy, yellow-brown droppings from 3 to at least 13 days after inoculation. At necropsy, the caeca were distended with fluid and gas. There was gaseous fluid in the intestinal tract, which also showed a loss of muscular tone. There was no mortality but infected poults showed decreased weight gain and a decreased ability to absorb D-xylose compared with uninoculated controls. Dual infection of poults with astrovirus and group D *Rotavirus* produced a more severe experimental disease than astrovirus alone. Intestinal maltase activity was decreased in experimentally infected commercial poults from 3–7 days after inoculation.

Turkey astrovirus type 2 has been associated with PEMS in the USA. This syndrome is characterized by enteritis, high mortality, growth depression, lymphoid atrophy and immunosuppression. Other viruses, including turkey enteric coronavirus, may be detected in poults with PEMS.

Pathogenesis

Turkey astroviruses grow primarily in enterocytes located along the sides and near the base of villi throughout the small intestine, producing lesions of mild crypt hyperplasia. Villous atrophy has not been observed. With *Turkey astrovirus* type 2 there was minimal death of enterocytes and an absence of inflammation. The mechanism by which diarrhoea is induced is unknown.

Turkey astrovirus type 2 has been isolated from the thymus, bursa, spleen and plasma as well as from the intestinal tract of experimentally infected poults. The relative size of the thymuses of experimentally infected poults was decreased but there was no difference in the sizes of the bursa and spleen. Also, the functional properties of the macrophages and lymphocytes exposed to *Turkey astrovirus* type 2 in vivo and in vitro were impaired, so the virus may play a role in producing the immunosuppression associated with PEMS.

Virus detection/isolation

Astroviruses can be detected in faeces by direct negative contrast or immunoelectron microscopy and until recently this was the only diagnostic method available. Turkey astroviruses have not yet been propagated in cell culture but there have been reports of isolation of the virus following inoculation and passage in 20-day-old SPF turkey embryos via the yolk-sac and in 22–25-day-old embryos inoculated by the amniotic route. More recently reverse-transcription polymerase chain reactions (RT-PCRs) have been described that are able to detect and identify astrovirus in faeces and homogenates of intestinal and lymphoid tissues from infected poults. These can distinguish between turkey astrovirus types 1 and 2. Antigen-capture enzyme-linked immunosorbent assays (ELISAs) have also been reported. No serological tests are available yet.

CONTROL

The general comments concerning control of *Rotavirus* infections (Ch. 32) apply equally to astrovirus infections. Because of the resistance of astroviruses to chemical and physical treatment, special emphasis needs to be placed on disinfection and good management practices in order to limit the spread of astrovirus infections between flocks of young turkeys. No vaccines are available.

DUCK VIRUS HEPATITIS TYPE II

EPIDEMIOLOGY

Cause

An astrovirus has been identified as the probable cause of DVH type II. This disease has been described only in East Anglia, England. It was widespread in 2–6-week-old ducks on fattening fields from 1963–1968. By 1969 the disease had disappeared but it reappeared in 1983–1984. Ducks are the only known hosts of the virus but as all outbreaks have initially involved fattening ducks kept in the open, it is possible that other wild birds act as vectors. Using cross-protection and challenge tests, the duck astrovirus was shown to be antigenically distinct from astroviruses isolated from chickens and turkeys and from the picornaviruses that cause DVH types I and III. The virus can be grown with difficulty in chick and duck embryos following amniotic sac inoculation. After 6–10 days' incubation, infected embryos may be inert and stunted, with green necrotic livers. Examination of affected livers by negative-contrast electron microscopy reveals the presence of large numbers of astrovirus particles. The isolated virus has been grown in a chicken hepatocellular carcinoma cell line (LMH) following serial passage. The virus is excreted in the faeces and appears to spread horizontally by contact with infected ducklings or fomites.

DIAGNOSIS

Clinical signs

The clinical signs are similar to those of DVH type I (see Ch. 29). Losses of between 10% and 25% in 3–6-week-old ducks and up to 50% in 6–14-day-old ducks were reported. Diseased ducklings were the progeny of parents that had received DVH type I vaccine. The clinical signs and lesions are highly suggestive, particularly if they occur in the progeny of parents that have been vaccinated against DVH type I.

The pathogenesis of astrovirus infection in ducks is unknown but the main target organs appear to be the liver and kidneys. As with DVH type I, adult ducks are refractory to disease.

Virus detection/isolation

Laboratory diagnosis is based upon direct electron microscopic examination of livers from dead ducks. Virus isolation can be attempted in chick or duck embryos. Serological diagnosis is not recommended because very low levels of antibody are often detected in convalescent sera.

CONTROL

An experimental live attenuated vaccine propagated in chicken embryos has been used successfully. This is administered by subcutaneous inoculation before the young ducks go out onto the fields. Inoculation of susceptible ducklings with convalescent serum has been used successfully on affected farms. Reducing contact with wild birds by rearing ducks indoors will reduce the incidence of the disease.

AVIAN NEPHRITIS VIRUS

EPIDEMIOLOGY

Cause

A virus designated *Avian nephritis virus* (ANV) was first described in Japan in 1979. It was isolated from the rectal contents of an apparently normal 1-week-old broiler chick. ANV was provisionally identified as an enterovirus on the grounds of morphology (30 nm small, round virus particles), RNA content, cytoplasmic replication, resistance to lipid solvents and acid, and partial stabilization to heat inactivation by magnesium chloride. However, following the complete sequencing of the viral genome ANV has been identified as an astrovirus. ANV is antigenically unrelated to DVH type II. At least two serotypes of ANV have been identified, designated ANV 1 and ANV 2.

Spread

Available evidence suggests that ANV is distributed worldwide in domestic fowl. Antibody to ANV has also been detected in flocks of SPF chickens. Antibody has also been detected in turkeys by indirect immunofluorescence but not by serum neutralization. As turkeys resist experimental infection with ANV, this suggests that turkeys are infected with a virus antigenically related to but distinct from ANV. It was not detected in 111 fertile eggs laid by SPF hens experimentally infected with the virus, indicating that, if it occurs at all, vertical transmission occurs at a very low frequency. ANV spreads readily to in-contact chickens, probably through ingestion of faecally contaminated material.

DIAGNOSIS

Clinical signs and lesions

The importance of ANV as an avian pathogen is not fully established. Following oral inoculation of 1-day-old SPF chickens with the G-4260 strain of ANV, diarrhoea was observed from 3–7 days after infection. Also, inoculated chicks showed 33% mortality and had significantly lower body weights 14 days after inoculation than uninoculated controls. Visceral urate deposition was observed in the dead chicks. Histologically, the kidneys of birds examined 14 days after infection showed interstitial nephritis of varying severity. Other isolates of ANV differed from the G-4260 strain in various aspects of their pathogenicity in the same disease model.

While chickens of any age can be infected with ANV, 1-day-old chicks are the most susceptible; there is a developing age resistance to disease.

Since the original isolation, viruses with similar morphology and physical characteristics and antigenically indistinguishable from ANV have been isolated in Japan and Europe. These include viruses associated with the runting stunting syndrome in Belgium and the UK. These produce depressions in weight gain of variable severity in orally infected broilers. Histopathological lesions in the small intestine include villous stunting and increased crypt depth.

Virus isolation

To isolate ANV, samples of faeces and/or kidney should be inoculated into cultures of chick kidney cells grown in serum-free medium or into chick embryos via the yolk sac or chorioallantoic membrane (CAM) routes. Some isolates of ANV produce a typical enterovirus rounded cell cytopathic effect. However, growth in cell cultures is more reliably detected by immunofluorescence. Infected chick embryos die, but signs of ANV infection are not pathognomonic. Immunofluorescent staining of yolk stalk or CAM preparations is required to demonstrate that ANV is present.

Serology

Antibodies to ANV have been detected by indirect immunofluorescence, serum neutralization tests and ELISA. Of these, serum neutralization is the most sensitive, but is costly and laborious.

CONTROL

Until the role of ANV is better defined, no control measures are recommended. ANV should, however, be eliminated from SPF flocks.

CHICKEN ASTROVIRUS

In recent years, isolations of three chicken astroviruses antigenically related to each other and antigenically and genetically distinct from ANV1 and DVH type 2 astrovirus have been described. These viruses have been designated chicken astrovirus. They were isolated in chick embryo liver cell cultures and also grew well in the LMH cell line. They caused mild diarrhoea and some distension in the small intestines of experimentally infected 1-day-old SPF chicks. Antibody to chicken astrovirus was widespread in broilers and broiler breeders and was also present in some turkey flocks. Their ability to cause disease in the field has not yet been investigated but the virus was isolated from chicks with runting stunting syndrome or enteric problems. The amino acid sequence derived from the relatively conserved nonstructural polyprotein of chicken astrovirus showed 55% identity with that of ANV1 and 58% identity with that of turkey astrovirus type 2. The antigenic relationship of chicken astrovirus to ANV2 remains to be investigated.

FURTHER READING

Baxendale W, Mebatsion T 2004 The isolation and characterization of astroviruses from chickens. Avian Pathol 33: 364–370

Gough R E, Stuart J C 1993 Astroviruses in ducks (duck virus hepatitis type II). In: McFerran J B, McNulty M S (eds) Virus infections of birds. Elsevier, Amsterdam, p 505–508

Guy J S, Miles A M, Smith L et al 2004 Antigenic and genomic characterization of turkey enterovirus-like virus (North Carolina, 1988 isolate): Identification of the virus as turkey astrovirus 2. Avian Dis 48: 206–211

Imada T, Yamaguchi S, Mase M et al 2000 Avian nephritis virus (ANV) as a new member of the family Astroviridae and construction of infectious ANVc DNA. J Virol 74: 8487–8493

Koci M D, Schultz-Cherry S L 2002 Avian astroviruses: Avian Pathol 31: 213–227

Reynolds D L, Schultz-Cherry S L 2003 Astrovirus infections. In: Saif Y M (ed) Diseases of poultry, 11th edn. Iowa State University Press, Ames, p 320–326

Woolcock P R 2003 Duck hepatitis. In: Saif Y M (ed) Diseases of poultry, 11th edn. Iowa State University Press, Ames, p 343–354

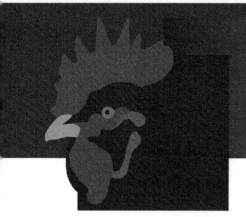

CHAPTER 34

Daniel Todd and
M. Stewart McNulty

Circoviridae

The family *Circoviridae* contains small, icosahedral, non-enveloped viruses with single-stranded, circular DNA genomes. On the basis of its larger virion and genome sizes and differences in genome organization, *Chicken anaemia virus* (CAV) has been assigned to the genus *Gyrovirus* of the *Circoviridae*, while other members of the family, which include *Psittacine beak and feather disease virus* (BFDV), *Pigeon circovirus* (PiCV), *Goose circovirus* (GoCV), *Canary circovirus* (CaCV), *Duck circovirus* (DuCV) and *Porcine circovirus* types 1 and 2 (PCV1, PCV2), belong to the *Circovirus* genus. Additional circoviruses likely to be assigned to the genus *Circovirus* include those from gouldian finch (*Chloebia gouldiae*) (FiCV) and herring gull (*Larus argentatus*) (GuCV).

CHICKEN ANAEMIA VIRUS

EPIDEMIOLOGY

Cause

An agent capable of causing increased mortality associated with anaemia, lymphoid depletion, liver changes and haemorrhages throughout the body in experimentally infected chicks was first described in Japan in 1979 and was designated chicken anaemia agent (CAA). CAA is now known to be a small (25 nm), non-enveloped icosahedral virus (Fig. 34.1) containing a single-stranded, circular DNA consisting of approximately 2.3 kb, and has been renamed *Chicken anaemia virus* (CAV). CAV is a remarkably resistant virus: its infectivity resists heating at 80°C for 15 min, treatment with chloroform and exposure to pH 3.

Available evidence suggests that only one serotype of CAV exists, although antigenic differences between isolates can be detected using monoclonal antibody reactivity. The existence of a second CAV serotype was suggested when an antigenically distinct agent was shown to cause similar pathogenic effects following experimental infection of specific-pathogen-free (SPF)

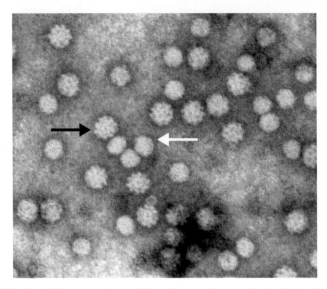

Fig. 34.1 Negatively stained *Chicken anaemia virus* (25 nm diameter; black arrow) and psittacine beak and feather disease particles (20 nm diameter; white arrow).

chickens. However, this agent needs to be isolated and molecularly characterized to confirm that it represents a second CAV serotype. All naturally occurring isolates of CAV appear to be pathogenic for experimentally infected chicks.

Hosts

CAV has been isolated from chickens in an increasing number of countries worldwide and serological surveys indicate that CAV infection is common in chickens throughout the world. In a small survey of UK turkey and duck sera, no antibodies to CAV were found. It is not known if avian species other than domestic fowl can be infected. Neutralizing activity against CAV has been reported in sera of Japanese quail, but it is not known if this is due to infection with CAV or to the presence of antibody to an antigenically related virus. On the basis of its narrow host range, CAV is very unlikely to have zoonotic potential.

Spread

There is both field and experimental evidence for vertical transmission of CAV. However, under normal circumstances, in which the majority of birds in a breeder flock have acquired antibody to CAV during the rearing period, this appears to be of minor importance. Serological evidence indicates that, in the UK at least, most breeders become infected before onset of lay with horizontally transmitted virus, probably by ingesting infected material.

DIAGNOSIS

Signs

Disease resulting from CAV infection occurs in the progeny of breeder flocks that are infected for the first time with the virus after they come into lay. In these circumstances, CAV is vertically transmitted to the progeny. No clinical signs are seen in the parents. However, around 2 weeks of age, the young chicks show variable mortality. This can be as great as 60% but usually averages around 10%. The most characteristic changes in infected chicks are anaemia, aplasia of the bone marrow and atrophy of the thymus, spleen and bursa of Fabricius. Haemorrhages may occur under the skin and throughout the skeletal muscles. Enlarged livers and gangrenous dermatitis may also be present. Synonyms for this condition include anaemia dermatitis syndrome, infectious anaemia syndrome, haemorrhagic syndrome and blue-wing disease. Most of the reported outbreaks of anaemia dermatitis syndrome have occurred in broilers but the condition also occurs in replacement pullets.

Subclinical infection of the progeny of immune breeder flocks is common and usually occurs soon after maternally acquired antibodies have disappeared at about 3 weeks of age.

Pathogenesis

Experimental studies have shown that anaemia and other pathological changes associated with CAV are produced only following parenteral inoculation of high doses of CAV into neonatal, fully susceptible (i.e. no maternal antibody) chicks. Chicks develop an age resistance to experimental disease, but not to infection, between 7 and 14 days of age. Chicks infected by contact with parenterally inoculated chicks are also resistant to experimental disease but become infected and shed virus. Maternal antibody is protective. Chicks with maternal antibody usually show no disease or anaemia following parenteral inoculation but may become infected and shed the virus. SPF chick embryos infected with CAV via the yolk sac hatch normally but show typical signs of disease around 1–2 weeks of age.

Experimental dual infection of CAV and immunosuppressive viruses such as reticuloendotheliosis virus, virulent *Marek's disease virus* and infectious bursal disease (IBD) virus enhances the apparent pathogenicity of CAV, resulting in greater mortality and more persistent anaemia and histological lesions. In such dual infections the protective effect of maternal antibody to CAV may be overcome. In chicks dually infected with CAV and IBD virus, the age resistance was overcome and contact-infected chicks also developed anaemia. The importance of this phenomenon under field conditions requires investigation. CAV has been shown to be immunosuppressive. Functional changes were detected in splenic lymphocytes and splenic and bone marrow macrophages from both clinically affected and subclinically infected chicks. Following intramuscular inoculation of susceptible day-old chicks, CAV was consistently recovered from all organs examined, including the brain, liver, bone marrow, rectal contents and lymphoid organs, for up to 21 days after inoculation. The principal sites of CAV replication are precursor T cells in the thymic cortex and in haemocytoblasts in the bone marrow. Destruction of these cells accounts for the immunosuppression and anaemia. However, the virus also replicates in all lymphoid aggregates throughout the body.

Virus detection and isolation

Outbreaks of clinical disease are normally diagnosed on the basis of the characteristic signs and pathology. There is also usually a history of a common breeder flock, which is often close to peak egg production. Laboratory diagnosis is based on immunofluorescent or immunocytochemical detection of CAV antigens in thymus or bone marrow from affected chicks. Viral DNA can also be detected in the same material by techniques such as in situ hybridization, dot blot hybridization or polymerase chain reaction (PCR).

Virus isolation is not recommended as a diagnostic method because it is slow and expensive. However, CAV can be isolated, either in cultured cells, including MDCC-MSB1 and MDCC-CU147, or by inoculation of susceptible 1-day-old chicks. Specimens of choice for CAV isolation are liver, thymus, spleen and buffy coat. Growth of CAV in experimentally infected chicks is detected by demonstration of anaemia (haematocrit below 27%) and other characteristic lesions, and by development of antibody. Growth in MDCC-MSB1 cells is detected by cytopathology and immunofluorescent staining. Up to 10 passages in MSB1 cells may be required to isolate the virus. The most sensitive PCR methods are likely to have greater sensitivity than virus isolation. However, given that low levels of CAV DNA can persist in chickens for months after infection, detection of virus DNA by a highly sensitive PCR technique may be of questionable value to the diagnostician faced with clinical disease problems.

Serology

Serum antibodies to CAV have been detected by a variety of serological tests, including serum neutralization, indirect immunofluorescence and enzyme-linked immunosorbent assay (ELISA). A number of ELISAs are commercially available. Serological screening is commonly undertaken to identify seronegative breeder flocks in whose progeny disease is likely to occur and to monitor the success of vaccination. Additionally, serological testing is used to monitor SPF chicken flocks that are used to supply eggs for vaccine production.

CONTROL

As CAV infection is very common, it is not practicable to maintain breeder flocks free of infection throughout their lifetime. Infection during the rearing period is subclinical and occurs in the majority of breeder flocks. However, isolated breeder flocks may not experience infection until they are in lay, with disastrous consequences for the progeny. Live vaccines are available for administration parenterally or via the drinking water to breeder chickens during the rearing period to protect against vertical transmission.

There is evidence that horizontally acquired, subclinical CAV infection of the broiler progeny of immune breeder flocks is associated with significantly impaired economic performance. At present, there are no means of controlling these losses by vaccination.

Because CAV is egg transmitted and has also been present in some SPF chicken flocks used for vaccine manufacture, there is a danger that the virus could contaminate avian vaccines. It is therefore important to ensure that SPF flocks are maintained free from infection with CAV.

CIRCOVIRUS INFECTIONS OF OTHER AVIAN SPECIES INCLUDING PIGEONS, GEESE AND DUCKS

EPIDEMIOLOGY

Cause, hosts and spread

Seven of the nine circoviruses currently or tentatively assigned to the genus *Circovirus* infect avian species, with the majority having been characterized as circoviruses on the basis of nucleotide sequence similarities shared with PCV1. PCV1, the most studied and type species of the genus, was first characterized in 1979. The PCV1 virions measure 20 nm in diameter and contain the smallest DNA genome (1.8 kb) possessed by an animal virus. PCV1 is resistant to high temperature and pH 3. Avian circoviruses have single-stranded DNA genomes ranging from 1.8 kb to 2.0 kb and are likely to resemble PCV1 in their physicochemical properties. Viruses from the genus *Circovirus* share very similar genome organizations but can be differentiated by comparison of their genome nucleotide sequences and the translated amino acid sequences of the two major *Circovirus* proteins. Avian circoviruses appear to have narrow host ranges. For example, geese and ducks, which are related anatid birds, are infected with different circoviruses. On this basis, cross-infection of other avian and mammalian species is considered unlikely.

PiCV infections have been reported in racing pigeons and/or in pigeons reared for meat in North America, Australia and a number of European countries. GoCV infections have been reported in farmed geese in Germany, Hungary and Taiwan, while ducks farmed in Germany, Hungary, France and the USA have been reported as *Circovirus*-infected. Serological tests are not yet available to assess levels of infection but it is probable that *Circovirus* infections of these domesticated avian species occur at a high prevalence worldwide. Interestingly, circoviruses have not yet been detected in chickens and turkeys. Similarly, gyroviruses have not been detected in those avian species in which circoviruses have been recognized.

Infections with avian circoviruses are generally diagnosed in juvenile birds; circoviruses have been detected in geese, ducks and pigeons as young as 1 week old. Findings with racing pigeons indicate that most birds aged 3–10 weeks are infected and that virus can frequently be detected in cloacal swabs for months thereafter. PiCV DNA has been detected in tissues from most adult (>1 year old) racing pigeons, suggesting that some adults may be carriers. The detection of PiCV DNA in embryos supports the view that vertical transmission is possible, but horizontal transmission to young birds through the ingestion of infected material is thought to be more common. It remains to be determined whether *Circovirus* infections of geese and ducks are similar in these characteristics.

DIAGNOSIS

Clinical signs

Circovirus infections of pigeons are associated with a variety of clinical signs, including weight loss, diarrhoea, respiratory distress and poor race performance, while infections of farmed geese and ducks are associated with growth retardation, developmental problems and feather disorders. *Circovirus*-induced immunosuppression can predispose some birds to secondary infections. For example, the immunosuppression induced by *Circovirus* infections of geese was considered to be a predisposing factor for other microbial pathogens, including *Reimerella anatipestifer* and *Aspergillus fumigatus*.

Pathogenesis

Information relating to pathogenesis is based on examination of field material, since there have been no reports describing experimental disease reproduction in pigeons, geese and ducks. *Circovirus* infections of clinically affected birds are associated with lymphocyte depletion and the detection of intracytoplasmic globular or botryoid inclusions, which are commonly found in macrophages within lymphoid tissue such as bursa of Fabricius (Fig. 34.2). These inclusions, which are characteristic of circoviruses, contain paracrystalline arrays of tightly packed virus particles. The target cells and major sites of virus replication remain to be identified for the circoviruses of pigeons, geese and ducks. In psittacine birds, BFDV replicates principally in the epithelial cells of the feather follicle. Circoviruses are highly dependent on the host cell

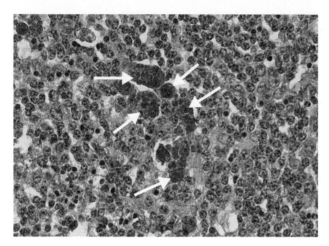

Fig. 34.2 Botryoid inclusions (arrows) in the cytoplasm of several cells in the bursa of Fabricius of a pigeon. Such inclusions are commonly seen in *Circovirus*-infected pigeons and are characteristic of viruses of the *Circovirus* genus. (Courtesy of Dr Joan A. Smyth, University of Connecticut.)

replication machinery, because of their small genome size, and virus will be produced in greater amounts in rapidly replicating cells. For this reason, macrophages are unlikely to support efficient virus replication and the appearance of circoviruses in the cytoplasm of these cells is probably due to their phagocytosing function.

Using bursa of Fabricius samples obtained from clinically affected and apparently normal racing pigeons, diagnostic testing showed that PiCV could be detected in a higher (84%) proportion of birds by PCR than by in situ hybridization (75%), dot–blot hybridization (63%) and histology (41%). Based on observations made with pigeons and with geese, it is likely that many birds experience mild, subclinical infections with no apparent associated histopathology. Semiquantitative dot–blot hybridization and real-time PCR tests indicate that very high virus loads can be detected in some pigeons, geese and ducks, and it is likely that such birds are the most severely affected by *Circovirus* infection. The factors that dictate whether infections are mild and subclinical or clinically severe are unknown but may include route of exposure, virus dose, virus strain, levels of maternal antibody and presence of other pathogens.

Virus isolation and detection

Avian *Circovirus* infections, including those caused by PiCV, GoCV and DuCV, were originally diagnosed by histology and electron microscopy. There have been no reports describing the isolation and propagation of such as viruses in cell culture or embryos. The lack of in vitro propagation methods has restricted attempts to produce virus-specific antibodies for use in antigen-detecting diagnostic tests such as immunohistochemistry or immunofluorescence. Attention has therefore focused on molecular diagnostics, including PCR, dot–blot hybridization and in situ hybridization, which depend on the ability to detect virus DNA. Successful PCR tests have been described for PiCV, GoCV and DuCV. However, the detection by PCR of PiCV DNA in samples from clinically normal pigeons suggests that PCR may be of questionable use as a disease indicator because of its high sensitivity. So far, there have been no reports describing the development of tests for detecting virus-specific antibody. Such tests are likely to depend on the use of virus antigen produced by recombinant DNA-based expression systems.

CONTROL

Because *Circovirus* infections of pigeons, geese and ducks are likely to be common and wide-spread, it is impracticable to attempt eradication. It is possible that the clinical effects in young birds might be reduced by increasing maternal antibody levels. This might be achieved by vaccinating breeding birds and, concomitantly, the levels of vertical transmission, should such occur, might be reduced. In the absence of a cell culture propagation method, vaccine development is likely to involve the use of recombinant DNA-based technologies. It is also possible that the implementation of thorough disinfection and hygiene procedures during the early rearing period will reduce the levels of infectious virus to which the young birds are exposed and that this will have a beneficial effect on clinical outcome.

FURTHER READING

Ball N W, Smyth J A, Weston J H et al 2004 Diagnosis of goose circovirus infection in Hungarian geese using polymerase chain reaction and dot blot hybridization tests. Avian Pathol 33: 51–58

Duchatel J P, Todd D, Smyth J A et al 2006 Observations on detection, excretion and transmission of pigeon circovirus in adult, young and embryonic pigeons. Avian Pathol 35: 30–34

Fringuelli E, Scott A N J, Beckett A et al 2006 Diagnosis of duck circovirus by conventional and real time polymerase chain reaction. Avian Pathol 34: 495–500

McNulty M S 1991 Chicken anaemia agent: a review. Avian Pathol 20: 187–203

McNulty M S, McIlroy S G, Bruce D W et al 1991 Economic effects of subclinical chicken anaemia agent infection in broiler chickens. Avian Dis 35: 263–268

Noteborn M H M, Koch G 1995 Chicken anaemia virus infection: molecular basis of pathogenicity. Avian Pathol 24: 11–31

Smyth J A, Moffett D A, McNulty M S et al 1993 A sequential histopathologic and immunocytochemical study of chicken anemia virus infection at one day of age. Avian Dis 37: 324–338

Soike D, Kohler B, Albrecht K 1999 A circovirus-like infection in geese related to a runting syndrome. Avian Pathol 28: 199–202

Todd D 2000 Circoviruses: immunosuppressive threats to avian species: a review. Avian Pathol 29: 373–394

Vielitz E, Landgraf F 1988 Anaemia–dermatitis of broilers: field observations on its occurrence, transmission and prevention. Avian Pathol 17: 113–120

Woods L W, Latimer K S 2000 Circovirus infection of non-psittacine birds. J Avian Med Surg 14: 154–163

Yuasa N, Taniguchi T, Yoshida I 1979 Isolation and some characteristics of an agent inducing anemia in chicks. Avian Dis 23: 366–385

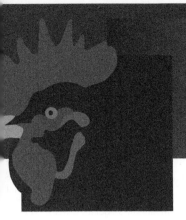

CHAPTER 35

Richard E. Gough

Parvoviridae

Although the small DNA viruses that make up the family *Parvoviridae* are further divided into two subfamilies and six genera, only viruses of subfamily *Parvovirinae*, genus *Parvovirus* are known to cause disease in poultry. There is an avian adeno-associated virus, subfamily *Parvovirinae*, genus *Dependovirus*, but its significance as a pathogen is unclear.

Goose parvovirus (GPV) infection, often referred to as Derzsy's disease, is a highly contagious disease of young goslings (subfamily Anatinae, tribe Anserini) and Muscovy ducks (*Cairina moschata*, also of tribe Anserini). The disease, also known as goose or gosling plague, goose hepatitis, goose enteritis or infectious myocarditis, can result in 100% mortality. GPV has been reported from all the major goose farming countries of Europe, including the former Soviet Union and Israel. The disease has also been reported from the People's Republic of China, Taiwan, Japan and south-east Asia. A similar disease caused by *Muscovy duck parvovirus* (MDPV) has also been reported from many of the above countries where Muscovy ducks are intensively farmed, and from California, USA.

Although vaccines are available the disease remains a serious problem in countries where geese and Muscovy ducks are farmed intensively.

Parvoviruses and parvovirus-like viruses have been reported in broiler chickens, associated with infectious runting disease. Parvovirus-like particles have also been detected by electron microscopic examination of intestinal contents from chickens, game birds and turkeys. The significance of the presence of these viruses in these species has yet to be confirmed.

EPIDEMIOLOGY

Cause

GPV and MDPV have been reported to show differences in host range, antigenicity and nucleotide sequences. Both viruses were originally classified as autonomous members of the

Parvoviridae on the basis of morphological, biochemical and culture characteristics. Intact virions are unenveloped and hexagonal in shape with an estimated 32 capsomere and a diameter of 20–22 nm. The density of the virus in caesium chloride is approximately 1.38 g/mL and the genome is composed of single-stranded DNA about 5–6 kb in length. Using a MDPV isolate three major proteins of 91 kDa (VP1), 78 kDa (VP2) and 58 kDa (VP3) and a fourth lighter protein of 51 kDa have been identified and those of GPV have been reported to be similar. The virus is very resistant to chemical and physical inactivation, with no significant loss of activity after 1 h at pH 3. No haemagglutinating activity has been reported for these viruses using a variety of red blood cells under various conditions.

Recently, partial nucleotide sequencing and DNA cross-hybridization studies have indicated that GPV is more closely related to the human *Dependovirus* genus than to other autonomous parvoviruses. It has been shown that human helper-dependent adeno-associated virus type 2 can enhance the replication of GPV under in vitro conditions. No antigenic relationship with chicken or mammalian parvoviruses has been reported.

There are thought to be no public health risks associated with GPV and MDPV.

Host

GPV infection occurs in all breeds of domestic goose and in Muscovy ducks. The disease has also been reported in wild geese following accidental infection and serological evidence suggests that the virus is present in several species of goose in Europe.

MDPV infection has been reported to occur in various genetic crosses of Muscovy ducks and several indigenous breeds of duck in the Far East. Geese appear to be much less susceptible to MDPV than to GPV.

In both geese and Muscovy ducks the disease is strictly age-dependent, with up to 100% mortality occurring in birds under 1 week of age. Progressive resistance to infection occurs, so that by the time the birds are 4–5 weeks old negligible losses occur. Following infection, older geese and Muscovy ducks show no clinical signs but respond immunologically. Other breeds of waterfowl and domestic poultry appear refractory to infection.

Spread

In susceptible goslings and Muscovy ducklings the most serious parvovirus outbreaks occur following vertical transmission of the virus. In breeding stock that become subclinically infected a latent infection may become established, with subsequent egg transmission of the virus. This may result in poor fertility or mortality of the embryo during incubation or in the neonatal bird. The severity of the infection in the newly hatched gosling or duckling will depend on the levels of maternally derived antibody. Horizontal transmission usually occurs via contaminated drinking water and feed. Once in the digestive tract the virus replicates in the intestinal wall and subsequently enters the blood. Following a viraemic phase the virus reaches various organs, including preferentially the liver and heart. Replication in these organs causes severe pathological changes and death within 2–5 days of showing clinical signs in susceptible neonatal birds. Infected birds excrete large amounts of virus in their faeces, resulting in transmission of the virus by direct and indirect contact.

Following infection, age-resistant birds may excrete virus in their faeces for several weeks. The site of viral replication is unknown but is thought to be in the intestinal mucosa.

DIAGNOSIS

Clinical signs

The course of the disease may be very rapid in goslings/ducklings under 1 week of age with anorexia, prostration and death in 2–5 days. In birds with variable levels of maternally derived antibody or 1–3-week-old birds the disease follows a more protracted course, with mortality levels below 10%, although morbidity levels may be high. In goslings there is often a nasal and ocular discharge with associated head shaking. The uropygial glands and eyelids are often red and swollen and examination of the birds may reveal a fibrinous pseudomembrane covering the tongue and oral cavity. A profuse white diarrhoea may also be evident in many of the birds. Young birds that survive the acute phase may develop a more prolonged disease characterized by loss of down, reddening of the skin and profound growth retardation. In goslings there may be an accumulation of ascitic fluid in the abdominal cavity, which causes the goslings to stand in a 'penguin-like' posture. Similar clinical signs may be seen in Muscovy ducklings, which also show pronounced locomotor problems. Some reports suggest that an enteric form of GPV exists that is not associated with classical signs of GPV.

Lesions

In acute cases gross lesions are frequently found in the intestinal tract and heart, which appears pale and is characteristically rounded at its apex. Congestion and enlargement of the pancreas, liver and spleen are often described. In cases with a more prolonged clinical course a variety of lesions may be present, including a serofibrinous perihepatitis and pericarditis, ascites, catarrhal enteritis, liver dystrophy and pulmonary oedema.

The main histopathological features are degeneration and infiltration of the myocardial cells and the presence of Cowdry type A intranuclear inclusions. Similar histological changes may be seen in the enterocytes and smooth muscle cells. Intranuclear and intracytoplasmic inclusion bodies may be found in the liver hepatocytes, which become vacuolated and infiltrated with fat. Similar changes occur in the spleen, kidney, pancreas, bursa and thymus. In Muscovy ducklings muscle fibre degeneration, mild sciatic neuritis and polioencephalomyelitis have also been reported. The pathological features will vary depending on the age of the birds at the time of infection.

Virus isolation

For attempted isolation of GPV a selection of 20% w/v tissue suspensions, including heart and liver, are prepared in antibiotic phosphate-buffered saline and inoculated into embryonated goose or Muscovy duck eggs or cell cultures derived from them. Following inoculation in the allantoic cavity of 10–15-day-old susceptible goose or Muscovy duck eggs, embryo mortality occurs 5–15 days later. The embryos appear haemorrhagic, particularly the liver and kidneys. A minimum of two blind passages should be undertaken before the isolation is considered to be negative. Further passage of isolated virus will result in consistent embryo mortality between 4 and 10 days after inoculation. Attempted isolation of MDPV should be carried out in susceptible Muscovy duck eggs of a similar age.

Parvovirus can also be isolated following the inoculation of primary cell cultures derived from 12–15-day-old goose or Muscovy duck embryos. Isolation is facilitated by inoculating cell cultures at the time of preparation and before they form a confluent monolayer. The virus produces a cytopathic effect consisting of rounded, refractile cells 3–6 days after inoculation. Several passages may be required before a cytopathic effect is detected, particularly when attempting to isolate the Muscovy duck parvovirus.

Characterization

The presence of the virus can be confirmed by electron microscopy examination of the egg or tissue culture concentrates. Neutralization tests using specific antisera to GPV and MDPV can also be used to identify the virus.

Various antigen detection techniques have been developed to detect and identify parvoviruses in post-mortem tissues, embryonated eggs and cell cultures. These include immunofluorescence, immunoperoxidase, antigen capture, enzyme-linked immunosorbent assay (ELISA), digoxigenin-labelled DNA probe and nucleic acid dot-blotting assay.

Agar gel immunodiffusion tests have also been described to identify parvoviruses in embryonic tissues and allantoic fluids from infected embryos.

The polymerase chain reaction (PCR) has also been developed to detect parvoviruses. Primers have been designed from conserved regions of the VP1 and VP2 genes that encode for the capsid proteins. These can be used to differentiate strains of GPV and MDPV following restriction fragment length polymorphism analysis. Phylogenetic analysis has been used to characterize the molecular properties of different isolates, and some differences between specific amino acids were found that could be used to differentiate vaccine and field strains of GPV.

Serology

Several serological techniques have been described to detect antibodies to parvovirus in submitted serum samples, including: virus neutralization, agar gel precipitin, ELISA, plaque reduction assay and a sperm agglutination-inhibition test. These serological tests can be used to confirm parvovirus infection and also to determine the immune response following vaccination. Demonstration of antibody in the yolk of eggs will provide information on the levels of maternal derived antibody in the progeny.

CONTROL

Many outbreaks of *Parvovirus* can be directly attributed to hatching goslings or Muscovy ducklings from eggs contaminated with the virus. This often results from the practice of incubating and hatching eggs that have originated from breeding flocks infected with *Parvovirus*. Only eggs from known *Parvovirus*-free flocks should be incubated and hatched together. This means that countries that are free of *Parvovirus* infection should import hatching eggs only from countries that can guarantee that their flocks are also free of this virus. Birds that survive an outbreak of disease should not be used for breeding as they are potential carriers of the virus.

Before vaccines became available passive immunization of young birds with hyperimmune serum was practised widely. However, this was found to be both time-consuming and expensive, particularly as two doses of serum were usually required to produce satisfactory immunity. Both live and oil-emulsion inactivated GPV and MDPV vaccines are widely available in countries where the disease is endemic. In some cases the vaccines are bivalent and contain both GPV and MDPV antigens. Live vaccines have been developed following attenuation of the virus by multiple passage in embryonated goose or duck eggs or cell cultures. These vaccines are administered by injection of neonatal birds or breeding flocks and have been shown to induce a good immune response. Inactivated vaccines are also used in breeder flocks, particularly those in which *Parvovirus* has not been diagnosed.

Good biosecurity is also an important factor in reducing the risk of infection by preventing contact between wild geese, which can be latently infected with GPV, and domestic geese and Muscovy ducks.

FURTHER READING

Gough R E 1998 Goose parvovirus (Derzsy's disease). In: Swayne D E, Glisson J R, Jackwood M W et al (eds) Isolation and identification of avian pathogens, 4th edn. American Association of Avian Pathologists, Kennett Square, p 219–222

Gough R E 2003 Goose parvovirus infection. In: Saif Y M (ed) Diseases of poultry, 11th edn. Iowa State University Press, Ames, p 367–374

Tatar-kis T, Mato T, Markos B, Palya V 2004 Phylogenetic analysis of Hungarian goose parvovirus isolates and vaccine strains. Avian Pathol 33: 438–444

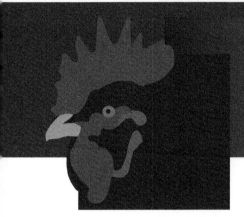

Richard E. Gough

Caliciviridae and hepeviruses

The virus family *Caliciviridae* is currently comprised of four recognized genera: *Vesivirus*, *Lagovirus*, *Norovirus* and *Sapovirus*. Formerly, it was considered that hepatitis E and related viruses, which form the *Hepevirus* genus, were members of the *Caliciviridae*. However, recent, more detailed molecular analysis has indicated that hepeviruses show sufficient divergence from caliciviruses for them to be assigned their own family. There is a proposal to create a new family, assigned the name *Hepiviridae*, of which *Hepevirus* is currently the sole genus.

Caliciviruses are non-enveloped viruses 27–40 nm in diameter and possess a single-strand positive sense RNA genome of approximately 7–8 kb. When observed by transmission electron microscopy, typical particles show cup-shaped depressions on the surface, from which the name calicivirus (from calix) is derived (Fig. 36.1).

Caliciviruses have been associated with diseases of mammals (seals, swine, cattle, various Felidae, canines, rabbits, primates and humans), reptiles (snakes), amphibia, fish and birds. The viruses show diverse tissue tropisms resulting in various disease conditions, such as blistering of the skin and mucosa, pneumonia, abortion, encephalitis, myocarditis, hepatitis, haemorrhage and enteritis. During the last 20 years particles showing the distinctive calicivirus morphology have been detected by negative-contrast electron microscopy infrequently in avian species, usually associated with enteric problems in commercial broiler chickens, game birds and guinea fowl. Caliciviruses have also been detected in goldfinches (*Carduelis carduelis*) and white terns (*Gygis albie Rothschildi*). In cases involving commercial poultry the aetiological role of the caliciviruses has not been established. While enteric problems feature in many of the cases, a variety of other pathogens have also been implicated in the disease outbreaks, including coccidiosis, colisepticaemia, aspergillosis, rotavirus, reovirus, adenovirus and enterovirus-like agents.

Recent studies have shown that the viruses associated with big liver and spleen (BLS) disease and hepatitis–splenomegaly syndrome (HSS) of chickens are genetically and antigenically similar and related to human and porcine hepatitis E viruses that make up the *Hepevirus* genus. On the basis of this similarity with mammalian hepeviruses it has been proposed that the viruses

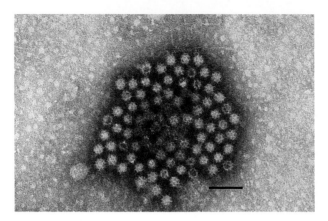

Fig. 36.1 Avian *Caliciviridae* particles detected in the intestinal contents of broiler chickens. Bar = 100 nm.

responsible for BLS and HSS be tentatively referred to as avian *Hepatitis E virus* (HEV) to distinguish them from human and porcine HEVs. The zoonotic risk of avian HEVs has not yet been determined.

BIG LIVER AND SPLEEN DISEASE

BLS was first described in Australia in the 1980s and subsequently in the UK and USA. Typically the disease affects broiler breeders and layer breeders and is characterized by drops in egg production, increased mortality and enlarged livers and spleens. In the USA the disease has been associated with 'primary feather drop syndrome', where broiler breeders fail to peak during production, show delayed sexual maturity and moult primary feathers. There is serological evidence that BLS is now widespread in commercial poultry in other parts of the world. The putative virus associated with BLS is a hepevirus genetically similar to the virus associated with HSS.

EPIDEMIOLOGY

Cause

Definitive identification of the etiological agent of BLS has not been possible following electron microscopy examination of tissues from infected chickens. Using molecular methods a cDNA clone representing a portion of the virus genome was sequenced and found to have over 60% similarity to human *Hepatitis E virus*. Further studies are required in order to fully characterize and determine the classification of the virus. Using suspensions of liver from infected birds the virus was shown to be resistant to treatment with ether and chloroform but not after heat treatment at 56°C for 1 h or 37°C for 6 h.

Spread

Horizontal transmission occurs between flocks on farms by the faecal–oral route, although spread within a flock may be relatively slow. Under experimental conditions aerosol transmission was not successful. Inoculation of chicken embryos with BLS-infected liver homogenates resulted in a state of persistent antigenaemia up to 11 months of age, at which time birds placed in contact also became infected. BLS antigen was detected in 1-day-old culled broiler chicks and in the livers of broiler chickens that were the progeny of a BLS-affected flock. This suggests that vertical transmission probably occurs following field infection. Chickens of all ages are susceptible to infection but clinical disease is only seen in birds over 24 weeks of age.

DIAGNOSIS

Clinical signs and lesions

Chickens of all ages are susceptible to infection but clinical disease is only seen in birds over 24 weeks of age. There is considerable variation in the severity of the clinical signs and morbidity and mortality is generally low. In Europe and the USA clinical signs are usually mild or inapparent compared to those seen in Australia. Sick birds are found sitting under nest boxes or along the sides of the houses, often with pale wattles and combs and soiling of the vent feathers. The first signs are usually a rapid drop in egg production lasting for up to 3–4 weeks with another 3–5 weeks before normal production is regained. In extreme cases egg drops of up to 20% have been reported, with poor eggshell quality. If the disease appears early in production a failure to attain peak production may be the first sign of BLS.

At postmortem examination birds are generally in good bodily condition but there are gross changes to the liver, spleen and ovaries. The liver is often enlarged and small subcapsular haemorrhages may be present. The spleen is two or three times larger than normal with a mottled appearance, and the pulp may contain numerous pale foci. Regression and rupture of the ovaries may occur, causing egg peritonitis. Other lesions include pulmonary congestion with oedema and enteritis, particularly in the duodenum. Histological lesions in the initial stages of the disease include lymphoproliferative changes in the liver and spleen, resulting in hepato- and splenomegaly followed by a pyknotic destructive phase that coincides with the onset of clinical signs. Two to three weeks later there is a macrophage responsive phase with marked infiltration of the macrophages, which is followed by a late response and recovery stages.

Haematological changes also occur with BLS; including reduced PCV values, small and damaged erythrocytes, enlarged vacuolated thrombocytes, occasional large blast-type cells and a leucocytosis.

Virus isolation and detection

Traditionally the agar gel immunodiffusion (AGID) test was used to detect BLS antigen in homogenates of liver and spleen during the proliferative stages of the disease using monospecific BLS antibody. More recently antigen-capture enzyme-linked immunosorbent assay (ELISA), which incorporates a monoclonal antibody, and immunofluorescence on frozen tissues, have been developed to detect BLS antigen.

The virus associated with BLS has not been propagated in a range of avian and mammalian cell cultures or embryonated eggs from several avian species.

Molecular techniques such as polymerase chain reaction (PCR) are being developed and have been used to detect the virus in samples of liver and faeces.

Serology

The AGID test has been used to detect antibodies in flocks with clinical BLS. Antigen detection usually precedes or is concurrent with the appearance of detectable antibody, which persists for the life of the chicken. Infection of young and immature chickens does not produce a detectable antibody response until the birds are sexually mature. Antibody-detecting ELISAs have been widely used and shown to be more sensitive than the AGID test.

CONTROL

There is no specific therapeutic or prophylactic treatment for BLS apart from good biosecurity and thorough cleaning and disinfection. The disease has a tendency to persist on affected sites. Commercial vaccines have not been developed because of the difficulty of propagating the virus.

HEPATITIS–SPLENOMEGALY SYNDROME

The disease was first recognized in chickens in North America during the late 1980s and has been variously called weeping liver syndrome, necrotic haemorrhage hepatitis–splenomegaly syndrome, chronic fulminating cholangiohepatitis, necrotic haemorrhagic hepatomegalic hepatitis, necro-haemorrhagic hepatitis and hepatitis–liver haemorrhage syndrome. The disease is similar to BLS but the various synonyms for HSS suggest that typically it is a more haemorrhagic disease than BLS with clotted blood or bloodstained fluid present in the abdomen of affected birds. The disease is found most commonly in 30–72-week-old broiler breeders and layers, associated with drops in egg production and increased mortality. The aetiological agent is thought be a hepevirus genetically similar to BLS but the clinical disease has not been reproduced in laboratory trials, although pathological changes and seroconversion were observed. Antibodies to HSS are widespread in both affected and clinically normal flocks in the USA.

EPIDEMIOLOGY

Cause

Electron microscopy examination of bile samples from chickens with HSS has revealed non-enveloped virus particles 30–35 nm in diameter. Molecular analysis of the viral genome has shown that it shares 50–60% nucleotide sequence identity with pig and human hepatitis E viruses and approximately 80% identity with an Australian strain of BLS virus. It has been proposed that the agent associated with HSS should be identified as an avian HEV.

Spread

Under commercial conditions the transmission and spread of HSS virus in chicken flocks is similar to BLS virus. In laboratory studies groups of 60-week-old SPF chickens inoculated by the oronasal and intravenous route shed virus in their faeces from respectively 10–56 days and 1–21 days post-inoculation. These results suggest that the primary mode of transmission is via the faecal–oral route.

DIAGNOSIS

Clinical signs and lesions

No particular clinical signs have been reported prior to death, although occasionally egg production drops of up to 20% occur. At post-mortem the gross pathology includes enlarged, friable, mottled livers containing numerous haemorrhages with subcapsular haematomas and attached blood clots. The abdominal cavity may contain both clotted and unclotted blood and the spleens are frequently enlarged, with amyloidosis present. Both active and regressive ovaries have been found in affected chickens. Microscopically, lesions in the liver vary from multifocal patches to extensive hepatic necrosis and haemorrhage. Lesions in the spleen consist of lymphoid depletion accompanied by an increase in mononuclear cells. Specific staining shows accumulation of amyloid in the liver and spleen.

Virus isolation and detection

The causative agent of HSS has not been successfully isolated and propagated in cell cultures or embryonated eggs. Electron microscopy examination of bile extracts from affected chickens has revealed virus particles 30–40 nm in diameter. Molecular diagnostic methods such as reverse-transcription PCR (RT-PCR) have been developed to detect HEV in faeces, serum, bile and liver homogenates from inoculated chickens.

Serology

An ELISA has been developed for testing poultry flocks in the USA using plates coated with purified avian HEV antigen. The results showed that, of 76 different flocks in five states of the USA, 71% of the flocks and 30% of the chickens were positive for HEV antibodies. In chickens less than 18 weeks of age 17% were considered ELISA positive compared with 36% of adult birds.

CONTROL

As with BLS disease, the only method of preventing and controlling HSS is by practising good biosecurity and enhanced hygienic measures.

FURTHER READING

Billam P, Huang F F, Sun Z F et al 2005 Systematic pathogenesis and replication of avian hepatitis E virus in specific pathogen free adult chickens. J Virol 79: 3429–3437

Gough R E, Drury S E, Collins M S 1997 Detection of avian enteric caliciviruses. In: Chasey D, Gaskell R M, Clarke I N (eds) First international symposium on caliciviruses. Proceedings of a European Society for Veterinary Virology Meeting, Reading, UK, p 83–87

Haqshenas G, Shivaprasad H L, Woolcock P R et al 2001 Genetic identification and characterization of a novel virus related to human hepatitis E virus from chickens with hepatitis-splenomegaly syndrome in the United States. J Gen Virol 82: 2449–2462

Huang F F, Haqshenas G, Shivaprasad H L et al 2002 Heterogeneity and seroprevalence of a newly identified avian hepatitis E virus from chickens in the United States. J Clin Microbiol 40: 4197–4202

Meng X J 2005 Hepatitis E virus: Cross-species infection and zoonotic risk. Clin Microbiol Newsl 27: 43–48

Payne C J 2003 Big liver and spleen disease. In: Saif Y M (ed) Disease of poultry, 11th edn. Iowa State University Press, Ames, p 1184–1186

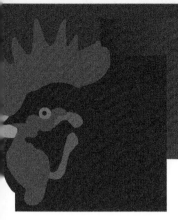

CHAPTER 37

Ilaria Capua

Arthropod-borne viruses

Arthropod-borne viral diseases are caused by viruses known as arboviruses (*ar*thropod-*bo*rne), which, although taxonomically placed in several virus families, share the common feature of being maintained in nature through biological transmission between vertebrate hosts by haematophagus arthropods. Arboviruses replicate in the tissues of the vertebrate host, multiply in the tissues of arthropods and are passed on to a new vertebrate host through the bite of arthropods after a period of extrinsic incubation. Therefore, by definition, arboviruses have a vertebrate host and an invertebrate host, although several arboviruses have very complex life cycles involving multiple vectors and hosts. Since arboviruses rely on high-titre viraemias for the perpetuation of their life cycle, they often do not cause disease or death in their vertebrate hosts. For several arboviruses, wild birds and small mammals such as rodents or lagomorphs are considered amplifiers of infection because of the asymptomatic high-titre viraemias they develop, their prolificity and behaviour.

A number of arboviruses are responsible for zoonotic diseases, and disease in humans or in domestic animals is often recognized as the only sign of the presence of infection in a given area.

At present, 535 viruses are listed in the *International catalogue of arboviruses including certain other viruses of vertebrates*. Among these, viruses belonging to six families (*Togaviridae, Arenaviridae, Flaviviridae, Bunyaviridae, Reoviridae* and *Rhabdoviridae*) contain arboviruses that have been isolated from birds or from ornithophilic arthropods. Nevertheless, viruses that appear to be arthropod-borne are constantly isolated by virologists worldwide, and the *Catalogue* is continuously updated.

Arthropods that may transmit arboviruses include ticks and dipterous insects of three families: mosquitoes, ceratopogonid midges (*Culicoides*) and phlebotomine flies (sandflies). The life cycle of the virus in the arthropod is characterized by active replication in the salivary glands, which allows the arthropod to transmit the infection by biting the vertebrate host. Some arboviruses infect the ovary of the invertebrate host, allowing transovarian infection, thus amplifying infection through the progeny.

Table 37.1 | Arthropod-borne viruses infecting poultry and other birds

VIRUS	TAXONOMY	VECTOR	DISEASE IN POULTRY
Viruses that cause disease in birds			
Highlands J	Family: *Togaviridae* Genus: *Alphavirus*	Mosquitoes (also via semen)	Weakness, depression egg production drops up to 70% in adult turkeys, high mortality in young turkeys
Turkey meningoencephalitis	Family: *Flaviviridae* Genus: *Flavivirus*	Mosquitoes	Neurological signs and egg production drops in turkeys >10 weeks old
Viruses that cause disease in birds and humans			
Eastern equine encephalitis	Family: *Togaviridae* Genus: *Alphavirus*	Mosquitoes: *Culiseta melanura*	Neurological signs with high mortality in pheasants, partridges and ducks
Western equine encephalitis	Family: *Togaviridae* Genus: *Alphavirus*	Mosquitoes: *Culex* spp.	Rare – nervous signs in turkeys, pheasants, partridges
Venezuelan equine encephalitis	Family: *Togaviridae* Genus: *Alphavirus*	Mosquitoes	None in poultry?
West Nile	Family: *Flaviviridae* Genus: *Flavivirus*	Mosquitoes	Infects a large number of wild and domestic birds, sometimes lethally
Viruses that infect birds and cause disease in humans			
Crimean–Congo haemorrhagic fever	Family: *Bunyaviridae* Genus: *Nairovirus*	Ticks, mainly *Hyalomma* spp.	Infections of ostriches, chickens and guinea fowl reported

Generally speaking, although birds are often involved in life cycles of arboviruses, outbreaks of arbovirus infections in domestic poultry appear to be rather infrequent. Nevertheless, the emergence of epidemics has occurred on several occasions, mainly related to climatic conditions that favour an increase of vector population.

Arboviruses that infect poultry must be considered under three divisions: arboviruses that cause disease in birds (Highlands J infection, turkey meningoencephalitis), arboviruses that cause disease in birds and in humans (eastern equine encephalitis, western equine encephalitis, west Nile viruses) and arboviruses that infect birds and cause disease in humans (*Crimean–Congo haemorrhagic fever virus*). The viruses in these categories discussed in this chapter are summarized in Table 37.1.

ARBOVIRUSES THAT CAUSE DISEASE IN BIRDS

HIGHLANDS J VIRUS

Highlands J virus (HJV) belongs to the *Alphavirus* genus of the *Togaviridae* family. It was first isolated from blue jays in Florida, USA, in 1960 and has been described as a cause of disease in chukar partridges and in intensively reared turkeys causing, in the latter, two distinct clinical diseases. It is responsible for poor egg production performance in turkey breeders and mortality in young poults. The infection is transmitted by mosquitoes, although transmission of infection via infected semen has also been reported in intensively reared turkeys.

HJV is similar to *Eastern equine encephalitis virus* (EEEV) in its natural cycle. For this reason HJV is often used as an indicator species in eastern equine encephalitis surveillance programmes. Exposure to HJV has not been directly associated with human illness.

DISEASE

In turkey breeders infection with HJV has been associated with dramatic drops in egg production (70%), accompanied by the production of whitish, fragile and shell-less eggs. The affected birds showed no excess mortality, although weakness and depression often accompanied the egg drops. Gross lesions were generally absent except for ovarian atrophy and regression associated with accumulation of peritoneal fluids in a limited number of birds.

On the basis of the evidence collected during field outbreaks, experimental work has shown that turkey stags may transmit infection to hens via infected semen. In fact, virus was recovered from the semen of infected males, which clinically exhibited transient weakness and depression associated with viraemia.

In young meat turkeys infection with HJV has been associated with high mortality. Clinical signs were characterized by weakness, somnolence, restlessness and acute death. On postmortem, birds exhibited enlarged livers, enlarged spleens and marked dehydration. Atrophy of the bursa of Fabricius was also observed in dead poults.

In chukar partridges, clinical signs are associated with neurological disorders. Affected birds exhibit depression, weakness and incoordination, which are associated with a viral encephalitis accompanied by myocarditis. Other pathological findings are represented by catarrhal enteritis and mottling of the spleen.

Natural infection in chickens has not been reported, although experimental infection of young broilers with HJV has shown that these birds are susceptible to infection.

DIAGNOSIS

HJV may be isolated in cell cultures such as Vero or BHK 21. The intracerebral inoculation of newborn mice has also been used successfully. An alternative method is the inoculation of specific-pathogen-free (SPF) eggs via the yolk sac. The virus may be identified by virus neutralization or complement fixation test, bearing in mind the possible cross-reactions with other arboviruses, particularly *Western equine encephalitis virus* (WEEV; see below). Other arbovirus infections should be considered in differential diagnosis aided by laboratory investigations.

A reverse-transcription polymerase chain reaction (RT-PCR) test is available to detect HJV RNA from infected cell culture supernatants, bird brain tissues and mosquitoes.

TURKEY MENINGOENCEPHALITIS VIRUS

The disease is also known as Israel turkey meningoencephalitis after its first description in Israel. It is caused by a member of the *Flaviviridae* family and is transmitted by various species of mosquito.

In turkeys, the clinical condition appears as a nervous disorder, affects birds older than 10 weeks of age and is characterized by somnolence, incoordination and paralysis of the wings and of the legs, which leads to the bird resting on the ground motionless. In laying turkey hens this disease has been associated with drop in egg production.

Gross lesions include atrophy or enlargement of the spleen, myocarditis and egg-yolk peritonitis in laying birds. Histologically, viral meningoencephalitis with cuff-like perivascular lymphocytic infiltration can be observed, often associated with myocardial necrosis.

DIAGNOSIS AND CONTROL

Diagnosis by virus isolation is achieved through inoculation of liver, spleen and brain suspensions into susceptible cells (chicken embryo fibroblasts), which readily develop a cytopathic effect. An alternative method is to inoculate the suspensions into the yolk sac of developing embryos, although several passages may be necessary to cause embryo mortality.

The intracerebral inoculation of newborn mice also represents a sensitive method for the isolation of this agent. Recently a RT-PCR test has been developed. Serological diagnosis may be achieved by means of virus neutralization or haemagglutination inhibition tests.

Other arbovirus infections must be considered in differential diagnosis since it is not possible to differentiate between them on the basis of clinical signs. In addition, Newcastle disease may also cause similar clinical signs and must also be excluded.

Live attenuated vaccines have been developed to control the disease, although control of the vector population is also of vital importance.

ARBOVIRUS INFECTIONS THAT CAUSE DISEASE IN BIRDS AND IN HUMANS

EASTERN, WESTERN AND VENEZUELAN EQUINE ENCEPHALITIS VIRUSES

Eastern, western and Venezuelan equine encephalitis (EEE, WEE, VEE) are caused by arboviruses belonging to the *Alphavirus* genus of the *Togaviridae* family. The viruses cause encephalitis in horses and humans, although generalized infections may also develop. The virus vectors are mosquitoes and in addition to horses and humans the transmission cycles involve birds and rodents. Clinical disease in horses, humans and birds generally occurs in midsummer or autumn, as a result of climatic conditions that favour the activity of vectors.

EASTERN EQUINE ENCEPHALITIS VIRUS

The virus (EEEV) is widespread throughout North and South America, including the Caribbean region; in this respect, the adjective 'Eastern' is misleading.

The primary vector, *Culiseta melanura*, is a highly ornithophilic mosquito that occasionally feeds on mammals. A great number of wild birds, mainly passerines, develop high-titre viraemias that amplify and perpetuate the infection without the host showing clinical signs. Because *C. melanura* feeds mainly on birds, other mosquitoes are considered to be responsible for the escape of infection from the *C. melanura*–avian cycle to mammalian hosts.

DISEASE

Major epidemics of EEE have been reported in pheasants, as well as fatal outbreaks in other birds such as turkeys, ducks and chukar partridges. Infection associated with a clinical condition has also been reported in emus.

Although *C. melanura* is responsible for the primary infection of an avian flock, behavioural habits of birds, such as feather plucking and cannibalism, have been shown to be a means of spread within a flock. In addition to this, transmission through the semen may occur and turkey semen collected during the viraemic phase has been able to infect artificially inseminated hens.

Clinical signs in pheasants are characterized by nervous disorders such as severe depression torticollis and tremors, incoordination and paralysis of the wings and legs. Mortality may reach 80%. At post-mortem, no gross lesions can be detected, while histopathology of the central nervous system (CNS) includes vasculitis, foci of necrosis and degeneration of the neurons. Meningitis is also often observed.

A similar condition has been reported in chukar partridges, in which nervous disorders were associated with high mortality rates. On post-mortem, spleens appeared mottled and hearts pale and discoloured. Histologically, myocardial necrosis and CNS lesions such as gliosis, satellitosis and perivascular lymphocytic cuffing could be seen.

Natural infection of Pekin ducks has resulted in a paralytic disease associated with mortality levels of 2–60%. Histopathologically, oedema of the spinal cord white matter, lymphocytic meningitis and microgliosis were observed.

Natural outbreaks reported in turkeys were characterized by a clinical condition that included somnolence, incoordination, tremors and paralysis of the legs and wings. Mortality rates were generally low ($\approx 5\%$). Similar to the disease in pheasants, no gross lesion could be detected while severe histopathological lesions could be detected throughout the CNS. Calcification of blood vessel walls in the cortex, in the cerebellar folia and in the basal part of the medulla was a consistent histopathological finding.

In turkey breeders EEEV infection has caused drops in egg production associated with a decrease in egg quality. Eggs appeared whitish, decoloured and with a fragile shell, some eggs being laid without the shell. No clinical signs attributable to disorders of the CNS could be seen and the only gross lesion observed was ovarian regression.

Experimental infection of chickens has shown that they are highly susceptible to the disease up to 14 days of age, subsequently becoming refractory to it. Clinical signs affected the CNS with depression, drowsiness and incoordination. Histologically, CNS lesions were inconsistent, although foci of necrosis and perivascular cuffing could be seen. The heart exhibited myocardial damage such as inflammation and necrosis.

A case of EEEV infection has also been reported in two emus, which exhibited diffuse severe haemorrhagic enterocolitis and necrosis of the spleen and liver. Experimental reproduction of the disease in two ostrich chicks showed that these birds are also susceptible to infection.

DIAGNOSIS

EEEV may be isolated on susceptible cell cultures (Vero, BHK 21, chicken embryo and duck embryo cells) in which cytopathic effects can be observed within 48–72 h. The intracerebral inoculation of newborn mice and subcutaneous or intramuscular inoculation of day-old SPF chicks has also been used. An alternative method is the inoculation of SPF eggs via the yolk sac. The virus may be identified by virus neutralization, complement fixation tests and RT-PCR assay.

Antibodies to EEEV may be detected by a variety of serological techniques (virus neutralization, haemagglutination inhibition, complement fixation and enzyme-linked immunosorbent assay (ELISA)), although the haemagglutination inhibition test using goose red blood cells appears to be the technique most widely used.

Other arbovirus infections, Newcastle disease, avian influenza, avian paramyxovirus type 3 and avian encephalomyelitis must be considered in the differential diagnosis. This should be supported by serological or virus isolation procedures.

CONTROL

Prevention is achieved by controlling vector populations, either by land reclamation or treatment of the environment with chemical agents. Inactivated vaccines developed for horses have been used in pheasant flocks, although their efficacy remains to be fully evaluated.

WESTERN EQUINE ENCEPHALITIS VIRUS

WEEV was first recognized in the western part of North America and was subsequently thought to be widely distributed throughout the Americas. However, it is now believed that infections that occur east of the Mississippi river are caused by a related arbovirus, known as HJV (see above).

The primary vectors of WEE are mosquitoes belonging to the *Culex* genus, particularly *Culex tarsalis*, which is scarcely present east of the Mississippi river. *C. tarsalis* is an ornithophilic mosquito that feeds prevalently on passerine birds (particularly nestling house sparrows, *Passer domesticus*), which are responsible for the amplification of infection. Other mosquito species become infected from feeding on viraemic passerines and are responsible for the transmission to other birds, lagomorphs such as the European hare (*Lepus europeus*) and the jack-rabbit (*Lepus californicus*), reptiles and amphibians. Most infections in vertebrate hosts are inapparent.

DISEASE IN BIRDS

WEEV infections have been associated rarely with disease in avian species. Limited evidence has been reported from a natural outbreak in a turkey flock, characterized by nervous disorders such as somnolence, tremors and incoordination. Isolation of WEEV has been reported from a pheasant and it has been considered as a cause of outbreaks of high mortality in chukar partridges.

DIAGNOSIS

Isolation of WEEV is achieved by the intracerebral inoculation of suckling mice or by the inoculation of susceptible cell cultures, such as Vero cells. The agent is commonly identified by virus neutralization tests and by RT-PCR test, which is the most sensitive assay.

VENEZUELAN EQUINE ENCEPHALITIS VIRUS

Although infection of domestic poultry has never been reported, *Venezuelan equine encephalitis virus* (VEEV) is known to infect over 100 species of bird. Among these, shorebirds, and particularly herons, appear to serve as amplifier hosts. The infection is present in the tropical areas of the Americas and is transmitted by a variety of mosquitoes, the majority of which belong to the *Culex* genus.

USUTU VIRUS

Usutu virus (USUV) is a relatively little known member of the genus *Flavivirus* (family *Flaviviridae*) and was originally isolated from mosquitoes in South Africa in 1959. It is closely related to human pathogens such as *West Nile virus* (WNV) and it is primarily transmitted between avian reservoir hosts and mosquitoes in a sylvatic transmission cycle, although mammals could be inadvertent hosts if bitten by infected mosquitoes.

This virus was known only in Africa prior to 2001 when it was isolated for the first time in Europe, causing fatalities among wild birds in Austria. Isolations of this virus have also been made from humans but there are no reports of severe disease.

DISEASE IN BIRDS

In the summer of 2001, USUV was responsible for an episode of mortality among Eurasian blackbirds (*Turdus merula*) and great grey owls (*Strix nebulosa*) in Austria. In the consecutive four summers numerous blackbirds again succumbed to USUV infection in the same area.

Pathological lesions include encephalitis, myocardial degeneration and necrosis of the liver and spleen.

USUVs do not cause clinical signs in intravenously inoculated chickens and pathologically the virus is responsible only for signs of stimulation of the immune system. Experimental USUV infection leads to inconsistent viraemia and seroconversion in chickens, suggesting that this species is unlikely to be useful for sentinel purposes in USUV surveillance programmes. At present nothing is known about the pathogenicity of USUV in naturally infected domestic poultry.

DIAGNOSIS

USUV can be isolated in cell cultures such as Vero cell culture and it can be identified by immunohistochemistry, in situ hybridization and RT-PCR. Serological diagnosis is achieved by means of haemagglutination inhibition tests.

WEST NILE VIRUS

West Nile fever is an arthropod-borne zoonosis transmitted by mosquitoes and caused by a virus belonging to the *Flaviviridae* family. WNV is one of the most widely distributed arthropod-borne viruses and has been isolated in several countries of Africa, Asia, Europe and recently in the USA. The natural life cycle of WNV involves the transmission of the virus from mosquitoes to wild birds. Infectious mosquitoes carry the virus in their salivary glands and infect susceptible birds during blood-meal feeding. Infection in wild birds produces a high viraemia for 1–4 days following exposure, allowing transmission of WNV to mosquitoes to complete the cycle. The virus has been identified in at least 43 mosquito species from 11 genera, although not all of these are competent vectors. Members of the *Culex* genus are thought to be the most efficient for spreading the virus among birds.

WNV has a wide host range, replicating in birds, reptiles, amphibians, mammals, mosquitoes and ticks. Among mammals, clinical illness has been documented most frequently in humans and horses.

Phylogenetic studies based on the sequence of the E glycoprotein gene of WNV have shown the existence of two lineages. Lineage II viruses comprise WNV strains only from Africa and these have not been associated with human encephalitis cases. Lineage I strains have been isolated from Africa, Europe, Asia, the Middle East and North America and have been responsible for disease in humans.

DISEASE IN BIRDS

Avian hosts are the primary vertebrate reservoir in the maintenance of WNV. Avian morbidity and mortality in outbreaks in North America and the Middle East is a new feature of WNV. Until recent times, natural infection of wild birds was associated with inapparent and subclinical conditions.

The emergence of a new and more virulent strain of WNV in Israel and in the USA has produced an unprecedented pattern of disease in wild birds. This new virus variant, Isr98 strain, has caused extensive mortality in captive and free-ranging birds in the USA. WNV has been detected in dead birds of almost 200 different species. Clinical signs following WNV infection are often nonspecific (anorexia, weakness, depression, weight loss) but some wild birds exhibit neurological signs such as circling, abnormal neck and head posture and ataxia. Brain haemorrhage, splenomegaly, meningoencephalitis and myocarditis can be found at necropsy.

Most reported fatal infections in birds in North America occurred in crows (*Corvus brachyrhynchus*) but WNV has been often recovered also from sick pigeons (*Columba livia*), domestic sparrows (*Passer domesticus*) and owls (family Strigidae). Experimental infection of wild birds with the New York 1999 strain demonstrated that birds of the orders Passeriformes and Charadriiformes are more efficient reservoirs than other species tested, such as those from the orders Columbiformes, Anseriformes, Psittaciformes, Piciformes, Gruiformes and Galliformes.

Experimental studies showed that most species of domestic birds are susceptible to infection with WNV but only young chickens (*Gallus domesticus*) and domestic geese (*Anser anser domesticus*) show clinical disease and mortality.

Young geese are very susceptible to infection with WNV and neurological signs including paralysis, opisthotonos and incoordination are the most frequent signs of WNV infection. Direct transmission has been reported between experimentally inoculated geese and contact geese, suggesting that horizontal transmission of WNV can occur in commercial flocks.

Young chickens and geese develop a high-titre viraemia and can act as amplifiers of infection for mosquitoes. Older chickens and turkeys do not undergo a high-titre viraemia and this feature makes older chickens ideal sentinels for surveillance efforts.

DISEASE IN HUMANS

WNV has emerged as an important human and animal (including wildlife) health threat. In a few years the virus spread in several countries, reaching the American continent. Humans are considered dead-end hosts since they generally do not develop significant viraemias and until recent times west Nile fever in humans was considered a mild disease with sporadic clinical cases. During the last 10 years there has been an increase in severity of disease in humans with the emergence of the new variant Isr98 strain. Since the emergence of this new variant of WNV in North America several human cases have been reported, sometimes causing severe and even fatal illness. Clinical manifestations associated with WNV infection in humans can vary from a mild disease with fever, headache and skin rash to a severe disease with neurological symptoms due to encephalitis and meningitis. In some instances the disease may be fatal.

Diagnosis and control

WNV may be isolated on Vero cells and by the intracerebral inoculation of suckling mice. WNV produces cytopathic effects or forms plaques in cell culture and is lethal in mice. The isolate can be identified with a monospecific antiserum by means of the virus neutralization test, by fluorescent antibody or by indirect fluorescent antibody tests with monoclonal antibodies, bearing in mind that cross-reactions with other members of the Japanese encephalitis serocomplex may occur. Viral RNA may be detected by means of RT-PCR or real time RT-PCR tests performed on infected tissues.

The plaque reduction neutralization test is the standard test for confirmation of virus-specific antibodies but some cross-reactivity still occurs with closely related virus. Serological assays can include detection of IgM antibodies by capture ELISA (MAC-ELISA). The presence of IgM indicates recent exposure to the virus. Other rapid tests are direct ELISA and haemagglutination inhibition tests, which are used to screen serum specimens for detection of antiflavivirus antibody. Another alternative is an epitope-blocking ELISA test, which is useful to monitor WNV activity in multiple avian species.

Prevention and control of WNV can be accomplished through vector control, preventive measures to decrease the risk of exposure and eventually by the use of vaccines to protect susceptible hosts from clinical disease and to reduce transmission of the virus.

ARBOVIRUSES THAT INFECT BIRDS AND CAUSE DISEASE IN HUMANS

CRIMEAN–CONGO HAEMORRHAGIC FEVER VIRUS

Crimean–Congo haemorrhagic fever virus (CCHFV) is a tick-borne zoonosis caused by an arbovirus belonging to the *Nairovirus* genus of the *Bunyaviridae* family. Infection is transmitted to vertebrate hosts by the *Hyalomma marginatum marginatum*, *Riphicephalus rossicus* and *Dermacentor marginatus*, ticks for which trans-stadial and transovarial infections have been described. Experimental evidence indicates that the most efficient vectors appear to be members of the genus *Hyalomma*. In fact, the world distribution of the virus coincides with the distribution of these ticks. The cycle of this infection includes: small mammals; free-living, ground-frequenting birds, including ostriches; ruminants; and occasionally humans.

The first outbreak of the disease was described in 1944 in the Crimean peninsula in people bitten by ticks while harvesting crops and sleeping outdoors, and therefore it was named Crimean haemorrhagic fever. In 1956 a virus named Congo was isolated from a sick child in what was then the Belgian Congo. In 1969 it was demonstrated that the two viruses were in fact identical and from then on the two names have been used in combination.

The virus is widely distributed in Asia, Africa, the Middle East and eastern Europe, and in the European Union evidence of infection has been reported in Greece, France and Portugal. Apart from field infections, occasional common source nosocomial outbreaks have been reported throughout the years.

INFECTION IN BIRDS

Little information was available on CCHFV infection of birds prior to 1984 when a worker contracted the disease at an ostrich abattoir in Oudtshoorn district, South Africa. Following this first report, further observations linked to ostrich husbandry have been described. Nevertheless, experimental infection of ostriches with CCHFV indicates that these birds develop transient viraemia but do not exhibit any clinical signs. Viraemia in birds has also been reported in domestic chickens and guinea fowl.

DISEASE IN HUMANS

The disease in humans is a haemorrhagic fever with a mortality rate of 30%. Humans become infected by direct contact with blood or other infected tissues from livestock or by tick bite. Clinical symptoms and signs result from liver and endothelial damage and impairment of hae-mostasis. Platelet counts drop dramatically and there is evidence of widespread haemorrhages such as petechial rashes, bleeding from the nose and internal bleeding. Disseminated intravascu-lar coagulopathy occurs and contributes to further tissue damage.

DIAGNOSIS AND CONTROL

Virus isolation from tissues or blood of human patients or viraemic birds should be performed in a maximum security laboratory and it may be achieved by intracerebral inoculation of suck-ling mice, although inoculation of susceptible cell lines such as Vero and CER may also be used. The virus does not cause cytopathic effect and it is commonly detected in infected cells by immunofluorescence tests. A RT-PCR test is available for the identification of CCHFV and recently a one-step real-time RT-PCR assay has been developed.

Antibodies (IgG and IgM) may be detectable by the indirect immunofluorescence technique or by ELISA. A competitive, monoclonal-based ELISA has been successfully used for the detec-tion of specific antibodies in ostriches.

No vaccines are available at present for disease control in humans or for the prevention of infection in animal hosts.

FURTHER READING

Blitvich B J, Marlenee N L, Hall R A et al 2003 Epitope-blocking enzyme-linked immunosorbent assays for the detection of serum antibodies to West Nile virus in multiple avian species. J Clin Microbiol 41: 1041–1047

Chvala S, Kolodziejek J, Nowotny N et al 2004 Pathology and viral distribution in fatal Usutu virus infec-tions of birds from the 2000 and 2002 outbreaks in Austria. J Comp Pathol 131: 176–185

Chvala S, Bakonyi T, Hackl R et al 2005 Limited pathogenicity of Usutu virus for the domestic chicken (*Gallus domesticus*). Avian Pathol 34: 392–395

Dauphin G, Zientara S, Zeller H et al 2004 West Nile: worldwide current situation in animals and humans. Comp Immun Microbiol Infect Dis 27: 343–355

Glaser A 2004 West Nile virus and North America: an unfolding story. Rev Sci Tech 23: 557–568

Johnson A J, Langevin S, Wolff K L et al 2003 Detection of anti-West Nile virus immunoglobulin M in chicken serum by an enzyme-linked immunosorbent assay. J Clin Microbiol 41: 2002–2007

Karabastos N (ed) 1985 International catalogue of arboviruses 1985 including certain other viruses of Vertebrates, 3rd edn. American Society for Tropical Medicine and Hygiene, San Antonio

Komar N 2000 West Nile viral encephalitis. Rev Sci Tech 19: 166–176

Kramer L D, Wolfe T M, Green E N et al 2002 Detection of encephalitis viruses in mosquitoes (Diptera: Culicidae) and avian tissues. J Med Entomol 39: 312–322

McLean R G, Ubico S R, Bourne D, Komar N 2002 West Nile virus in livestock and wildlife. Curr Top Microbiol Immunol 267: 271–308

Monath T P 1989 The arboviruses: epidemiology and ecology, vol. III. CRC Press, Boca Raton

Swanepoel R 1994 Classification, epidemiology and control of arthropod borne viruses. In: Coetzer J A W, Thomson G R, Tustin R C (eds) Infectious diseases of livestock with special reference to Southern Africa. Oxford University Press, Oxford, p 103–120

Swanepoel R 1994 Crimean–Congo haemorrhagic fever. In: Coetzer J A W, Thomson G R, Tustin R C (eds) Infectious diseases of livestock with special reference to Southern Africa. Oxford University Press, Oxford, p 723–729

Thomson G R 1994 Equine encephalitides caused by alphaviruses. In: Coetzer J A W, Thomson G R, Tustin R C (eds) Infectious diseases of livestock with special reference to Southern Africa. Oxford University Press, Oxford, p 636–641

Wages D P, Ficken M D, Guy J S et al 1993 Egg production drop in turkeys associated with Alphaviruses: Eastern Equine Encephalitis virus and Highlands J virus. Avian Dis 37: 1163–1166

Weissenbock H, Kolodziejek J, Url A et al 2002 Emergence of Usutu virus, an African mosquito-borne flavivirus of the Japanese encephalitis virus group, central Europe. Emerg Infect Dis 8: 652–656

Whitehouse C A, Guibeau A, McGuire D et al 2001 A reverse transcriptase-polymerase chain reaction assay for detecting Highlands J virus. Avian Dis 45: 605–611

Yapar M, Aydogan H, Pahsa A et al 2005 Rapid and quantitative detection of Crimean–Congo haemorrhagic fever virus by one-step real-time reverse transcriptase-PCR. Jpn J Infect Dis 58: 358–362

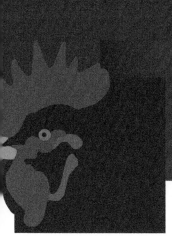

SECTION 4

Paul F. McMullin

FUNGAL DISEASES

Chapter **38**   Fungal diseases   **428**

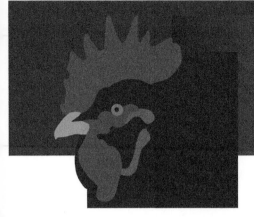

Thomas Brown and
Frank T. W. Jordan with
Alisdair M. Wood

Fungal diseases

Fungi are 'heterotrophic' eukaryotes with an absorptive nutrition and, unlike plants, are unable to make their own food by photosynthesis. They are classified in the separate kingdom Fungi. They may occur as both single-celled and multicelled organisms, and their cell walls contain chitin (which is also the main constituent of arthropod exoskeletons) and β-glucans. Those of greatest importance in causing disease in poultry do so either by tissue invasion and damage or by producing toxins in grain or finished feeds, which, when ingested by the host animal, cause toxicosis (mycotoxicosis).

INVASIVE FUNGI

The respiratory tract, nervous system and eyes of commercial poultry are commonly infected by fungi worldwide and cage, wild and zoo birds (particularly penguins) are also affected. Infections are most frequently caused by *Aspergillus* species. Other similar but less common fungal infections are caused by *Mucor, Penicillium, Rhizopus, Absidia, Dactylaria, Paecilomyces* and *Alternaria*.

ASPERGILLOSIS (BROODER PNEUMONIA)

Respiratory aspergillosis is a common mismanagement problem in commercial and backyard poultry.

EPIDEMIOLOGY

Aetiology

Organisms cultured from affected organs in decreasing frequency are: *Aspergillus fumigatus, Aspergillus flavus, Aspergillus niger, Aspergillus glaucus* and *Aspergillus terreus*. These organisms are common soil saprophytes worldwide and grow on organic matter in warm (>25°C) humid environments including damaged eggs in hatcheries, ventilation systems, poultry litter and feed. Fungal hyphae are 4–12 μm in diameter and bear conidiophores producing conidia (spores) 2–6 μm in diameter that are easily spread in air.

Host

Newly hatched turkeys, chickens and ducks are highly susceptible to infection but disease also occurs frequently in neonates of other avian species.

Influencing factors

Influencing factors on incidence and severity include cold stress, high ammonia concentrations, dusty environments, concurrent debilitating factors and immunosuppression. Older poultry are constantly exposed from the environment but rarely develop clinical disease. Concentrated exposure to spores, immunosuppression, concurrent physiological stressors or infectious, nutritional or toxic disease increase the risk and severity of disease.

Spread

Exposure is by inhalation of spores. These often originate from infected eggs that are opened during incubation or hatching, releasing large numbers of spores and contaminating hatch-mates. Infection within the hatchery may also occur from contaminated air ducts or other equipment. Particular care in egg sanitation and avoidance of in-hatchery *Aspergillus* challenge is required where in-ovo vaccination is in use, as the shell puncture facilitates entry and dissemination of spores. After infection in the hatchery, lateral transmission after placement is not usually a significant source of new infections. Aspergillosis can also be produced by inhalation of spores from contaminated feed or poultry house litter. Fungal growth in wet litter produces large numbers of spores that become aerosolized as this litter is dried. In such instances, new cases may continue to appear for some time after placement.

Pathogenesis

Airborne conidia ('spores') come to rest on conjunctival, nasal, tracheal, parabronchial and air sac epithelium, where they may germinate and initiate granulomas at these sites. They are rapidly disseminated haematogenously to other tissues and this is the likely route of exposure producing lesions in the brain, pericardium, bone marrow, kidney, and other soft tissues. Fungal proliferation tends to be confined within the expanding granulomas and is rarely able to invade adjacent tissues in immunocompetent birds. Chronic disease, especially in turkeys, often terminates in impedance of pulmonary blood flow caused by enlarging pulmonary granulomas and this causes right-ventricular dilatation and ascites. Another cause of mortality is aspergillosis-induced exudate that becomes lodged in the trachea or syrinx, producing acute respiratory embarrassment and sometimes asphyxiation in chronically infected individuals.

DISEASE

Clinical signs

Infected poultry flocks often exhibit a biphasic mortality pattern. Acute respiratory disease may cause 5–50% mortality in the first 1–3 weeks of age. Survivors often develop chronic disease with up to 5% mortality due to chronic pulmonary insufficiency, ascites, blindness or neurological fungal metastasis. Within the first 3–5 days neonates infected in the hatchery become dyspnoeic, polypnoeic, with open-mouthed breathing (gaspers) due to progressive airway obstruction. Survivors may become lethargic and stunted, develop conjunctival swelling and blindness and exhibit torticollis and other central nervous system abnormalities. Older individuals may remain subclinically affected for some time, only to develop slowly progressive respiratory embarrassment as their increasing body weight places demands on a reduced functional pulmonary mass. They may also become asphyxiated as a result of blockage of the airways. A common feature of dyspnoea associated with aspergillosis is the lack of rales or other respiratory noises.

Lesions

Lesions are found in the respiratory tract, including particularly the trachea, bronchi, lungs and air sacs. Occasionally lesions are seen in the viscera, the eye and the brain. The lesions appear as white or pale yellow granulomatous, discrete nodules of 1–9 mm in the lungs, often surrounded by pneumonic tissue, as plaques in the air sacs, as caseous exudate in the trachea, as focal plaques on the surface of the brain and meninges and as fungal keratoconjunctivitis or panophthalmitis in the eye. The lesions that develop in the air sacs are often dark green-brown because of the development of fungal conidiophores, which are pigmented.

DIAGNOSIS

Neither clinical signs nor lesions can be accepted as specific for aspergillosis. Clinical signs of respiratory disease in the first 2 weeks of life with air sac plaques or intrapulmonary nodules are highly suggestive but similar neonatal dyspnoea and similar lesions may be caused by certain viral or viral vaccine infections. Furthermore, similar pulmonary or ocular granulomas are indistinguishable grossly from those produced by some other fungal, coliform, *Staphylococcus*, *Salmonella*, *Mycoplasma* or mixed infections. Slowly progressive respiratory disease in adults is similar to many other chronic respiratory diseases. Pigmented older lesions in air sacs are strongly suggestive of aspergillosis. However, diagnosis is dependent on the demonstration in lesions of 4–12 μm diameter, of branched, septate *Aspergillus* hyphae. They may be seen microscopically in smears or imprints of lesions after the addition of one or two drops of 10% KOH and heating to clear. Also, hyphae are routinely observed in microscopic haematoxylin/eosin-stained sections, but special fungal stains (periodic acid–Schiff, Grocott's methenamine-silver (GMS) or calcofluor white) may be required in some cases. For demonstration of conidiophore morphology and speciation, granulomas or plaques may be cultured on Sabouraud dextrose agar with antibiotics and the fungus distinguished on morphology.

CONTROL

There is no current commercial treatment available for aspergillosis but in an outbreak every effort should be made to reduce or eliminate exposure to spores. Removing infected litter or covering it with fresh material, and use of an appropriate disinfectant spray (to control dust and target germinated spores) may be helpful in some circumstances. Clinically affected birds should be culled. After flock depletion, the premises should be cleaned and disinfected, the ventilation investigated and an effort made to determine the source of infection so that it may be avoided n future. For individual pet or hobby birds, or rare and valuable birds in zoological collections, reatment with antifungal medicines such as itraconazole may be attempted.

Prevention by vaccination is also not commercially practicable and therefore control is depend-nt on reducing exposure to the fungus and associated risk factors. Eggs for hatching should be ollected and stored so as to reduce sweating and exposure to spore-laden dust. Hatchery equip-nent, ventilation and air ducts should be cleaned, disinfected and monitored by periodic cul-ures. During brooding, in particular, management should avoid wet litter or soil and mouldy or lusty feeds and should provide adequate ventilation and disinfected feed and water lines.

DACTYLARIOSIS

This is a relatively rare, mainly neurological, disease of chickens and turkey poults. Less frequently, pulmonary lesions indistinguishable from those of aspergillosis are seen, usually in addition to nvolvement of the nervous system.

EPIDEMIOLOGY

Aetiology

The causative organism is *Dactylaria gallopava*, an opportunistic, phaeohyphomycotic (forming pigmented hyphae and yeastlike cells in tissue), weakly dematiaceous (having dark-coloured, brown or black conidia and/or hyphae), thermophilic fungus. It grows well on organic matter t 25–37°C but optimally at 45°C. Hyphae are brown, 1.2–2.4 µm in diameter, and bear two-elled brown conidia (spores) averaging 15 × 3 µm. Spores are released into the air and spread.

Host

Outbreaks occur in birds between 1 and 5 weeks of age.

Spread

The sources of infection are environments characterized by high temperatures (>43°C) and low pH (<5). Such conditions exist in piles of wet shavings and poultry litter that have undergone natural heating process. Hardwood shavings and sawdust are frequently incriminated. Lateral ransmission is not usually significant, although new cases will continue to occur as long as oung birds remain on the contaminated litter.

Pathogenesis

Exposure of birds is by inhalation of spores but disease is produced by penetration of blood ves-els and haematogenous spread to the central nervous system.

DISEASE

Clinical signs

Mortality may be up to 10%, predominantly as a result of neurological disease. Infected poults nd chicks develop torticollis, paresis and incoordination. In a minority of cases ocular lesions develop and produce blindness and, in rare cases, pulmonary granulomas develop and cause dyspnoea as in aspergillosis.

Lesions

The principal lesion in dactylariosis is a meningeal or encephalitic necrosis that is grey or yellow and well delineated. This lesion is most commonly seen in the cerebellum or caudal cerebral cortex but can appear anywhere in the brain. Gross ocular and pulmonary lesions appear similar to those for aspergillosis.

DIAGNOSIS

Clinical signs and gross lesions are insufficiently specific to allow diagnosis. Rapidly progressive nervous system disease in young birds can also be seen with vitamin-E-deficiency-induced encephalomalacia, Newcastle disease, infectious avian encephalomyelitis, bacterial meningitis or aspergillosis.

Brain lesions should be examined microscopically. The lesions differ from the mycotic encephalitis of aspergillosis by having more malacia and haemorrhage, and a far larger number of giant cells. Brown hyphae less than 3 μm in diameter may be seen in unstained sections but fungal stains (GMS) are routinely required for diagnosis. Microscopic sections must be examined carefully as the narrow hyphae of *Dactylaria* are nearly identical in width to capillaries. Those containing pigmented 2 μm diameter hyphae and large numbers of giant cells are strongly suggestive of dactylariosis. The fungus may be cultured from brain lesions or litter on Sabouraud dextrose agar with added antibiotics at 45°C. Colonies produce brown pigment that diffuses into the surrounding medium, and have characteristic two-celled brown conidia.

CONTROL

Prevention, as outlined for the management of litter and feed for aspergillosis, is the only satisfactory procedure.

CANDIDIASIS (CROP MYCOSIS, THRUSH)

Oral, oesophageal or crop candidiasis occurs very frequently but only rarely causes clinical signs. The condition is associated with concurrent disease, nutritional deficiency, immunosuppression or altered microflora, and is more probably the result of an opportunistic than a primary infection.

EPIDEMIOLOGY

Aetiology

The most frequent causal agent is *Candida albicans*, a dimorphic yeast that appears as round to oval 3–4 μm budding yeasts (blastospores) on epithelial surfaces, or 3–5 μm diameter branching septate hyphae or pseudohyphae in deeper tissues. *Oidium pullorum* and *Candida krusei* are isolated less frequently from typical cases of crop mycosis and may not be involved in lesion development. *C. albicans* is ubiquitous in the environment and is often present in the upper gastrointestinal tract of normal birds.

Host

Disease is more common in birds under 3 weeks of age, suggesting acquired or age resistance.

Influencing factors

One of the most common predisposing factors is prolonged antibiotic administration, which suppresses normal bacterial flora and competition for nutrients, thus allowing *Candida* to proliferate. Other risk factors include highly contaminated drinkers or feeders, eating litter, concurrent immunosuppression, environmental stress or nutritional disease.

Pathogenesis

Candida is acquired by ingestion and probably becomes part of the resident flora of the mouth, oesophagus and crop; under predisposing conditions it proliferates on the surface and hyphae or pseudohyphae invade superficial epithelial layers. This invasion stimulates epithelial hyperplasia and pseudomembrane or diphtheritic membrane formation.

DISEASE

Clinical signs

Mortality directly caused by candidiasis is low to nonexistent and most signs are referable to other concurrent diseases or reduced growth due to reduced feed intake. In rare cases there is systemic invasion and signs of neurological, renal or intestinal disease may be present.

Lesions

The surface of the crop and, less frequently, the oesophagus and pharynx are coated with multifocal or confluent mats of white cheesy material. Candidal mats and membranes are often adherent and cannot be washed away like normal accumulations of mucus. A distinct 'yeasty', beer-like smell is sometimes noticed. An inflammatory response to mucosal candidiasis is mild unless ulceration is produced.

DIAGNOSIS

Pseudomembranes and diphtheritic membranes in the crop, oesophagus and mouth are highly suggestive of candidiasis but can be produced after ingestion of caustic substances, trichothecene mycotoxins and in severe cases of oral trichomoniasis. Visualization of yeasts, hyphae and pseudohyphae microscopically in either scrapings (mixed with KOH 10% and heated to clear) or histological sections will confirm candidiasis. Speciation requires culture on Sabouraud dextrose agar or other fungal culture media, but many normal birds may be positive.

CONTROL

Crop mycosis is best prevented by controlling predisposing factors, including excess use of antibiotics, and encouraging cleanliness and sanitation. Candidiasis can be temporarily controlled with dietary gentian violet (8 mg/kg) or nystatin (142 mg/kg) but use of these compounds may not be approved in some countries. Effective water sanitizers may be helpful in maintaining sanitation. Acidification of drinking water with organic acids may also be helpful but careful attention to dose is required – inadequate doses of organic acids stimulate the growth of yeasts and moulds in drinker systems.

FAVUS (WHITE COMB, RINGWORM)

This disease is no longer economically significant in commercial poultry but is occasionally seen in backyard or hobby chickens and more rarely in turkeys. Infections are superficial, chronic and either self-limiting or slowly progressive.

EPIDEMIOLOGY

Aetiology

Infections are usually caused by *Trichophyton megninii* (*Trichophyton gallinae*), a dermatophytic fungus that produces macro- and microconidia in culture but not in infected tissues. *Microsporum gypseum* and *Trichophyton simii* have also been isolated. Favus usually affects only individual animals within a group. It is transmissible to other animals by contact or fomites but only rarely to humans. It spreads very slowly but premises can become contaminated.

Pathogenesis

Lesions are produced initially in unfeathered skin (comb, wattle, shanks) by superficial invasion of the stratum corneum by hyphae and result in epidermal hyperplasia and hyperkeratosis. They tend to slowly expand concentrically and infection is contained within the nonviable superficial layers of the skin and thus inflammatory reaction to infection is minimal.

DISEASE

Signs and lesions

Lesions occur on the comb, wattles and less frequently the shanks, initially as a few grey cup-like spots that increase in size and coalesce to form a wrinkled crust; they are dry and scaly. With time lesions may regress, become static or progress to adjacent superficial feathered skin. Lesions in feathered skin may develop depressions around follicles (favus cups). No significant systemic invasion or signs are routinely encountered other than loss of feathers and scaliness of the skin.

DIAGNOSIS

Trichophyton infections are diagnosed by histological visualization of hyphae or spores in skin lesions and feather follicles, followed by culture on Sabouraud dextrose agar or selective dermatophyte media.

CONTROL

Many infections resolve spontaneously with time. If treatment of individual animals is required, crusts should be removed and infected sites dressed with topical antifungals. Systemic antifungal therapy may also be attempted in valuable individuals. Infected individuals should be removed and sites disinfected.

MYCOTOXICOSES

Mycotoxicoses (see also Ch. 44) are diseases of animals caused by ingesting toxins produced by fungi growing on grains or feed or contaminated litter. They are seen worldwide. Growing fungi produce a vast array of complex chemicals as by-products and elaborate them into surrounding substances. Some are toxic to animals (mycotoxins), some to bacteria (antibiotics) and some to both. Fungal growth is required for mycotoxin production in grain but this growth may or may not produce visible damage to the grain. Fungi can infect and grow in grain prior to harvest, during storage or after inclusion in finished feeds. Many mycotoxins are stable during milling processes that reduce microbial loads and improve digestibility, such as steam pelleting and cooker-extrusion pelleting, and during storage of feed and feed ingredients storage, so that toxins can be present in grains and finished feed after the fungi that produced them are dead.

Thousands of chemically distinct mycotoxins exist. The strain of fungus, temperature, moisture, grain substrate and degree of stress on the host plant all determine whether toxins will be produced and in what amounts. Individual fungal strains often synthesize more than one mycotoxin, and these toxins often act synergistically so that the toxicity of the toxins together is much greater than the sum of their individual toxicities. This should be kept in mind when setting acceptable toxin levels in grains used in animal feeds. Toxin levels listed below are those experimentally associated with specific clinical signs.

Aflatoxicosis, ochratoxicosis and trichothecene mycotoxicosis are the most commonly seen mycotoxicoses in commercial poultry.

AFLATOXICOSIS

Aflatoxin is the most prevalent and economically significant mycotoxin to be consumed by poultry.

EPIDEMIOLOGY

Aetiology

Aflatoxin is found in corn (maize), peanuts, cottonseed, millet, sorghum and other feed grains. *A. flavus* produces the majority of the toxin and gives it its name, but aflatoxin is also produced by *Aspergillus parasiticus*. Both fungi are ubiquitous in the environment, contain toxigenic and nontoxigenic strains, and produce aflatoxin in warm (30–35°C), high-humidity (0.90–0.99 water activity) conditions. Aflatoxin contamination is thus more likely in grains grown or handled in the tropics or subtropics. Handling or storage of grains in these conditions anywhere may also stimulate production. Stressing host plants by insect damage, drought, poor nutrition or delayed harvest increases aflatoxin production.

Naturally occurring aflatoxin contains aflatoxins B_1, B_2, G_1 and G_2, but aflatoxin B_1 is usually in the highest concentration and is the most toxic. Aflatoxin is stable once formed in grain, and is not degraded during normal milling and storage. Other toxins produced with aflatoxins under field conditions may play a synergistic role in toxicity.

Host

Young poultry are more sensitive to aflatoxin than adults. There are also large species differences, with ducks being 10 times more sensitive than chickens, and turkeys intermediate between the two.

Pathogenesis

After ingestion, aflatoxin B_1 undergoes biotransformation to numerous highly reactive metabolites with diverse adverse effects on metabolism. Metabolites bind to DNA and RNA, reduce protein synthesis and decrease cell-mediated immunity and to a lesser extent humoral immunity. With continued exposure intrahepatic biliary epithelial hyperplasia and extramedullary haematopoiesis occur, the latter in response to a toxin-induced anaemia. Aflatoxin is rapidly excreted in the bile and urine and does not accumulate or persist in body tissues. This perhaps explains the rapid recovery of egg production and hatchability after cessation of toxin ingestion.

DISEASE

Clinical signs

Aflatoxicosis does not usually induce mortality directly, although high levels (>10 ppm) may be lethal. The most economically significant effects of aflatoxicosis on growing birds are decreased growth and poor feed conversion (>1 ppm). There is also a marked decrease in resistance to infections such as salmonellosis, coccidiosis, infectious bursal disease and candidiasis, with resultant increased condemnations at processing (>0.5 ppm). Poultry manifesting aflatoxicosis may also have failure of normal pigmentation and increased bruising (>0.5 ppm). Intoxicated adult hens have decreased egg production and the hatchability of those eggs that are produced is reduced (>2 ppm). In adult breeder males testicular weights and sperm counts are reduced. Insemination of hens with semen from affected males has shown decreased fertility in some studies and no significant reduction in others.

Lesions

Lesions will depend on the age of the host and the dose of toxin and can include enlarged livers which become friable and yellow with increasing dose, kidney and spleen enlargement, and diminution of the bursa of Fabricius, thymus and testes. Petechial haemorrhages or bruises after trauma are also increased because of decreased clotting factor synthesis and increased capillary fragility.

OCHRATOXICOSIS

EPIDEMIOLOGY

Aetiology

Ochratoxicosis occurs less frequently in poultry than aflatoxicosis but is more lethal because of its acute toxicity. Its name derives from *Aspergillus ochraceus*, the first fungus shown to produce it. Most naturally occurring cases have been associated with ochratoxin produced by *Penicillium veridicatum* but five other species of *Aspergillus* and six other species of *Penicillium* produce it as well. Ochratoxin is a dihydroisocoumarin derivative linked to L-β-phenylalanine. Ochratoxin A and the dechlorinated B form occur naturally but ochratoxin A is the most toxic and is produced in greater quantities.

Host

Young poultry are most sensitive to ochratoxin ingestion and ducks are seven times more sensitive to the acute effects than chickens. Quail and turkeys are also more sensitive to ochratoxicosis than chickens.

Spread

Environmental conditions favouring ochratoxin production are similar to those for aflatoxin, and simultaneous contamination with both is common.

Pathogenesis

Ochratoxin A inhibits protein synthesis, produces acute proximal tubular epithelial necrosis in the kidneys and inhibits normal renal uric acid secretion.

DISEASE

Signs

Acutely intoxicated birds are depressed, dehydrated and often polyuric (>4 ppm) and die in acute renal failure. Survivors will be stunted, poorly feathered, and have increased clotting times, anaemia and immunosuppression (>0.6 ppm). There may be loss of pigmentation and reduced weight gain (>2 ppm). Laying hens may have delayed sexual maturity, or develop wet droppings, causing increased numbers of stained eggs. There is also a decrease in egg production and hatchability (>2 ppm), and poor performance in progeny derived from intoxicated hens.

Lesions

Affected kidneys are white to tan, swollen, hard and may have white pinpoint urate crystals. If damage is extensive enough to cause renal failure there is dehydration, hyperuricaemia and visceral urate deposition. Pasty white urates are deposited on pericardial, perihepatic, peritoneal and articular surfaces. These deposits may be mistaken for inflammatory exudate but their true nature can be determined by microscopic examination of impressions or smears, or histological sections. More commonly, birds survive in compensated renal failure and kidneys appear enlarged, fibrotic and pale.

In addition to the renal lesions there is mild to moderate fatty change and glycogen deposition in hepatocytes, resulting in yellow enlarged livers. There is also some mild decrease in bursal and thymic size consistent with immunosuppression.

TRICHOTHECENE MYCOTOXICOSIS

Trichothecene mycotoxicosis occurs fairly frequently in commercial poultry but at naturally occurring levels does not usually cause mortality. Losses result from reduced feed intake, decreased growth and immunosuppression.

EPIDEMIOLOGY

Aetiology

Trichothecene mycotoxins occur frequently in wheat, corn (maize) and other grains used for poultry feed production and are produced by many species of *Fusarium*, *Stachybotrys* and at least three other genera. They also produce many nontrichothecene mycotoxins, some of which may exacerbate the clinical effects of the trichothecenes present.

Fusarium and *Stachybotrys* grow at many temperatures but toxin production is highest in cold (<20°C), moist conditions. Trichothecenes are therefore associated with cool climates, particularly when grain harvests have been delayed into the winter months or infected grain has been stored in cold conditions. This is distinct from aflatoxin or ochratoxin production and thus simultaneous contamination with these toxins is rare. There are approximately 80 chemically related sesquiterpinoid trichothecene mycotoxins described, but most is known about the effects of the 12,13-epoxytrichothecenes T-2, hydroxy T-2 (HT-2), diacetoxyscirpenol (DAS, anguidine) and deoxynivalenol (DON, vomitoxin). It is not known if these four compounds cause most field cases of trichothecene mycotoxicosis. Zearalenone (F-2) also falls in this category but its effects in commercial poultry are minimal.

Host

Young birds are more susceptible than older ones.

Pathogenesis

Trichothecene mycotoxins of significance in poultry produce their pathogenic effects by two mechanisms: direct epithelial necrosis and radiomimetic effects that destroy rapidly dividing cells. T-2 causes epithelial necrosis of mucous membranes on contact. Ulcers occur where this contact is frequent or where contaminated feed becomes lodged. Thus erosions and ulcers on the hard palate, tongue and rostral oropharynx, and chemical burns of the rostral tip of the tongue are due to the direct caustic effects of T-2. DAS is also epithelionecrotic but its effects are slightly less severe than those of T-2. Depending on the dose, ulcers appear 3–4 days after initial toxin intake and continue to worsen as long as exposure persists. The radiomimetic effects result from trichothecenes severely inhibiting protein synthesis and tissues with short cellular life spans and high turnover rates are affected in trichothecene mycotoxicosis. This accounts for the suppression by T-2 of haematopoiesis, lymphopoiesis, normal immune responses and normal replication of feather follicle epithelium and, in severe cases, replication of enterocytes. Individual trichothecenes differ in their production of the above effects. T-2 very effectively produces oral ulcers at low doses and produces the radiomimetic effects at slightly higher doses. DAS produces systemic radiomimetic effects at low doses but is an inefficient producer of oral ulcers. In contrast, DON is relatively nontoxic in poultry and produces no oral ulcers, no feed refusal and no radiomimetic effects at naturally occurring doses.

DISEASE

Signs

There is reduced feed intake, weight gains and feed efficiency, also, anaemia and poor feathering with broken feather shafts. Affected adult birds will develop oral ulcers, decreased egg production, decreased shell quality and hatchability (>20 ppm T-2).

Lesions

Ulcers are found at the commissures of the mouth, on the hard palate adjacent to the beak and the palatine cleft, and on the dorsal surface of the tongue (>2 ppm T-2). Ulcers are not usually produced further down the oesophagus unless the birds eat large amounts of feed rapidly. There may be reduction in size of the bursa of Fabricius and thymus glands of young birds and birds may show anaemia and pale bone marrow.

It should be noted that oral ulcers are not specific, since dietary copper sulphate (>200 ppm) and other caustic or traumatic dietary ingredients induce identical lesions.

OTHER MYCOTOXICOSES

Several other mycotoxicoses have been rarely described in poultry but the overall economic significance of these toxicoses is low.

CITRININ

Citrinin is a nephrotoxin produced in a variety of cereal grains by *Penicillium citrinum*. During citrinin toxicosis, mortality is rare but water consumption is increased and there is diffuse polyuria manifested as wet droppings (>300 ppm). Clinical signs begin within hours after initial exposure, persist as long as toxin-containing feed is consumed and stop 8–10 h after cessation of exposure. Grossly kidneys are slightly swollen but there are no microscopic lesions except at very high dosages.

OOSPOREIN

Oosporein is a nephrotoxic mycotoxin produced by *Chaetomium trilaterale*. Ingestion by chicks (>300 ppm) or turkeys (>500 ppm) produces acute proximal tubular nephrosis and acute renal failure in severe cases. Effects are particularly severe in poultry less than 1 week old and lead to visceral and articular urate deposits and mortality up to 20%.

FUSARIUM FUNGI

Fusarium fungi produce a wide variety of other mycotoxins. Some strains of *Fusarium moniliforme* produce fumonisins, a group of water-soluble mycotoxins associated with equine encephalomalacia and swine pulmonary oedema. Poultry are apparently more resistant. Ingestion of 325 ppm by turkey poults and 250 ppm by broiler chicks is required to decrease feed intake and body weights.

MONILIFORMIN

Moniliformin is another mycotoxin produced by some *F. moniliforme* strains as well as by *Fusarium fujikuroi*. It has been associated with acute myocardial necrosis and death in ducks, chickens and turkey poults. Decreased feed intake and reduced body weights are seen in poults fed 50 ppm, and in broiler chicks fed 100 ppm.

FUSAROCHROMANONE (TDP-1)

Fusarochromanone (TDP-1) is a rarely encountered mycotoxin produced by multiple isolates of *Fusarium*. It produces leg deformities and tibial dyschondroplasia in chicks fed 20 ppm, although the majority of naturally occurring tibial dyschondroplasia does not appear to be due to this toxicosis.

ERGOTISM

Ergotism is caused by the alkaloid toxins produced by *Claviceps* species, particularly *Claviceps purpurea* ('ergot of rye'). The fungi grow on wild grasses and common cereal grains, including wheat, barley and, more rarely, oats. Rye is most frequently affected. The acute disease takes the form of convulsions, ataxia and coma followed by death. In the chronic form there is reduced growth or reduced egg production, poor feathering, diarrhoea and gangrene affecting the comb, wattles, beak and feet and sometimes vesicles and ulcers on the shanks and feet.

DIAGNOSIS OF MYCOTOXICOSES

The clinical signs, gross and histopathological lesions may be helpful but not specific. The results of feeding trials with the suspect feed to reproduce the field toxicosis is also of value but it may be difficult to obtain replicate feed samples. Samples of suspect feed and mouldy clumps for feeding trials and chemical analysis should be collected directly from the trough in the poultry house. Samples can be rapidly screened for aflatoxin, ochratoxin, T-2, DON and fumonisin with commercially available solid or liquid phase competitive enzyme-linked immunosorbent assay (ELISA) tests. These inexpensive rapid tests can be done in minutes with material on the farm or in the feed mill and yield generally excellent results. Positive tests should be confirmed by more rigorous analytical chemical methods, including thin layer chromatography, high-performance liquid chromatography, gas chromatography, mass spectrophotometry, or monoclonal antibody technology. Such confirmation requires the capability of the diagnostic laboratory for both analysis and interpretation.

The identification of significant levels of mycotoxins in sick birds or fresh carcasses from the field is often precluded because most mycotoxins and their metabolites are rapidly excreted or broken down so tissue residues cannot be detected. In some rare cases, however, analysis of crop or intestinal contents of acutely affected birds, or fresh droppings from poultry houses may be of assistance.

CONTROL OF MYCOTOXICOSES

Prevention of mycotoxicoses is dependent on adherence to quality assurance applied to grain supplies, feed manufacture, feed delivery, storage and presentation to stock. Tolerance levels for specific mycotoxins should be set and grain suppliers should be informed of these limits. Mycotoxins are considered undesirable substances in feeds and regulated under EU Directive 2002/32/EC.

Incoming grain shipments should be probed and tested for moisture and mycotoxin levels using either ELISA, affinity columns or other appropriate chemical assays. Shipments falling outside acceptable levels should be rejected. Grain storage bins and feed mill equipment (i.e. pellet mills, pellet coolers, augers and feed trucks) should be inspected and cleaned on a routine schedule. Feed preservatives and antifungals may be added to prevent fungal growth in storage bins or finished feeds and pelleting feed can reduce fungal spores. Poultry farms should have two bins per house to allow rotation and cleaning. Feed mills and farmers should hold back samples of each finished feed for future analysis if warranted.

Detoxification including ammoniation and the application to feed of non-nutritive clays have been used in order to reduce or prevent the absorption of toxins. However, it is important to appreciate that their effectiveness may vary or be limited to certain toxins. Over the last 10 years particular studies have assayed the value of non-nutritive clays, especially against aflatoxicoses. They include aluminosilicates, zeolites, bentonites and clinoptilolites. They have high binding capacity against aflatoxin, reduce its absorption from the gastrointestinal tract and are generally inert, nontoxic and economical in use.

FURTHER READING

Bailey R H, Kubena L F, Harvey R B et al 1998 Efficacy of various inorganic sorbents to reduce the toxicity of aflatoxin and T-2 toxin in broiler chickens. Poult Sci 77: 1623–1630

Blalock H G, Georg L K, Derieux W T 1973 Encephalitis in turkey poults due to *Dactylaria gallopava*: a case report and its experimental reproduction. Avian Dis 17: 197–204

Brown T P, Rottinghaus G E, Williams M E 1992 Fumonisin mycotoxicosis in broilers: performance and pathology. Avian Dis 36: 450–454

Diaz D E (ed) 2005 The mycotoxin blue book. Nottingham University Press, Nottingham

Englehardt J A, Carlton W W, Tuite J F 1989 Toxicity of *Fusarium moniliforme* var. *subglutinans* for chicks, ducklings, and turkey poults. Avian Dis 33: 357–360

Hoerr F J 2003 Mycotoxicoses. In: Saif Y M (ed) Diseases of poultry, 11th edn. Iowa State University Press, Ames, p 1103–1132

Kubena L F, Harvey R B, Phillips T D et al 1990 Diminution of aflatoxicosis in growing chickens by dietary addition of hydrated, sodium aluminosilicate. Poult Sci 69: 727–735

Kunkle R A 2003 Fungal infections. In: Saif Y M (ed) Diseases of poultry, 11th edn. Iowa State University Press, Ames, p 883–902

Kunkle R A, Rimler R B 1996 Pathology of acute aspergillosis in turkeys. Avian Dis 40: 875–886

Leeson S, Diaz G, Summers J D 1995 Aflatoxins. In: Leeson S, Diaz G, Summers J D (eds) Poultry metabolic disorders and mycotoxins. University Books, Guelph, p 248–279

Oguz H, Kurtoglu V, Coskun B 2000 Preventive efficacy of clinoptilolite in broilers during chronic aflatoxicosis (50–100 ppb) exposure. Res Vet Sci 69: 197–201

Spooner B, Roberts P 2005 Fungi. The New Naturalist Library. Harper Collins, London

Walser M M, Allen N K, Mirocha C J et al 1982 *Fusarium*-induced osteochondrosis (tibial dyschondroplasia) in chickens. Vet Pathol 19: 544–550

Weibking T S, Ledoux D R, Brown T P et al 1993 Fumonisin toxicity in turkey poults. J Vet Diagn Invest 5: 75–83

Wyatt R D 1991 Poultry. In: Smith J E, Henderson R S (eds) Mycotoxins and animal foods. CRC Press, Boca Raton, p 553–605

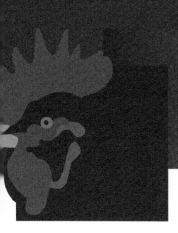

SECTION
5

Paul F. McMullin

PARASITIC DISEASES

Chapter **39**   Parasitic diseases   **444**

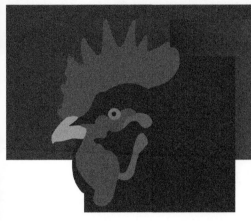

CHAPTER
39

Alexander J. Trees

Parasitic diseases

COCCIDIOSIS

Coccidiosis is one of the most important diseases of poultry worldwide and most forms are characterized by enteritis. It is caused by protozoa of the phylum Apicomplexa, which undergo a direct life cycle with transmission between hosts by way of a resistant oocyst. In the host, the parasite grows and multiplies intracellularly in epithelial and subepithelial cells usually in the gut but, in a few species, in other organs. Most coccidia in poultry belong to the genus *Eimeria*.

The *Eimeria* are highly host-specific. Within each host there may be several species of varying pathogenicity, which are, however, unique to it. *Eimeria* spp. infections are ubiquitous and it has been said that the only limit to their distribution is the distribution of their hosts. However, disease is likely to occur only under conditions of high stocking density on litter, which favour the build-up of potentially pathogenic populations of the parasite. Thus, coccidiosis is especially important in intensive broiler poultry operations. Apart from causing disease, subclinical infections cause impaired feed conversion and since feed costs comprise some 70% of the cost of producing broiler chickens, the economic impact of coccidiosis is considerable. For example, it has been estimated that the total cost of chicken coccidiosis in the UK in 1995 was £38.5 million (Williams 1999).

LIFE CYCLE/BIOLOGY

The life cycle of a typical *Eimeria* sp., illustrated in Figure 39.1, comprises a parasitic and a nonparasitic phase. The infective stage – the sporulated oocyst – is ingested and the action of mechanical and chemical factors in the gut (bile salts and trypsin) leads to the release of sporocysts and then sporozoites in the duodenal lumen. The sporozoites invade the mucosa, sometimes

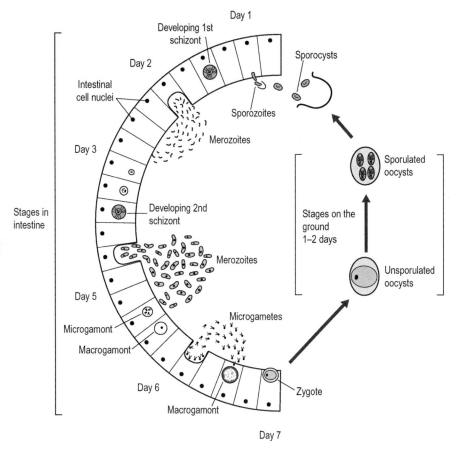

Fig. 39.1 Life cycle of *Eimeria tenella*, typical of the genus *Eimeria*.

passing down the whole length of the alimentary tract before doing so. There follow phases of intracellular growth and asexual multiplication with periodic release of merozoites back into the gut lumen. After a number of such schizogonous cycles (the number is primarily a genetically determined characteristic of a given species or strain), sexual forms – the gametocytes – develop intracellularly. These differentiate into macro- and microgametocytes. The microgametocyte releases many microgametes, which are flagellated and motile and migrate to the macrogametocytes. The macrogametocyte develops into a single macrogamete, which, after fertilization, develops into a zygote and thence an oocyst. During this process, large intracytoplasmic granules appear peripherally and eventually coalesce to form the oocyst wall. In histological sections these are very characteristic and clearly identify the macrogametes (Fig. 39.2). An important feature is that this cycle is quite rapid, with a prepatent period of about 4–5 days (which varies slightly with species), and involves colossal multiplication. The degree varies with species but optimally may result in hundreds of thousands or even millions of oocysts produced from one ingested oocyst.

When oocysts are passed in faeces they contain an undifferentiated spherical body. These oocysts only become potentially infective after undergoing sporulation. This entails subdivision into

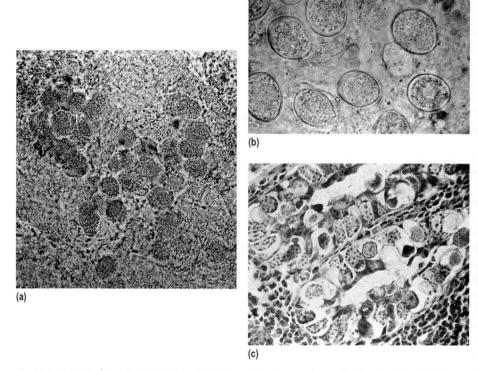

Fig. 39.2 Diagnosis of coccidiosis; *Eimeria tenella* in tissues. (a) Wet smear, clumps of schizonts, × 140. (b) Wet smear, unsporulated oocysts, × 1120. (c) Caecal section, macrogametes and oocysts in epithelial cells. Haematoxylin/ eosin, × 512.

four sporocysts, each of which contains two sporozoites. (In genera other than *Eimeria* there may be a different arrangement.) Sporulation requires three conditions: warmth, moisture and oxygen. Under optimal conditions, around 25–30°C, this takes 1–2 days. Sporulated oocysts, protected by the thick oocyst wall, are resistant to a fairly wide range of normal environmental conditions and the ability of at least some to survive for months or years is a key factor in the epidemiology of coccidial infections. Temperatures above 56°C and below freezing are lethal, as is desiccation, but oocysts are able to tolerate most disinfectants. Only low-molecular-weight compounds, such as ammonia and methyl bromide, effectively kill oocysts and these gases are used to decontaminate experimental facilities. Under practical farm conditions it is more common to use proprietary products that release ammonia in a controlled manner – even then special care is required to protect the operator.

The identification of different species of *Eimeria* in a given host necessitates consideration of a number of characteristics. Oocyst morphology may be useful, especially if length:width ratios are determined, but will not distinguish many species. The site and nature of lesions are valuable practical criteria. In a research context, identification may be definitively determined by cross-immunity experiments, electrophoretic analysis of isoenzymes or DNA-based methods.

IMMUNOLOGY

Day-old chicks do not normally derive passively transferred protective immunity from the hen (but see below) and birds of any age are susceptible to coccidiosis. In practice, most acquire infection in the first few weeks of life and this infection induces a good immunity. In most situations this persists for life because of frequent low-grade re-exposure to infection but, in the absence of infection, immunity may wane. A cardinal feature is that immunity is species-specific. Thus in chickens, for example, immunity to *Eimeria maxima* does not confer complete resistance to *Eimeria tenella*, and so on. Within species, there appears to be remarkably little strain variation and strains of the same species isolated from widely separated locations will provide substantial cross-protection. However, important exceptions are *E. maxima* and *Eimeria acervulina*.

Immunity is best engendered by repeated exposure to low numbers of oocysts, so-called 'trickle' infection, and this, of course, is the usual situation in the wild. Immunity is manifest as a reduction in lesions and a marked reduction in oocyst output due to both a reduction in the number of sporozoites that successfully invade host cells and an inhibition of intracellular development of those that do. The mechanisms of immunity are not yet fully established but cell-mediated responses appear to be crucial. Secretory IgA may also contribute to protective immunity but circulating antibodies, although produced in response to infection, normally play only a minor role. However, if antibody levels in laying hens are high as a result of challenge infections while laying, antibodies may be passively transferred to chicks in sufficient quantity to inhibit oocyst output. This effect is particularly due to antigametocyte antibodies and has been exploited to produce a transmission-blocking vaccine (see below). In this, maternal IgG antibody is transferred via the yolk and can protect not only against the homologous species but against other species too.

EPIDEMIOLOGY

The severity of disease is dependent on both the species of *Eimeria* and the size of the infecting dose of oocysts. It is impossible under farming conditions to produce a coccidia-free environment. Oocysts will remain in buildings from previous crops of birds and will also be carried in on two legs (the dirty feet of *Homo sapiens*!) or possibly by other vertebrate and invertebrate agencies. From whatever source, chicks introduced to buildings quickly become infected. Because of the short prepatent period of the parasite and its high biotic potential, the number of oocysts in the litter rises rapidly (Fig. 39.3). A dynamic interaction ensues between the acquisition of flock immunity by 'trickle' infection and the amplification of the parasite population. Usually, immunity will be acquired without clinical disease occurring; oocyst output will be reduced and litter oocyst populations fall rapidly. However, if the balance is disturbed by factors that favour the parasite, such as an initial high degree of environmental contamination and/or ideal sporulation conditions (e.g. wet litter), pathogenic numbers of infective oocysts will be ingested by nonimmune birds and disease will result. In chickens on litter, this typically occurs at 3–6 weeks of age but may occur in older birds, especially with certain species, e.g. *Eimeria necatrix*, or under conditions in which immunity has waned or has never been fully acquired. This may happen, for example, if floor-reared birds are caged for laying, thus preventing reinfection, and are subsequently re-exposed to infection. Certain anticoccidials are so effective in preventing infection that they inhibit the acquisition of immunity. Thus, after drug withdrawal, birds may be fully susceptible at an age when they might normally be expected to be immune.

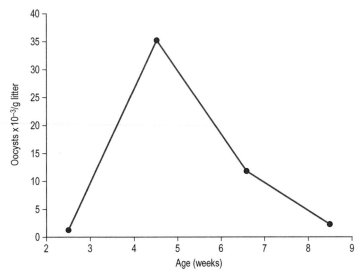

Fig. 39.3 Oocyst counts ($\times 10^{-3}$) per g of litter during the growth of broiler chickens. (Drawn from mean data from 47 houses supplied by Long & Rowell 1975.)

For this reason, many outbreaks of coccidiosis follow errors in the inclusion of prophylactic drugs in feed, or inadvisable programmes.

It is important to appreciate that, irrespective of the occurrence or nonoccurrence of clinical disease, coccidial infection (subclinical coccidiosis or coccidiasis) always occurs in birds reared on litter and this may have important economic consequences by impairing performance and feed conversion.

To summarize, the key factors in the epidemiology of coccidiosis are as follows:
- Oocysts persist in the environment
- There is normally no maternally derived protective immunity in chicks
- The parasite has a short prepatent period and a high biotic potential
- Disease is a function of host numbers and immunity, oocyst dose and coccidial species
- Immunity is acquired by infection and maintained by continual reinfection.

CHICKEN COCCIDIOSIS

There are seven important species, detailed in Figure 39.4. In addition, *Eimeria hagani*, first described in 1938, has only rarely been described since. *Eimeria mivati*, described in 1965, is now considered to be a spurious species comprising a mixture of *E. acervulina* and *Eimeria mitis*. All seven species appear to be distributed throughout the world. *E. acervulina* and *E. maxima* are the most prevalent, with *E. tenella* the commonest of the highly pathogenic species.

The sites and nature of lesions vary between species. In the duodenum only *E. acervulina* is likely to cause lesions. These are characteristically white, irregular linear lesions ('zebra striping') associated with gamonts and oocysts. In heavy infections these may coalesce and become less obvious. Oocysts of *Eimeria praecox* and *E. mitis* can also be found in the

Characteristics	High pathogenicity; dysentery, high mortality, high morbidity		
	E. brunetti	*E. necatrix*	*E. tenella*
ZONE PARASITIZED		Large schizonts, no oocysts 	
MACROSCOPIC LESIONS	Coagulation necrosis, mucoid, bloody, enteritis	Ballooning, white spots (schizonts), petechiae, mucoid blood-filled exudate	Onset: haemorrhage into lumen Later: thickening, whitish mucosa, cores, clotted blood
(x 10^{-9} m) OOCYSTS REDRAWN FROM ORIGINALS	10 20 30 	10 20 30 	10 20 30
LENGTH x WIDTH (μm) LENGTH = WIDTH =	24.6 x 18.8 20.7–30.3 18.1–24.2	20.4 x 17.2 13.2–22.7 11.3–18.3	22.0 x 19.0 19.5–26.0 16.5–22.8
OOCYST SHAPE AND INDEX – LENGTH / WIDTH	Ovoid 1.31	Oblong ovoid 1.19	Ovoid 1.16
SCHIZONT MAX (μm)	30.0	65.9	54.0
PARASITE LOCATION IN TISSUE SECTIONS	2nd generation schizonts subepithelial	2nd generation schizonts subepithelial	2nd generation schizonts subepithelial
MINIMUM PREPATENT PERIOD (h)	120	138	115
SPORULATION MINIMUM (h)	18	18	18

Medium pathogenicity; lesions, but low mortality, high morbidity		Low pathogenicity; no lesions	
E. acervulina	*E. maxima*	*E. mitis*	*E. praecox*
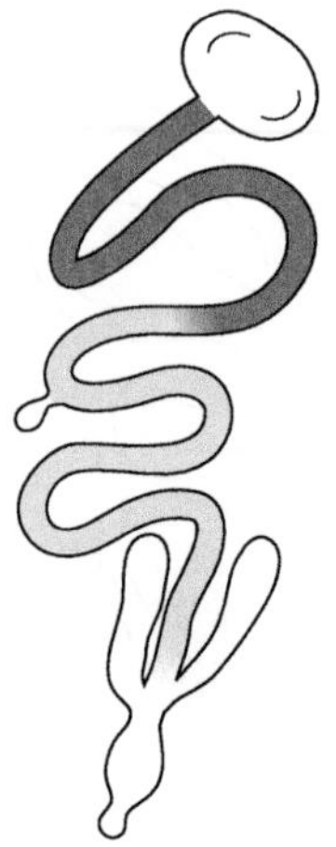	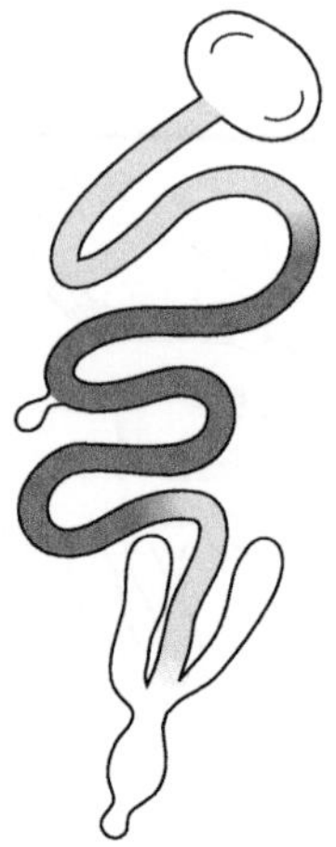	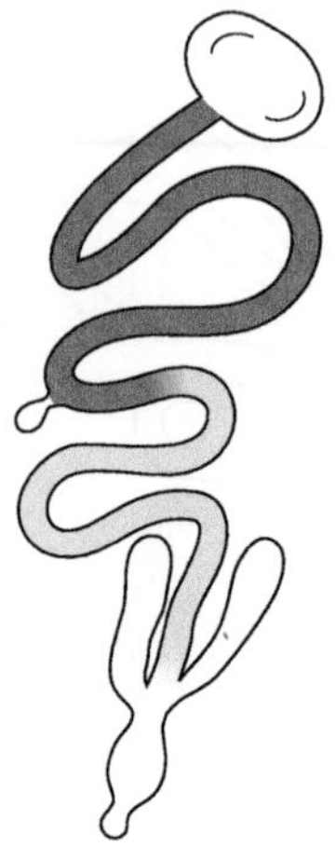	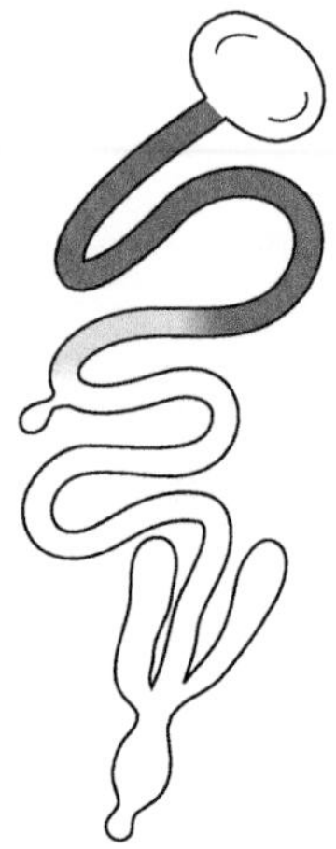
Light infection: transverse, whitish bands of oocysts. Heavy infection: plaques coalescing, thickened wall	Thickened walls, mucoid blood-tinged exudate, petechiae	No lesions, mucoid exudate	No lesions, mucoid exudate
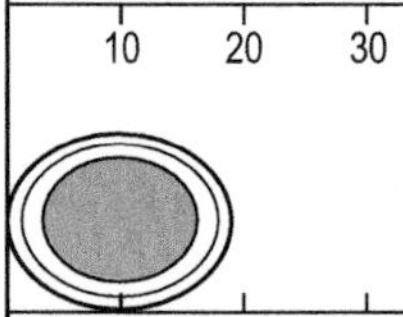 10 20 30	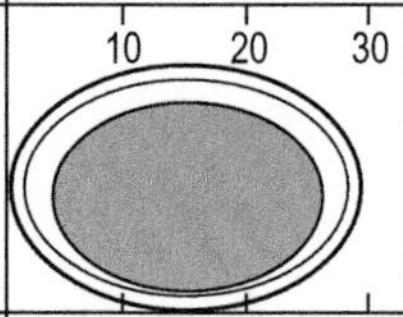 10 20 30	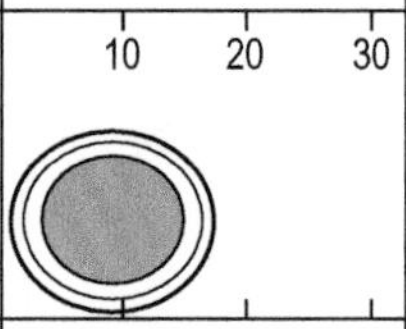 10 20 30	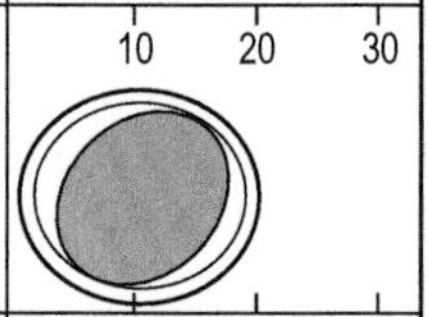 10 20 30
AV = 18.3 x 14.6 17.7–20.2 13.7–16.3	30.5 x 20.7 21.5–42.5 16.5–29.8	16.2 x 16.0 14.3–19.6 13.0–17.0	21.3 x 17.1 19.8–24.7 15.7–19.8
Ovoid	Ovoid	Subspherical	Ovoid
1.25	1.47	1.01	1.24
10.3	9.4	11.3	20
Epithelial	Gametocytes subepithelial	Epithelial	Epithelial
97	121	99	83
17	30	18	12

Fig. 39.4 Characteristics of *Eimeria* spp. of the fowl.

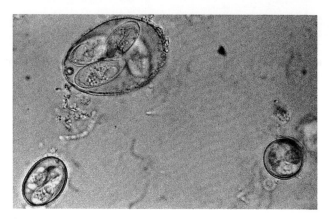

Fig. 39.5 Oocysts of *Eimeria maxima* and *Eimeria acervulina* (× 1300).

duodenum. In the mid-intestine *E. necatrix* causes both white and red focal lesions with ballooning of the intestinal walls and an accompanying dysentery. The white lesions are clumps of schizonts. Gametogeny and oocyst formation take place in the caeca but without lesions. *E. maxima* causes discrete focal, haemorrhagic lesions. The pathology is associated with the particularly large gamonts of this species. Soft, mucoid, salmon-pink-coloured faeces are typical. The oocysts are the most distinctive of those of all chicken *Eimeria* spp., being much the largest (although oocysts of *Eimeria brunetti* do overlap in size) and with a golden-brown-tinted oocyst wall (Fig. 39.5). *E. maxima* is highly immunogenic and flock immunity will be quickly established following infection. In the lower intestine *E. brunetti* causes haemorrhagic lesions. *E. tenella* causes caecal coccidiosis, initially with blotchy haemorrhagic lesions, accompanied by haemorrhage into the caecal lumen and dysentery. The second-stage schizonts in their deep, subepithelial position are responsible for the lesions. This phase resolves in 1–2 days and the caeca become pale and shrunken, with a thickened wall. A core of cellular debris and oocysts forms in the lumen. With *E. tenella* and *E. necatrix* there may be massive haemorrhage into the gut and high mortality. Increased mortality may also be associated with *E. brunetti*.

TURKEY COCCIDIOSIS

Five species have been described that may cause lesions in turkeys (Table 39.1). They are thought to be widely distributed. Disease is confined to young poults, with older turkeys very resistant. Dysentery is rarely associated with any of the infections, a watery diarrhoea being more typical. *Eimeria adenoeides* is the most pathogenic of the turkey coccidia and causes high mortality in very young poults. Faeces may be fluid and blood-tinged and contain mucoid casts. *Eimeria meleagridis*, although much less pathogenic, also causes lesions in the caecum and is distinguished on the basis of a lower shape index (length/width). *E. gallopavonis* parasitizes a similar region but primarily infects the rectum, with limited involvement of the caecum. *Eimeria meleagrimitis* is a pathogenic species infecting the upper intestine. In all these species, gamonts and oocysts are the stages most likely to be associated with lesions.

Table 39.1 | Some characteristics of the important *Eimeria* spp. infecting turkeys

	HIGH PATHOGENICITY			LOW PATHOGENICITY	
	E. adenoeides	*E. meleagrimitis*	*E. gallopavonis*	*E. meleagridis*	*E. dispersa*
Site of lesions	Caecum	Anterior and mid-intestine	Rectum	Caecum	Anterior and mid-intestine
Type of lesion	Possibly petechial haemorrhages, mucoid exudate. Caecal cores	Haemorrhagic lesions, dilation of jejunum, casts	Ulceration, yellow exudate	Creamy exudate, caseous core	Watery or mucoid exudate; yellowish faeces
Mean oocyst size (μm)	25.6 × 16.6	19.1 × 16.2	27.1 × 17.2	24.4 × 18.1	24.2 × 19.3
Shape index (L/W)	1.54	1.17	1.52	1.35	1.25

Authority: *E. dispersa*, Long & Millard 1979; all other species, Moore & Brown 1951.

COCCIDIOSIS IN OTHER SPECIES

Geese

Intestinal coccidiosis can be a severe problem in goslings. Although a number of species have been described, *Eimeria anseris* is the most pathogenic, with *Eimeria nocens* also a frequent con-current infection. *E. anseris* causes a haemorrhagic enteritis in the small intestine, with diarrhoea. Oocysts are colourless, distinctly pyriform, measuring $22 \times 27\,\mu m$. Those of *E. nocens* are brown, thick-walled, $31 \times 22\,\mu m$, with a micropyle. Also highly pathogenic in goslings is the species *Eimeria truncata*, the cause of renal coccidiosis. *E. truncata* is one of the few eimerian parasites that has forsaken the gut, parasitizing epithelial cells in the kidney tubules. Severe infection in 3–12-week-old birds causes depression, emaciation, diarrhoea and mortality. There are macroscopic pale focal lesions on the kidneys and parasites are found in the kidneys or cloaca near the junction of the ureters. The distinctive oocysts are oval ($21.3 \times 16.7\,\mu m$ average size) with a polar cap at one end.

Ducks

Probably the most pathogenic coccidial infection is *Tyzzeria perniciosa*. This can cause severe disease in ducklings under 7 weeks of age, with a haemorrhagic enteritis of the anterior small intestine, dysentery and a high mortality. Both haemorrhagic and pale focal lesions are present. The sporulated oocysts contain eight sporozoites free within the oocysts, so that *T. perniciosa* may be readily differentiated from other less pathogenic *Eimeria* spp. in the same host.

Game birds

In pheasants the major species are *Eimeria colchici*, *Eimeria duodenalis* and *Eimeria phasiani*, the first probably being the most pathogenic. The initial stages of these infections occur in the intestine with gametogony and oocyst formation in the lower small intestine and caeca.

With *E. colchici* there is an enteritis and cores may form in the caeca where the oocysts are produced. Acute disease with mortality may be associated with caecal coccidiosis caused by *Eimeria legionensis* in red-legged partridge and by *Eimeria tsunodai* in Japanese quail. In young guinea fowl, coccidiosis caused by *Eimeria numidae* and *Eimeria grenieri* may be a severe problem.

Pigeons

Coccidiosis caused by *Eimeria labbeana* and *Eimeria columbanum* may be a problem in pigeon lofts.

CLINICAL SIGNS AND DIAGNOSIS

The presence of dysentery, diarrhoea or soft, mucoid faeces will alert the vigilant farmer to problems, although with less pathogenic species the only signs will be poor growth and impaired feed conversion. The earliest signs with the pathogenic species may be a sudden increase in daily mortality.

Post-mortem examination is essential to confirm diagnosis and a few sick birds should be sacrificed for this purpose so that fresh material is available. Lesions may be noticeable from the serosal surface but the mucosal surface should be examined carefully. It is important to demonstrate the parasite in association with lesions by examination of mucosal scrapings. Examination of wet smears diluted with isotonic saline under a coverslip with appropriate lighting will normally be sufficient to detect schizonts, gamonts and oocysts (Fig. 39.2). At higher power, merozoites can be distinguished. If required, thin smears can be stained to identify all stages. The causal species will usually be identifiable by such examination but diagnosis may be complicated by a number of factors:

- Multiple species infections are common
- Heavy infections lead to 'overflow' of parasites and lesions beyond their predilection site and also may cause lesions to coalesce and, ironically, be less obvious (e.g. *E. acervulina*)
- Birds in the field are being continuously infected, so that parasites at all stages in the life cycle may be found
- Heavy infections may occur secondarily to other primary disease conditions (e.g. salmonellosis, infectious bursitis or clostridial disease).

In birds receiving anticoccidial prophylaxis, investigation of an outbreak of disease should also include the submission of feed samples for drug assay. Samples should, of course, be representative of the feed used 5–10 days prior to the outbreak. This analysis will reveal whether or not the outbreak was associated with the accidental omission of drug or its inclusion at a suboptimal dose, or whether drug resistance is occurring.

CONTROL OF COCCIDIOSIS IN CHICKENS

Control in broilers relies principally on drugs. Effective live attenuated vaccines are now available and are particularly used for breeders or layer replacements, and a similar vaccine has been developed specifically for meat-type chickens. A succession of anticoccidial agents has been introduced since the 1940s and has been crucial in controlling coccidiosis during the development of the broiler industry. However, the emergence of coccidial drug resistance has cut short the useful life of successive drugs. Together with the fact that the cost of drug development has escalated as a result of increasingly demanding registration requirements, this has meant that the commercial incentive to develop new anticoccidials has been much reduced. The possibility that drugs may not indefinitely be relied upon to control coccidiosis has led to an increase of interest in alternative means of control. The possibilities for control are considered under four headings: hygiene, genetics, immunization and drugs.

Hygiene

It is impossible under commercial farming conditions to prevent infection. In the case of game birds, ducks and geese, wild birds may contribute infection but the major source in all species is likely to be residual environmental contamination from previous crops. For reasons previously discussed, it is impossible to chemically eliminate coccidial oocysts from a farm environment. Good hygiene, however, can substantially reduce the numbers of oocysts contaminating the environment and, most importantly, can ensure that litter is kept dry so as not to provide good sporulation conditions. Attention should be paid to prevention of overflowing waterers and leaking water pipes. By maintaining birds on perforated floors, coccidiosis infection is vastly reduced. This is one of the major advantages that would accrue if broilers were so reared but, for a variety of reasons, this is not yet commercially feasible. Layers are often kept on wire floors without access to litter, although the proportion of layers kept on deep litter with or without access to free range is steadily increasing. Cage housing can occasionally be disadvantageous in that any immunity to coccidiosis that birds may have acquired during rearing on litter may wane.

Genetics

This is a theoretical strategy not in practical use. It has been known for many years that strains of fowl can be bred that are less susceptible to coccidiosis. This approach to control has not been developed, partly because of the efficacy and availability of drugs and partly because of other overriding priorities in breeding programmes. However, interest in this strategy is increasing as modern technologies of genetic manipulation develop.

Immunization

Live vaccines

A number of commercial vaccines have been introduced that use wild (i.e. nonattenuated) isolates. These depend on the precise delivery of low numbers of oocysts, such that immunity is engendered but disease does not occur. Importantly, all seven *Eimeria* spp. of chickens have been attenuated by rapid passage in vivo, selecting so-called 'precocious' strains. Although these precocious strains have lost virulence, they retain immunogenicity. Several commercial vaccines are available in the UK and elsewhere, using live attenuated oocysts, and can be used for broilers, broiler-breeders, breeders and layer replacements. Some vaccines comprise all the chicken *Eimeria* spp.; others include a more restricted range and most include two lines of *E. maxima* to provide good immunity to heterologous challenge with that species. Birds are vaccinated through drinking water between 5 and 9 days of age or by spraying on food at 1 day old. Good efficacy against field challenge has been reported and millions of doses of these vaccines have now been used (Shirley et al 2005).

Subunit vaccine

A nonliving subunit vaccine has been developed and is available in several countries (CoxAbic® – www.coxabic.com). This so-called transmission-blocking vaccine utilizes native gametocyte antigens of *E. maxima*, which are administered to breeding hens. This maternal immunization confers antibody-mediated passive protection on the broiler chick offspring. By reducing their oocyst shedding, it reduces the build-up of environmental infection and allows the acquisition of active immunity.

Drugs

Drugs are used primarily prophylactically. The term 'coccidiostat' specifically describes compounds that inhibit but do not kill the parasite, in contrast to coccidiocides. The term anticoccidial agent is to be preferred to describe all drugs with activity against coccidia. Most anticoccidials are formulated as feed additives and broiler feed almost always contains an anticoccidial agent, except during the mandatory withdrawal period prior to slaughter. Apart from preventing disease, the inclusion of drugs will usually prove economically beneficial because of the control of subclinical coccidiosis. The main drugs currently used are summarized in Table 39.2. The most widely used drugs in the USA and Europe are the ionophores. Monensin was the first example, introduced in the early 1970s. Ionophores are fermentation products that affect ion transport across cell membranes. This action is quantitatively selective but the drugs are potentially toxic to both target and nontarget species of animal. Moreover there are potentially toxic interactions between some ionophores and certain antibiotics (e.g. tiamulin). The inclusion rates of anticoccidials in feed are crucial, both to ensure efficacy and to

Table 39.2 | Some drugs used for coccidiosis control

TYPE OF COMPOUND	GENERIC NAME	TRADE NAME(S)	NOTES
Ionophorous antibiotics	Monensin	Coban, Elancoban	The first of the ionophores
	Lasalocid	Avatec	
	Salinomycin	Sacox, etc.	
	Narasin	Monteban	
	Maduramicin	Cygro	
	Semduramicin	Aviax	
Pyridones	Clopidol	Coyden	
Quinolones	Decoquinate	Deccox	
Guanidines	Robenidine	Cycostat, Robenz	
Thiamine analogues	Amprolium	Amprol, Amprolmix	Also in various combinations with ethopabate, sulfaquinoxaline and pyrimethamine. In water or feed
Carbanilide	Nicarbazin	Nicarb, Nicrazin (with narasin, Maxiban)	Synergistic with narasin
Sulphonamides	Various	Various	Water-soluble. Mainly used for treatment or strategic dosing in water, for prophylaxis or treatment
	Diclazuril	Clinacox	
	Toltrazuril	Baycox	

prevent toxicity, and the feed mill is an integral part of the process of coccidiosis control. It is also important, especially where nonintegrated systems are prevalent, that the instructions for correct and safe product usage printed on the anticoccidial premix bags are conveyed to farmers.

The efficacy of many anticoccidials has been reduced by drug resistance. The speed at which this occurs, as a result of selection, varies greatly between compounds. It has been very slow to emerge against the ionophores but some degree of resistance has been reported in both Europe and the USA. Moreover, side resistance (to other compounds in the same chemical family) has been described.

In order to combat resistance, drug programmes involving changing compounds during the grow-out of a crop ('shuttle' programmes), or at less frequent time intervals for an entire operation (switching or rotation), have been advocated. There is no scientific evidence to suggest that shuttle programmes delay the emergence of resistance.

Outbreaks of disease are usually treated with water-soluble drugs, such as sulphonamides or toltrazuril. Water medication is convenient and can be rapidly given – an important consideration. Toltrazuril can also be used to support prophylactic measures. In broiler operations, the cost of an outbreak of disease will be substantial, even if therapy is effective, and prophylactic measures should be reviewed.

CONTROL OF COCCIDIOSIS IN OTHER BIRDS

In turkeys in-feed prophylaxis is generally used for the first few weeks of life (Table 39.3). Fewer drugs are registered for turkeys than chickens and some ionophores are toxic to turkeys (particularly older turkeys), even at doses recommended for chickens. Vaccines are being commercially developed, using live, nonattenuated isolates of turkey *Eimeria* spp. analogous to the chicken vaccines.

In other species, control is more dependent on hygiene and treatment with sulphonamides. Care is required in the use of other anticoccidials, which should only be used if they are known to be safe for the target species. In game birds, lasalocid can be used in feed. For pigeons, sulfadimethoxine is specifically available.

Table 39.3 | Main methods of coccidiosis control in different classes of poultry

CLASS	STRATEGY	COMMENTS
Chicken broiler	Chemoprophylaxis	From 1 day old to 3–5 days before slaughter
	Vaccination	See text
Chicken layer/breeder replacements	Immunization by natural infection with partial drug control	Drugs withdrawn before lay
	Vaccination	See text
Turkey meat birds	Chemoprophylaxis	To 6–8 weeks of age
Turkey breeder replacements	Immunization by natural infection with partial drug control	
Others	Chemotherapy	Drug treatment as and when required
	Chemoprophylaxis	Few drugs approved

CRYPTOSPORIDIOSIS

Cryptosporidiosis is caused by apicomplexan protozoa of the genus *Cryptosporidium* which have affinities with *Eimeria* but also a number of notable dissimilarities. In mammals, enteric infections and diarrhoea are characteristic but in birds disease is more usually associated with infection of the respiratory tract.

C. baileyi causes respiratory disease and *C. meleagridis* has been described in association with enteric disease in birds. The avian cryptosporidia do not normally infect mammals and mammalian isolates do not easily infect birds. Within avian hosts, cryptosporidia have been found infecting chickens, turkeys, game birds, geese, ducks, cage birds and others and isolates do not have rigid host specificity.

In their parasitic phase, cryptosporidia parasitize the margin of epithelial cells, appearing in conventional histological sections to be extracellular, although electron microscope studies have revealed them to be enclosed within the host epithelial cell membrane. In this site, phases of asexual multiplication (schizogony) followed by gametogeny occur, with the extracellular release of merozoites and microgametes respectively. Following zygote formation, oocysts are shed already sporulated. The prepatent period is very short (3 days). Oocysts have a tough wall and are environmentally resistant. Experimentally, infection can be achieved readily by intratracheal as well as oral routes and oocysts will excyst on mucous membranes.

Infections can occur in very young chicks. Disease has been reported in chickens, turkeys, ducks, pheasant, quail, peafowl and others at a wide variety of ages from 2–11 weeks or older. It is apparent that chickens can be a source of infection for turkeys. Disease associated with enteric infection appears to be rare. By contrast, respiratory infection may produce a variety of clinical signs depending on the particular sites involved. There may be air sacculitis, pneumonia, sinusitis or conjunctivitis, with coughing, dyspnoea, nasal discharges and mortality. Respiratory cryptosporidiosis may be quite common in some parts of the world. For example in Georgia, USA, it accounts for 1–5% of all diagnostic submissions.

Diagnosis is based on the demonstration of organisms in sections of the relevant mucosal epithelium (Fig. 39.6) and of oocysts in stained smears from the respiratory mucosa. With a modified

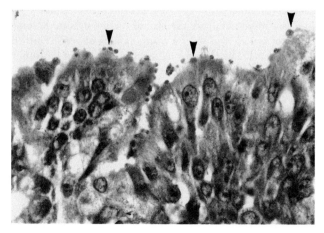

Fig. 39.6 Cryptosporidiosis. Organisms are visible on the mucosal margin. Section of conjunctival mucosa from a pheasant with conjunctivitis. Haematoxylin/eosin, × 1000. (Courtesy of C. J. Randall.)

Ziehl–Neelsen stain, the oocysts stain red, are 4–6 μm in diameter, subspherical and should be sought using a high-power objective. There is no specific therapy. Oocysts are resistant to most chemical agents, except ammonia, 10% formalin or hydrogen peroxide.

HISTOMONIASIS (BLACKHEAD)

Also known as infectious enterohepatitis, histomoniasis is caused by the protozoan *Histomonas meleagridis*, a parasite that has affinities with the amoebae and the flagellates. It infects a variety of gallinaceous birds throughout the world but is primarily a cause of disease in turkey poults, although occasionally disease is reported in game birds, chickens and guinea fowl. In the USA, this disease was formerly much more important than it is now.

BIOLOGY/LIFE CYCLE

The parasite invades the caecal mucosa and then spreads via the blood to the liver. In tissues of the gut and liver the parasite grows and multiplies intercellularly, leading to the formation of necrotic foci surrounded by colonies of organisms. In the gut lumen the parasite is flagellated and pleomorphic, 3–16 μm in diameter, but in tissues it rounds up and loses its flagellum. *Histomonas* is a delicate organism. It does not form cysts and direct faeco–oral transmission can only be achieved experimentally, with difficulty. The most important natural route of transmission is within the egg of the caecal nematode *Heterakis gallinarum*. Parasites are ingested by worms in the caecal lumen. In females, they gain access to the nematode eggs, which are ultimately shed in host faeces and are available to infect further hosts. The earthworm may also intervene in this cycle as a transport host in which *Heterakis* larvae may hatch but remain viable and infected with histomonads in the earthworm tissues. Once infection has established in a flock transmission may occur by direct cloacal invasion by freshly excreted parasites in the litter.

EPIDEMIOLOGY

The role of *H. gallinarum* and the earthworm are crucial in the epidemiology of histomoniasis. As well as providing safe passage through the gizzard for the delicate histomonad, their role ensures the persistence of infection in soil for many months or years. Furthermore, the wide host range of both histomonad and *Heterakis* means that a variety of birds (but notably chickens) may provide a source of infection. It follows that this infection has been especially important in outdoor-reared turkey enterprises. It can also occasionally cause clinical disease in adult chickens, both housed breeding chickens and free range layers.

CLINICAL SIGNS/DIAGNOSIS

In turkeys, signs become apparent 7–12 days after infection and include anorexia, depression and sulphur-yellow droppings. Blackhead is an imprecise colloquialism, since a cyanotic head is neither invariable nor unique to histomoniasis. Mortality may be high, reaching a peak about a week after the onset of signs. Lesions occur in the caeca and then in the liver. The typhlitis may be accompanied by severe ulceration and the exudate, at first serous or haemorrhagic, becomes caseated and may form a core. In the liver, the focal pale lesions that appear from days 10–12 of infection are pathognomonic. Diagnosis can usually be made on the gross post-mortem lesions, which remain conspicuous long after death. If parasitological confirmation is required, stained sections from the periphery of liver lesions will reveal rounded-up organisms, each surrounded by a space. Identification of living organisms in wet preparations from caecal lesions is less easy and requires fresh material and a heated microscope stage.

CONTROL

Now that the particular role of carrier chickens, *Heterakis* and earthworms is known, control based on appropriate management has reduced the incidence of disease. Turkeys should not be reared with chickens or on ground that has carried chickens, even several years before. Prophylactic medication has been used, even in indoor-reared turkeys, for the first few weeks of life. Note that the compounds used for histomoniasis control are different from those for coccidiosis control. Dimetridazole has been used for prophylaxis or treatment in turkeys or game birds but has been withdrawn from use in many countries for food-producing poultry. Drug resistance has not been a problem.

DISEASES DUE TO OTHER FLAGELLATED PROTOZOANS

A variety of flagellated protozoa are common commensals of the avian gut but *Spironucleus* (formerly *Hexamita*) *meleagridis* and *Trichomonas* sp. may occasionally cause disease in turkey poults or young game birds. Spironucleosis is a particular problem in pheasants and partridges.

S. meleagridis can cause a watery diarrhea due to reduced water absorption from the gut. Postmortem, the intestine, especially in its anterior parts, is distended with watery contents, which contain the organisms. *S. meleagridis* is 6–12 μm long and carries six anterior and two posterior flagella. In stained smears two nuclei may be seen. In tissue sections, the organism may be found in large numbers in the lumina of mucosal crypts. The organism is excreted in the form of cysts which facilitate transmission. Furazolidone, tetracyclines and dimetridazole have been used as treatments.

Trichomonas gallinae is an important pathogen of the mouth, crop and oesophagus of pigeon squabs, causing 'oral canker' with yellow necrotic lesions and a sometimes profuse caseous exudate. Sometimes there is systemic spread with involvement of the viscera, including the liver. Rarely, this disease has been reported in turkey poults. Other trichomonads are commensals of the large bowel and may occasionally be associated with disease in game birds or turkey poults. In young game birds, outbreaks have been characterized by foamy yellow droppings and mortality. At post-mortem examination, the caeca are distended with foamy, light-coloured contents. The causal organisms are typified by four anterior flagella and a single recurrent posteriorly directed flagellum, which encloses an undulating membrane. No cysts are formed by trichomonads and transmission is by the direct faeco–oral route via contaminated feeders and waterers. Wet, crowded conditions will favour transmission.

Diagnosis of these flagellate infections is best made by demonstration of the living organisms in wet smears of intestinal contents prepared from freshly dead carcasses and examined with a heated microscope stage. Stained thin smears can also be prepared; dilution of gut contents in serum will reduce distortion on drying and make it easier to see morphological detail.

459

LEUCOCYTOZOONOSIS

Leucocytozoon spp. are arthropod-transmitted protozoa related to *Plasmodium* spp. Disease has been described in ducks and geese caused by *Leucocytozoon simondi*, in turkeys by *Leucocytozoon smithi* and in chickens by *Leucocytozoon caulleryi*. These species appear to be widely distributed in many parts of the world although they are only locally of major importance (e.g. *L. caulleryi* in South East Asia). Leucocytozoonosis has not been reported in poultry in the UK, but a number of fatal outbreaks have occurred in captive psittacine birds exposed to vectors in outdoor aviaries. These have been due to transmission of a *Leucocytozoon* sp. from wild birds.

In the avian host, asexual multiplication occurs in cells of various organs such as liver, lung, heart, brain and spleen and gamonts occur intracellularly in blood cells. Gamonts are ingested by the blood-feeding vectors (*Simulium* spp. in the case of *L. simondi* and *L. smithi*; *Culicoides* spp. for *L. caulleryi*) and undergo further development in them, resulting in sporozoites in the vector salivary glands, which are infective at a subsequent blood meal. Chronic subclinical infections provide a source of infection for the seasonally active vectors leading to epidemic outbreaks in the summer. Clinical signs include inappetence, weakness, anaemia and mortality. Diagnosis is by demonstration of gamonts in stained blood smears. Gross lesions in the musculature may be caused by large tissue schizonts of *L. caulleryi*.

Control depends on limiting exposure to the vectors. Simuliids (blackflies) breed in fast-flowing rivers and feed by day; *Culicoides* midges breed in damp mud and manure and are crepuscular in activity. Screening poultry houses will reduce exposure to bites. The infections are difficult to treat. Most success has been achieved using clopidol or sulphonamide/pyrimethamine combinations as treatments or prophylactics.

SPIROCHAETOSIS (BLOOD SPIROCHAETES)

This disease is caused by the spirochaete *Borrelia anserina* and is transmitted by the soft tick *Argas persicus*. It is thus limited in distribution to areas where the tick is common. The disease is particularly important in North Africa, the Middle East and Asia. It is uncommon in the USA (although the tick is present) and is absent from the UK.

The spirochaete can infect a wide variety of birds but disease mainly occurs in young fowl. Signs include anorexia, fever, depression, cyanosis of the head and anaemia. Affected birds pass bile-stained faeces and may become paralysed before death. On post-mortem examination, the most characteristic sign is an enlarged and mottled spleen. The mottling is due to ecchymotic haemorrhages. The liver may be similarly affected.

The spirochaete may be found in stained blood smears or in wet blood films examined by dark-field illumination. Detection may be aided by examining the interface between the buffy coat and plasma after microhaematocrit centrifugation of heparinized blood. In birds in the late stages of disease, spirochaetes may be difficult to find. Subinoculation into young chicks or embryonating eggs, or serological tests have also been described to assist diagnosis. Penicillin and a number of other antibiotics are very effective therapeutically. Tick control measures are also indicated. Vaccines comprising inactivated organisms have been used effectively, but many serotypes may exist.

HELMINTH PARASITES

A great variety of helminths infect birds. In free-ranging waterfowl, for example, there are many helminth infections with intermediate invertebrate hosts. The host parasite lists of Soulsby

(1982) will be useful in studying parasitism of less-commonly encountered host species. The following account is selective and concentrates on the helminths of chickens and turkeys. In these hosts, helminths are not usually a major cause of disease or economic loss where indoor rearing prevents access to intermediate hosts and because of the relatively short life span of broilers.

NEMATODES OF THE RESPIRATORY TRACT

Syngamus trachea causes the condition of 'gapes' in gallinaceous birds; the related *Cyathostoma bronchialis* causes a similar condition in geese.

Syngamus parasitizes the trachea of a variety of wild as well as domestic birds. Disease is due to physical blockage of the airway, leading to dyspnoea, typified by an outstretched neck with open mouth (Fig. 39.7) but may also manifest as lack of condition and mortality. The life cycle may be direct or, more usually, indirect, involving the earthworm. As a result, soil can remain infected for years. The disease is now most usually seen in birds reared in outdoor pens, such as game birds and ornamental or zoo birds. *Syngamus* eggs must be distinguished from those of *Capillaria* spp. (Fig. 39.8).

INTESTINAL NEMATODES

There are three main genera of significance: *Capillaria* spp., *Heterakis* and *Ascaridia*, which can readily be distinguished by gross differences in size (Fig. 39.9).

Capillaria spp., while the smallest of these nematodes, can be highly pathogenic when present in large numbers. Different species parasitize different parts of the alimentary tract and may have direct or indirect life cycles (Table 39.4). Probably the most common and pathogenic in modern units is *Capillaria obsignata*, which has a direct cycle and can be a problem in birds on litter. Post-mortem, worms are found by careful examination of mucosal washings under a dissecting microscope. The adult male worms have a single spicule enclosed by a spicule sheath, and the eggs are distinctive (Fig. 39.8).

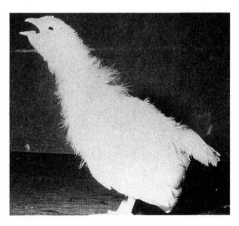

Fig. 39.7 A chick with 'gapes' caused by *Syngamus trachea*.

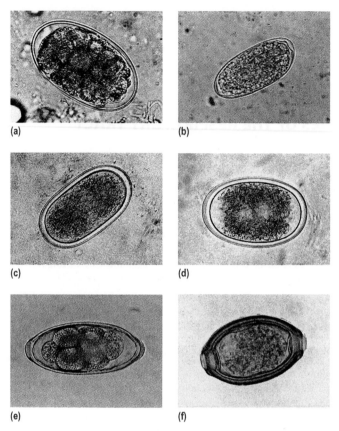

Fig. 39.8 Some helminth eggs of poultry. (a) *Amidostomum anseris*. (b) *Trichostrongylus tenuis*. (c) *Heterakis* sp. (d) *Ascaridia* sp. (e) *Syngamus trachea*. (f) *Capillaria* sp. × 640. (Courtesy of Janssen Pharmaceutical.)

Heterakis gallinarum is commonplace in the caecum of chickens, turkeys and many other species. It is probably never pathogenic but is important because of its role in the transmission of histomoniasis. However, the related *Heterakis isolonche* invades the caecal mucosa of pheasants and can cause a severe or fatal nodular typhlitis. *Heterakis* spp. have a direct life cycle.

Ascaridia are the largest nematodes of birds. The adults live in the lumen of the small intestine but the larval stages invade the mucosa. *Ascaridia galli* may cause ill-thrift, enteritis or intestinal impaction, the degree of effect being related to the number of worms present. The life cycle is direct, so debilitating infestations can occasionally occur in birds on litter, especially if the litter is reused in the case of broilers.

In the caecum, apart from *Heterakis* spp., infestations with the much smaller *Trichostrongylus tenuis* may occur in a variety of domestic and wild birds. *T. tenuis* is especially important as a pathogen of grouse in the UK and has also been reported as causing disease in goslings.

The most important nematode in geese is *Amidostomum anseris*, which can cause severe disease in goslings, with anorexia, emaciation, anaemia and death. The nematode parasitizes the gizzard, where it causes erosions. It has a direct life cycle.

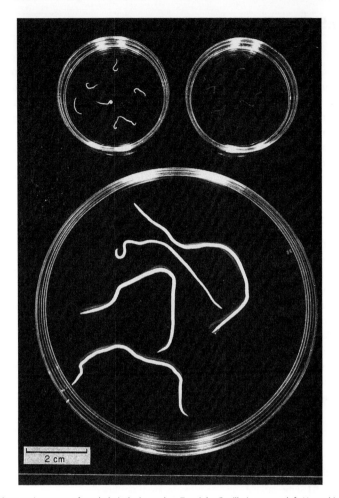

Fig. 39.9 The three main genera of gut helminths in poultry. Top right *Capillaria* sp.; top left *Heterakis* sp.; bottom *Ascaridia* sp.

Table 39.4 | *Capillaria* species of poultry

SPECIES	PREDILECTION SITE	INTERMEDIATE HOST	COMMENTS
Capillaria annulata	Oesophagus, crop	Earthworms	Turkeys, game birds
Capillaria contorta	Oesophagus, crop	None or earthworms	Turkeys, game birds
Capillaria bursata	Small intestine	Earthworm	Chickens and others
Capillaria caudinflata	Small intestine	Earthworm	Various hosts
Capillaria obsignata	Small intestine	None	Various hosts
Capillaria anatis	Caecum	?	Mainly ducks

CESTODES AND TREMATODES

A large number of cestodes and trematodes have been described in birds. Most are of low pathogenicity. All require intermediate hosts and are of negligible importance in modern poultry operations. Trematodes utilize molluscan intermediate hosts and are especially prevalent in free-ranging waterfowl. Cestodes utilize arthropod and other invertebrate intermediate hosts. Some of the more significant (relatively speaking) species are listed in Table 39.5. They parasitize the digestive or reproductive (*Prosthogonimus*) tracts. Their principal definitive hosts are shown but other hosts are also parasitized. Probably the commonest to occur in modern poultry operations is *Raillietina cesticillus*.

CONTROL OF HELMINTHIASES

Management practices largely determine the extent and types of helminthiases. Modern intensive poultry systems preclude infestations from older birds, wild bird reservoirs or most intermediate hosts, and pathogenic populations of helminths cannot usually build up in broiler chickens with a short life span. However, for species that produce highly resistant eggs (e.g. *Ascaridia*), the reuse of litter, or inadequate cleaning between crops, may allow a sequential build-up of potentially harmful parasite numbers.

These remarks do not apply to free-range rearing, as is used for game birds and show collections and is widely employed for some types of poultry in many parts of the world. There are relatively few anthelmintics licensed for use in birds. Flubendazole can be given in feed to chickens, geese, turkeys and game birds to control intestinal nematodes and *Syngamus trachea*. For cestodes and trematodes, control measures are best directed against the intermediate hosts.

Table 39.5 | Some tapeworms and trematodes of poultry

TAPEWORMS	PRINCIPAL DEFINITIVE HOST	INTERMEDIATE HOSTS	LENGTH OF MATURE WORM (MM)
Amoebotaenia cuneata	Chicken	Earthworms	3
Choanotaenia infundibulum	Chicken	Housefly, beetles	50–200
Davainea proglottina	Chicken	Slugs, snails	4
Echinostoma revolutum	Duck, chicken, turkey	Various species of water snail	10–22
Hymenolepis cantaniana	Chicken	Beetles	20
Hymenolepis carioca	Chicken	Stable fly, dung beetles	40
Prosthogonimus macrorchis	Chicken, duck	Water snail and then dragonfly	5–7
Raillietina cesticillus	Chicken	Beetles	50–150
Raillietina tetragona	Chicken	Ants	100–250
Raillietina echinobothrida	Chicken	Ants	200–340

ECTOPARASITES

LICE

Several species of biting (chewing) lice (order Mallophaga) may infect poultry. They spend their entire life cycle on the host and cause irritation by feeding on skin and feather. *Menocanthus stramineus* is probably the commonest in chickens and it may also infect turkeys. It is found on the skin, especially around the cloaca and on the breast and thighs, laying eggs on the base of the feathers. Lice infestations tend to increase in autumn and winter.

Other species in chickens include *Lipeurus caponis* in the wing and tail feathers, *Cuclotogaster heterographus* on feathers of the head and *Goniocotes gallinae* on down feathers. In turkeys, in addition to the foregoing, the large turkey louse, *Chelopistes meleagridis*, may be found.

MITES

Two species of nonburrowing mite can be serious pests because of their blood-sucking habits: *Dermanyssus gallinae* (the red mite) and *Liponyssus* (*Ornithonyssus*) *sylviarum* (the northern fowl mite). Heavy infestations, especially of *Dermanyssus*, can cause reduced egg production and anaemia. *Dermanyssus* can also transmit *Borrelia anserina*.

D. gallinae is widely distributed throughout the world and infests chickens and other birds. It feeds mainly at night, retiring by day to cracks and crevices in cages and buildings where the eggs are laid. As a result, inspection of birds during the day may not reveal infestation. The red mite is serious economically, particularly in adult breeding and laying chickens. *Liponyssus* may be common in caged layers and also infests turkeys and other birds. It never leaves the host and in heavy infestations causes blackening of feathers due to excreta and dark egg masses. Differentiation of these two mites is important because their differing habits require different approaches to control. *Dermanyssus* has a D-shaped ventral anal plate (Fig. 39.10) compared with the oval plate of *Liponyssus* and the mouthparts are also different.

Burrowing mites of the genus *Cnemidocoptes* may cause feather loss (depluming itch mite, *Cnemidocoptes gallinae*) or excessive scaliness of the skin, leading to thickening and even deformity

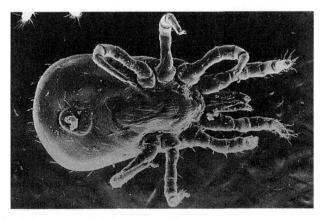

Fig. 39.10 Scanning electron micrograph of *Dermanyssus gallinae*.

of the legs (scaly leg mite, *Cnemidocoptes mutans*). Diagnosis is confirmed by examining skin scrapings cleared in 10% potassium or sodium hydroxide.

Other mites that may cause problems include some invasive species that may be found in air sacs (*Cytodites nudis*) or subcutaneously (*Laminiosioptes cysticola*).

FLEAS

Several species of flea have been reported from poultry worldwide. Fleas breed off the host and can remain infesting the environment for many months. The sticktight flea (*Echidnophaga gallinacea*) is unusual in that it remains attached to the host for days or weeks. It parasitizes a variety of birds and the irritation and blood loss can be severe. The adult fleas are vulnerable to treatment but reinfestation can occur from the environment where, as is normal for fleas, the eggs and larvae develop.

TICKS

The most important tick is the soft tick *Argas persicus*, which is widely distributed in tropical and subtropical areas. The instars blood feed for short periods at night, spending most of their time off the host, hidden in cracks and crevices. Apart from causing anaemia, anorexia, weight loss and depressed egg output, *Argas* transmits *Borrelia*.

CONTROL OF ECTOPARASITES

Good hygiene and the use of specific chemicals form the basis of control. Consideration of the parasite habits will indicate whether chemicals are best applied to the birds, to the environment or to both. For lice, *Liponyssus* and burrowing mites, treatment of the birds is appropriate. For scaly leg mite, dipping the legs alone in acaricide may be sufficient. For *Dermanyssus*, fleas and *Argas* ticks it is necessary to apply chemicals to buildings as well as birds.

A variety of chemicals have been used, including pyrethroids, organophosphorus compounds (malathion, coumaphos) and the carbamate carbaryl. Malathion is very safe in poultry and may be applied to housing with birds still present. Some products are not readily available or are banned. This may create difficulties in treating egg-laying hens and in red mite control. It is important to use only compounds that are approved for poultry and to use them in the approved manner. Some other acaricides/insecticides, which are used in mammals, may be dangerous to use in poultry, either because they are toxic or because they may lead to unacceptable residues in meat or eggs.

Different formulations are provided for specific purposes. Sprays are convenient for treating birds or buildings. Dusts are convenient for treating litter or providing dust baths.

REFERENCES

Long P L, Millard B J 1979 Studies on *Eimeria dispersa* Tyzzer 1929 in turkeys. Parasitol 78: 41–51

Long P L, Rowell I G 1975 Sampling broiler house litter for coccidial oocysts. Br Poult Sci 16: 583–592

Moore E N, Brown J A 1951 A new coccidium pathogenic for turkeys, *Eimeria adenoeides* n.sp. (Protozoa: Eimeriidae). Cornell Vet 41: 125–136

Shirley M W, Smith A L, Tomley F M 2005 The biology of avian *Eimeria* with an emphasis on their control by vaccination. Adv Parasitol 60: 285–330

Soulsby E J L 1982 Helminths, arthropods and protozoa of domesticated animals, 7th edn. Baillière Tindall, London

Williams R B 1999 A compartmentalised model for the estimation of the cost of coccidiosis to the world's chicken production industry. Int J Parasitol 29: 1209–1229

FURTHER READING

Long P L 1981 The biology of the coccidia. University Park Press, Baltimore

McDougald L R 2003 Coccidiosis. In: Saif Y M (ed) Diseases of poultry, 11th edn. Iowa State University Press, Ames, p 974–991

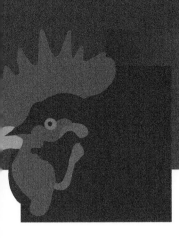

SECTION

6

Mark Pattison

DISEASES OF BODY SYSTEMS

Chapter **40**   Diseases of the musculoskeletal
                  system   **470**

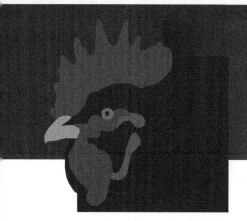

CHAPTER 40

Barry H. Thorp

Diseases of the musculoskeletal system

Musculoskeletal diseases in poultry are typically identified by the presence of lameness and are often called 'leg weakness'. Lameness is a consequence of biomechanical or neural dysfunction or pain and is usually a welfare concern. In most cases severely lame commercial poultry should be culled. Musculoskeletal disorders are often multifactorial and result from nutritional, husbandry, infectious or genetic factors. Production characteristics of modern poultry lines (e.g. growth rate in broiler chickens, egg production in laying hens) place great demands on the musculoskeletal system, and inadequacies in nutrition or husbandry will often result in musculoskeletal diseases.

For the last 30 years concerns have been expressed about leg weakness in broilers, although the incidence has probably improved over the same time frame. Within northern Europe changes in the incidence of lameness disorders in broilers reflect changes in genetic selection, disease challenge, husbandry practices and the use of antibiotic growth promoters.

In the 1980s bone deformities and tibial dyschondroplasia were considered the main cause of lameness in broiler chickens. The incidence of these diminished as genetic selection strategies against these disorders improved. The emergence of virulent Gumboro disease in the early 1990s caused immunosuppression and a high incidence of bacterial infections in bones and joints. This was brought under control by an effective vaccine strategy. Then in the mid 1990s the removal of meat and bone from poultry diets contributed to calcium and phosphorus requirements not being met and rachitic type disorders, particularly in growing turkeys and broilers. In the late 1990s the removal of antibiotic growth promoters then increased the incidence of mild enteritis and associated malabsorption of calcium and phosphorus, leading to bone growth disorders. In addition a 'new' bone disease emerged in broilers, resulting from infection of the air sac of the free thoracic vertebrae with *Enterococcus caecorum*, leading to spinal cord damage and paralysis.

Husbandry systems also influence bone disorders; for example, in layers the change in recent years from caged systems to barn and free-range systems has changed the incidence and pattern of bone fractures.

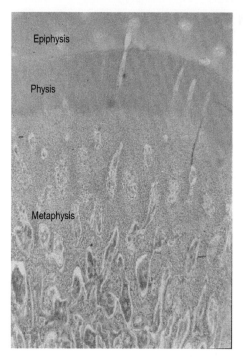

Epiphysis

Physis

Metaphysis

Fig. 40.1 Histological section of the growth plate from a 21-day-old broiler chicken. The cartilaginous epiphysis contains no secondary ossification centre but the epiphyseal vascular canals can be seen. These penetrate the underlying physeal cartilage but do not extend through to the metaphysis. The metaphyseal cartilage is composed of mineralized cartilage and hypertrophic chondrocytes. The metaphysis is penetrated by metaphyseal vessels, which contain osteoclasts that remove the cartilage and osteoblasts, then lay down bone. Haematoxylin/eosin, ×25.

Knowledge of normal bone morphology and how it changes during growth is required before abnormalities can be fully understood. The terminology applied to skeletal tissues and their pathology is detailed in Appendix 1. A long bone consist of a shaft or diaphysis with, at each end, a metaphysis, growth plate (physis) and epiphysis that is covered in a layer of articular cartilage. Only some avian epiphyses contain a secondary ossification centre: many of them remain purely cartilage until the end of growth. For example the proximal and distal tibiotarsus contain secondary ossification centres from approximately 3 weeks of age, whereas there are no secondary ossification centres in the proximal or distal femur. Long bones grow by endochondral ossification: within the growth plate chondrocytes proliferate and then hypertrophy (Fig. 40.1). The cartilage matrix of the hypertrophic chondrocytes is then mineralized, removed and replaced by bone. The width of a long bone increases by appositional bone growth. There is marked variation in the histology of skeletal tissues in poultry, dependent on breed (strain), age, sex and nutrition. The normal growth plate of the proximal tibiotarsus is about 0.5–2 mm thick, reflecting the rate of growth. The diaphysis should be composed of cortex containing haversian systems of lamellar bone. In the young broiler the cortex is rapidly forming (modelling) and then remodelling. It often therefore appears poorly organized compared to the cortical bone of slow-growing layer-type poultry or adults.

POST-MORTEM EXAMINATION

Before post-mortem examination there should be an assessment of the flock. This entails gathering a full history, identifying and examining live, lame birds and forming an opinion as to general flock health, litter quality and management. Investigations must extend to all factors present during the initial development of the pathology. This approach requires an estimate of the likely time-course of bone diseases but ensures a comprehensive and correctly focused investigation. Gross pathology may be inadequate for an accurate diagnosis, and histopathology is usually necessary. In some instances further specialist skills, such as the preparation and examination of undecalcified tissue sections to investigate calcium deposition in cases of rickets, may be required. Investigations may include microbiology, bone ashing and analysis of feed samples. Serum samples may be collected for viral and mycoplasma serology.

An assessment of the likely cause of the lameness of the live birds enables the post mortem to be more focused. Table 40.1 indicates the clinical and pathological features of some common lameness disorders. During the post-mortem examination the general health status of the bird should be assessed but particular attention should be given to the legs and spine. The birds should be killed without introducing further musculoskeletal abnormalities and ideally by gently restraining the bird and injecting an overdose of a barbiturate. Holding a bird by the legs for cervical dislocation will result in musculoskeletal damage that may complicate further examination.

For a comprehensive musculoskeletal investigation in broilers the following protocol should be considered:

1. **Initial dissection**: The legs should be skinned and the spine transversely sectioned anterior and posterior to the hip joints.
2. **Spinal pathology**: Where leg weakness is attributed to possible spinal pathology the thoracic spine should be dissected. Examination of the ventral surface of the thoracic spine will probably show abscessation associated with the air sac of the free thoracic vertebrae. The thoracic section of the spinal cord can then be sectioned in the midline for further examination (Fig. 40.2). Where osteomyelitis is detected a swab should be taken for bacteriology. Deformation and displacements of the vertebrae may also cause spinal cord damage. For a definitive diagnosis it may also be required to take samples of thoracic vertebrae and spinal cord for histological assessment.
3. **Identify bone deformities**: The symmetry of the right and left legs should be examined and torsional or angular leg deformities noted.
4. **Identify gross tendon or muscle lesions**: The gastrocnemius tendon is exposed and rupture or tenosynovitis is easily identified by thickening of the tendon, plus local bruising if the lesion is recent. Also, gross pathology of any of the main leg muscles should be readily apparent.
5. **Examination of stifle and hock joints**: The legs can now be dissected, muscles should be removed, joints opened aseptically and tendons and ligaments examined. Where excessive or turbid synovial fluid indicates the probability of infection, suspect joints can be directly swabbed and cultured for bacteria.
6. **Examination of hip joints**: In broilers there can be disintegration of the femoral head due to bacterial infection (femoral head necrosis) (Figs 40.3 and 40.4) but separation of the cartilaginous epiphysis from the underlying bone is a common post-mortem artefact. Artefact is minimized by careful sectioning of the muscles round the hip joint prior to disarticulating the joint. Where infection is obvious, swabs can be used to sample for bacteria. Histopathology of the affected tissue can assist with the diagnosis (Fig. 40.5). To isolate

Table 40.1 Diagnostic guide to some common lameness disorders

CLINICAL SIGNS	GROSS AND HISTOPATHOLOGY	LIKELY CAUSE	AETIOLOGICAL FACTORS	DIAGNOSTIC METHODS
Sitting back on hocks and cannot rise; on examination there is no obvious lesion in the legs and no pain response in the legs	1. Deformity of thoracic spine – causing spinal cord compression	Spondylolisthesis (kinky back)	Genetic	Histopathology of thoracic vertebrae and spinal cord
	2. Bacterial or fungal infection of thoracic spine (osteomyelitis)	Scoliosis Infectious spondylopathy	Environmental contamination	Bacteriology of spinal abscess Histopathology of thoracic vertebrae and spinal cord Mycology
As above in breeders/layers	Demyelination of sciatic nerve	Riboflavin deficiency Marek's disease	Dietary	Histology of nerve Analysis of diet Gross pathology Diet analysis
	Collapse of thoracic spine because of osteopenia	Severe osteomalacia/porosis (cage layer fatigue)	Incorrect calcium/phosphorus in rear, prelay or lay	
Birds appear to be uncomfortable walking, with bilateral lameness. The bones of the hock joint may appear thickened, and a lot of mild bone deformities may be present. Bones and beak are more malleable than normal	Thickening of all long bone growth plates due to an accumulation of nonmineralized cartilage. Accumulation of proliferating and/or hypertrophic chondrocytes	Rickets	Hypophosphataemic Hypocalcaemic Vitamin D malabsorption Genetic	Histopathology of growth plates and metaphyseal bone Undecalcified histology Bone ash and mineral Diet analysis
Bone deformity – bowing of the proximal tibiotarsus, with thickened tibiotarsal growth plates	Thickening of growth plates in proximal tibiotarsus and/or proximal tarsometatarsus due to an accumulation of nonmineralized cartilage composed of transitional chondrocytes	Dyschondroplasia	Marginal hypocalcaemia Genetic	Histopathology of proximal tibiotarsi, tarsometatarsals Undecalcified histology Bone ash and mineral Diet analysis
Bone deformity in the absence of growth plate thickening, sometimes tibiotarsus or tarsometatarsus with displacement of the gastrocnemius tendon	Valgus (lateral), varus (medial) and/or torsional deformity of a long bone, frequently tibiotarsus or tarsometatarsus in the absence of growth plate abnormality	Previous period of rickets or dyschondroplasia Long bone deformity	Genetic Exercise Diet Growth rate Unknown	Estimates of bone torsions and angulations Bone ash and mineral Diet analysis
Long bone deformity with shortening and no thickening of growth plates	Tibiotarsus and tarsometatarsus shortened with no defect in growth plate mineralization or appositional bone growth	Chondrodystrophy – but not very common	Deficiencies, including: manganese, choline, niacin, vitamin E, biotin, folic acid, pyridoxine	Histopathology of growth plates and metaphyseal bone Undecalcified histology Bone ash and mineral

Table 40.1 (Continued)

CLINICAL SIGNS	GROSS AND HISTOPATHOLOGY	LIKELY CAUSE	AETIOLOGICAL FACTORS	DIAGNOSTIC METHODS
			Mycoplasma Genetic Mycotoxins	Analysis of diet for mineral and mycotoxins
Severely lame, difficulty in rising, wings used for support, possible pain on palpation of medial aspect of femur	Disintegration of proximal femur – must be confirmed histologically as can be confused with post-mortem artefact	Bacterial infection of proximal femur and/or tibiotarsus, so-called femoral head necrosis	Immunosuppression through agents such as IBD (including vaccine strains) Bacterial challenge Staphylococci Reovirus *Mycoplasma* Bacterial infection secondary to immunosuppression through stress or other disease	Histopathology – Gram stain Bacteriology
Severely lame – hot, swollen joints and/or tendons	Synovitis/tenosynovitis with marked local inflammation and where there is joint involvement mucopurulent synovial fluid	Infectious synovitis/ tenosynovitis		Histology Bacteriology Virology Mycoplasmology Serology Feeding and water management
Hopping lame; on physical examination there is palpable thickening of the gastrocnemius tendon above the hock joint	Tendon rupture	Synovitis/tenosynovitis in the absence of infection	Insufficient exercise in rear for proper tendon development to meet the demands of production	Histology Bacteriology Virology Mycoplasmology Serology Feeding, water and lighting management
Bone fractures	Inadequate structural bone	Osteodystrophies Dyschondroplasia Osteomyelitis Bone marrow lymphoma Vitamin C deficiency	Trauma Nutritional	Histopathology of diaphysis Undecalcified histology Bone ash and mineral Bone strength Analysis of diet
Nonspecific lameness	Muscle necrosis/degeneration	Poorly defined	Genetic Conformation Ionophores	Histopathology Plasma creatine kinase Feed analysis

IBD, infectious bursal disease.

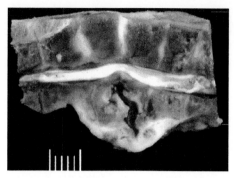

Fig. 40.2 Thoracolumbar spine from a 35-day-old broiler chicken. There is a spinal osteomyelitis (spinal abscess) of the free thoracic vertebrae. (Courtesy of Dr John Barnes.)

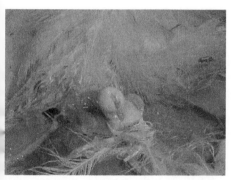

Fig. 40.3 The proximal femur from a 35-day-old broiler chicken. The articular cartilage is a shiny white colour and no abnormalities can be seen.

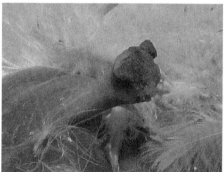

Fig. 40.4 The proximal femur from a 35-day-old broiler chicken. There is a complete disintegration of the proximal femur and much of the cartilaginous tissue is retained within the hip. This can be femoral head necrosis or in some instances a post-mortem artefact. Histopathology or bacteriology can be used to confirm the diagnosis.

bacteria from samples of bone is more difficult. A method that works is to dissect the bone extremity, flame it to kill any surface contamination introduced during dissection and place it in a small plastic bag containing 0.01 M phosphate buffered saline and crush it. Pliers work well. The crushed suspension is then swabbed, inoculated on to blood agar and cultured in aerobic conditions at 37°C.

7. **Bone deformities**: The most commonly deformed bone is the tibiotarsus. This can be dissected free of muscle and assessed. Tibial torsion around the long axis should be between 0° and 15° external and there should be little or no valgus (lateral) deformity (Figs 40.6 and 40.7). Varus (medial) deformity is abnormal. Tibial bowing is the most common deformity and this can be assessed by measuring the tibial plateau angle, which should be about 20°.

8. **Rickets and tibial dyschondroplasia**: These are assessed by looking at the thickness of the tibiotarsal growth plate. If this is thickened, then other growth plates should also be examined. Rickets affects all growth plates evenly whereas dyschondroplasia is usually localized to the proximal tibiotarsus (Fig. 40.8), although in some cases small focal lesions may be seen in

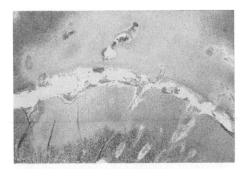

Fig. 40.5 A histological section from the proximal femur of a 35-day-old broiler chicken. There is extensive necrosis, seen as an area of pale staining. Blood vessels are occluded by thrombi and strongly basophilic bacterial colonies. This is typical of femoral head necrosis. Haematoxylin/eosin, ×25.

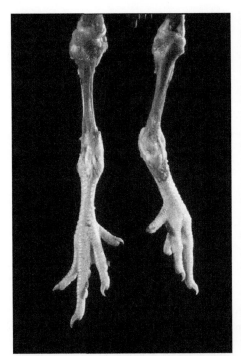

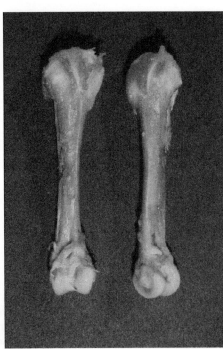

Fig. 40.6 Dissected right and left hind limbs from a 42-day-old broiler. There is lateral twisting and/or valgus of the left leg and the right leg appears normal. Further assessment is easier once the bones are individually dissected (see Fig. 40.7).

Fig. 40.7 The tibiotarsi from Fig. 40.6 further dissected. The lateral torsion of the left tibiotarsus is now obvious by comparing the locations of the proximal and distal articular surfaces. There is no valgus or varus deformity of either bone.

the proximal tarsometatarsus. It must be remembered that the growth plate responds very rapidly to changes in available calcium or phosphorus. A rachitic growth plate can, within 24–48 h, assume a 'normal' appearance if the dietary calcium or phosphorus imbalance is corrected. Where rickets has been prolonged there will be an increased flexibility of all the bones of the skeleton.

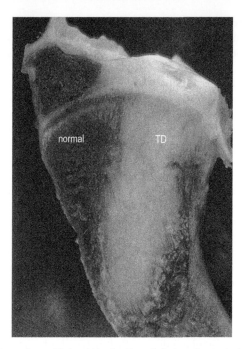

Fig. 40.8 The proximal tibiotarsus from a 35-day-old broiler. Normal physis and metaphysis are present on the left of the growth plate. An extensive plug of nonmineralized cartilage (TD) extends from the physis to occupy the right side of the metaphysis. As the growth plate of the proximal tibiotarsus of a broiler grows about 1 mm per day and the cartilage plug extends over 15 mm this lesion must have been initiated more than 15 days previously. A normal finding is the presence of a secondary ossification centre present in the cartilaginous epiphysis.

9. **Bone mineral content**: The assessment of cortical bone ash values for calcium and phosphorus will give a more accurate 'history' of the calcium and phosphorus status of the skeleton. Ashing of similar but 'normal' bones by the same laboratory may be required to establish baseline values. In growing bones with rickets it can be convenient and practical to send the proximal tibiotarsus for histopathology and a section of the shaft for ashing. For a reliable analysis of the ashing data a minimum sample size of bones from at least 10 birds should be used. See Appendix 2 for details of a methodology for bone ashing and estimation of calcium and phosphorus content.

The methods and thoroughness of investigation of individual birds will be modified depending on the number of birds available for post-mortem and the nature of the musculoskeletal diseases encountered. The methods of investigation will be influenced by the history and by the clinical examination of a flock. Table 40.1 gives indications as to likely diagnoses.

INFECTIOUS SKELETAL DISORDERS OF MEAT-TYPE FOWL

Femoral head necrosis

Femoral head necrosis is one of the most common causes of severe lameness in broilers. The pathology is a bacterial osteomyelitis. It is more common in older broilers and is typically seen from 22 days of age. Birds are characterized by a severe lameness that may be unilateral; frequently the wing tip will be used for support during rising and sitting. Also, on gross examination there are no obvious limb pathologies, although the birds may vocalize on manipulation of the hip joint. Lesions are most common in the proximal femur but are also seen in the proximal tibiotarsus.

The initial site of the bacterial infection is at the tips of the blood vessels of the growth plate. These vessels are end-arterial systems with a very sluggish blood flow. The incomplete basement membrane causes the blood, and any bacteria present, to be in direct contact with the cartilage of the growth plate. The consequence of a bacterial focus in these vessels is the formation of thrombi that occlude the vessel – thereby preventing the invasion of white cells to 'remove' the infectious foci. The bacteria flourish and the toxins they produce diffuse into the surrounding cartilage, killing the cells and resulting in disintegration of the tissue.

In the same way as the bacteria have created a site safe from the body's normal defence systems, they are also protected from any antibiotic medication. The initial infection is dependent on a bacteraemia and is influenced by the status of the target tissue. Also, some strains of staphylococci have a predilection for establishing this sort of infection, probably because of an ability to adhere to the cartilage. The route for bacteria getting into the blood-stream is probably via the respiratory tract, although alternatives include the skin route, the intestine following coccidial challenge, or the footpads. In some instances bacterially contaminated vaccines are responsible. In these cases there may be an abscess at the site of injection. The longer bacteria survive in the circulation the greater is their opportunity to localize to the growth plate. Immunosuppression may prolong bacteraemia. This may be through infection with immunosuppressive viruses such as Gumboro disease. Rickets can also be associated with an increased incidence of femoral head necrosis.

Specific typed strains of staphylococcus are frequently found in cases of bacterial infections in the bones of broilers. Floor eggs have been shown as common carriers of staphylococci, and the use of floor eggs for hatching should be minimal. There is the potential for surface carriage of staphylococci on eggshells. In some hatcheries the dust and fluff samples from hatchers frequently have significant staphylococcal counts of types found in bacterial infections in the bones of broilers. A high standard of egg grading and hatchery hygiene can reduce the risk. Precautions include setting floor eggs separately or on the lower trays. Formaldehyde fumigation within the hatchers is also likely to help. In addition, the examination of hatchery fluff samples can be used to monitor for contamination with staphylococci.

Spinal osteomyelitis

The abdominal air sac associated with the free thoracic vertebrae is also the site of initiation of a focal osteomyelitis. This leads to collapse of the spinal cord and paralysis due to spinal cord compression (Fig. 40.2). Bacteria isolated are usually *Staphylococcus* sp. or *Enterococcus caecorum*. This condition is seen clinically in broilers after about 35 days of age, although the local infection probably starts prior to that. There is the possibility that these bacteria may localize in the air sacs at hatching or soon after. Control is then through egg and hatchery hygiene, with effective fumigation of hatchers with formaldehyde. On farms with a persistent problem of a high incidence some degree of control may be achieved by using antibiotics at about 25–30 days of age.

Hock joints and gastrocnemius tendons of broiler breeders

Commonly, most lame breeders show damage of the gastrocnemius tendon and/or inflammation and swelling of the hock joint. This area is easily examined in the live bird. Staphylococci are commonly isolated from these tissues, although sterile gastrocnemius tendon rupture can also be common. Typically, outbreaks of this type of lameness in breeders are associated with:

- Management practices that cause chronic stress leading to immunosuppression, and/or joint and tendon trauma
- Diseases that chronically debilitate the flock, an example being coccidiosis
- Inadequate skeletal growth in the first 6 weeks leading to poor conformation and incorrect load on the tendons and joints.

Problems are most common during maximum feed restriction in rear (11–14 weeks), when the birds are coming into production (22–25 weeks of age) and at peak production. Probably the most common stressor is inadequacies in feed administration. Problems include poor feed distribution and inadequate feed space per bird, resulting in competition-induced stress in the birds. This may be caused by prolonged feed distribution times (more than 3 min with frequent interruptions in feed availability), feed tracks having to run more than twice during feeding, or inadequate feed space (minimum 15 cm) for every bird, with poor and uneven feed distribution. Frequently there are too few audits to ensure that the feeding system is running to specification, for example having three feed tracks but only two that are working properly. In addition, there may be a combination of the above problems.

Immunosuppressive stress can also be induced when there are problems with the water supply to the stock. Other stressors during rear can also contribute to an increased incidence of bacterial infections in bones and joints, for example a heavy coccidiosis challenge. In addition, where the rearing environment does not provide sufficient physical activity for the birds, the tendons will be structurally underdeveloped and prone to tendonitis and tendon rupture when the birds are exposed to the physical demands of the laying house. This situation may develop where there is insufficient lighting during rearing and/or an absence of perches or slats.

In the majority of outbreaks of tendinitis in flocks the evidence for a consistent and clearly defined viral involvement is poor. Tendon pathology will occur in the presence and absence of both live and killed reovirus vaccinations.

Reovirus

The role of reovirus in leg disorders is often difficult to assess. The finding of reoviruses and positive serology may be an incidental finding unrelated to the pathology. On other occasions, reoviruses may localize in already damaged tissues but may not have been part of the initial pathology. In some parts of the world, reoviruses are considered a major cause of tenosynovitis and rigorous vaccination programmes use live and killed reoviruses. In some cases multivalent vaccines are used. Despite the prevalence of vaccines there are few examples of fully documented cases of reovirus as the cause of lameness disorders and few where the reovirus has adequately fulfilled Koch's postulates. In my experience, injection with some live reovirus vaccines in the first few days of life may be associated with subsequent tendon problems. Ideally, chicks should have maternally derived antibodies against reoviruses. This is achieved by monitoring the antibody status of parent stock and, when required, using killed vaccines in patent stock.

Mycoplasma

Mycoplasma synoviae obviously has a role to play in infectious bone disorders and can be monitored serologically. Although there is variation in the pathogenicity of different strains, mycoplasma does not survive well in the environment. The key to mycoplasma control is buying negative stock. Then there is a requirement to ensure good biosecurity, the provision of a high standard of clean-out, no multiage sites and effective control of the movement of stock, people and equipment. If *Mycoplasma* is endemic through a vertically integrated organization with less than ideal biosecurity, vaccination may be a sensible control option.

Control of common infectious bone and tendon disorders

In all cases of bacterial bone and joint infections the response to antibiotic treatment is poor to variable. These infections, once established in skeletal tissues, cannot be cured using the methods of medication available on a poultry farm. Individual lame birds should be culled: they are a source of infection and will not improve. The possible use of antibiotics is to control the bacteraemia contributing to new cases and to modify the bacterial flora within the flock. Where individual birds are of high value the use of injections of long-acting antibiotics may result in improvement in some of the less severe cases.

Control within a commercial company should include reducing the sources of infection and minimizing the susceptibility of the stock. Minimizing potential sources of infection requires:
- A high standard of hygiene throughout the egg production and handling chain
- Not using floor eggs or other bacteria-contaminated eggs, with good egg-handling practices
- Ensuring that water and feed are not contaminated.

Feeding and other management practices should be designed to minimize stress caused to the chicken. In some parts of the world, skip-a-day feeding has been shown to be of value in preventing leg disorders during rear. For rearing birds, management practices should encourage physical activity to strengthen tendons and bones, and during production the equipment in laying houses should be designed and laid out to minimize the potential for physical damage and stress to bones, joints, tendons and feet. There is a requirement to monitor for and prevent clinical and subclinical rickets to ensure good-quality skeletal growth. It is also necessary to minimize exposure to immunosuppressive viruses such as infectious bursal disease.

NONINFECTIOUS SKELETAL DISORDERS OF MEAT-TYPE FOWL

Spondylopathies

Vertebral deformities and/or displacements (spondylopathies) are seen most frequently in the thoracic vertebrae and may be seen clinically as a paralysis due to spinal cord compression. There are five thoracic vertebrae in the fowl; the third is fused to the notarium and the fifth is fused to the lumbosacral vertebra. This leaves the fourth as the free thoracic vertebra. It is at this site that deformity and displacement most frequently occurs, with spinal cord compression. At post-mortem examination visually assessing the vertebrae for deformity can be difficult but lesions can be confirmed by a histopathological assessment of the spinal cord. Spinal osteomyelitis has been described in the previous section.

Rotational (torsional) and angular (valgus/varus) deformity

Long bones are not perfectly straight. They all exhibit some degree of lateral, medial, anterior or posterior bend. They also show some torsion (rotation) about their long axis. The normal bend and twist in long bones reflects the organization of the collagen fibres within the bone and enables them to bend or twist under load rather than fracture. The quantity of 'normal' torsions and angulations is partly defined by the loads applied and by the mechanical properties of the growing bone. If either of these is abnormal then bone deformity is likely to result. This is most common in the tibiotarsus as valgus deformity and excessive external rotation (Figs 40.6 and 40.7). Poor mineralization of the bone, as in rickets, will alter the mechanical properties of the bone, increase the ease of deformation and lead to deformities. Altered loading may be a consequence of abnormal physical activity, deformity in other bones or abnormal conformation.

Clinical and subclinical rickets may be the cause of increased incidence of long bone deformities in older birds long after the growth plate abnormalities associated with rickets have gone. As in all cases of all skeletal pathology, investigations must go back to the estimated start date of the insult. In broilers the most common age for rickets is between 10 and 18 days of age.

Rickets

Rickets is usually seen in rapidly growing chicks. In all forms of rickets a failure of mineralization leads to flexibility of long bones. Rickets is caused by a deficiency of calcium or phosphorus or insufficient vitamin D. The deficiency may be in the diet, due to malabsorption or a consequence of an imbalance between dietary calcium and phosphorus. Marginal or subclinical rickets may frequently go unreported but may be associated with poor chick performance, a poorer gait and an increase in bone deformities.

Specific calcium and phosphorus deficiencies experimentally result in distinct histopathology but the histopathological picture in field material can be more confusing. In rickets attributed to a relative or absolute deficiency of calcium there is thickening of the epiphyseal plate due to an accumulation of proliferating chondrocytes and this is accompanied by an increase in the length of the perforating epiphyseal vessels. In rickets attributed to a relative or absolute deficiency of phosphorus there is an accumulation of hypertrophic chondrocytes. Vitamin D deficiency effectively results in hypocalcaemic rickets.

The incidence of hypophosphataemic rickets has increased in some parts of Europe in recent years. This is due to a tendency to keep dietary phosphorus low to reduce costs and to reduce environmental contamination by poultry litter. There is therefore more reliance placed on dietary plant sources, where the availability of phosphorus may be highly variable. Bacterial infections are more common in bones with hypophosphataemic rickets. The accumulated hypertrophic chondrocytes in hypophosphataemic rickets result in a marked increase in the length of metaphyseal vessels. These very long metaphyseal vessels are likely to have a sluggish circulation and a greater cartilage surface area. Circulating bacteria will therefore be even more able to attach to the cartilage walls and establish infectious foci.

To investigate rickets, especially subclinical rickets, it is useful to do bone ashing and get estimates of the calcium and phosphorus content (see Appendix 2). Deviation from the 'normal' ratio of calcium to phosphorus in the bone of 2:1 suggests an episode of calcium or phosphorus deficiency. Evidence of a previous rachitic episode can also be established if the relative lengths and widths of long bones from 'normal' and 'affected' flocks are compared. The bones from the rachitic flocks will tend to be relatively short.

Rachitic episodes due to low calcium may respond to vitamin D_3 or its metabolite 25-hydroxy vitamin D_3 added to the water. This is also true of rickets associated with malabsorption.

Dyschondroplasia

Dyschondroplasia occurs as a focal thickening of the bone growth plate and is most common in the proximal tibiotarsus (Fig. 40.8) and tarsometatarsus. The typical lesion is in the proximal tibiotarsus and is called tibial dyschondroplasia. The accumulated mass of cartilage is vascular and nonmineralized and composed of small round chondrocytes that have not hypertrophied. This is unlike rickets, where the accumulated cartilage is always across the full width of the growth plate and is still penetrated by vessels.

A wide variety of factors have been shown to influence the incidence and severity of dyschondroplasia. These include genetic selection, calcium/phosphorus ratios in feed, metabolic acidosis through excess chloride in feed, and incorrect acid–base balance. Other conditions that severely affect the health of the bird, such as mycotoxicosis, will also cause tibial dyschondroplasia. In a normal flock of broilers, clinical tibial dyschondroplasia will only be seen in a small proportion of the birds, although subclinical lesions may be more common. When a high clinical incidence is apparent then a dietary cause should be suspected. This is most commonly a relatively low calcium to phosphorus ratio or an elevated chloride relative to sodium and potassium, disrupting the acid–base balance. The dietary electrolyte balance (DEB) is the principal factor in acid–base regulation and for growing broilers should be about 200–230 mEq/kg and probably not above 250 mEq/kg. This can be calculated using Mongin's equations using the quantity of Na, K and Cl in the diet $(434.8 \times \%Na) + (255 \times \%K) - (281.7 \times \%Cl)$ (Mongin & Sauveur 1977).

The development of a tibial dyschondroplasia lesion takes time and the size of the lesion is proportional to the rate of long bone growth; therefore a tibial dyschondroplasia lesion of 1 cm has taken at least 10 days to form. Investigation of causal factors must extend back to the time the initial lesion started to develop.

The most common cause of an 'outbreak' of dyschondroplasia in a flock of modern broilers is marginal inadequacies in dietary calcium or a marginal calcium/phosphorus imbalance at about 2 weeks of age preceding dyschondroplasia at 4 weeks of age. Any rachitic growth plate pathology which may have been associated with the initial development of dyschondroplasia will probably have disappeared by 4 weeks of age. However, diagnosis may be assisted by looking at calcium and phosphorus values in bone ash samples and in the relevant diets.

Chondrodystrophy

Chondrodystrophy is rarely perceived as a problem in modern flocks. Chondrodystrophy results in short, thick and usually misshapen long bones and often an apparent enlargement of the hock joints. Displacement of the gastrocnemius tendon may occur. Chondrodystrophy is a generalized disorder of the growth plates of long bones such that linear growth is impaired and appositional growth remains normal. It is distinct from rickets in that mineralization is not impaired. Histologically there is a lack of columnar organization in the proliferative zone of the growth plate and a very narrow hypertrophic zone. The term perosis, at one time used for this and other conditions, is confusing and ambiguous and should not be used.

Manganese deficiency results in chondrodystrophy, which has been confirmed by histopathological studies. The following deficiencies have also been reported to contribute to chondrodystrophy: choline, niacin, vitamin E, biotin, folic acid and pyridoxine.

Chondrodystrophy may be a consequence of mycoplasma infections. Turkey syndrome 65 was attributed to *Mycoplasma meleagridis* and infection of young birds with *Mycoplasma gallisepticum* or *Mycoplasma iowae* can also lead to chondrodystrophy. The skeletal changes have been likened to a nutritional chondrodystrophy, possibly because the mycoplasma impairs the supply of nutrients to the growth plate cartilage.

In turkeys chondrodystrophy may be inherited as a single autosomal recessive gene causing galactosamine deficiency. Very high brooding temperatures have been associated with chondrodystrophies.

Fracture

Fractures may be attributed to trauma or are secondary to other disorders, such as nutritional and metabolic osteodystrophies, dyschondroplasia, some forms of mycotoxicosis and osteo-myelitis. Transverse fractures of the proximal tibiotarsus in growing turkeys may occur as a consequence of bone marrow lymphomas. Metaphyseal fractures in proximal tibiotarsi of 5–8-week-old pullets were attributed to a possible vitamin C deficiency, because of similarities with Moller–Barlow disease in mammals. Excess aluminium reduces bone ash, weight gain and feed efficiency and could contribute to fractures.

Foot-pad dermatitis (pododermatitis)

Foot-pad dermatitis is a type of contact dermatitis that starts as hyperkeratosis, erosions and dis-coloration of the skin and may progress to ulcers. The pathology appears to be triggered by litter conditions and is influenced by diet and dietary factors (methionine, biotin deficiency, protein digestibility and high unsaturated fats) and enteric health. Litter will deteriorate in poultry houses with poor environments (poor ventilation, inadequate insulation, uneven heating), with excessive drinking and with enteric conditions that cause diarrhoea and poor-quality droppings. Wet litter will soften the foot pads and make them more susceptible. A high or low litter pH will also contribute to lesions. High pH arises through ammonia in the environment and low pH may occur through the addition of high levels of acid in feed. Insufficient litter may con-tribute to foot pad dermatitis, as will poorly absorbent materials. Wood shavings appear to be the litter of choice, but good litter management is also critical.

Degenerative joint disease

Degenerative joint disease can cause lameness in adult broiler strain fowl. The histopathology of avian degenerative joint disease, which typically shows areas of cartilage thinning, surface fibril-lation and necrosis, is similar to that seen in osteoarthrosis in other species. The common prac-tice of weight control in broiler breeding stock significantly reduces the incidence and severity of degenerative joint disease to the point where significant lesions are rarely reported. The degen-erative changes seen in the joints of some caged layers are likely to be a primary osteoarthrosis. Osteoarthritis could also be a sequel to an infectious joint condition such as *Mycoplasma*, result-ing in an inflammatory arthropathy.

Articular/epiphyseal osteochondrosis

Osteochondrotic lesions are most frequently seen in turkeys and heavy broiler breeders approaching maturity. Lesions are most common in the hip joint, the distal tibiotarsus and the epiphyses of the synovial joints adjacent to the sixth thoracic vertebra. Where osteochondrotic lesions involve the articular surface they are likely to contribute to the development of osteoar-throsis within the joint. This is a pathology reported in the trochanter and antitrochanter of the hip joint of the mature turkey.

Deep pectoral myopathy

This lesion, seen in broilers and sometimes regularly in broiler breeders, is in the supracoracoid muscle and appears to be due to an ischaemic necrosis caused by a disruption in the blood sup-ply. It may be attributed to:

- **Wing flapping and subsequent tissue damage and necrosis**: When birds are handled or caught by their feet they may flap their wings violently. This may sever the blood vessels that irrigate the deep pectoral muscles. More commonly, the muscle may swell during exercise and there is insufficient space for its expansion because of its tight, inelastic aponeurosis. The resulting increase in intramuscular pressure and the development of oedema causes blood supply restriction, ischaemic necrosis and tissue degeneration. Weighing broilers towards the end of growth can cause sufficient flapping to produce these changes. Also, inadequacies of the harvesting process can result in excessive flapping. There is a theory that improved exercise in the young, up to 3 weeks old, reduces the incidence in older birds.

- *Infectious bronchitis virus* (**IBV**) **variant**: An association has been suggested between deep pectoral myopathy in meat-type chickens and infection with the IBV variant 49/1 (793B). This type of lesion in the pectoral muscles (pectoralis major) seems to be different from the deep pectoral myopathy where the supracoracoid muscle goes through a necrotic process that is thought to be caused by a disruption in the blood supply. This is best checked by IBV variant serology, although 49/1 infection in an integrated company would also often be associated with egg drops and shell quality issues in breeders.
- **Mycotoxins**: There may be a relationship between mycotoxin problems and 'green muscle'. The suggestion is that some mycotoxins, e.g. aflatoxin, may cause capillary fragility, in which case it is important to collect liver and kidney samples from affected birds and submit them for histopathological assessment.
- **Deficiency in antioxidants**: Another potential problem is that stress caused by products of oxidative processes can cause capillary fragility and haemorrhaging. These are associated with fat, meat and bonemeal quality problems (rancidity), lack of antioxidant in the feed and marginal deficiencies of vitamin E and/or selenium. Some improvements may be seen by boosting the levels of vitamins E and C in the feed or by administering these in the drinking water prior to when lesions are first observed and until the birds are processed.

Ionophore toxicity

Ionophore toxicity causes a severe myodegeneration of the adductor leg muscles, resulting in a reluctance to walk, gait abnormalities and lameness. Problems are most frequently seen when a broiler premix, containing ionophore-based coccidiostats, is added to broiler breeder, turkey or guinea fowl diets. Ionophore toxicities may also be a consequence of feed mixing errors, when excessive ionophore-based coccidiostats are added to a diet. Tiamulin may potentiate the myodegeneration properties of ionophores.

Other focal myopathies have also been seen in growing turkeys. Little is seen grossly but muscle degeneration is evident histologically and plasma levels of creatine kinase are elevated. Damaged muscle fibres are seen in the superficial pectorals, gastrocnemius and other muscles of the legs.

SKELETAL DISORDERS OF LAYER-TYPE FOWL

Osteopenia (cage layer fatigue)

The total calcium held in the skeleton of a layer is about 40 g; every egg requires 4 g of calcium. The skeleton serves as a flexible reserve to meet these demands but has to be adequately and correctly replenished by dietary calcium. This requires a high degree of management and nutritional skill.

The most frequent skeletal pathology in layer-type fowl is bone fracture due to osteopenia. The condition is frequently termed cage layer fatigue. In a typical severe case the long bones and

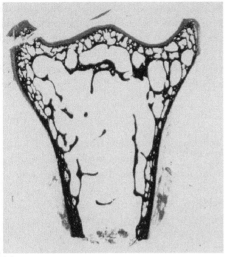

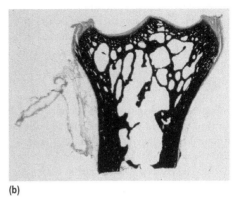

(b)

(a)

Fig. 40.9 (a) The toe (first phalanx) from a 72-week-old female layer. The section shows thin cortical and subchondral bone, full of large cavities (osteoporosis). The overlying articular cartilage is red. (b) The toe (first phalanx) from a 72-week-old male layer. The section shows far thicker cortical and subchondral bone with fewer and smaller spaces. The overlying articular cartilage is red. Von Kossa, ×5.

vertebrae fracture and the sternum and ribs may be deformed. Posterior paralysis may result through collapse of thoracic vertebrae and spinal cord compression. Most commonly, the osteopenia is a consequence of osteoporosis, a deficiency in the quantity of fully mineralized, structural bone (Fig. 40.9). Where osteomalacia is also a feature (seen as deformed sternum and ribs), there are likely also to have been inadequacies in the supply of calcium and/or phosphorus during growth.

Skeletal integrity is determined by structural bone: compact, cortical bone and cancellous, trabecular bone, both of which are lamellar. The reproductively active fowl has two forms of bone: structural and medullary. Medullary bone is rapidly produced, highly labile, woven bone and has no structural role but simply provides calcium for shell formation. From the onset of lay, high oestrogen levels cause the bone cells to form medullary bone and not lamellar (structural) bone. However, if medullary bone is inadequate, the hen will use both bone types to meet the demands of eggshell formation. Structural bone lost during lay will not be replaced and the bone will be weakened and will remain weakened until the end of lay.

There is a large variation in the bone status of individual hens from a flock. Calcium requirements during growth, prelay and lay vary markedly. Changes from grower to prelay diets and then to layer diet result in changes in available calcium, phosphorus and vitamin supplements. Thus individual variation in a flock may result in the mineral requirements of some birds being compromised at a critical point in skeletal development. Flock uniformity in skeletal and reproductive development tying in with the correct levels of dietary calcium is vital to the prevention of osteopenia in fowl.

Good skeletal development should be encouraged in layers and replacement breeding stock, particularly important is achieving a good skeletal frame in the first 6 weeks of life. There is some evidence to suggest that, if excessive calcium is provided in advance of when it is required, the metabolism of the bird may, for a period of time, be refractory to calcium absorption when it is required. Therefore, calcium must not be excessive during rear. The calcium demands to produce medullary bone should be met from 2 weeks before first egg (coinciding with the onset of follicular activity and the rise in oestrogen levels). Calcium levels should be further increased with the commencement of egg production. Sources of calcium that enable the slow release of mineral, such as oyster shell, appear to give the best results.

Osteopetrosis

Osteopetrosis is characterized by abnormal growth and extensive modelling (formation) of bone. In mammals it results in a metaphyseal sclerosis. In chickens and guinea fowl, osteopetrosis is attributed to strains of avian leukosis/sarcoma virus and results in a mid-diaphyseal, pericortical accumulation of highly cellular immature bone and a marked rise in serum alkaline phosphatase activity. The condition is bilaterally symmetrical and involves the tarsometatarsus and tibiotarsus particularly. The natural disease is uncommon but has been reported in turkeys.

Amyloidosis

Deposits of amyloid found in the joints of chickens are usually attributed to the amyloidogenic potential of arthrotropic bacterial species (*Staphylococcus aureus*, *Escherichia coli*, *Salmonella enteritidis* and *Enterococcus faecalis*). Extensive amyloid arthropathy is usually primarily caused by *E. faecalis*, but not by all *E. faecalis* isolates. Experimental evidence and clinical cases indicate that joint amyloidosis attributed to *E. faecalis* is a consequence of joint or tendon sheath injection with *E. faecalis*. Clinical cases are most frequently seen unilaterally in the hock joint of individual replacement pullets or broiler breeders. These were attributed to contamination with *E. faecalis* during intramuscular administration of a previously sterile vaccine diluent, for example Marek's vaccine in day-old chicks.

REFERENCE

Mongin P, Sauveur B 1977 Interrelationship between mineral nutrition, acid-base balance, growth and cartilage abnormalities. In: Boorman K N, Wilson B J (eds) Growth and poultry meat production. British Poultry Science, Edinburgh, p 235–247

FURTHER READING

Randall C J 1991 A colour atlas of diseases and disorders of the domestic fowl and turkey. Wolfe Publishing, London, p 114–116

Whitehead C C (ed) 1992 Bone biology and skeletal disorders in poultry. Poultry Science Symposium 23. Carfax Publishing, Abingdon

APPENDIX 1: GLOSSARY OF MUSCULOSKELETAL TERMS

Abnormal angulation

The bone is abnormally bent medially (varus), laterally (valgus), dorsally or ventrally

Appositional growth

Growth on the surface of bone or cartilage within the periostial or perichondrial tissue

Arthropathy
Pathology within a joint or joints

Avulsion
A tendon or ligament has been forcibly detached from a bone

Bone modelling
Initial bone formation

Bone remodelling
Sequential resorption and re-formation of bone

Bowing
Usually refers to an angular deformity of the tibiotarsus, along a ventral–dorsal plane

Cancellous bone
Spongy bone forming a network in the medulla, consist of trabeculae of lamellar bone

Chondroblast
Cells producing cartilage

Chondroclast
Multinuclear cell that resorbs cartilage, probably an osteoclast

Chondrocytes
Mature cartilage cells

Chondrodystrophy
A failure of growth plate cartilage proliferation, resulting in shortening of the long bones

Compact bone
Lamellar bone organized into sheets, cylinders (haversian systems)

Cortical (diaphyseal) bone
Compact bone

Diaphysis
Shaft of long bone

Dyschondroplasia
A failure of growth plate chondrocyte differentiation, resulting in an accumulation of avascular growth plate cartilage within the metaphysis

Endochondral ossification
Bone formation preceded by a cartilage model

Endosteum
Thin connective tissue lining of bone

Epiphysis
At each end of a long bone, between the articular cartilage and the growth plate of a growing long bone; may contain an ossification centre

Free thoracic vertebra (FTV, T4)
The 4th thoracic vertebra, between the 5th, which is fused to the synsacrum, and the 3rd, which is fused to the notarium

Growth plate (physis)
Site of long bone growth where cartilage is produced to be replaced by bone

Interstitial growth
Cartilage growth by cell division and matrix production

Intramembranous ossification
Bone formed directly within connective tissue

Kyphosis
Posterior curvature of spine

Lamellar bone
Highly organized structural bone

Lordosis
Anterior curvature of the spine

Medullary bone
Temporary, small spicules of woven bone attached to trabecular and cortical bone. A source of calcium for egg shells

Metaphysis
Between growth plate and diaphysis, consist of newly formed bone that has replaced cartilage produced by the growth plate

Notarium
Fused thoracic vertebrae (T1, T2, T3)

Osteoarthritis
Inflammatory synovial joint abnormality in which cartilage and bone disorders culminate in joint malfunction

487

Osteoarthrosis

Noninflammatory synovial joint abnormality in which cartilage and bone disorders culminate in joint malfunction

Osteoblast

Bone forming cell

Osteochondrosis

Foci of chondrocyte degeneration and death resulting in the failure of the replacement of cartilage by bone during endochondral ossification

Osteoclast

Multinuclear cell that resorbs bone

Osteocyte

Mature bone cell within bone

Osteodystrophy

Bone pathology of nonspecific cause; includes osteoporosis and rickets

Osteoid

Nonmineralized bone matrix

Osteomalacia

Incomplete mineralization of bone, resulting in increased osteoid

Osteomyelitis

Bacterial infection within the bone

Osteopenia

A reduction in the quantity of normal bone tissue

Osteopetrosis

Increased skeletal density, due to abnormal bone growth and modelling

Osteoporosis

A reduced quantity of fully mineralized structural bone

Periosteum

Outer layer of dense connective tissue on the surface of bone

Physis

Growth plate

Rickets

A failure of growth plate cartilage and bone mineralization, resulting in an accumulation of vascularized cartilage within the metaphysis

Scoliosis

Lateral curvature of the spine

Spondylolisthesis

Anterior displacement of vertebrae relative to adjacent vertebrae

Spondylopathies

Vertebral pathologies

Synsacrum

Fused thoracic, lumbar and sacral vertebrae

Tarsometatarsus

The fused metatarsal and tarsal bones of avian species

Tibial plateau angle

Angle between the proximal articular surface of the tibia and the long axis of the tibia

Tibiotarsus (tibia)

The fused tibia and tarsal bones of avian species

Torsion

The twist within the long axis of a bone, which, if outside the normal range, results in torsional deformity. Torsion can be external, where the bone is twisted so the anterior surface of the distal end is rotated away from midline, or internal, where the anterior surface of the bone is rotated towards midline

Trabecular bone

Fine sheets or struts of lamellar bone crossing between cortices

Valgus

Lateral angular deviation

Varus

Medial angular deviation

Woven bone

Poorly organized, highly cellular, rapidly produced bone, usually in response to fracture, or as medullary bone in reproductively active birds or as a consequence of some forms of tumour

APPENDIX 2: OBTAINING ESTIMATES OF BONE ASH, CALCIUM AND PHOSPHORUS

Samples

A mid diaphyseal cylinder of cortical bone from the tibiotarsus makes an excellent sample. The remaining bone extremities can then be used for histopathology.

Determination of bone ash, calcium and phosphorus

The fat is extracted by placing the cortical bone samples in petroleum spirit (bp 40–60°C) for 8h. The samples are then dried at 100°C for 16 h or until a constant weight. The weight of the dry, fat-free bone is then recorded. The samples are then ashed in a muffle furnace at 550°C for 12h or until a constant weight, cooled and reweighed. The result is reported as percentage bone ash of dry, fat-free weight.

For calcium and phosphorus analysis 10ml of 6N hydrochloric acid is added to the cooled bone ash within the crucible. This solution is then evaporated to dryness on a hotplate. The precipitate is dissolved by adding 20mL of deionized water and heating. The resulting solution plus washing from the crucible are filtered through no. 40 ashless filter paper into a 100mL volumetric flask. Phosphorus is determined colorimetrically using the TRAACS 800 automated chemistry system or equivalent. The extracted bone solution is mixed with molybdovanade reagent and the resulting yellow solution measured at 420nm. Calcium is determined by atomic absorption spectrophotometry at a wavelength of 422.7nm. A lanthanum salt is added to eliminate the interference of other elements.

Using this method, typical ash values for broilers would be about 45–50% and calcium and phosphorus of 18% and 9%, respectively. The ratio of calcium to phosphorus should also be noted, although, to properly evaluate suspect samples, there should be comparison with the results from known normal samples processed in the same laboratory using the same methodology.

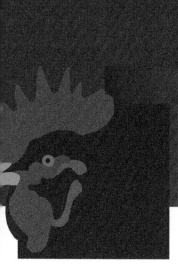

Paul F. McMullin and
Mark Pattison

OTHER DISEASES, POISONS AND TOXINS

Chapter **41**   Practical epidemiology of
poultry disease and
multifactorial conditions   **492**

Chapter **42**   Nutritional disorders   **510**

Chapter **43**   Management as a cause
of disease in poultry   **536**

Chapter **44**   Toxicants in poultry   **548**

Chapter **45**   Diseases of game birds   **560**

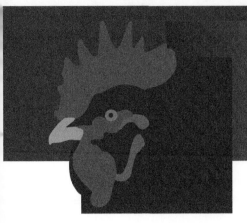

J. J. (Sjaak) de Wit

Practical epidemiology of poultry disease and multifactorial conditions

Epidemiology is usually defined as the study of disease in populations and of the factors that determine its occurrence. The term 'disease' is used broadly here, its meaning ranging from a subclinical disease or infection to severe illness. The term 'population' defines a group of animals. Its size may vary greatly depending on whether it refers to a pen, a house, a farm, a region, an integrated production system, a country or the international poultry industry. The manifestation of an infection can vary from subclinical to serious disease, depending on many factors such as virulence of the agent, climate, nutrition, housing, secondary infections, growth rate, sex, age, protection by vaccinations, etc. Identifying all factors that influence the occurrence and manifestation of a disease is the ultimate goal of an epidemiological study, so that preventive measures can be developed and implemented based on objective data rather than on guesswork. Epidemiology tries to find answers to specific questions. Why is a specific disease present on a specific farm, or in a specific kind of chicken house or region? Why is it increasing? Why do we find it mainly in a certain breed or kind of chicken? How often does it occur in this region, and what are the costs? What can we do to prevent or control it and would the benefit justify the cost? The reward of good epidemiological knowledge is improved understanding of 'what is going on' and 'what we can do about it'.

Good veterinary epidemiological studies require knowledge of a variety of fields beyond veterinary science per se. They require knowledge of diseases, infectious agents, noninfectious causes, interactions of potential causes, potential relevant factors, diagnostic techniques, management, breeding, economics, feed, housing, mathematics, statistics, etc. This often makes epidemiological studies complicated, and they are always challenging.

DEFINITIONS

In order to avoid confusion as to the meaning of frequently used terms in epidemiology, the most important ones are defined here.

- **Types of disease occurrence**: An outbreak of a disease is *sporadic* when it occurs occasionally in a limited area, in a limited time, and then disappears again. An *endemic* occurrence is when the disease is normally present in the population. Usually this means it is occurring quite often (many affected flocks) or even constantly. An *epidemic* is when there is a rapid increase in the number of cases of an infectious disease in a population. For an epidemic to occur, something new or unusual has to be introduced to the population. A *pandemic* is a widespread epidemic that affects a large proportion of an international population.
- **Incidence** is the number of new cases that occur in a population over a certain time (e.g. a day, a week, a month). Usually, incidence is expressed as a percentage of the total population. The length of time an individual case survives or takes to recover has no effect on incidence.
- **Prevalence** is the percentage of diseased or infected birds in a (certain) population at a certain time or time-period. No distinction is made between acute and chronic cases, so disease of longer duration tends to show increased prevalence.

The cause of disease

A disease can be caused by a single factor or a combination of different factors. Robert Koch has defined a single cause of disease by the use of the following postulates: a pathogen is causal if:

- It is present in all cases of the disease
- It does not occur in another disease as a fortuitous and nonpathogenic parasite, and
- It is isolated in pure culture from an animal, is repeatedly passaged and induces the same disease in other animals.

There are many examples of diseases that are caused by single, infectious or noninfectious factors. Infectious bronchitis, Newcastle disease, laryngotracheitis, Gumboro disease, Marek's disease and coccidiosis can all be reproduced by inoculating a chicken with a single agent. However, even in these single-cause diseases there can be a wide variation in the severity of the disease in response to other factors. So, from an epidemiological point of view, the factors that influence the severity of the disease in the field are at least as important as the 'single cause' itself.

For other diseases, it is clear that there is no such thing as a single cause. These multifactorial diseases are much more difficult to reproduce. Hence, for these diseases epidemiological studies are also much more complicated.

Multifactorial diseases can be divided into several groups:

- **Diseases that are caused by combinations of well-known causes**: for example, *Clostridium perfringens* does not normally cause necrotic enteritis and neither does coccidiosis. However, the combination can
- **Diseases that are caused by different combinations of partly unknown causes**: for example infectious stunting syndrome (ISS) and poult enteritis and mortality syndrome (PEMS)

- **Syndromes, such as respiratory disease or drops in egg production, that can be caused by more than one specific (combination of) cause(s)**: Several strains of *Infectious bronchitis virus* (IBV), *Avian pneumovirus* (APV), low-pathogenic *Avian influenza virus* (LPAIV), *Newcastle disease virus* (NDV) and *Mycoplasma gallisepticum* can all be involved with respiratory disease complex (RDC) and drops in egg production.

Statistical association

Association is the degree to which two variables interdepend or co-vary. Variables are statistically positively associated when they co-occur more frequently than would be expected by chance. Variables are statistically negatively associated when they co-occur less frequently than would be expected by chance (e.g. the application of an effective vaccine and the presence of outbreaks). The *level of significance* of an association denotes the chance that the detected statistical association (in the selected samples) is actually not present in the whole population. A generally accepted significance level is 5% ($p < 0.05$). It is very important to realize that the calculation of the statistical level of significance is based on the data that are put in the formulas. When the data themselves are not correct or not representative for the population, because of bias, the statistical calculations cannot correct for this. By selecting data or using nonrepresentative data, an effect can be highly significant but still be irrelevant for the whole population.

However, there is also a risk that there is a certain association between variables in the population but that it is not detected in the study. This risk is usually denominated the β-error. The *power* of a study is the complement to the β-error $(1-β)$: the probability that an effect that is really present in the population is detected (statistically significant) in the study. A generally accepted level of power to aim for in a study is 80% or higher. Both level of significance and power do have a major influence on the required sample sizes (birds or flocks). Increasing the power of a study from 80% to 95% about doubles the required number of samples.

For example, within a broiler integration Meat-XXL a study is designed to determine the role of *M. gallisepticum* in RDC in their broiler flocks. In the last year, 25% of their broiler flocks had shown respiratory problems. It is suspected by the management of the integration that the presence of *M. gallisepticum* would increase the risk of getting RDC from 20% to 30%. In this situation, comparing the occurrence of RDC in about 240 *M. gallisepticum*-infected flocks and 240 *M. gallisepticum*-free flocks would be required to achieve a power of 80% (80% chance that the detected percentage of RDC would be significantly ($p < 0.05$) higher in the *M. gallisepticum*-infected flocks). Increasing the power of this study to 95% would require 420 flocks in each group.

It is important to realize that a (significantly) positive association of a factor with a disease, does not necessarily mean that it is a causal relationship. For example, if factor A causes a disease that results in manifestations B and C, there will be a statistical causal association between A and B, and between A and C. However, there will also be a statistical association between the two response variables, B and C, arising from their separate associations with A, but this is a noncausal association.

For example, it is likely that farmers in an area with an endemic occurrence of very virulent *Infectious bursal disease virus* (vvIBDV) (causal factor A) will use more intermediate plus (or hot) IBDV vaccines (response factor B). On average, they will suffer higher losses due to respiratory diseases (response factor C) than farmers in other areas that are free of immunosuppressive viruses. As a consequence, you may find a positive association between the use of these IBDV vaccines and the presence of respiratory diseases (and use of antibiotics – response factor D) on farms in the endemic area. However, this association is noncausal, as IBDV vaccines do not cause an increase in respiratory diseases. On the contrary, without the use of IBDV vaccines, the problem would even be greater because of clinical infection with vvIBDV.

When attempting to establish a causal association, the following principles should be considered.

- **The time sequence of the events**: A cause has to be earlier in the flock than the disease. The time between introduction of the cause and disease (incubation time) has to be biologically explainable. When serology is used for diagnosing the infection, the relation between the seroconversion and disease has to be biologically explainable.
- **The statistical significance and strength of the association**: If a factor is causal and the study size was valid, there will be a strong statistically significant association between the factor and the disease.
- **Biological gradient**: If a dose–response relationship can be found between a factor and a disease, the plausibility of a factor being causal is increased.
- **Consistency**: If an association exists in a number of different circumstances, a causal relationship is more likely.
- **Compatibility with existing knowledge or common sense**: It is more reasonable to infer that a factor causes a disease if a plausible biological mechanism has been identified than if such a mechanism is not known. Although this may sound very logical and acceptable, there are many examples in the poultry industry that show otherwise. Many products are sold and applied in poultry flocks on the basis only of information provided by the supplier. When a product or manipulation is applied at the time of peak expression of a disease, it is easy to assume that it has had a curative effect. Subsequently, this observed 'positive effect' is communicated to others. When an effect of a product is claimed that cannot be explained by existing scientific knowledge or common sense, it does not necessarily mean that it is nonsense but that it does require much more research. This will show whether the claim was wrong or help expand our knowledge in the search for the explanation of the effect.

Risk factor

A risk factor has a significant positive or negative association between the presence of the factor and the disease. This association can be either causal or noncausal.

Knowledge of risk factors, even of noncausal factors, is useful in identifying populations to which veterinary attention should be directed. For example, it would not be surprising to find that the prevalence of *M. gallisepticum*-infected flocks was higher on multiage layer farms than on single-age farms. Although the multiage system is not itself the cause of the *M. gallisepticum* infections, it still is relevant information in the prevention of *M. gallisepticum* infections.

When developing preventive measures it is important to identify those risk factors that are causal, against which control should be directed. For example, in well-managed broiler flocks sudden death syndrome (flip-over) can be the major cause of death. It is positively associated with high-quality management, unlimited feeding, the sex of the broilers (mainly males are affected) and high-intensity light. In other words, the presence on the farm of these factors increases the risk of having sudden-death syndrome as a main cause of mortality. Reduction of the noncausal risk factor 'high-quality management' will not be the best approach to reducing the number of flip-overs. Reduction of the growth rate by feed management or reduction of light intensity in the broiler house might be, if they are, in fact, risk factors on that farm.

DIAGNOSTIC PITFALLS

In epidemiological studies, birds or flocks are divided in different groups based on a diagnostic process. This makes the diagnostic approach an integrated part of the study. When the diagnosis is wrong, the results of the epidemiological study will be useless.

Table 41.1	Relation between sensitivity, specificity, predictive value and prevalence to Infected (or diseased) bird		
		YES	**NO**	
Test result	**Positive**	a	b	a + b
	Negative	c	d	c + d
		a + c	b + d	n = a + b + c + d

For a good diagnosis, proper sampling, proper sampling size, proper tests and proper interpretation of the results is essential.

Tests

There are no perfect tests (sensitivity and specificity of 100%; see below). Within one test, sensitivity and specificity compete. Increasing the sensitivity of a test will decrease the specificity in that test. Therefore, the cut-off of a test is always a compromise.

The relation between sensitivity, specificity, predictive value and prevalence is explained in Table 41.1.

- **Sensitivity** (diagnostic): The percentage of the infected animals that are detected by the test (positive), $a/(a + c)$. False-negative results (the sample from a diseased/infected animal that is negative in the test) can have several causes, such as the design itself, inappropriate sample size or timing of sampling (too soon after the infection in serology, or too late in virology), very low level of humoral immune response (noninvasive *Salmonella* spp., IBV or NDV vaccination in the presence of high maternal immunity, or immunosuppression). For diagnostic work at flock level, false-negative results are usually not a problem, as not all samples have to be identified as positive in order to find the flock positive.
- **Specificity** (diagnostic): The percentage of the noninfected animals that have a negative test result, $d/(b + d)$. Possible reasons for false-positive results are the test design or reagents used, poor quality of the sample, cross-reactions caused by infections by other agents that share common antigens (e.g. *Salmonella enteritidis* and *Salmonella typhimurium* in lipopolysaccharide, *M. gallisepticum* and acute phase *Mycoplasma synoviae*, IBV serotypes, paramyxoviruses 1, 3 and 7) and cross-reactions by shared factors in e.g. vaccine and test (temporary false positives in the *M. gallisepticum* serology after the recent application of inactivated, non-*M. gallisepticum*, vaccines).

NB: Sensitivity and specificity have nothing to do with mistakes made by the laboratory.

- **Predictive value of a positive test result**: The percentage of the positive test results that originate from infected animals, $a/(a + b)$.
- **Predictive value of a negative test result**: The percentage of the negative test results that originate from noninfected animals, $d/(c + d)$.

NB: The predictive value depends very much on the prevalence of the infected animals.

The field veterinarian often has to deal with the predictive value of test results. To demonstrate the influence of the prevalence of the disease on the predictive value of a test result we will take the following example:

Suppose the sensitivity of an enzyme-linked immunosorbent assay (ELISA) for the detection of p27 antigen of *Avian leukosis virus* (ALV) (J-subtype) is 90% and the specificity 99%. This means that 1% of noninfected breeders will have a (false-)positive test result. Now suppose that farmer X owns 1000 breeders, of which 40% were infected in 1996, 1% in 2002, and 0% in 2006.

Table 41.2	Influence of the prevalence of the disease on the predictive value of a test result: 1996 figures			
		AVIAN LEUKOSIS VIRUS INFECTION		
		YES	NO	
P27 ELISA result	Positive	360	6	366
	Negative	40	594	634
		400	600	1000

→ predictive value of a positive p27 ELISA result in 1996: 360/366 = 98%.

Table 41.3	Influence of the prevalence of the disease on the predictive value of a test result: 2002 figures			
		AVIAN LEUKOSIS VIRUS INFECTION		
		YES	NO	
P27 ELISA result	Positive	9	10	19
	Negative	1	980	981
		10	990	1000

→ predictive value of a positive result in 2002: 9/19 = 47%.

Table 41.4	Influence of the prevalence of the disease on the predictive value of a test result: 2006 figures			
		AVIAN LEUKOSIS VIRUS INFECTION		
		YES	NO	
P27 ELISA result	Positive	0	10	10
	Negative	0	980	990
		0	990	1000

→ predictive value of a positive result in 2006: 0/10 = 0%.

Tables 41.2–41.4 illustrate how these figures would affect the results of the ELISA test.

So, the predictive value of a test result depends heavily on the prevalence of the disease: the higher the true prevalence the greater the positive predictive value. So, one (infected) farm can be very happy with the test, while its (noninfected) neighbour is not.

Sample size

Sensitivity and specificity as discussed so far are based on a diagnostic approach for individual animals. In the poultry industry, we are not interested in one chicken but in groups, houses or flocks. As it is not possible or desirable to sample all birds in a flock, a certain number of samples are taken and tested. Based on the results of these selected birds, a diagnosis is made for the whole flock. This makes the number and selection of birds to be sampled important. Selection of the wrong birds or collecting the wrong number of samples increases the risk of arriving at a wrong conclusion for the whole flock and also, therefore, the wrong conclusions in the epidemiological study.

Number of birds sampled

Flock sensitivity

Flock sensitivity is the chance that a disease/infection is detected because at least one sample is positive. It is obvious that more samples results in a greater chance of detection. The flock sensitivity can be estimated using the formula:

flock sensitivity $= 1 - (1 - p)^n$,

where $n =$ number of samples and $p = $ [(prevalence $\times$ sensitivity) $+ (1 -$ prevalence) $\times (1 -$ specificity)].

For example: sensitivity (for one sample) 90%, specificity 99%, 10 samples and a prevalence of 10%: flock sensitivity $= 0.65$ (65%).

Flock specificity

The flock specificity is the chance that all tested samples of a group of noninfected (nondiseased) show a negative result. However, the more samples are taken, the greater the chance that we will find one or more false-positive results. The flock specificity can be estimated using the formula:

flock specificity $=$ (specificity)^n,

where n is the number of samples.

Example: specificity (for one sample) 99%: flock specificity for 60 samples $= 0.99^{60} = 55\%$.

Conclusion: taking more samples increases the chance of detecting the infection but also increases the chance of false-positive results. When the prevalence of the infection within the flock is low, many samples have to be taken (unless the sampling can be based on certain 'signs') and this will in turn decrease the flock specificity.

Therefore the number of samples has to be carefully considered: not too few, not too many. This is easy to say yet difficult to achieve in practice.

The formula to calculate the required number of samples (random sampling) to obtain a 95% certainty (level of confidence) to detect the infection in a flock (one or more positive samples) is:

$n = [1 - (1 - 0.95)^{1/D}] [N - 0.5(D - 1)]$,

where $n =$ required number of samples, $D =$ number of infected animals, $N =$ total number of animals (group, house, farm).

Table 41.5 shows the required sample sizes for 95% certainty of detecting infections for certain flock sizes and prevalences.

Using appropriate software, such as the freely available software program EPISCOPE, one can calculate the required sample size (within a flock) for a known flock size, estimated prevalence and required level of confidence.

	Required sample size for 95% certainty of detection of the infection (one or more positive test results) when using a test with 100% sensitivity											
Table 41.5												

FLOCK SIZE	PREVALENCE (%)											
	50	**40**	**30**	**25**	**20**	**15**	**10**	**5**	**2**	**1**	**0.5**	**0.1**
20	4	6	7	9	10	12	16	19	20	20	20	20
100	5	6	9	10	13	17	25	45	78	96	100	100
500	5	6	9	11	14	19	28	56	129	225	349	500
1000	5	6	9	11	14	19	29	57	138	258	450	950
5000	5	6	9	11	14	19	29	59	147	290	564	2253
10000	5	6	9	11	14	19	29	59	148	294	581	2588
∞	5	6	9	11	14	19	29	59	149	299	596	2995

Selection of birds for sampling

In the case of a clinical disease, birds should be sampled that are representative of the clinical signs. It is best to take birds from the different stages of the disease (if present). Birds that represent the early stage of the disease usually have more virus than birds that have been sick for a week. Certainly, for diseases with a short period of infectivity, such as APV, birds in the early stage of the infection (first clinical signs) are needed in order to be able to detect the virus. In other cases, it could be that the detection of the causative virus is easier in early birds than in the later stage of infection because of the damage to the target organ. For example, the detection of *Infectious larynotracheitis virus* (ILTV) in the trachea is much easier in birds with the first signs (wet eyes) than in birds with a severe haemorrhagic tracheitis. In those birds, most of the epithelium (carrying the virus) is already destroyed. On the other hand, selection of birds that are in the early stage of infection only can mask the clear clinical signs or lesions that are important in making the differential diagnosis.

When sampling a healthy flock (to monitor freedom from certain subclinical diseases), it is advisable not to sample birds which have a problem that is certainly not related to the infection one is sampling for. For example, a flock of young layers was moved to the layer house 5 days ago, and 1% of the birds are strongly dehydrated because they were not able to find the drinking system. When this flock is sampled to check the level of antibodies to NDV, it is advisable not to sample the dehydrated birds, as they are not representative for the flock and they might show artificially raised NDV titres because of the dehydration.

FORMULATING A CAUSAL HYPOTHESIS

The first step in any epidemiological or diagnostic investigation is descriptive. Usually, the time, place, population, age, housing system, feed mill, etc. are described first. A detailed description of the time of occurrence of disease may provide information on, for example, climatic influences, incubation periods and sources of infection. The distribution of a disease within the poultry population may indicate an association with type of chicken or a specific breed of chicken, feed mill, housing system, etc.

Based on all the data, a hypothesis of the potential cause or causes of the disease can be formulated. When there are some clear, well-defined potential causes, direct diagnostic research can be performed. When the initially available data provide information that suggest that a certain

Table 41.6	Results of epidemiological data presented in a 2 × 2 table where calculations can be made to decide whether there is a statistically significant association between the presence of the factor and the disease

		INFECTED (OR DISEASED) FLOCK		
		YES	NO	
Factor X	**Present**	a	b	$a + b$
	Absent	c	d	$c + d$
		$a + c$	$b + d$	$n = a + b + c + d$

number of factors might be of importance or that the role of certain factors is unknown, we may have to decide that we need to collect more data from the population at risk.

Observational studies are used to identify risk indicators and to estimate the quantitative effects of the various component causes that contribute to the occurrence of disease in the field. The studies are performed using field data. Observational studies are much more subject to bias than experimental studies, in which there are usually only a few variables. In the field, however, there are many variables that can have an influence on the data. This makes it difficult to come to conclusions about one of the variables specifically.

TYPES OF OBSERVATIONAL STUDY

In an epidemiological study, a comparison is made between two or more groups for the frequency of disease or exposure. With a few exceptions, epidemiological studies in the field are usually observational studies. This is in contrast to experimental studies, in which the researcher can control the experiment and variables, including the addition of positive and negative controls, excluding external factors that could complicate the results.

There are three types of observational study: cross-sectional, case-control and cohort.

In a *cross-sectional study* a certain number of birds or flocks are selected randomly from the total population and studied for the presence or absence of factor A (a certain disease) and the simultaneous presence or absence of factor B (potential cause). In a cross-sectional study, only the total number of selected birds or flocks is predetermined. In Table 41.6 this is represented as $(n = a + b + c + d)$. The number of a, b, c and d are unknown at the start of the study. For a cross-sectional study, the prevalence of the disease should preferably be high if we are to avoid the costs of a very large study.

In a *case-control study*, the number of cases ($a + c$ in Table 41.6) and the number of controls ($b + d$ in Table 41.6) are predetermined.

In a *cohort study*, the number of exposed (to a certain factor) birds or flocks ($a + b$ in Table 41.6) and the number of non-exposed birds or flocks ($c + d$ in Table 41.6) are predetermined.

After collection of the epidemiological data, the results can be presented in a 2 × 2 table like Table 41.6 and calculations can be made so as to decide whether there is a statistically significant association between the presence of the factor and the disease. From this 2 × 2 table, the value of relative risk or odds ratio can be calculated. The *relative risk* is the ratio between the ratio of diseased flocks in the factor-X-exposed flocks $[a/(a + b)]$ and the ratio of diseased flocks in the flocks that are not exposed to factor X $[c/(c + d)]$. When the relative risk is significantly greater than 1, this indicates a positive statistical association (which could be causal but could also be noncausal) between the presence of factor X and disease. When the relative risk is

Table 41.7	Results of a cohort study for the presence of respiratory disease in flocks with an *Infectious bronchitis virus* (IBV) infection		
		RESPIRATORY DISEASE COMPLEX	
		YES	**NO**	
IBV detection	**Positive**	21	7	28
	Negative	5	17	22
		26	24	50

significantly less than 1, this indicates a negative statistical association (which again could be either causal or noncausal) between the presence of factor X and disease. An example of a negative association between factor X and the presence of disease could be where factor X was the application of a protective vaccine.

Table 41.7 presents the results of a cohort study for the presence of respiratory disease in flocks with an IBV infection. Here the relative risk ratio would be (21/28)/(5/22), i.e. 3.3. This means that the presence of IBV in a flock increases the chance of having a respiratory disease by a factor of 3.3. It must be realized that the significance and confidence interval of the detected ratio must also be determined.

The *odds ratio* is another way of expressing the degree of association between the factor and disease. It expresses the ratio between the ratio of the presence of factor X in diseased flocks (a/c) and the ratio of the presence of factor X in healthy flocks (b/d). This can be rewritten as ad/bc. In Table 41.7 the odds ratio would be (21/5)/(7/17), i.e. 10.2. Once again, the significance and confidence interval of the detected ratio must be determined.

In many cases, simple statistical methods are not sufficient for epidemiological studies. Therefore, it is advisable to include a professional statistician in the team that is performing the study. It is highly recommended to involve the statistician when designing the study, rather than waiting until afterwards. This increases the chance of obtaining useful results. The freely available software program EPISCOPE can be a great help for making calculations.

STUDY PITFALLS

The most important pitfalls of epidemiological studies are bias, inaccurately identifying non-causal associations as causal, inappropriate study size and poor statistics.

Bias

Bias is a distortion of the results of the epidemiological study caused by a systemic error in the protocol of the study or of the data collection. Because of this bias, the results of the epidemiological study are not representative for the real situation of the entire population. Common causes of bias are described below.

Selection bias

Here, the selected groups of birds or flocks are not representative of the situation of the whole population. For example, when a new anticoccidiosis product is being tested and compared with an existing product on a number of farms, the houses and farms should be divided randomly between the two products. When this is not done, the results of the study (efficacy of the new product) may be not representative of the effect in the entire population.

Another example might involve a new breed of layer (LoTE = lots of table eggs) that is introduced into the market and gets a market share of 10% in a few years. After some time there are rumours (most probably initiated by the competition) that the LoTE layers are performing less well than the competition. A feeding company collects all the data of all their customers and shows that the LoTE layers produced on average 5 eggs fewer during the laying period than other breeds. So, the conclusion might appear simple: do not choose LoTE hens. However, there might be a different reason for the lower production. Which farmers are most willing to buy a new breed? – the farmers who were not satisfied with the performance of the previous flock. On average, this could well be the farms with poor management. If the technical data of the previous flocks had been taken into account, it might have shown that the LoTE flocks had produced on average 20 eggs per hen more than the previous flocks. In this case, the conclusion would have been: buy more LoTE hens. This example shows that a comparison of technical performance of breeds in the field can only be done when all other variables are evenly divided over the breeds that are being compared.

For each epidemiological study, we must question whether there has been a potential selection bias. This requires thorough knowledge of the field situation and epidemiology.

Diagnostic bias

This occurs where the selected groups of birds or flocks are not divided into the diseased group and healthy (control) group on the basis of the same diagnostic approach. For example, in a certain number of layer flocks with high feed consumption, poor feathering and decreased egg production, a chronic enteritis of unknown aetiology is diagnosed by histology. It is suspected that the chronic enteritis caused by unknown factor(s) is the cause of the poor performance of the flocks. In search for potential causal risk factors, it is decided that the history of those flocks (parents, breeds, rearing, feed, vaccinations, etc.) will be compared with the data of an equal number of well-performing flocks of the same age. If this study selects its diseased flocks on the basis of clinical signs in combination with the histological diagnosis of chronic enteritis and the control flocks only on the basis of the performance of the flocks, there is a diagnostic bias in the study protocol. To avoid this bias, the healthy flocks would need a histological check for the absence of chronic enteritis.

Confounding

Confounding is the situation in which the effect of a factor is confused with the effect of a second factor (the confounder). A confounding factor is associated with, but not the consequence of, the first factor. The magnitude of the effect of the confounding factor is unknown and may vary from minimal to large, and it can lead to underestimation or overestimation of the factor of interest. Confounding is of considerable importance in epidemiological studies and one of the major pitfalls in field studies.

An example of confounding would be a study of the effect of *Ascaridia galli* infections on the feed conversion of layer flocks. Suppose that it was found by a feed company that *Ascaridia*-infected hens needed 5 g extra feed per day compared to the uninfected flocks. There could have been at least two confounders in this study. A first confounder could be the effect of *Capillaria obsignata* infections on the feed conversion of the same hens. It would not be surprising to find that *Ascaridia* and *Capillaria* infections were positively associated. Therefore, flocks that were infected with *Ascaridia* would show a higher prevalence of *Capillaria* infections than the flocks that were free of *Ascaridia*. The detected difference of 5 g per day between *Ascaridia*-infected and uninfected flocks might be partially due to the *Capillaria* infection.

A second confounder could be the housing system. If part of the flock was housed in cages and part was housed in a free-range system, it would be very likely to find a positive association between uninfected flocks and the cage system. The detected difference of 5 g per day between *Ascaridia*-infected and uninfected flocks might be partially due to the difference in housing systems.

Interaction

This is where the effect of a risk factor depends (partly) on the presence of another factor. For example, when broilers are immunosuppressed by a combination of *Chicken anaemia virus* (CAV), Marek's disease and variant IBDV, the effect of a better Marek's vaccination might be less than in a situation without IBDV and CAV.

As another example, a single reovirus infection in young commercial layers will normally be subclinical. However, when the reovirus infection co-occurs with a CAV infection in young layers without antibodies against CAV, the mortality due to 'blue wing disease' will most probably be higher than that due to the CAV infection alone.

Detection of bias

Detection of bias can be very difficult and requires a critical mind and thorough knowledge of the factor itself, the pathogenesis, the bird and its environment. This is different from statistics, in which we are only working with figures.

Study size

In epidemiology, there is a simple basic rule for the preferred size of the study to get the best results: the bigger, the better. However, as costs and time are also important, compromises have to be made. Several formulae can be helpful in deciding for an appropriate study size (within flocks and number of flocks to be studied). In order to be able to use these formulae, assumptions have to be made as to the magnitude of the effect (expected difference between groups), percentage of diseased or healthy birds or flocks and the required statistical significance and power. It is important to realise that the outcome of these formulae depends very considerably on these subjective assumptions. This can easily make the results look better and more precise than they are in reality.

MULTIFACTORIAL CONDITIONS

Because of the possible complex aetiology of, in particular, respiratory and enteric disease, it is important to understand the role of the different agents in the disease process. Such understanding should be helpful in designing logical control or prevention strategies.

INFECTIOUS STUNTING SYNDROME

ISS is a transmissible disease that is seen worldwide and results in a variable percentage of runted and stunted birds. It is also sometimes known as 'pale bird syndrome', 'malabsorption syndrome', 'infectious runting' and 'runting and stunting syndrome'. The financial losses are caused by an increased number of culled birds, poor feed conversion, reduced weight (increased fattening period) and lower uniformity at slaughter causing financial losses for the processor. There may also be increased costs from treatments with vitamins, important trace elements and, sometimes, antibiotics.

EPIDEMIOLOGY

Cause

The clinical disease can be reproduced by feeding young chickens bacteria-free intestinal or proventricular homogenates obtained from affected chickens, suggesting a viral aetiology. Many viruses, such as *Calicivirus*, *Enterovirus*, *Parvovirus*, toga-like particles, picorna-like viruses, reoviruses and *Rotavirus*, have been detected in affected flocks, but none of them has been shown to be capable of causing the disease on its own. This strongly suggests that ISS has a multifactorial cause. As ISS shows itself in at least three different forms (main problem in small intestines, pancreas or proventriculus), it seems very likely that several combinations of etiological agents can be involved in an infection of the intestinal tract, resulting in a clinical manifestation that is called ISS.

Predisposing factors

The disease can be seen in all kind of chickens but shows itself mostly, and most severely, in broilers. The severity of ISS is age-dependent. Clinical signs are most severe after infections of 1-day-old chickens. Many cases have been linked to certain, mostly young breeder flocks, suggesting a vertical transmission or low level of maternal immunity against the causative agents of ISS. Poor cleaning and disinfection or short down-time periods have been shown to increase the severity of ISS in subsequent flocks.

Usually, successive flocks show improvements possibly due to a decreased level of vertical transmission, a protective effect of maternal immunity and/or changes in cleaning and disinfection and management practices.

The severity of ISS is also dependent on the feed quality. High-nutrient-density feed, marginal dietary vitamin concentrations and mycotoxins can increase the damage.

DIAGNOSIS

As there does not seem to be a single cause for ISS, but many, there is no diagnostic test for ISS. The diagnosis mainly depends on the clinical signs and gross lesions.

Clinical signs

The percentage of affected chickens in a flock with ISS can vary from a few percent to more than 90%. All three forms of ISS are clinically and epidemiologically similar and may occur concurrently in the same flock. However, it can also happen that only one or two forms are seen in a flock or a region at a certain time. Usually, within the first week of life, there are signs such as ruffled feathers, reluctance to move, coprophagia and mucoid diarrhoea with pasting of faeces around the cloaca. Growth retardation can be significant at 1 week of age. Poor feathering, resulting in retained down feathers on the head and neck (yellow heads) and broken and displaced primary wing feathers (helicopter feathering), can be seen subsequently. A varying percentage of birds can show lameness due to secondary osteodystrophy. In the most severe cases some of the smallest birds can even show opisthotonos due to a secondary encephalomalacia. Affected birds given high-carotenoid diets can be relatively pale in their skin pigmentation compared with unaffected or less affected birds.

Gross lesions

Affected birds can be relatively small for their age and pale. Distension of the intestinal lumen with poorly digested contents can be observed in chickens given food a few hours before being killed and necropsied. In chickens that have not recently eaten, the intestines contain clear watery or mucoid fluid. Depending on the form of ISS, the pancreas can be hard, atrophic and very pale. In the proventriculus form, the proventricular wall will be thickened and mottled because of pallor of the underlying affected lobules. Ulcers and haemorrhages can be seen in the mucosa.

In all forms of ISS, osteodystrophy is commonly seen in the affected birds of a few weeks of age. Because of the osteodystrophy, the disarticulation of the hips during the necropsy can easily result in a separation of the femoral head from the femur. This can also happen during catching, transport and handling of the birds for slaughter.

CONTROL

There is no vaccination schedule that prevents ISS. On several occasions, it has been shown that reovirus strains are likely to be a part of the cause, and vaccination of the breeders can be helpful in preventing or reducing the damage of ISS.

Prevention of infection of the next flock requires the basic disease prevention principles: use of all-in/all-out production together with thorough cleansing and disinfection of the broiler houses and their immediate surroundings, preferably with formaldehyde or an equivalent. This should reduce the infectious load in the environment. Another part of prevention or damage control is maternally derived immunity. In general, progeny of young breeder flocks appear to be more affected than progeny of other breeders. Where possible, it would be preferable to place progeny from older breeders on farms with an increased risk of ISS. These breeders should preferably be located in the same area as the broiler farm to have the highest chance of having relevant maternally derived immunity against the combination of etiological agents that is involved in ISS in that local situation.

Vertical transmission of ISS itself has not been shown but there is little doubt that certain agents that can be involved in ISS, such as reovirus, can be vertically transmitted. Because of the robustness of the viruses that may play a role in inducing ISS, vertical transmission could also happen through faecal contamination of hatching eggs. For this disease, as for hatchery hygiene in general, a dirty egg should not be considered as a hatching egg.

As the function of the gut is decreased, feed quality can play an important role in the severity of the manifestation of ISS. A feed that is already digested with difficulty by healthy chickens will increase the severity of ISS. Feeds with relatively low amounts of vitamins and other essential components will result in deficiencies because of the decreased efficacy of the digestion and absorption of the feed components.

Treatment with antibiotics can have a temporarily positive effect on the accompanying dysbacteriosis but does not cure the disease.

Supplementation with extra vitamins and trace elements may be effective in reducing the severity of ISS. However, a treatment of a few days might be less effective as a longer treatment, as the nutrient absorption is disturbed for a longer time in ISS.

POULT ENTERITIS MORTALITY SYNDROME

PEMS is a highly infectious disease of young turkeys that is defined as a clinical syndrome characterized by excessive to spiking mortality profiles, diarrhoea, growth depression, stunting and immunosuppression. The most serious clinical signs are seen in 1–4-week-old turkeys. It is mostly seen in multiage meat-turkey production systems, either through there being multiple ages on the same farm (particularly where the difference in age is 6–10 weeks) or because of a very high density of turkey farms in a local area. Some multiage breeding farms where the gap in age between subsequent flocks is around 14 weeks have remained unaffected over long periods.

PEMS has been shown to be a very difficult disease to control and prevent. Depopulation of PEMS-affected flocks and thorough cleaning of contaminated houses have failed to prevent PEMS in the next flock, especially on multiage farms.

Although many viruses, bacteria and parasites have been detected in PEMS-infected birds, the inciting agent remains unknown. Vertical transmission of PEMS has not been shown. Infections with *Turkey coronavirus* (TCV) have been linked to PEMS, as areas having a higher prevalence of TCV also had an increased level of PEMS. TCV alone, however, does not cause PEMS and PEMS can be seen in TCV-negative flocks. At the moment TCV is considered to be one of the components that can play a role in the syndrome of PEMS. Several strains of *Turkey astrovirus* and *Turkey reovirus* are also considered to play a role in PEMS.

As with ISS, PEMS can be reproduced experimentally by exposing naive poults to the intestinal contents of infected birds. The disease has also been reproduced by inoculating naive turkey poults with a bacteria-free filtrate from the thymus from PEMS-infected birds.

CONTROL

It seems likely that several combinations of etiological agents can be involved in an infection of the intestinal tract and other organs, resulting in the clinical manifestation that is called PEMS, so there is no general vaccination schedule that prevents it. Specific vaccines are not available for any of the infectious agents that have been found in PEMS. There is some circumstantial evidence that a PEMS problem has been controlled by periodic depletion of the whole multiage site, associated with application of multivalent commercial inactivated vaccines intended for breeding chickens (containing NDV, two strains of IBV and turkey rhinotracheitis virus). Although these field experiences are very interesting, there needs to be further investigation. When a TCV-like strain would be involved (in that area), it would not be totally unexpected to find a certain level of cross-protection by inactivated IBV vaccines, as IBV and TCV do have some antigens in common. Further study of these findings, either by further epidemiology or preferably in an experimental setting, would be needed to confirm the results before they could be recommended in general.

Prevention of infection of a next flock requires, therefore, the basic disease prevention principles: use of all-in/all-out production and thorough cleansing and disinfection of turkey houses as well as immediate surroundings, preferably with formaldehyde or an equivalent. A review of the epidemiology in a particular production setting may also suggest other control measures, such as the rescheduling of production to reduce the 'multiage-ness' on each farm or, where feasible, in the local area. When the multiage system cannot be avoided, try to increase the difference in ages between the flocks.

It has been shown that the brooding temperature has an influence on PEMS-associated mortality. A higher brooding temperature reduced the mortality.

As the function of the gut is decreased, the feed quality can play an important role in the severity of the manifestation of PEMS. A feed that is, in any case, digested with difficulty by healthy turkeys will increase the severity of PEMS.

Treatment with antibiotics will reduce mortality but does not cure the disease itself.

Supplementation with extra vitamins and trace elements may be effective in reducing the severity of PEMS. However, a treatment of a few days might be less effective than a longer treatment, as the nutrient absorption is disturbed for a longer time in PEMS.

RESPIRATORY DISEASE COMPLEX

The severity of the clinical signs after a respiratory infection vary markedly, depending on the pathogenicity of the strain of the pathogen, the age of the birds, the bird species, the presence of other primary or secondary pathogens, active immunity, maternally derived immunity, climate, immunosuppression, etc. Under field conditions, it is more commonly the case than not to have at least two or more variables that play a role in a respiratory disease. Therefore, the best approach to deal with respiratory diseases is to consider them to be a RDC. This decreases the risk of underestimation of the problem, leading to a less efficient treatment of the diseased flock or approach for the next flock.

Well-known examples of multiple respiratory infections are those involving mycoplasmas and respiratory viruses in chicken and turkey. A single *M. gallisepticum* or *M. synoviae* infection in chickens often results in subclinical disease. Interactions with NDV, IBV, APV, infectious laryngotracheitis or LPAIV, such as the H9N2 strain, are known to increase the severity of *M. gallisepticum* and *M. synoviae* infections (and the other way around). Combinations of more than two agents or factors usually cause even more damage. The increasing number of countries that have to deal with the LPAIV H9N2 have found that a single infection of H9N2 or in combination with *E. coli* will show itself as an infection with low-pathogenicity avian influenza. However coinfection with H9N2, *Escherichia coli* and a second virus such as IBV, perhaps in combination with a poor climate, can show itself as a respiratory disease with a much higher percentage mortality.

The virulence of each of the infectious agents involved will influence the severity of the respiratory disease. A more virulent *M. gallisepticum* strain will cause more respiratory distress than a mild strain when combined with the same IBV strain. In this respect, it has to be realized that all live respiratory viral vaccines, even the mild ones, do cause some degree of damage. Under the wrong conditions, live respiratory vaccines can increase the susceptibility to and incidence of colibacillosis or infections with *Ornithobacterium rhinotracheale*. Improper application of live vaccines, either by spray or drinking water, can result in a major part of the flock not receiving an immunizing dose of vaccine, leading to circulation of the live vaccinal virus within the flock. This can cause a 'rolling' vaccination reaction. This delays the protection and makes the flock more susceptible to RDC.

EPIDEMIOLOGY

Effects of immunosuppressive agents

Immunosuppressive agents, especially infectious bursal disease in chickens and haemorrhagic enteritis virus in turkeys, are known to increase susceptibility to respiratory infections. They also can decrease the efficacy of vaccinations or cause increased vaccine reactions. Therefore, the control and monitoring of these immunosuppressive agents are an essential factor in controlling respiratory disease.

Role of environmental factors

Environmental factors play a significant role in interacting with infectious agents in the production of respiratory disease in poultry. Environmental factors that are known to be an important component of the climate in the chicken house include atmospheric ammonia (NH_3), dust, humidity, draught and temperature. Exposure of chickens and turkeys to 10–20 ppm of NH_3 is enough to cause damage to the respiratory tract. The damage to the mucociliary system in the respiratory tract increases with higher concentrations and longer exposure times. The clearance of *E. coli* and other agents from the respiratory tract will be impaired and this will increase the risk of the flock getting air sacculitis if challenged with IBV or another pathogen.

The presence of dust in the air has a negative effect on the health of the respiratory tract for at least two reasons. The dust itself can irritate the respiratory tract but, perhaps more importantly, a significant proportion of dust consists of dried faeces. Therefore, dust contains many bacteria, including *E. coli*.

Humidity, either too high or too low, can play an important role as an additional factor for a respiratory disease. Very low humidity can have a dehydrating effect on the respiratory tract, especially in very young birds. Also the vaccination reaction after a spray application (e.g. in the hatchery) with a respiratory virus can be increased because of the dehydration of the droplets, causing a deep respiratory application of the vaccine instead of upper respiratory application. High humidity can have a negative effect on the respiratory tract also. A fast-growing chicken such as the broiler has to get rid of much heat, largely via the respiratory tract. Where humidity is high, it is more difficult to excrete the heat by breathing. In these conditions, the bird has to breathe more and harder, meaning that it inhales more dust, bacteria, irritating chemicals, etc., and that panting overcomes some of the bird's natural defences.

CONTROL

Control and prevention of RDC depends on several factors. Whatever the cause or causes of RDC, a good climate (avoiding cold and heat stress, draught, ammonia, etc.) is always essential to prevent RDC or to minimize the losses.

As RDC can be caused by many infectious agents in all kind of combinations, control and prevention of RDC needs a good diagnostic approach of the problem, which might be a combination of virology, bacteriology, molecular biology and serology. The most direct approach is sampling the birds at the beginning of the clinical signs. In prolonged cases, it can be advisable to sample birds at a later phase of the infection too. It is advisable not only to look for the most common viruses and bacteria, such as IBV and *E. coli*. Quite often, people are reluctant to look for the presence of unwanted viruses such as LPAIV strains, because of the possible consequences. If virus tended to 'die out' because it was ignored, this might be wise. However, most viruses like to be ignored, as that increases the chance of more replications of themselves in more susceptible birds. In epidemiology, this is called 'spread' and may become an 'epidemic'.

When a virus is being detected, further typing is desirable. This will help with decisions about the vaccination programme of the next flock. When the typing of the detected strain shows that it is very related to a vaccine that was used in the flock, the vaccination procedure should be checked thoroughly, as there may have been a rolling reaction due to improper vaccination procedure. It must be appreciated that the effect of mass application of live respiratory vaccines is easily underestimated. Another important issue is to check the flock with RDC for the presence of immunosuppression.

FURTHER READING

Episcope: http://www.clive.ed.ac.uk/winepiscope/

Gerstman B 2003 Epidemiology kept simple: an introduction to traditional and modern epidemiology, 2nd edn. John Wiley, New York

Thrusfield M 2007 Veterinary epidemiology, 3rd edn. Blackwell Publishing, Oxford

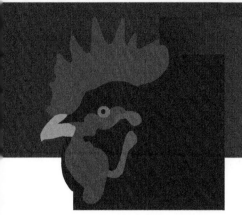

CHAPTER

42

Patrick W. Garland and
Steven Pritchard

Nutritional disorders

INTRODUCTION

There are a great variety of clinical conditions that are induced by nutritional deficiencies and imbalances. These may arise from gross deficiency in the ration supplied to poultry, antagonism between nutrients, destruction or inactivation during feed manufacture, impaired absorption or metabolic disorder that renders supply inadequate.

However, it should be noted that, with the vast improvement in knowledge of precise requirements for specific nutrients and the better characterization of feed ingredients along with the commercial availability of manufactured micronutrients, the occurrence of such disorders is now fortunately rare. The occurrence of simple deficiencies is unlikely and this makes any clinical diagnosis difficult, as the true cause is probably a complex interaction of a number of factors and nutrition may well not be the predisposing element.

A specific mineral or trace element deficiency generally produces characteristic signs, reflecting specific metabolic functions; for example, fat-soluble vitamins A and E are involved with membrane integrity; water-soluble vitamins and trace elements with enzyme systems. Very profound effects may be brought about by a deficiency of minute amounts of these nutrients at the site required.

Supplementation

It is usual to incorporate feed supplements of vitamins and trace elements to give levels permitting adequate safety margins, in order to allow for such factors as higher than average requirements or losses during manufacture (resulting from instability), i.e. 'allowance' vs 'requirement'. This has become important with the use of high temperature and dwell time processing of feed that is intended to eliminate *Salmonella*. Processing techniques introduced mainly in the mid-1990s have resulted in the use of temperatures as high as 120°C for expanded feeds and more commonly 80–85°C for 2 min. Table 42.1 shows the typical losses of vitamins to be expected

Table 42.1 Average vitamin retention after feed processing (%)		
VITAMIN	**PELLETING AT 81–85°C**	**EXPANDING AT 116–120°C**
A – beadlet	95	94
D₃ – beadlet	94	96
E – acetate	94	95
K – (MSBC)	70	52
Thiamine HCl	86	84
Riboflavin	91	87
Pyridoxine	90	90
Cobalamin	97	95
Pantothenate	91	91
Folic acid	90	89
Biotin	90	90
Niacin	91	87
Ascorbic acid	50	46
Choline chloride	98	98

MSBC, menadione sodium metabisulphite complex.

through different processing techniques, which need to be accounted for when determining supplemental levels.

Physical form

The physical form in which the mill presents the feed may be of importance with respect to feed intake, feed wastage and environmental dust pollution. Consistent physical quality is the key. Mashes should be formulated and manufactured to minimize the risk of physical separation of different particle fractions. Slight variations in nutrient intake caused in this way are of no real significance if the bird is healthy with good body reserves, because the duration of undersupply of a nutrient will be relatively short.

With pelleted or crumbed feed the bird has little opportunity to feed selectively or to supplement its diet in the event of any nutritional imbalance. This places a heavy responsibility on the diet formulator to provide adequate nutrients in the correct balance with one another. This has become further complicated by the practice of adding whole-grain cereals to compounded broiler feeds in Europe. This can lead to dilution of micronutrients and permits some selective feeding, which may be detrimental to bird performance if not carefully managed.

Antinutritional factors

Feed ingredients can act as a carrier for antinutrients (enzyme inhibitors, lectins, goitrogens, etc.), contaminant toxins (including alkaloids, mycotoxins, heavy metals, etc.) and pathogenic microorganisms. Suitable systems for raw material quality control should be in place to minimize such risks to bird health and performance, since the above can overcome the generous use of added micronutrients and lead to the clinical signs associated with a classical deficiency syndrome.

A high standard of feeding management on the part of the farmer is equally important to ensure that every bird has an adequate and consistent supply of fresh feed and water.

Enzymes

The poultry industry has come to rely on the use of exogenous enzymes in feeds to improve the nutrient digestibility of raw materials, increase energy yield from cereals, improve litter quality and reduce waste excretion. Most laying hen and meat bird rations now contain enzymes to aid digestion of nonstarch polysaccharides and improve release of phosphorus from phytate.

The benefits of these additions, either as powders added to the feed mix or liquids applied to pelleted feeds, have been considerable.

Problems of overdosing of enzymes are not reported but inconsistent addition or omission will cause problems. In the case of those enzymes targeted at carbohydrates their absence will affect energy yield and hence feed intake but more importantly there is the potential to increase digesta viscosity and faecal moisture content. Where phytases are used to increase phosphorus availability the consistent addition of the intended amount is important to prevent mineral imbalances and suboptimal phosphorus uptake.

Nutrient deficiencies

It is a matter of fact that today simple uncomplicated nutrient deficiencies are rarely encountered in the field. Experience, however, teaches us not to be complacent in the light of, for example, fatty liver and kidney syndrome (FLKS) in fast-growing broilers. Similarly, ascites and leg problems in fast-growing broiler chickens have been an issue but changes in management practice, breeding and nutrition have greatly reduced the incidence of these syndromes. Therefore it is prudent to be aware that new problems can develop.

In feeding the breeding hen, it is necessary to allow for an adequate carry-over of micronutrients into the egg and hence into the hatched chick/poult, in order to achieve maximum hatchability and chick vitality. Some vitamins (including riboflavin) are transported into the egg by means of a specific binding protein; this places a limit on the amount that it is possible to transfer into the egg naturally. Egg injection techniques are now available commercially for vaccination and some work on injecting vitamins has been conducted. The age of the breeder flock (broilers and turkeys) appears to have an influence on the efficiency of carry-over of vitamins into the egg.

Field conditions affecting hatchability do exist, which can be wrongly attributed to a vitamin deficiency, for example the depressed hatchability and defective down syndrome in broiler breeders that Whitehead et al (1993) concluded was not due to a riboflavin deficiency.

It should be borne in mind that nutritional deficiency conditions arising in the first week after hatching generally reflect the food reserves in the yolk sac, derived from the maternal diet, rather than the nature of the starter feed.

Alternative management systems

The keeping of poultry in extensive management systems and applying rules relevant to specific marketing labels such as 'free-range', 'traditional free-range', 'free-range total freedom' and 'organic' means that nutritional disorders may arise specific to these systems.

It is well established that free-range laying hens benefit from higher sodium levels in the diet in relation to the incidence of aggressive behaviour. Typically levels of 0.16–0.18% are employed, compared with cage birds where 0.14% would be used. Of increasing interest are the constraints applied in meeting organic regulations and the requirement of individual sector bodies. Potential problems arise from the limitations placed on the raw materials that can be used in these rations and the fact that the proportion of conventional materials is being progressively reduced with the aim of achieving 100% organic materials of agricultural origin. The inability to use synthetic sources of amino acids means that methionine can be marginal in organic rations, to such an extent that pecking can occur in layers or meat birds. Prevention depends upon the ability to source and use materials with better protein quality, such as potato protein or pea protein extracts. There is less safety margin in such rations and therefore prevention of other predisposing factors, such as marginal sodium, vitamins or management, is important.

A practical consideration is that the use of oils in organic rations is limited, since it must be expeller oil from organic sources. Therefore mash diets may be dusty and lead to low feed and hence nutrient intakes, thereby exacerbating marginal nutrient intakes.

Interactions

Fat-soluble vitamins are absorbed with the fat component of the diet mediated by bile salts in mixed micelles. Any factor that interferes with normal fat absorption may induce a fat-soluble-vitamin deficiency.

Antagonisms can occur between the different fat-soluble vitamins because of competition at the point of absorption. Excessive levels of an individual vitamin should therefore be avoided (see vitamin A, below). Where the dietary fat contains a high proportion of polyunsaturated fatty acids, the need for vitamin E will be increased as a result of the increased oxidation potential.

B vitamins act in the regulation of intermediary metabolism and overlapping of some of these pathways occurs. Thus, for example, choline, cobalamin and folic acid interact directly in the metabolism of methyl groups, and a deficiency in one of these vitamins can lead to an increased requirement for the others. In other cases, an excess of some vitamins can induce a deficiency of others; for example, the biotin status of the chick can be depressed by oversupplementation with a wide range of other B vitamins. Excessive choline supplementation has a similar effect on biotin requirement; in addition, high levels of choline chloride in feed supplements can significantly increase the rate of loss of other constituent vitamins during product storage.

Some vitamins can interact with amino acids where the amino acid exerts a vitamin-sparing effect, for example tryptophan with niacin and methionine with choline.

Other aspects of the diet can affect the requirements for certain vitamins involved in metabolic interconversions; for example, high dietary protein levels increase the requirements for pyridoxine, folic acid and biotin, and low-fat/high-starch diets increase the needs for thiamine and biotin.

Table 42.2 provides some vitamin information relative to poultry and gives units of measurement as well as principal commercial forms.

VITAMIN A

The term vitamin A covers a number of physiological forms (retinol, retinoic acid, retinaldehyde and retinyl ester). Retinol is the most common form in nature. It is a fat-soluble vitamin found primarily in animal products such as liver and fish oils. As a result, background levels in raw materials are generally low. Some plant materials (e.g. maize) do however contain beta carotene, which is described as 'provitamin A' and can be converted to vitamin A by the bird. Wheat-based diets are assumed to have no background vitamin A activity.

Key functions

Vitamin A is concerned with the maintenance of epithelial structure and function.

Table 42.2 | Some vitamin information relative to poultry

VITAMIN	PRINCIPAL COMMERCIAL FORM	MEASUREMENT	PRINCIPAL ACTIVITIES
A	Vitamin A acetate Vitamin A palmitate	iu	Epithelial tissue structure and function/egg production
D	D_3 (cholecalciferol)	iu	Calcium and phosphorus absorption and translocation
E	D- and DL-α-tocopherols D- and DL-α-tocopherol acetate	1 iu vitamin E = 1 mg DL-α-tocopherol acetate	Inter- and intracellular antioxidant/cell membrane integrity
K	K_1 (phytomenadione) K_3 (menadione)	No standard	Antihaemorrhagic/prothrombin
B_1	Thiamine hydrochloride Thiamine mononitrate	mg thiamine hydrochloride/kg	Enzyme systems/carbohydrate metabolism/antineuritic
B_2	Riboflavin Sodium riboflavin phosphate	mg riboflavin/kg	Enzyme systems/nutrient and cellular metabolism/production and hatchability
B_6	Pyridoxine hydrochloride	mg pyridoxine/kg	Enzyme systems/amino acid metabolism
Niacin	Nicotinic acid Nicotinamide	$mg\,kg^{-1}$	Enzyme systems/metabolism
Pantothenic acid	Sodium D-pantothenate Calcium D-pantothenate	mg D-pantothenic acid/kg	Coenzyme A/metabolism/neural pantothenate function
Biotin	Biotin	$\mu g/kg$	Epidermal maintenance/bone/scleroprotein/carboxylation enzymes, notably pyruvate carboxylase and acetyl CoA carboxylase
Folacin	Folic acid	mg folic acid/kg	Amino acid metabolism
B_{12}	Cyanocobalamin	$\mu g/kg$	Protein, carbohydrate and fat metabolism

Deficiency

Deficiency of this vitamin in isolation is unlikely, since practical allowances are generous and the bird will maintain vitamin reserves in the liver, which will cover any short-term deficit. Deficiency signs are as follows:

- Epithelial/mucous membrane metaplasia, with secondary infection, particularly of respiratory and intestinal tracts; the kidneys are affected, with impacted ureters (nutritional nephropathy) and visceral urate deposition
- Reduced production and hatchability, production ceasing before hatchability is severely affected
- Reduced appetite and growth, rough plumage
- Corneal hyperkeratosis, central and peripheral nerve lesions and hyperkeratosis of mucous membranes of mouth and oesophagus (Fig. 42.1), which is the usual pathognomonic sign.

Laboratory confirmation of deficiency is obtainable by assay of the vitamin content of liver. This is best achieved by removal of a whole liver from a freshly killed bird, the liver being stored at 4°C or below (depending on time interval) until assay. There are standard tests for determination of the vitamin A content of feeds.

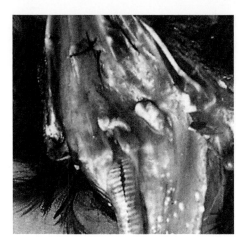

Fig. 42.1 Vitamin A deficiency. Hyperkeratosis of the exits of the mucous glands in the chicken oesophagus.

Excess

Because of the relatively low cost of this vitamin and the use on farm of vitamin preparations that are high in vitamin A, excess supplementation can occur. It has been clearly demonstrated that excess levels have interfered with absorption of vitamins E and D_3 (Whitehead 1998). This is of particular concern with young birds or those undergoing disease challenge, since a lack of vitamin E is detrimental to the immune response.

VITAMIN D

The term vitamin D covers two main forms; ergocalciferol (vitamin D_2), which is poorly utilized by poultry, and cholecalciferol (vitamin D_3). Vitamin D_3 is a fat-soluble vitamin and is only found at any appreciable level in very specific tissues such as fish liver oils. Common feed ingredients contain little or no vitamin D and the required supplement should be incorporated as cholecalciferol (vitamin D_3).

Key functions

Vitamin D, as the renal metabolite 1,25-dihydroxycholecalciferol (following initial hydroxylation in the liver to the 25-hydroxy product), has the main function of inducing the synthesis of calcium-binding proteins and of controlling intestinal absorption and blood translocation of calcium; it has similar effects, but to a much lesser extent, on phosphorus.

Deficiency

- Rachitic deformities (caused by inadequate dietary calcium, phosphorus or vitamin D3 or calcium:phosphorus imbalance) develop, especially in the legs, producing painful, hard joint swelling and lameness, abnormality being most clearly seen in the structure of the proximal tibiotarsus. The tubercula and capitula (i.e. the head) of the ribs may be enlarged and occasionally the costochondral junctions (Fig. 42.2). The bones, beak and claws become soft and pliable. Growth is retarded; feather development is poor.

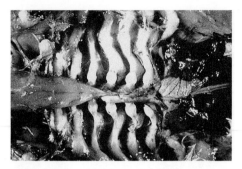

Fig. 42.2 Rickets caused by vitamin D deficiency affecting the ribs.

• In the laying bird, moderate deficiency causes osteomalacia, giving rise to brittle bones of reduced density and cortical strength (osteoporosis) – such bones are light, porous and fragile. As the deficiency progresses, eggshells become thinner, before soft shells occur and then production falls. Hatchability also suffers and embryonic abnormalities are seen. In severe deficiency, egg production stops rapidly, thereby sparing the hen from the effects of calcium deficiency.

The majority of the vitamin D_3 supplement is normally added to feed in a stabilized standard preparation with vitamin A. It is impossible, practically, to assess the vitamin D status of an animal but biological samples, such as feeds, can now be assayed by high-performance liquid chromatography (HPLC), provided that the analyst takes extreme care with extraction and separation and that there are no interfering factors present. Otherwise, a frequently used method of vitamin D determination in feedstuffs is to measure the level of vitamin A and from this to extrapolate the level of D from the standard A and D vitamin that was added. Assay of high-potency substrates (such as vitamin premixes for supplementing compounded feeds) may be carried out by several laboratory procedures.

Excess

Grossly excessive levels are toxic, leading to tissue calcium deposition. This is rarely seen in practice and there is growing interest in higher supplementation levels, as detailed below.

Additional information

In Europe the maximum permitted level in feed is limited to 3000 iu/kg for layers and 5000 iu/kg for meat birds. However recent work by Whitehead et al (2004) has questioned the validity of these levels by demonstrating that tibia breaking strength and bodyweight of 14-day-old broilers were maximized at 10 000 iu/kg. Tibial dyschondroplasia was also minimized at this higher level. Responses to vitamin D_3 appear to be strongly influenced by the relative levels of dietary calcium and digestible phosphorus.

While the typical supplement provides vitamin D_3 (cholecalciferol), there has also been growing interest in the use of vitamin D metabolites as a result of concerns over skeletal integrity and certain specific issues such as tibial dyschondroplasia. This is a condition seen in meat poultry and is characterized by the presence of uncalcified masses or 'plugs' of avascular cartilage composed of prehypertrophic chondrocytes. These develop in the proximal metaphyses, particularly of the tibiotarsi and less frequently in other bones, and appear to be caused by a slowing of the normal processes of chondrocyte differentiation. The lesion can lead to angular deformity of the tibiotarsus and may be an important contributor to lameness. Dyschondroplasia has a strong genetic component and severe lesions can be detected by radiological imaging devices in live birds and selected against.

Experimentally complete prevention of tibial dyschondroplasia by including 1,25-dihydroxyvitamin D has been reported and 1-hydroxyvitamin D appears effective at similar dose levels of $5 \mu g/kg$. Because of the strong interaction of these metabolites with dietary calcium there is a risk of hypercalcaemia and growth depression when higher concentrations of both nutrients occur. As a result of these difficulties, commercial development work has concentrated on 25-hydroxyvitamin D_3. This metabolite has a much higher safety margin and is being successfully used in combination with cholecalciferol although the results are less consistent than with 1,25-dihydroxyvitamin D (Whitehead 2000a).

Chapter 40 contains further information on skeletal disorders.

VITAMIN E

The term vitamin E covers a range of tocopherols and tocotrienols that all have vitamin E activity. The key form for poultry is the α-tocopherol. Like A and D, vitamin E is a fat-soluble vitamin that is quite widely distributed in plant materials such as cereal germs, most oilseeds and leafy plants. These naturally occurring tocopherols are easily oxidized in air, or by peroxides of polyunsaturated fatty acids. Hence, the amount of fat or oil (particularly polyunsaturated fatty acids) present in feed plays a part in determining the amount of vitamin E that should be included. Vitamin E may be described as a naturally occurring antioxidant. Feed is normally supplemented with synthetically produced DL-α-tocopherol acetate but recent work by Lauzon et al (2006) has shown that in excess of 50% of supplementary vitamin E can be excreted. This has led to interest both in new commercial synthetic forms and the use of naturally extracted E.

Key functions

Vitamin E has several different, though related functions; most important is as an inter- and intracellular antioxidant, preventing oxidation of unsaturated lipids within cells; deficiency allows abnormal formation or accumulation of excessive lipid hydroperoxides, with resulting cell tissue damage. The more active the cell, the more lipid is required for activity and the greater the risk of damage. This protective role ensures erythrocyte stability and capillary blood vessel integrity. In this antioxidant role vitamin E cannot be considered in isolation because there is a close working relationship between vitamin E and selenium in their functions within tissues.

There are a range of other functions, in many of which the mode of action is unclear – among them regulation of the pituitary–midbrain system (thus influencing thyroid and adrenal hormone output), nucleic acid metabolism, involvement in fertility and prevention of degenerative change in muscle and liver.

Deficiency

Vitamin E occurs in most body tissues, with no major storage sites and, although blood level varies with recent feed absorption, it is a reasonable indicator of body status. Inadequate vitamin E levels give rise to several conditions in poultry, which may occur separately or together depending on age, degree of deficiency and other factors.

The importance of the biological function of vitamin E is demonstrated by the several syndromes that may appear in its absence. As a fat-soluble intracellular antioxidant, a primary function of tocopherol is a protective effect on cell membranes; hence, deficiency results in damage to

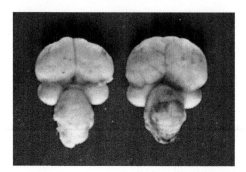

Fig. 42.3 Vitamin E deficiency. Nutritional encephalomalacia. Left: normal; right: cerebellar haemorrhages.

blood vessels and changes in capillary permeability. Deficiency in breeders may give rise to early embryonic mortality associated with vascular lesions (usually around day 4 of incubation).

In young growing birds deficiency conditions include encephalomalacia, exudative diathesis and nutritional muscular dystrophy. However, the role of vitamin E in a bird's immune status is probably more important since it has been shown that responses in this area occur at much higher concentrations of E than are required to eliminate classical deficiency symptoms.

Encephalomalacia (crazy chick disease)

Encephalomalacia (Fig. 42.3) is seen in birds (usually in good condition) up to the age of 5 weeks or so (commonly weeks 2 and 3). Clinical signs are of muscular weakness, progressive ataxia with frequent falling, spasmodic violent incoordination, head retraction and/or torticollis, paralysis and death.

Vascular lesions give rise to oedema and petechial and larger haemorrhages in the cerebellum, with ensuing neurone degeneration. Such gross lesions, seen in fresh brains in association with appropriate clinical signs and history, are virtually pathognomonic. That the cerebellum constitutes the target organ, while the cerebrum is not affected, is perhaps related to increased polyunsaturated fatty acid levels, which appear to occur in the second and third weeks in the cerebellum but not in the cerebrum.

On gross examination it may be necessary to examine numerous birds for typical 'diagnostic' cerebellar lesions to be found.

The condition is prevented by adequate vitamin E; selenium is said to have some prophylactic effect. The usual treatment is vitamin E given via drinking water.

Exudative diathesis

Capillary wall lesions lead to increased vascular permeability, with resulting blood and plasma leakage; this accumulates subcutaneously, particularly over the breast and under the wings, also intermuscularly and in the pericardial sac.

The condition is prevented by and responsive to vitamin E and selenium. The usual treatment is vitamin E via drinking water.

Nutritional muscular dystrophy

Nutritional muscular dystrophy frequently occurs with exudative diathesis and tends to occur when vitamin E deficiency is accompanied by a deficiency of sulphur-containing amino acids (methionine and cysteine) in chicks, turkey poults and ducklings.

Microthrombosis of arterioles and smaller capillaries causes occlusion, which gives rise to degeneration and necrosis of muscle fibres, seen as pale streaks mainly in breast and thigh muscles (hence the reference to white muscle disease).

Prevention and treatment are by vitamin E supply, as previously described.

VITAMIN K

The antihaemorrhagic vitamin K occurs in a number of forms as derivatives of naphthoquinone. The most important, vitamin K_1, is present in green plants, fruits and liver oils; vitamin K_2 is present in animal and microbial materials. The essential structure in all vitamin K analogues is menadione (known also as vitamin K_3), which has vitamin K activity. Vitamin K_3 is qualitatively different in that it is not an antagonist of the anticoagulant drugs (e.g. dicoumarol, warfarin) and is water-soluble, whereas vitamins K_1 and K_2 are fat-soluble.

Vitamin K_3 or menadione acts as a provitamin and must be converted in the liver to menaquinone before it can exert a biological effect; however, since it is more readily manufactured than the other forms it is the basis for most commercial preparations. The various forms used tend to incorporate a bisulphite substituent and this confers greater potency than menadione. The forms used include menadione sodium bisulphite (MSB), menadione sodium bisulphite complex (MSBC), menadione dimethylpyrimidol bisulphite (MPB) and menadione nicotinamide bisulphite (MNB). These forms are also more stable, which is an important factor when considering feed processing conditions, as shown in Table 42.1. Even then there are considerable losses, which have to be accommodated for by higher allowances.

Key function

Vitamin K is indispensable for blood coagulation, and participates in prothrombin formation. It also plays a role in calcium metabolism. Vitamin-K-dependent proteins are found in bones, shell gland and eggshell.

Deficiency

Microbial synthesis occurs in the caecum and large intestine and as a result deficiency is very rare, especially in adult birds, although the supply of vitamin derived from microbial synthesis is thought only to be of benefit if faeces are consumed.
- Chicks can exhibit delayed blood clotting as a result of deficiency.
- Oral administration of antibacterial drugs such as sulfaquinoxaline and some other sulpha drugs are stated to be antagonistic to vitamin K activity.

The only real measurement of activity is the biological response in prothrombin production (by chick assay).

VITAMIN B₁ (THIAMINE)

The name is derived from the thiazole and pyrimidine rings in the structure; the synonym 'aneurin' relates to antineuritic properties, reflecting its important function in carbohydrate metabolism (via several enzyme systems).

Vitamin B_1 is present in almost all living tissues, plant and animal. Brewers yeast and cereal germs are good sources. Synthetically produced B_1 is usually in the form of thiamin hydrochloride or mononitrate.

Key function

Carbohydrate metabolism.

Deficiency

Deficiency signs in poultry are not seen in the field, though theoretically it is possible that the condition could occur in the presence of thiamine-splitting enzymes (thiaminases) in feed ingredients such as fishmeal.

- A deficiency will impair carbohydrate metabolism due to the role that thiamine plays as a cofactor and therefore a reduction in energy availability will arise, thereby affecting performance.
- A number of factors will influence the thiamine status of birds: high temperatures increase requirement and it has been shown that the level required to prevent polyneuritis is three times higher at $32°C$ than at $21°C$.
- The anticoccidial amprolium blocks thiamine metabolism while coccidia are competitors for thiamine.
- In experimentally induced deficiency the signs are dramatic: loss of appetite and growth, weakness, polyneuritis, opisthotonos and paralysis.

There are numerous methods of assay; measurement in practice is by weight unit (mg), although an international unit is defined. Thiamine is broken down in hot, humid conditions; breakdown is accelerated by high pH.

VITAMIN B2 (RIBOFLAVIN)

Historically known by various names, such as lactoflavin and ovoflavin, riboflavin is in fact a single compound that consists of a ribose sugar unit attached to a three-ring flavin structure.

Milk and yeast products are good sources of vitamin B_2. However, these are not commonly used as raw materials in poultry feeds and therefore supplementation with synthetic vitamin B_2 is required.

Key function

Present in virtually all living cells, vitamin B_2 derivatives function in several enzyme systems as coenzymes that unite with specific protein elements to form flavoprotein enzymes, involved in oxidation reduction, dehydrogenation, the metabolism of carbohydrate, amino acid and fat, and the regulation of cellular metabolism. Hence, the vitamin is essential for growth and health.

Deficiency

The vitamin is synthesized at sites of microbial activity in the gut of the adult bird (not in the young chick) but, as these sites are the caecum and large intestine, they are beyond the specific absorption site in the small intestine – hence, coprophagy appears to be a beneficial behaviour.

Following absorption, riboflavin is transported to various tissues for elaboration into enzymes and excess is excreted via the kidneys. The vitamin is not stored in the body but is stored in eggs, particularly the yolk. Absence of body storage means that daily provision in feed is required.

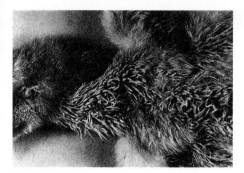

Fig. 42.4 'Clubbed down' in an embryo affected with vitamin B₂ deficiency.

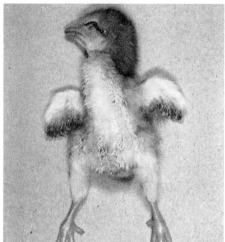

Fig. 42.5 Riboflavin deficiency – clubbed down.

The use of high-energy poultry diets, with ingredients low in vitamin B_2, necessitates additional feed supplementation. The appearance of signs of vitamin B_2 deficiency indicates a lack of available riboflavin but does not always necessarily imply inadequate feed supply of the vitamin, as antagonists (e.g. mycotoxins, notably aflatoxin) may interfere with absorption or body transport (as also may nonavailability of carrier protein); in certain poultry a recessive gene has been implicated in antagonism.

For quantitative determination of riboflavin in feed or tissue, direct fluorometry may be used. For tissue, concentration in erythrocytes is the most sensitive indicator. Recently, the measurement of a flavin-dependent enzyme (erythrocyte glutathione reductase, EGR) has been utilized as an indicator of riboflavin status.

In general terms, a lowered vitamin B_2 supply will lead to reduced growth rate and nonspecific conditions, such as dermatitis and nervous disorders, but the signs of severe deficiency in poultry depend on age.

Breeding poultry, including game birds, are particularly susceptible to marginal levels of riboflavin, which is required for optimum hatchability. Reduced egg production occurs in severe deficiency but with marginally low deficiency there is greatly reduced hatchability, with embryonic death peaks in mid and late incubation (dead-in-shell). Hatched chicks may be dwarfed and oedematous, show 'clubbed down' (Fig. 42.4), poor feathering and leg paralysis, often with inward curling of the toes and resting on the hocks (the so-called 'curled toe paralysis' and with similar degenerative changes in nerve trunks to those found in older chicks with 'curled toe') (Figs 42.5 and 42.6).

Taken together, curled toe paralysis and clubbed down are diagnostic of lack of available riboflavin in the yolk of the incubated egg.

Clubbed down is produced by a failure of the feathers to rupture their sheaths, producing a club shape. It should be noted that, even at acceptable hatchability levels, a small percentage of dead-in-shell chicks may be seen with clubbed down (and other 'nutritional' signs) not necessarily associated with breeder flock riboflavin deficiency. The condition is more often seen in embryos with black down, as vitamin B_2 is required for melanin production. Clubbed down may sometimes be seen in normal chicks from a normal hatch.

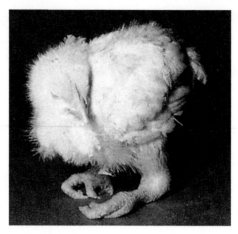

Fig. 42.6 Riboflavin deficiency – curled toe paralysis.

There is a field condition giving rise to depressed hatchability and a defective down syndrome in chicks that is not attributable to a dietary or metabolic lack of riboflavin (Whitehead et al 1993). The cause is unknown but field incidences have been severe with no response to additional supplementary riboflavin provided via water.

Curled toe paralysis may be seen in chicks and poults (sometimes around 10–14 days of age) if their feed has been low in available riboflavin. Birds may be unable to rise from their hocks (but remain alert), the legs being outstretched, with flaccid paralysis and frequently incurling of the toes, which is not maintained after death. The sciatic (and brachial) nerves are swollen and discoloured, histologically showing Schwann cell proliferation. Being reluctant or unable to move to feed, the bird's head, wings and tail feathers droop (in some chicks these may be the first signs observed); growth retardation, recumbency, emaciation and death follow. As indicated, signs may vary, some birds showing more severe paralysis without marked curling of the toes.

If nerve damage has not been irreversible, response to a potent riboflavin source (e.g. autolysed yeast or sodium riboflavin phosphate) is rapid. Very mild cases may recover without treatment if there is access to faeces.

(Note: curled toe paralysis should not be confused with the so-called crooked toe deformity associated with brooding under electric infrared lamps, in which the bird walks with toes turned out because of malformation of distal metatarsals and phalanges.)

VITAMIN B$_6$ (PYRIDOXINE)

There are three compounds that have vitamin B$_6$ activity: pyridoxine, pyridoxal and pyridoxamine. Each of these has similar biological activity, although pyridoxine is the most stable form. Sources include red meat and tissue, egg yolk, yeast and cereals.

Key function

Vitamin B$_6$ is involved in amino acid metabolism via numerous enzymes.

Deficiency

There are no pathognomonic signs and a clear-cut deficiency syndrome is not recognized in the field. Because of the multiplicity of metabolic functions, wide-ranging effects may be produced in deficiency, including reduced appetite, growth and production, deficient skin and plumage, anaemia, demyelination, weakness, paresis and chondrodystrophy.

Analytical detection of vitamin B_6 is very difficult.

NIACIN

Niacin (sometimes called vitamin B_3) comprises nicotinic acid and nicotinamide, both derived from pyridine. Appreciable quantities of this vitamin occur in cereals but are in a bound form and poorly utilized.

Key function

Niacin in its nicotinamide form is a critical part of the coenzymes involved in the metabolism of proteins, fats and carbohydrates.

Deficiency

Niacin can be synthesized by microbial action in the caecum and large intestine but, as there is little absorption beyond this level, this is of limited value. In avian tissues a certain amount is synthesized from tryptophan.

Many B complex vitamins work closely together in metabolism, either having a sparing action or increasing requirement, depending on individual functions. Vitamins B_1 and B_2, pantothenic acid, folic acid and vitamin B_{12} have a sparing and synergistic action on niacin, both in alleviating deficiency and in carbohydrate metabolism. In addition, vitamins B_1, B_2 and B_6 are required for conversion of tryptophan to niacin and a shortage of any of these can prevent it.

In deficiency there is loss of appetite, poor growth, skin and feather disorders, inflammation of the mucous membranes of the alimentary tract and nervous degeneration (i.e. a variety of nonspecific abnormalities). However, in young growing birds, niacin is one of the primary nutritional deficiencies (along with manganese, zinc, choline, biotin, folic acid and pyridoxine) that can cause chondrodystrophy. This is a generalized disorder of the epiphyseal growth plates of long bones that impairs linear growth but allows normal appositional growth and mineralization. This gives rise to bowing of the rapidly growing long bones with shortened tibiotarsal bones, enlarged hocks and slipped gastrocnemius tendon in severe cases. There are characteristic changes in the growth plates (see Ch. 40).

There has been some commercial interest in the strategic use of high levels of niacin as a cure for feather pecking in free-range layer flocks in the UK. Practical experience has been inconsistent in this regard and this is supported by the work of Hansen (1976), where high supplemental levels failed to prevent hysteria developing in white Leghorn hens. Responses to nicotinic acid by birds under stress conditions have however been recorded and therefore the requirement for physical performance appears to be greater when adverse conditions prevail.

PANTOTHENIC ACID

Pantothenic acid has been referred to as vitamin B_5 (USA) and also as the 'chick antidermatitis factor'. Pantothenic acid is an unstable hygroscopic oil and is widely distributed in plant and animal tissues.

Key function

Pantothenic acid is an essential part of coenzyme A (CoA), a vital element of energy and fatty acid metabolism, the citric acid cycle, antibody formation and neural function (via acetylcholine) and a precursor of cholesterol and thus of steroid hormones.

Deficiency

As with most B group vitamins, deficiency leads to loss of appetite and reduced growth; severe deficiency leads to dermatitis, with inflammatory changes in the corners of the beak and the eyelids, vent and feet, depigmentation, and roughening and loss of feathers.

Deficiency in breeder feed leads to lowered egg production and impaired hatchability, with embryo death peaks in early, mid or late incubation, depending on the extent of deficiency. Embryos are oedematous and haemorrhagic, those which hatch being stunted and weak. The above signs have all been determined experimentally – it would appear that pantothenic acid deficiency in poultry is rarely if ever seen as a clinical condition in the field.

Poultry do not benefit from its bacterial synthesis in the intestine.

Copper is the only common feed microingredient to antagonize pantothenic acid activity, affecting the rate of production or function of CoA.

There is no satisfactory method of determining body status of the vitamin: microbiological methods are used for feed assay, which is imprecise and with a wide variation between sample values, even from the same feed.

BIOTIN

Sometimes called vitamin H, biotin has a double ring structure with a number of isomers. The D isomer is the biologically active form. Most feed components contain biotin but much is organically bound and biologically unavailable. Such availability of biotin to poultry varies very widely between raw material feed ingredients; for example, from maize it is 100%, from wheat, 5%. The biotin molecule is sensitive to heat.

Key function

In general, biotin is essential for growth, food utilization, epidermal tissue maintenance, bone development and reproduction.

It is a cofactor for various carboxylation enzymes, two of the most important being pyruvate carboxylase (gluconeogenesis) and acetyl CoA carboxylase (lipogenesis), i.e. biotin is essential in carbohydrate and lipid metabolism, as well as in protein synthesis, where, via effects on RNA formation, it is particularly important in the control of scleroproteins (hard proteins such as keratin).

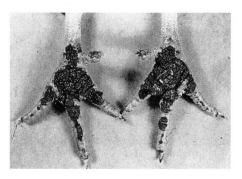

Fig. 42.7 Biotin deficiency – severely affected feet.

Deficiency

In poultry, biotin deficiency leads clinically to reduced growth, epidermal and sometimes bone lesions and, at the biochemical level, reduced biotin-dependent enzyme activity. The complete biochemical role is not fully understood.

Requirement of biotin may be correlated with the metabolic activity of tissues or sometimes of the whole animal. It may be increased for feather, skin and claw replacement, for high egg production and for optimum broiler growth.

Biotin is synthesized by microorganisms in the caecum and large intestine but this source (by coprophagy) is inadequate, supplying only up to about 10% of a growing bird's requirement and making an insignificant contribution to the breeder.

In addition, antagonists or interfering substances (biotin binders), including avidin (from egg albumen), streptavidin (from streptomycin moulds), peroxidizing fats, mycotoxins (notably aflatoxin) and possibly metabolic products from, or tissue damage by, *Mycoplasma meleagridis*, as in the TS65 (turkey syndrome 1965) condition in turkeys, cause signs consistent with biotin deficiency.

It is very difficult to determine accurately the biotin content of feeds, both because the amounts are very small and also because of the question of availability. Analysis is by bioassay and the typical range of results is of the order of 30–150%. In poultry, the liver level of biotin appears to be a good indicator of intake, as does blood, where analysis of the pyruvate carboxylase present is closely correlated to biotin supply in feed.

In growing chickens and turkeys the first signs of biotin deficiency occur in epidermal tissues. There is impaired feathering, periocular dermatitis, encrustations and fissures in the angles of the beak and eyelids and on the foot pads and toes (Fig. 42.7). Severe deficiency leads to growth depression, dry, sometimes villous, encrusted, fissured, haemorrhagic skin on the feet, notably the plantar surface, poor feathering, deformed 'parrot' beak and, sometimes, bone abnormality (chondrodystrophy), leading to shortened, bowed legs with enlarged hocks. High doses of supplemental biotin have recently been used as a means of reducing footpad dermatitis (Mayne 2005), although results are not consistent.

The occurrence and age incidence of this condition in the young bird, due to biotin deficiency, may be influenced by the biotin level in the egg (which in turn is influenced by the dietary status of the hen), high levels having an ameliorating or delaying effect.

Dietary biotin content is not considered to be important in nutrition for egg production but in breeder chickens and turkeys moderate deficiency will lead to impaired hatchability, with malformation of the embryonic skeleton (shortened and deformed lower leg and wing bones) and parrot beak. Biotin present in the egg (principally the yolk) is fundamental to hatchability and chick viability, these parameters improving with higher levels in the egg.

FLKS is a metabolic disorder causing death of young broilers (and sometimes layer pullets) commonly 10–30 days of age. FLKS is a condition that is described as biotin responsive, rather than one of uncomplicated biotin deficiency. It is usually associated with diets that have marginal levels of biotin and there may be no evidence of the signs of true biotin deficiency, as previously described. The syndrome is triggered by environmental factors rather than by nutrition.

FLKS arises from a failure of hepatic gluconeogenesis (i.e. the metabolic synthesis of glucose) and results in extensive fatty infiltration of body tissues, with enlarged liver, kidneys and heart but with no inflammatory or degenerative changes. Decreased hepatic gluconeogenesis caused by decreased pyruvate carboxylase activity leads to severe hypoglycaemia. Biotin is a cofactor for both pyruvate carboxylase (gluconeogenesis) and acetyl CoA carboxylase (lipogenesis). High-protein, high-fat feed decreases the need for lipogenesis (and hence for biotin by acetyl CoA carboxylase), so that biotin is available for pyruvate carboxylase and gluconeogenesis (acetyl CoA carboxylase is thought to have greater access to biotin than pyruvate carboxylase), which may be adequate unless the bird is stressed. However, on low-fat feed there may be insufficient biotin for both the enzymes and so, if normal feed intake is interrupted for even a short period of time, hypoglycaemia ensues and this is exacerbated by the very low glycogen reserves of the young chick. Following hypoglycaemia there is damage to the nervous system and death. As a response to low blood glucose, mobilization of free fatty acids occurs, with lipid infiltration into tissue.

The amount of biotin required for prevention of FLKS may be greater than that required for maximum growth rate. The condition can involve an interaction of nutritional, environmental, stress and maternal factors, which may act in the following way:

- **Biotin**: the single most important nutritional factor
- **Fat and protein**: high levels offer protection by depressing the need for lipogenesis (acetyl CoA carboxylase, which more readily sequesters biotin than pyruvate carboxylase); decreased lipogenesis means more biotin available for pyruvate carboxylase
- **Other vitamins**: elevated levels increase the incidence of FLKS
- **Pelleted feed**: more rapid growth occurs than with mash feed
- **Floor rearing**: faecal biotin is available; not so on wire floors (e.g. in cages)
- **Starvation and stress**: deplete glycogen (glucose) reserve
- **Age and biotin status of parent**: eggs from older hens have more biotin
- **Other diseases**: cause stress and/or depress intestinal absorption.

Clinical signs are of sudden onset, with well-grown birds becoming lethargic, aphagic and recumbent. Mortality may range from below 5% up to 30%.

Post-mortem findings are enlarged, pale, fat-infiltrated liver and kidneys, pink adipose tissue (due to capillary congestion) and often blackish fluid (due to blood content) in the crop and intestinal tract. The pallor of the liver and kidneys results from the presence of excessive amounts of fat (two to five times normal). This is mostly triglyceride with a high palmitoleic acid content. In the liver it accumulates in the intercellular spaces as well as in the hepatocytes but is not usually accompanied by disorganization of the cell contents or by degenerative or inflammatory changes. Large amounts of fat are deposited in the epithelial cells of the proximal convoluted tubules, causing swelling of the tubules and compression of renal structures. There are degenerative lesions in the tubules and these, together with the very conspicuous amounts of fat, are diagnostic. Fatty infiltration is widespread but less marked in other tissues, including cardiac and skeletal muscle and the central nervous system.

Inadequate biotin can therefore have two very different manifestations in young chickens: clinical skin and bone lesions or FLKS. The balance between these two forms is determined by the balance between the metabolic needs for different biotin-dependent enzymes. This balance is dependent in turn upon the dietary content of other nutrients, principally protein and fat.

FOLACIN (FOLIC ACID)

Several related compounds (pteroylglutamic acids) with similar activity in amino acid metabolism are grouped under this heading. Folic acid occurs in nature chiefly as a conjugate in virtually all living cells and is particularly abundant in green leaves.

Key function

The vitamin acts as a coenzyme carrying single carbon units, such as the methyl group, in many biochemical reactions, including the synthesis of specific amino acids (e.g. threonine, histidine, choline, purines) and is therefore required for nucleic acid synthesis and cell mitosis.

The molecule contains *para*-aminobenzoic acid (PABA), which few microorganisms can synthesize but, given supplies of PABA, caecal and colonic bacteria may do so, although there are doubts concerning efficacy and absorption. There is a close relationship between folacin and vitamin B_{12}, both being involved in the transfer of one-carbon groups.

Deficiency

As with other B group vitamins, reduced folic acid intake leads to nonspecific conditions, such as poor appetite and growth, diarrhoea, etc. More specifically, with greater deficiency a severe macrocytic megaloblastic anaemia develops caused by reduced erythrocyte formation; growth ceases and defective feather development and pigmentation occur. Leg deformities appear, due to chondrodystrophy, a generalized disorder of the growth plates of long bones, leading to shortened, bowed tibiotarsals and enlarged hock joints, with slipped tendon in more severe deformity. Folic acid is one of the numerous nutrients a deficiency of which may lead to this condition.

In addition, cervical paralysis may occur in turkey poults and young broiler birds; extreme light sensitivity has been reported in goslings. In each case these have been accompanied by whitish diarrhoea.

In breeding birds, production and hatchability are reduced and embryonic mortality increases. In slight deficiency, embryos may be of normal appearance but die soon after pipping. Severe depletion leads to short, bent tibiotarsus and, to a lesser degree, tarsometatarsus; syndactyly (fused claws) and parrot beak may also occur in embryos.

Several compounds interfere with the synthesis or metabolism of folacin, sulphonamides being accepted by many organisms as PABA alternatives. Thus, folic acid biosynthesis and bacterial growth are inhibited, one of the principal modes of action of sulphonamides.

Liver and blood serum levels of folate have been used to assay vitamin status by biochemical methods that are also used for feeds, although HPLC techniques are now more commonly used. However, while improved methods of folate extraction have been developed, these are not yet accepted as analytical standards. As with biotin, therefore, the range of values to be expected in feed assays is wide, 30–150%.

VITAMIN B$_{12}$

With the most complex structure of all the vitamins, the most important part of vitamin B$_{12}$ is cyanocobalamin. Vitamin B$_{12}$ is generally only found in ingredients of animal origin such as meat and fish meals.

Key function

Vitamin B$_{12}$ is involved in the metabolism of protein, carbohydrate and fat, and physiologically closely associated in this with folic acid.

Deficiency

In poultry the main importance of vitamin B$_{12}$ relates to embryonic death and hatchability. If laying birds are deficient, hatchability may drop to zero in about 6 weeks; mortality in chick embryos is likely, for the most part, to peak around 16–18 days with malposition, myoatrophy and chondrodystrophy. Embryos are oedematous and haemorrhagic, with an irregularly shaped heart. Chicks will show poor growth, feed conversion and feathering.

It is exceedingly difficult to make an accurate assessment of the vitamin B$_{12}$ status of an animal – the most accurate assay methods are biochemical, based on test microorganisms. Results are usually quoted as µg/kg feed or µg/100 mL blood.

CHOLINE

Choline forms part of the actual cell structure (in lecithins) and is sometimes classed as an accessory food substance rather than as a vitamin; choline may be synthesized in the liver and is required in considerably greater quantities than the other vitamins. It is occasionally referred to as vitamin B$_4$ or B$_7$. Most feed ingredients contain some choline. Fishmeal, soya and cereals are good sources but bioavailability is thought to be lower in vegetable materials than ingredients of animal origin; because of this, diets for growing and breeding birds are generally supplemented with choline chloride. In maize diets levels of supplementation need to be increased because background levels are approximately half that found in wheat.

Key function

Choline has a number of key functions:
- It forms part of various phospholipids (e.g. lecithin), which have essential roles in fat metabolism and cartilage structure
- In nerve transmission as acetylcholine
- As a methyl group donor (e.g. required to convert homocysteine to methionine for protein synthesis).

In this last role choline is first converted to betaine and as a result there has been interest in the replacement of choline supplements with betaine as a more efficient provider of methyl groups. Betaine cannot, however, totally replace choline in its other roles in metabolism.

Deficiency

The main signs of deficiency are as follows:
- Reduced growth rate
- Reduced hatchability in breeders
- Chondrodystrophy, although this is not a specific deficiency sign as a number of other nutrients are associated with this condition
- Increased fat deposition in the liver, leading to fatty liver.

VITAMIN C

Under normal conditions vitamin C (ascorbic acid) is not required by poultry as they are able to synthesize it directly themselves. However, there has been interest in the use of this vitamin in stress situations and in particular at high temperatures, when normal synthesis is believed to be inadequate. Whitehead & Keller (2003) thoroughly reviewed both scientific and practical studies, confirming positive but variable results. The commercial availability of both protected, heat-stable and standard forms has led to increased usage in the field.

CALCIUM AND PHOSPHORUS

About 99% of body calcium and 80% of the phosphorus are present in the skeleton, mainly as calcium hydroxyphosphate, which not only gives bones their mechanical strength but also acts as a mineral reserve. Calcium carbonate is the major constituent of eggshells. Calcium and phosphate have important functions as electrolytes in body fluids, calcium ions activating several hydrolytic enzymes and acting in nerve cell excitation, neuromuscular transmission, muscular contraction and blood clotting. Phosphate is a component of nucleic acids, phospholipids and certain proteins and coenzymes, as well as part of acid–base balance and other biochemical processes, such as metabolic energy transfer, protein synthesis and carbohydrate metabolism. Except for animal products (e.g. meat and/or bonemeal and fishmeal), the raw material ingredients of poultry feeds are low in calcium; hence, supplementation (e.g. with limestone) is included. Phosphate is mainly present in cereals and other plant products, largely as phytate (i.e. bound by phytic acid) and is poorly utilized. Phytate will also bind other minerals strongly, making them unavailable. Phosphorus in animal byproducts is almost completely available but plant phosphorus has a low biological availability for poultry, with only a minor part of the total phosphorus present being inorganic and thus fully available to birds. The majority, some 60–70%, is in the phytate form.

There is a lack of phytase in the avian intestine, especially in young chicks, but phytase is present in some grains. For these reasons, poultry feeds require supplementation with phosphate, although the use of supplementary phytase enzyme is becoming widespread in layer, broiler and turkey rations. This has reduced the reliance upon mineral phosphate in the diet, since a greater proportion of phytate phosphorus is utilized by the bird. A consequence of this is that total phosphorus levels in diets are lower than would be expected where a ration is not supplemented by enzyme, and this should be borne in mind when reviewing diet analytical data.

Some commercial phytase enzymes are heat-labile and should only be used where heat treatment of feed is not carried out, or they must be applied after the product has been processed.

Heat-stable products have been developed in recent years and will tolerate temperatures up to 80–85°C; beyond this they are affected and the same precautions should be applied.

It is not so much the absolute levels of calcium or phosphorus that are important but the relationship between them. Historically the ratio for growing birds was in the range of 1.8–2.0:1. This has progressed to 2.2:1 and now there is evidence to suggest that, for the fastest-growing strains of broiler chicken, wider ratios may be appropriate in the starter ration to avoid abnormal bone growth plates and hence tibial dyschondroplasia (Whitehead 2000b). A minimum 1.00% calcium and 0.45% available phosphorus may now be expected for the starter period. There is considerable debate about the phosphorus availability of individual feeding stuffs and there is not a good common database used by feed formulators within geographical regions. This means that individual companies will have developed their own database in this regard. Add to this the increasing use of phytase and it can be seen that interpretation of feed assays will be difficult without dialogue with those responsible for the ration formulation.

There are numerous interactions or interrelationships between the major mineral elements, i.e. calcium, phosphorus, magnesium, sodium and potassium; certain bone abnormalities (e.g. tibial dyschondroplasia) may be partly implicated in these relationships.

If a deficiency of either mineral occurs in a growing bird, rickets will be the consequence; the growth plate lesions seen will depend upon which is lacking. Also, the severity of the lesions will depend on the degree of deficiency and the amount of the other mineral present, since excess of one will increase the severity of deficiency of the other. Therefore hypocalcaemic or hypophosphataemic rickets will be more severe when diet phosphorus or calcium levels, respectively, are in excess.

Even when adequate calcium and phosphorus, in the correct ratio, is fed there can be instances of rickets due to metabolic disturbances or malabsorption arising from disease. Field experience has shown that on broiler farms where better than average physical performance is the norm there is an increased risk of rickets-like signs. The same feed used elsewhere has no adverse effect. In these cases water supplementation with vitamin D may help, as may the use of a vitamin D metabolite in the feed, but more probably a review of mineral supply is required. A change in management to achieve slower initial growth rates has also been shown to be effective in preventing the occurrence of these problems.

In mature birds where the growth plates have calcified, the skeletal abnormality arising from a deficiency of either calcium or phosphorus will be osteomalacia, leading to osteoporosis.

An early sign of calcium deficiency in the laying hen is the production of thin or soft-shelled eggs, which is typically noted as an increased incidence of second-quality eggs. However this alone is not definitive since the predominant causes of shell quality problems are disease- and stress-related.

Cage layer fatigue is seen in caged hens that are producing well, in fair bodily condition, and suddenly become recumbent (sometimes paralysed) with legs extended. The bones are brittle, with thin cortices; ribs and sternum are frequently deformed and skeletal fractures are common. Spinal compression is the cause of the paralysis. These problems are attributable to osteoporosis, which arises from a generalized loss of cancellous bone throughout the skeleton. During egg laying, there is a continual turnover of medullary bone, with resorption of existing bone and formation of new bone. However, cancellous bone cannot be formed while hens are in lay and the continuing processes of bone resorption mean that the amounts of cancellous bone decline during the laying period. The increased time during which modern strains of hen are continuously in lay leads to older hens becoming severely depleted in amounts of structural bone and developing osteoporosis. The relative inactivity of caged birds accelerates these processes. Giving birds more exercise can considerably improve bone quality. Nutrition, in contrast, is relatively ineffective in preventing osteoporosis, although poor nutrition such as deficiencies of calcium, phosphorus or vitamin D can accelerate the onset of osteoporosis.

Excess levels of phosphorus are detrimental to eggshell strength, so this mineral is reduced in rations as lay progresses. Early use of low-phosphorus diets will increase bone fragility in later lay and a careful balance is needed to optimize shell strength without compromising skeletal strength and hence welfare.

Excess calcium in the feed of young, growing birds (e.g. broilers or young pullets) will give rise to nephropathy. Feeding pullets on layer rations (i.e. about 4% calcium instead of about 0.8%) more than 10 days before the onset of lay is likely to cause problems: lesions arising are renal fibrosis, atrophy and failure, together with visceral gout.

SODIUM CHLORIDE

Sodium and chloride ions in the body perform vital functions in the maintenance of osmotic pressure, water and acid–base balance. The sodium ion is the principal cation of extracellular fluid and is involved in metabolite transfer across membranes and nerve impulse transmission. Chloride is a component of intra- and extracellular fluids and occurs as hydrochloric acid in proventricular gastric secretions. Deficiencies of these ions therefore produce widespread disturbances in cellular function and water distribution. Depending on the degree of shortfall, signs resulting will include retarded growth, reduced egg production, dehydration, neuromuscular dysfunction and death.

Poultry feeds must be supplemented to meet sodium requirements and this is usually done by adding common salt (sodium chloride) and/or sodium bicarbonate. Formulation for poultry is to a minimum sodium level of around 0.15–0.2%, the minimum requirement being about 0.12%. Below this level (e.g. at 0.10%), broiler chicks fail to grow optimally. In controlled environment housing it is necessary to maintain constant dietary levels of sodium and chloride, since variations will result in changes in water consumption that may lead to wet litter if the ventilation management is not altered quickly enough to accommodate the additional moisture in the atmosphere.

In commercial layer feeds the balance between potassium, sodium and chloride ions is very important in determining optimum egg-laying performance and also shell formation and quality. The bicarbonate ion is extremely important for the latter, both in its interaction with phosphorus (permitting mobilization and excretion of excess) and also in its role in blood pH control. Hence, today some sodium contribution to layer feed may come from sodium bicarbonate; similarly it is also used to optimize the electrolyte balance in broiler feeds.

Deprivation of sodium in laying hens causes an abrupt fall in egg production but, if the deprivation is only marginal and some laying continues, the fall in production is accompanied by greatly increased bird activity, with much increased pecking behaviour and cannibalism, especially at the everted cloaca of other birds ovipositing. In free-range and barn-laying flocks, where pecking can be more of a problem, it is standard practice to use 0.18–0.20% sodium in the ration while for caged birds 0.14% is adequate. The higher level does not prevent pecking completely but it reduces the susceptibility of the flock to developing the vice, which is usually triggered by management factors.

If greatly excessive amounts of salt are fed, frank signs of toxicity may develop, especially in young birds and if drinking water is also restricted. Clinical signs include diarrhoea, excessive thirst, loss of appetite, progressive muscular weakness, inability to stand, convulsions and death. Ascites may be present. Severe kidney damage occurs in young birds, with renal failure and death; post-mortem findings include visceral gout and urate-impacted ureters. Less severe toxicity results in cystic testes in young chicks. Older birds are more tolerant of raised salt levels, provided that adequate water is available, but feed intake and egg production are depressed by 5% sodium chloride in laying hen diets. The toxicity of salt is much greater when delivered via water, being approximately five times more lethal.

MANGANESE

This trace mineral has a close working relationship with magnesium in a number of body systems (e.g. in some enzymes and in DNA complexes).

Animal tissues fairly constantly contain about 500 µg/kg, which is not much affected by diet in adults. The greatest concentration is in the skeleton. Birds are much more susceptible to deficiency than mammals because their requirement is much higher (up to 100-fold in some cases). This is attributable to relatively poor duodenal absorption, which in poultry is only about 2–5% of the ingested manganese. Absorption is also inhibited by excessive dietary calcium and phosphorus.

Manganese activates several enzyme systems and is an essential component of pyruvate carboxylase, which also contains biotin and controls the rate of gluconeogenesis. It affects bone and eggshell formation, probably via alkaline phosphatase and acid mucopolysaccharides used in the organic matrix of bone, such as chondroitin sulphate. Consequently, skeletal deformities occur and eggshells become thin, porous and soft when manganese intake is inadequate.

When young growing birds are reared on a manganese-deficient diet, growth is retarded and there is a deformity of bone growth, i.e. chondrodystrophy.

In the laying or breeding bird, manganese deficiency causes a marked fall in egg production, with greatly reduced hatchability (e.g. down 50%) in incubated eggs. Embryos frequently die in the last third of incubation, showing gross skeletal and other defects including chondrodystrophy, micromelia, globular head, parrot beak, oedema of the cervicothoracic region and retarded down, feather and body growth. In newly hatched chicks, ataxia, tetanic spasms and head retraction may be evident. In compounded feeds manganese is frequently used as a marker to identify inclusion of the vitamin and mineral premix on assay. Therefore levels of 80–100 mg/kg are routinely added, which is above the requirement of birds.

ZINC

Zinc affects growth, development, reproduction and, through its involvement in many enzymes, is concerned with almost every metabolic function. A daily supply is required because of utilization and excretion. Efficacy of absorption is relatively low and the presence of phytic acid depresses uptake (by formation of an insoluble zinc complex), as does a high calcium level, excess calcium reducing the availability of phytate-bound zinc. In addition, high calcium levels in feed exacerbate the effects of zinc deficiency, although the mechanism of this effect is not understood. Zinc is stored in various mucosal cells, which, being continually shed, probably function as part of the homeostatic mechanism. The main reserves in bone can be mobilized for metabolic use even when calcium intake is high.

Of raw materials commonly used in poultry feeds the richest sources of zinc are animal protein ingredients (e.g. meat and fish meals). To ensure adequate intake, supplementation with a zinc compound (usually inorganic) has long been standard practice in feed manufacture. Zinc is required primarily for skeletal growth and development, for epithelial tissue formation and maintenance, and for egg production. Deficiency gives rise to poor growth and appetite, poor feathering and feather fraying, scaly skin, especially on the legs and feet, and, in young growing birds, the generalized growth plate disorder of chondrodystrophy described earlier.

Reduced egg production occurs in deficiency and hatchability is impaired. Embryonic mortality peaks around mid-incubation, with faulty trunk, spine and limb formation and abnormal beak, head, brain and eye development, presumably caused by zinc-dependent metabolic processes involved in the development of skeletal mesoderm.

SELENIUM

A metabolic role for selenium was found in 1973, when it was shown to be present in the cell enzyme glutathione peroxidase (GSH-Px), involved in the active removal of peroxides from cells. A close correlation generally exists between selenium and GSH-Px levels. The linkage between the biochemical roles of selenium and vitamin E was found to be that cell damage by lipid hydroperoxides (formed by the action of active peroxides on unsaturated fatty acids) could be prevented either by peroxide removal by GSH-Px or by the antioxidant activity of vitamin E (tocopherol) in competing with the unsaturated fatty acids and preventing hydroperoxide formation. Both functions are required when cells have heavy loads of active oxygen or unsaturated fatty acids. Selenium has other independent body roles.

Lack of dietary selenium limits production and function of GSH-Px, leading to lipid hydroperoxide production in oxygen-laden cells with subsequent cell wall damage, the clinical effects including myopathy, microangiopathy and capillary fragility. In poultry, the well-recognized clinical conditions arising from these defects include nutritional muscular dystrophy, exudative diathesis and encephalomalacia. Exudative diathesis is known to respond clinically to selenium supplementation in the presence of adequate vitamin E.

FATTY LIVER SYNDROME IN LAYING HENS

There are very important basic differences in carbohydrate and lipid metabolism in birds and mammals. Birds have blood glucose levels that are several times higher than mammals and mammalian embryos obtain glucose via the placental circulation, whereas the avian embryo develops on yolk nutrients, the energy source being almost all fat, not carbohydrate. The avian embryo must therefore have high levels of gluconeogenic enzymes, which decrease after hatching as carbohydrate intake becomes available. Furthermore, in contrast to mammals, where lipogenesis is mainly in adipose tissue, in birds it nearly all occurs in the liver, increasing in the first week or two after hatching from almost zero in the embryo (because of high yolk fat content) to much higher levels.

As hens approach lay and sexual maturity, there is a further and much more dramatic increase in liver lipogenesis, with very high blood plasma lipid levels available to supply the developing ova. Hepatic fat storage likewise increases enormously at this time.

It is this lipogenic liver function in birds that forms the keystone for the occurrence of conditions involving excessive accumulation of liver fat, e.g. FLKS in young birds and fatty liver haemorrhagic syndrome (FLHS) in older laying hens.

FLHS is characterized by very fatty liver accompanied by haemorrhage, the condition occurring sporadically, particularly in older caged hens of heavier breeds in hot weather. There is usually a fall in egg production in the affected flock. There is an increased fat (mostly triglyceride) content of the liver, which becomes putty-coloured and very friable, the fat content sometimes exceeding 70%. Death only occasionally occurs and is due to massive liver haemorrhage; the kidneys are pale and swollen and the abdomen contains large accumulations of fat, usually yellow and almost liquid at room temperature. Most of the flock are affected subclinically but the livers of these birds show subcapsular haemorrhages (mostly at liver lobe margins), long-standing haematomas, organizing blood clots, necrotic areas and other evidence of recent minor haemorrhage.

The exact cause of FLHS is not known but contributory factors include:

- Feed, especially high-carbohydrate, low-fat feed, given ad libitum (i.e. high-energy diets for increased egg production), leading to obesity; linoleic acid and selenium shortfalls exacerbate occurrence
- High temperature (which discourages movement that would reduce heat loss), lack of exercise (i.e. caged birds), stress
- High-oestrogen, low-thyroid blood hormone levels
- Strain of bird – the average liver lipid in different strains of layer may vary from about 25% to about 50% (NB: higher lipid levels are not linked to increased egg production).

A high percentage of liver fat (i.e. a fatty liver) is not in itself sufficient to cause FLHS but it does predispose the liver to haemorrhage, which mostly occurs in heavier birds in the latter half of the laying period.

Histologically, hepatocytes are grossly distended with fat globules, which disorganize internal structure and eventually rupture cell membranes. There is disintegration of pericellular reticulin and breakdown of vascular integrity, also evidence of secondary inflammation, necrosis and regeneration.

It seems that haemorrhage results from the steatosis but the exact pathogenesis is not understood; it is suggested that it is associated with overloaded normal tissue repair mechanisms, particularly GSH-Px.

NUTRITION IN RELATION TO IMMUNE STATUS AND DISEASE

The action of the immune system has been shown to be undermined by a variety of nutrient deficiencies. Supplementation with higher than normal levels of certain vitamins (e.g. vitamin A and vitamin E) has been shown to enhance the immune competence of poultry. A good example of this is the large-scale field study by Kennedy et al (1992), in which elevated vitamin E in broiler rations improved net financial returns from flocks with subclinical infectious bursal disease compared with flocks fed standard levels of vitamin E. There is also an effect of immune response upon nutrient requirements, with repartitioning of nutrients leading to impaired physical performance as a consequence of disease or vaccination challenge.

Modern parent stock management often relies upon maternal antibodies being passed to the chick or poult via the yolk sac for protection from disease. Work by Dibner (2000) has shown that these proteins will be used by the neonate for energy metabolism at the expense of immune function if diet energy relies upon added fat rather than digestible carbohydrate as an energy source. Therefore it is necessary to formulate diets with immune response in mind as well as growth requirements. The choice of feeding strategy is also important and must be selected in the light of a good understanding of the management and disease factors present on a given farm.

REFERENCES

Coelho M 1991 Vitamin stability in premixes and feeds: a practical approach. BASF Technical Symposium, Bloomington

Dibner J 2000 Early nutrition in young poultry. In: Garnsworthy P C, Wiseman J (eds) Recent advances in animal nutrition: Nottingham University Press, Nottingham

Hansen R S 1976 Nervousness and hysteria of mature female chickens. Poult Sci 55: 531–543

Kennedy D G, Rice D A, Bruce D W et al 1992 Economic effects of increased vitamin E supplementation of broiler diets on commercial broiler production. Br Poult Sci; 33: 1015–1023

Lauzon D, Johnston S, Southern L et al 2006 The effect of source of vitamin E on growth performance and vitamin E excretion in broilers. In: International Poultry Science Forum, Atlanta, 23–24 January 2006, M71, p 23

Mayne R K 2005 A review of the aetiology and possible causative factors of foot pad dermatitis in growing turkeys and broilers. WPSA J 61: 256–267

Whitehead C C 1998 Vitamin interactions and requirements in poultry. In: Proceedings of the 7th International Symposium on Animal Nutrition, Kaposvar, Hungary, p 3–31

Whitehead C C 2000a Recent developments in vitamins and broiler nutrition. In: Proceedings of the Maryland Nutrition Conference, Baltimore, p 41–57

Whitehead C C 2000b Recent developments on the effects of nutrition on skeletal disease. In: Proceedings of the 21st World's Poultry Congress, Montreal, 20–24 August 2000

Whitehead C C, Keller T 2003 An update on ascorbic acid in poultry. WPSA J 59: 161–184

Whitehead C C, Rennie J S, McCormack H A, Hocking P M 1993 Defective down syndrome in chicks is not caused by riboflavin deficiency in breeders. Br Poult Sci 34: 619–623

Whitehead C C, McCormack H A, McTeir L, Fleming R H 2004 High vitamin D_3 requirements in broilers for bone quality and prevention of tibial dyschondroplasia and interactions with dietary calcium, available phosphorus and vitamin A. Br Poult Sci 45: 425–436

FURTHER READING

Klasing K C, Johnstone B J, Benson B N 1991 Implications of an immune response on growth and nutrient requirements of chicks. In: Haresign W, Cole D J A (eds) Advances in animal nutrition. Butterworths, London, p 135–146

Leeson S, Summers J D 1997 Commercial poultry nutrition, 2nd edn. University Books, Guelph

Leeson S, Summers J D 2001 Scott's nutrition of the chicken, 4th edn. University Books, Guelph

Leeson S, Diaz G, Summers J D 1995 Poultry metabolic disorders and mycotoxins. University Books, Guelph

Randall C J 1985 A colour atlas of the diseases of the domestic fowl and turkey. Wolfe Medical, London

Recent developments in poultry nutrition 1989 (Derived from recent University of Nottingham Feed Manufacturers Conferences.) Butterworths, London

Scott M L 1987 Nutrition of the turkey. M L Scott, Ithaca

Whitehead C C (ed) 1992 Bone biology and skeletal disorders in poultry. In: Proceedings of Poultry Science Symposium 1992. Carfax, Abingdon

Whitehead C C, Portsmouth J L 1989 Vitamin requirements and allowances for poultry. In: Haresign W, Cole D J A (eds) Advances in animal nutrition. Butterworths, London, p 35–86

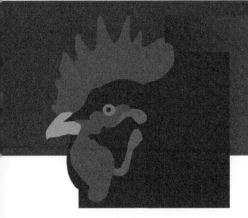

CHAPTER 43

Chris Morrow

Management as a cause of disease in poultry

Normally an animal maintains homeostasis by physiological adjustments to its metabolism or by moving to find food, water, a more comfortable temperature or shelter, better quality air, etc. Management is the control of the environment of an animal, consequently restricting the ability of the animal to move to adjust its physiological state.

Management may act as a primary cause of disease by active management or passive management factors: in other words, the stock keeper or farmer may have made a deliberate decision in setting a parameter (active management) or may have just let a parameter float (passive management). Good management must provide solutions for every bird in the population to be able to maintain homeostasis and achieve production goals. The focus on the management of a population requires a novel approach. For example: body weight uniformity is the key factor in successful management of a breeder flock. The more uniform a flock the more predictable the response of the flock to various management inputs. For example, increasing feed allocations at the beginning of lay will stimulate more birds in the same direction if the birds are at the same stage with regards to sexual development. This is the essence of population management rather than individual bird management.

It is easy to see how the manager must provide feed (of suitable quantity, quality and distribution), water, light, fresh air, heat control and space for each individual bird. It is more difficult to see how subtle adjustments in these inputs can cause or prevent major production and health problems. Often an input can be optimized for one output parameter but may cause problems with other parameters. For example, maximizing early fertility may mean that cockerels are overweight during later production periods and cumulative hatchability may be adversely affected.

Management can certainly be a secondary factor modulating the effect of infectious agents or other insults but the following discusses common conditions/diseases where management can be considered the primary cause or a major factor.

GENERAL

Hyperthermia

As temperatures increase birds will seek shelter, pant with mouth breathing though a wide-open beak, stand with wings outstretched, increase water intake and decrease feed intake. In severe hyperthermia death is by circulatory and/or respiratory collapse and/or metabolic imbalance.

The effect of heat depends on the age of the stock, past temperatures experienced by the stock and many other factors. High humidity and stagnant air will aggravate heat stress by decreasing the efficiency of heat dissipation. The longer the duration of a heat insult the more permanent the effect on production, although acclimatization can occur. Currently, best practice for preventing hyperthermia is implemented through engineering solutions. Housing design, ability to move air and evaporative cooling (misting or cooling cells) are effective strategies. Tunnel ventilation needs to achieve air speeds of 2–3 m/s at bird level for maximum effect. Baseline water consumption in commercial birds is roughly 1.8 times the amount of feed ingested. This can be expected to increase by 6% for every 1°C rise in temperature above 27°C.

In young chicks transient hyperthermia may cause high mortality as a result of chicks becoming depressed and dehydrated, but the surviving flock may rapidly recover from the effects. The ability to regulate body temperature is immature in young birds. For embryos and young poultry, coping with heat stress may alter the partitioning of nutrients and be immunosuppressive, delay gut development and decrease satellite cell proliferation in muscle tissue (thus potentially decreasing total breast yield in broilers).

In broilers, growth will be retarded in intensive rearing systems if heat generated by the birds is not removed. Broiler houses in all areas of the world need to be designed to remove this heat, especially after birds are 30 days of age. Regular walking by the stockman through the houses can get broilers to stand and help dissipate heat. Feather development can be altered by chronic heat stress. Feathering will be delayed and the shaft may be crooked or the plume may have breaks in more severe cases. Broilers can suffer acute heat stress during equipment failure or during transportation to or holding at the slaughterhouse. The coccidiostat nicarbazin makes broilers more susceptible to heat stress.

In older birds acute heat stress may cause temporary egg production drops. As a general strategy, poultry decrease the total heat to be dissipated by suspending production (and reducing feed intake, extending the feed consumption time and increasing water intake). Poultry start panting about 27°C but egg size in layers will start to decrease over 24°C. Temperatures over 43°C are lethal for chickens in as short a time as 3 h.

At post-mortem there is cyanosis of the featherless parts of the head and marked venous congestion throughout the whole carcass. In laying birds flaccid paralysis or ruptured ova will often be observed.

No nutritional adjustment will completely prevent the effects of high temperatures. Although many water additives have been suggested to help prevent the effects of high temperatures, most of these may have their effect by increasing water consumption. Additives to feed and water are often suggested and may be beneficial. Inappropriate nutrition and feeding can certainly aggravate the effects of heat stress – excess energy or unbalanced protein will increase the metabolic heat being generated. The provision of cool water may also be beneficial by insulating or shading tanks or feeding direct from mains. Feeding pellets and feeding during cool periods of the day can increase feed consumption.

Hypothermia

Young chicks will initially huddle and start making a different noise. Mortality may be marked, with birds failing to start feeding and exhausting the yolk. On post-mortem the crop is usually empty. Humidity and ventilation (and shelter for free-range production systems) are important components that need to be considered in estimating the effect of temperatures on poultry. Low brooding temperatures (<26°C) will trigger ascites later in the life of the broiler. Brooding temperatures will influence the development of feathers, and thus also the ability of the bird to cope with low temperatures later in life, and susceptibility to scratching-associated problems.

In older birds more energy will be used to maintain body temperature during winter if the housing and heating cannot maintain house temperature. In this case it is usual for more feed to be needed to maintain production during these periods.

Dehydration (acute and chronic)

In young chicks the vein on the metatarsus will become more prominent as the subcutaneous tissues shrink. The birds will display signs of thirst and may jump into drinkers and drown if water is suddenly introduced into the surround. Water loss from young chicks can be aggravated by holding them in an environment where temperature, ventilation and humidity are fluctuating. On post-mortem the carcasses will be dry, the kidneys may be pale and urates may be seen in the ureters. There may even be signs of visceral gout with urates in the pericardium.

In older chicks and adults, excessive water restriction may limit the amount of feed ingested. The normal ratio of feed to water is 1:1.8 but this should be increased as ambient temperature increases above 27°C. Birds tend to drink when they eat. Thirsty birds will focus on the drinkers. Their crops may be filled with hard feed that has not been softened by water. Water shortage may limit egg production, especially at peak production. This may be due to an inability of the drinker system to deliver enough water at peak demand periods. Drinking does not take place during the night. Nipple drinkers set too high may cause many birds to have a callus on the upper side of the base of the beak ('unicorns'), presumably in response to jumping to activate the nipple and hitting the line.

Chronic undersupply of water will limit egg production of hens and may trigger mortality-associated urolithiasis. These birds will have sharp urate accretions in the ureters, and urates covering the heart and other body linings, and may have complete atrophy of some kidney lobes and compensatory hyperplasia of remaining lobes. Death occurs when the ureter draining the remaining kidney tissue is occluded. Other causes of urolithiasis include infectious bronchitis infection and feeding high calcium rations (laying rations are typically 4% calcium) to birds for extended periods before the beginning of lay.

Emaciation

In some populations small birds continue to be identified, in spite of regular removal of affected birds. On post-mortem examination, serous atrophy of the fat around the heart is often noted and no body fat can be seen. This is common in large pens and is a deficiency in the evenness of feed distribution. Pan feeders set too high can also cause this.

Starve out

Failure to find feed at placement in the house will see mortality increase to a peak around day 4 as the yolk reserves are exhausted. Small dead birds or live birds will be found with little or no feed in the crops. Shavings or other material may distend and impact the crops. Gall bladders will be distended. Similar problems can occur in older birds when they are changed from one feeding system to another (house transfer, etc.) and the birds have difficulty finding the new source of food or water. Birds should be watched carefully at transfer time and the placing or initial confinement of birds on to slats is often practised.

Obesity

In broilers this can be caused by feeding unbalanced feeds. Feeds with too much energy or unbalanced protein may cause the deposition of a lot of fat. In the case of excess protein, excess amino acids are deaminated and this causes a lot of metabolic heat, and panting may start at a temperature lower than normal (27°C).

Asphyxiation (smothering)

Hysteria or piling up of birds in response to a perceived shock can cause sudden high mortality. Although some hysterical behaviour can be modulated by additions of some vitamins (especially B group), it is more usual that the previous experience of the birds has a greater effect. This is not as common in modern bird genotypes as in the past. Some panics may be caused by inputs that mimic predators while others may be novel stimuli (dressing the veterinarian up in a white coat where previously all staff wore dark clothes). On post-mortem it is usual to find pale areas in the breast muscle. This is an agonal change associated with other birds on top of the carcass pushing the blood out of these areas. Survivors may be seen gasping.

Splayed legs

Day-old chicks need to be delivered on rough textured paper to allow the development of standing. Turkey poults appear more susceptible to this and are commonly transported with fibre pads. Incorrectly chopped straw (too long) as litter in houses can also aggravate this condition. Once legs start to be affected the bird should be culled, as it will not recover.

Oral lesions from powdery feed

Oral lesions in poultry may be caused by any feed material that is traumatic or caustic (certain forms of calcium, copper sulphate and trichothene mycotoxins). They may also be caused by finely-ground feed lacking larger particles. It has been suggested that the large particles in feed clean the lining of the mouth. Affected birds develop bilateral lesions, initially under the tongue and then on the soft palate and sometimes further extensions. The lesions are covered with adherent feed dust. When healing or debrided an ulcer may be apparent. In contrast to T2 and similar toxins, no lesions are seen at the commissures of the beak or in the crops and performance is not markedly affected. Peak lesions are at the time of peak feed intake. The lesions usually take many weeks to develop. Prevention is by changing the feed form.

Beak necrosis

Various forms of beak necrosis have been described but usually no aetiology has been suggested. Low nipple lines may see birds drinking from the side of the beak and may cause this condition, but sometimes female breeders will be seen pecking at the side of the beak of male birds.

Mating damage

Mating damage to females may be caused by digit 1 (the hallux) of males and by the spur of some male strains. In broiler breeders, females can be seen with large unilateral lacerations on the flank, often with no apparent effect on health. Male broiler breeders often have the halluxes trimmed in the hatchery. Remnants of the nail on poorly trimmed halluxes or males that have not been trimmed (commonly incorrectly sexed as females) may also damage females.

Overmating is seen if mating ratios are inappropriate with males in excess or if the males are more sexually developed than the females at the time of mating up. Excessive wear of the feathers on the back and sides of the female will be seen, although sometimes damage to males from fighting with other males is seen. More subtle signs may be damage to the head and upper neck of females or loss of feathers from these areas.

Grille damage

Separate-sex feeding equipment, especially exclusion grilles, can sometimes cause traumatic lesions (especially if welding slag is still on the wires) or swelling of the head of breeders mimicking swollen head syndrome. If a flock suffers swollen head syndrome (*Avian pneumovirus* infection) and swelling of the head occurs then this will be aggravated by separate sex feeding equipment and it should be removed. Grille width needs to be at the current recommendations of the breeding companies supplying the stock.

Damage caused by equipment

New houses are prone to 'hardware disease', with birds ingesting nails and other pieces of metal. These often puncture the gizzard and may cause associated local peritonitis.

Equipment in houses can cause trauma when birds move over or under the equipment. Typically hock bruises and tenosynovitis can be caused by feeder tracks with grilles being set too low and birds having to jump over them rather than go under them.

Problems secondary to mutilations

Beak trimming must be done early (at less than 2 weeks of age) to prevent neuroma formation. It needs to be uniform or it will generate uniformity problems. Grading of flocks that have been poorly beak-trimmed will see the small pen containing the most severely beak-trimmed birds. The use of a hot blade at the correct temperature is needed to make sure that open wounds are not generated on the truncated beak, as these can be a portal of entry for bacteria.

Toe trimming of breeder males should be uniform if done to prevent damage to females. (See section above on mating damage.)

Vaccination hygiene is important to prevent bacteria from being injected. Killed vaccines should not be kept between batches of birds. Spray vaccines need to be made with fresh sterile water. Other sprays need to have hygiene programmes to stop spraying of bacteria on to the birds including in the hatchery and cooling systems.

BROILERS

Ventilation is extremely important in broilers, providing oxygen and removing volatile waste products of metabolism, moisture and heat (and wastes of gas combustion for heating houses).

It is important to implement the concept of minimum ventilation, especially where the economics of heating houses may be pushing to decrease ventilation.

Ammonia blindness

High ammonia levels from poor litter and poor ventilation will cause keratitis and blindness in broilers. Dust from dried litter will also cause keratitis.

Ascites

Ascites is a collection of fluid in the abdomen of the bird and is often seen with hydroperi-cardium and liver changes. In early cases hydropericardium may be the only finding in dead, well-grown birds. The heart is usually in systole. Fibrin clots may be present in the ascitic fluid. It occurs when the metabolic demands on the cardiovascular system are chronically greater than it can deliver. Genetic selection for increased muscle and growth rate increases metabolic demand in broiler stock. In response to the appearance and understanding of this condition, primary breeders of broiler stock have been successful in selecting for cardiovascular fitness, making birds more resistant to ascites. Factors that decrease the ability of the cardiovascular system include decreased oxygen tension in inspired air (high altitude, poor ventilation) and increased oxygen demand from increased metabolism due to hypothermia. Respiratory disease can also decrease lung efficacy and trigger ascites.

Ventilation is particularly important in broiler health and minimum ventilation needs to be defined for flocks on the basis of metabolic need (to supply oxygen and remove metabolic waste products), including allowing for the waste gas production from gas heaters and litter. These requirements change rapidly with the rapid growth of the bird and the build-up of waste in the litter.

Sudden death syndrome of broilers

This has been shown to be associated with spontaneous ventricular fibrillation in affected broil-ers. Mortality starts in the first week and broilers can be observed to flip over and flap before death. It is the major cause of death in well-managed broiler flocks, with deaths peaking from 1–3 weeks. Dead birds are often found on their backs with their legs extended. They appear to be bigger birds (compared with other birds being examined, although not necessarily the flock) and males are more commonly affected. On post-mortem examination the heart is found in diastole and the lungs are congested if examination is delayed. The abdomen is distended as the intestines contain ingesta. The electrolyte balance of feed may be important in minimizing mor-tality from sudden death syndrome. Lowering the energy intake of the birds will often decrease mortality from sudden death syndrome and this may be achieved by a number of management strategies, including feed formulation, changing from pellet to mash and feed restriction by lighting programmes. Genetic selection in environments using nutritionally dense pelleted feeds with long day lengths has been beneficial in reducing losses from sudden death syndrome.

Spiking mortality of broilers

This syndrome is observed as transient increased mortality of broilers, typically lasting 1–3 days in the second to fourth week of life. No visible lesions are present on post-mortem examination (which is typical of a metabolic problem). In the UK in the 1990s this was particularly associ-ated with coccidiostat programmes using 120 ppm nicarbazin for the first 12–16 days. Mortality was triggered by a stress episode, for example running out of feed or heater failure. In North America spiking mortality in chickens and turkeys appears to be different and although a viral aetiology has been proposed other management factors may be important.

Cellulitis

This is also called inflammatory process and is usually caused by a bacterial infection under the skin of birds in the lateral and ventral abdominal regions. In the slaughterhouse birds will be condemned for sheets of purulent material in the abdominal areas or skin scratches. In this multifactorial disease, management factors affecting the occurrence include scratching, extent of feather cover and immunosuppression (from nutritional or infectious causes). Factors that increase the incidence of broilers scratching each other include feeding programmes with insufficient feed space and rodents in the house. A common cause of immunosuppression is chicken anaemia virus infection. Maternal antibody appears protective for broilers, and breeders should be vaccinated. Nutritional strategies that use feeds with compositions below that recommended by the supplying genetics company can be immunosuppressive even though growth may be satisfactory.

Other management-influenced diseases of broilers include hock burn, foot pad dermatitis and deep pectoral myopathy. See Chapter 40 for a discussion of these conditions.

BREEDERS – BROILER PARENTS

Gorging

Breeders are feed-restricted to control body composition. Even allocation of feed to each bird is achieved by a distribution system that allows mild competition between birds for feed. (They need to eat feed when it is in front of them or there will be none for them later). If greater access to feed is accidentally allowed then some birds may eat too much feed. Typically this arises from access to too much feed, introduction of pellets or unevenly distributed feed (especially when feed was previously well distributed). This is seen as mortality with distended crops and occasionally dyspnoea. The presentation of this problem may be as a primary respiratory problem. Failure of water supply can also cause a similar problem. Mild gorging can trigger necrotic enteritis or intersusscaption in young birds.

Tenosynovitis from feed distribution problems

Morbidity and mortality from tenosynovitis, often with staphylococcal infection, is a common problem with feed restriction programmes. It appears that bird feeding behaviour is very important in the genesis of the problem. This can be a significant cause of culling, often starting at 10 weeks and continuing to 15 weeks or more. Observation of the birds during feeding will often find excitement and scrambling for feed. Feed quantities/volumes during this period are relatively small and an even distribution of the feed is needed so all birds can get their allocation. Failure to achieve these aims trains birds to fight for their food. This will also adversely affect body weight uniformity and the loss of uniformity will aggravate these problems and make feed distribution even more difficult.

The actual feeding equipment and its management will vary from farm to farm but the aim of having all birds calm during feeding is the same. Typical strategies include dividing the total feed of the week to be fed not all days of the week (so-called 'skip a day' – although this is not permitted in all countries), feed dilution, hand feeding or spin feeding on floor (this requires good, consistent pellet quality).

The use of track feeding during rearing poses special problems. Breeder feed track is usually narrower than broiler track so that less quantity of feed is in each feeder space at the same depth. It is important that the whole track is full of feed as soon as possible. Distribution can be improved by the installation of high-speed feeding systems, satellite bins, managing the feed depth, distributing the feed while the track is elevated and/or turning the lights off. It is important that feed is distributed within a maximum of 2–3 minutes. Mash feed is sometimes used to extend feeding up time. Twenty minutes would be the minimum. Uniformity will improve as the feed management is improved.

Tenosynovitis induced by rearing at low light intensity

Lame birds appearing at 6–8 weeks of age with secondary staphylococcal infection of tendons has been associated with rearing replacement broiler breeders at low light intensities (<1 lux). It is hypothesized that low light intensity leads to low levels of activity, with the result that the body 'miscalculates' how strong to make bones and tendons. This condition can be prevented by increasing rearing light levels.

Sudden death syndrome of broiler breeders

This appears to be an electrolyte imbalance which precipitates acute heart failure (probably ventricular fibrillation). At the beginning of lay mortality increases with hens flipping over at feeding time and convulsing before death. Dead birds have severely congested combs, wattles, ova and cloaca and this may extend to the oviduct and lungs. The heart is grossly enlarged. The stockman will, by walking up and down the house at feeding time, find new mortalities. Although the mortality usually ceases after peak of lay, the condition can be treated by potassium supplementation in the water. Potassium is usually added as $KHCO_3$ or KCl at 0.6 g per bird per day to the water. The cessation of deaths after supplementation is diagnostic.

The cause of the problem is often associated with electrolyte imbalance and careful attention to phosphorus levels and availability can usually prevent the problem. This problem can appear when large changes in diet raw materials occur, for instance the removal of meat and bone meal from the diet or a change to a vegetarian diet. Some breeds appear to be more prone to sudden death syndrome of broiler breeders than others and therapy may have to increase potassium supplementation for a response.

Spiral fractures of the femur in adult female breeders

This is seen in North American management systems in houses with slats at the beginning of lay. Affected females are overweight. It is thought that bone strength may be poor, possibly due to calcium in feed being finely ground for feed processing (extrusion) and therefore not retained in the gizzard and subsequently poorly solubilized and absorbed. The fractures occur as the hens jump down from the slats.

Calcium tetany in hens

This disease is often associated with increased mortality at the beginning of lay in broiler parent chickens in the USA, although it is probably more widespread. Paralysed or dead birds are found on the nest, with a partially formed shell in the oviduct. Sometimes weak birds are found on the litter; it is presumed that they are too weak to jump up to the slatted area to get to the nest box.

These birds may be mistaken for hens suffering from overmating. Changing birds on to a breeder diet before beginning of lay appears to predispose to this condition. Other factors include stimulation of poorly uniform flocks and the use of calcium that is very finely ground (pulverised limestone or preparation for use in extruders). There may be an interaction with high environmental temperatures (and consequent depression of appetite). The condition can be treated with vitamin D and extra calcium. Prevention is by supplementation of calcium in the form of shell grit from first egg. Extra calcium supplementation before this time can aggravate the situation.

Calcium tetany is also seen in commercial layers, particularly in noncage systems from the mid-lay period. Affected birds show marked leg weakness but many recover if removed to a recovery pen, usually after they have laid an egg. Cage layer fatigue is another similar condition that is caused by spinal or other fractures in osteoporotic birds (see Ch. 42).

Peritonitis and associated egg production problems

The aims of management at the beginning of lay in broiler breeders are to control ovarian function in the female so that maximum lifetime production can be achieved and to minimize stress. Laying usually starts in the 23rd week of life in European management systems and at 25 weeks in North American management systems, although this depends mainly on body composition and lighting stimulation.

Peritonitis (not associated with recognized bacterial infections such as *Pasteurella multocida*) is caused by a gross failure to control ovarian activity in broiler breeders. It is probably the most extreme aberration seen in erratic ovulation and deformed egg syndrome (EODES). An understanding of the management aims of bodyweight control in females is needed. The aim of restrictive feeding is to delay the first egg until the hen is mature enough for sustained egg laying. This delay allows for the prime sequence of egg production to be maximal. Without restrictive feeding the first egg would appear at 16 weeks but production would rapidly decrease. Other symptoms sometimes associated with failure to control ovarian function include increased double yolks (although these are not always present), increased erratic laying (individual birds) appearing as lower peaks, increased shell quality problems and decreased total egg production.

The mortality is usually twice to four times the usual mortality (normal mortality coming into lay is about 1% per month) experienced at the beginning of lay. It will often settle down after peak of lay but in some cases the mortality from peritonitis can continue through the total laying period.

Other observations include early first egg, early 5% egg production and putting on weight when coming into lay instead of producing eggs. Sometimes failure to respond to feed increases at 15 weeks, with corresponding body weight increase, is associated with flocks that go on to have peritonitis problems.

At post-mortem examination peritonitis or yolk material in the abdomen is the usual finding. When this is cultured a variety of organisms may be recovered but *Escherichia coli* is the most common. Analysis of the *E. coli* isolates made does not usually support a clonal infection and suggests that the infection is opportunistic. Salpingitis may also be observed. Ovaries comprising numerous ova will be seen in randomly selected birds.

The final part of sexual maturity begins at about 15 weeks and more food is allocated at this time to hens to stimulate and support the maturation and development of the reproductive organs. The current recommendation to change to a prebreeder ration at this time is to make the body weight response more predictable. If there is a large check in growth around 15 weeks (e.g. because the flock is moved) and the first egg is then at the usual time, this appears to shorten this final sexual development and peritonitis may be observed.

Birds can be light-stimulated at any time from 18–23 weeks of age but the closer to 18 weeks they are lit up the more likely it is that they will go on to develop peritonitis. This can be aggravated where composite flocks are managed to an average age (or worse still the oldest age) of components of the flock or if lightproofing is poor with in-season flocks. Production systems that utilize early eggs in the analysis of performance will over time tend to bring birds into lay earlier and then they may develop a peritonitis problem.

Factors such as high environmental temperatures (>27°C) will increasing panting and decrease nose-filtering of air and may increase bacterial deposition in air sacs and possibly peritonitis.

Situations where peritonitis may be seen include precocious stimulation or late checks in growth before lay. Poor body weight control, especially when out-of-season body weight profiles are being used, can precipitate peritonitis, with heavier birds being precocious. This may cause a seasonal problem with peritonitis in an organization. Artificial insemination, even when done well, will increase total in lay mortality by approximately 3%. Overweight birds may also be more prone to fatty liver haemorrhagic syndrome. Turkeys also appear to be susceptible to peritonitis and this may be by similar mechanisms.

Treatment with antibiotics is rarely successful, although it may decrease mortality during the treatment period. Note that birds dying of acute heat stress will often have burst and flaccid ova at post-mortem examination but will also have decomposition of the lungs and the flock will show acute reduction in feed intake and production.

Ascites in lay

This is a rare condition that can be triggered by having high sodium levels in laying feeds. It is quickly reversed by reducing the sodium levels. At post-mortem there is an accumulation of fluid in the abdomen and other features similar to those seen in broilers.

Cannibalism

Beak trimming practice, light intensity, stocking density and nutrition are considered significant variables influencing cannibalism. Other factors, such as body weight and/or acquired behaviour in pullets, are likely to be major variables in the induction of cannibalism in barn egg production systems. Feather sucking can often be a prelude to cannibalism. Carcasses are found without viscera and with wounds around the vent. Birds with blood on their beaks will be seen. Treatment is usually to decrease light intensity and check for other contributing factors such as pica, high humidity or excessive light intensity. In some areas treatment is practised by the introduction of meat meal into diets. In areas where light control in laying houses is poor, there may be more cannibalism in summer, with increased double-yolked eggs (usually associated with overfeeding when coming into lay). Here the focus of the birds is the everted vagina during oviposition. There are often a lot of bloodstained eggs seen in flocks with high double-yolks. Control of cannibalism is by prevention. Once established, light intensity may be decreased and in extreme cases emergency beak trimming may be justified.

LAYERS

Fatty liver haemorrhagic syndrome

Fatty liver haemorrhagic syndrome (FLHS) appears to be an expression of obesity in layers and breeders. Sometimes this is associated with egg production drops, the primary cause not being evident but secondary FLHS probably related to the continued consumption of feed at the expected level without production. Livers become enlarged, pale and friable and mild trauma causes rupture of the liver. At post-mortem examination clotted or unclotted blood is found in the abdomen of the birds that have died. Evidence of previous nonfatal haemorrhage may also be seen, with subcapsular haemorrhages also being present in the liver. Prevention and treatment is by trying to work out if any primary causes have been present and the adjustment of feed quantities (see Ch. 42). Differential diagnosis needs to include hepatitis splenomegaly syndrome, seen with avian hepevirus infection (see Ch 36).

Peritonitis, salpingitis and salpingoperitonitis

Peritonitis is the commonest post-mortem finding in commercial layers in the laying phase in many surveys. In some studies it has been suggested that low pullet bodyweights (in comparison to the breed standard) increases the incidence of cloacal haemorrhage, and that this tissue haemorrhage can act as a significant predisposing factor in the induction of cannibalism. Both cannibalism and vent trauma appear to be strongly correlated with the incidence of oviduct impaction, egg peritonitis and salpingitis. Mortality due to these oviduct dysfunctions, combined with cannibalism, explains up to 90% of mortality in barn egg-laying flocks. Uneven and underweight pullet flocks subsequent to low bodyweights during the rearing period may be predisposed to both cloacal haemorrhage and picking behaviours. It is not clear what the proximate cause of cloacal haemorrhage is, but it can be seen in single-bird cages and may be due to early large eggs. Excessively bright or prolonged usage of nest box lights increases vent damage, probably through pecking. *M. synoviae* may also play a part in layer peritonitis.

TURKEYS

Hepatic lipidosis in turkeys

This condition seems to affect only breeder females in rear from 12–24 weeks of age. The onset is acute with mortality of 2–15% in a particular house occurring within 4–5 days. This suggests something is 'synchronizing' the disease. At post-mortem the hens are in good body condition, dark breast muscles, straw-coloured transudate in abdominal cavity, enlarged mottled liver with numerous small haemorrhages and occasional large pale areas of lipid accumulation. There may be petechial and ecchymotic haemorrhages on the epicardium and fat around the gizzard, lung congestion and oedema and uncoagulated blood in larger vessels and heart. Histologically the liver structure is distorted by large vacuoles in the hepatocytes with displaced and degenerating nuclei. There are dilated central veins surrounded by degenerating and necrotic tissue and small to massive haemorrhages. The primary factor appears to be excessive weight gain between 10 and 20 weeks in rear. The condition is still poorly understood.

Aortic rupture

Typically, this affects fast-growing male turkeys over 6 weeks of age, with mortality peaking between 12 and 16 weeks. Death is sudden and a large clot of blood can be found in the abdomen. There is a rupture in the aorta; usually a longitudinal split between the external iliac and sciatic arteries. Other rupture sites include the thoracic aorta dorsal to the heart and the left atrium. Many clinicians approach this disease in a similar way to broiler ascites. Attention to details of ventilation and growth control can be effective in controlling the incidence of this disease. Control of excitement also appears to be important.

CONCLUSION

One of the main aims of management is to minimize stress on the birds. An understanding of the physiology of growth and reproduction in birds will help the manager modify the bird's environment to minimize stress. This needs to be done to supply the resources to each and every bird in the quantities they require (e.g. males may need more than females!). Heat needs to be uniform throughout houses, feed and water delivery systems need to give all birds approximately the same amount of food or water. Supplying averages without taking into account variation will generate variation in the birds and then this variation will create more variation and generally decrease production and profit.

Failure to maintain homeostasis is a disease state. This is a gross aberration but suboptimal performance may be an intermediate stage. Management may cause disease either as a primary cause or by potentiating the pathogenic effect of infections. It is in the farmer's interest to actively manage birds to prevent welfare problems and minimize the impact of infections and disease.

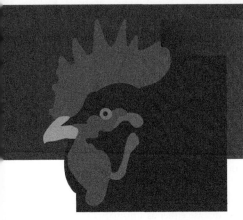

CHAPTER 44

Alan Shlosberg

Toxicants in poultry

Veterinary toxicology is the section of veterinary science of most complexity from a diagnostic viewpoint, mainly because of the existence of an immense number of potential causes of toxicosis. It is a fact that, with nearly all substances, dosage determines toxicity and thus very many added feed constituents, therapeutic agents and other apparently innocuous substances in the birds' environment have at some time induced toxicoses. Poultry toxicology is a particularly difficult subsection of veterinary toxicology. Species differences in response to toxicants, marked in mammals, are much in evidence in poultry and are even manifested between production types of a species (e.g. broilers, layers and breeding birds) mainly because of differing susceptibility and feed composition. About 95% of toxicoses are feed-related and the first response of poultry to most toxicants in the feed is to reduce feed intake. This may be sudden, when it is termed feed refusal, or gradual, when it is often difficult to distinguish whether it is a primary effect or secondary to sickness induced by another cause, including infectious disease. If contaminated feed is given to hatchlings, only reduced feed intake is seen. The typical signs of a toxicant (e.g. with ionophore coccidiostats), which would be the case in older birds, may not be apparent. In poultry, reduced performance (diminished bodyweight or gain, poor feed conversion, reduced egg production) is a very common consequence of exposure to toxicants, as well as being seen to some degree in most other infectious and metabolic diseases.

Diagnosis of toxicoses in poultry is best conducted by a combination of compiling a good history, field visits, the identification of clinical signs, necropsy findings and examination of samples in various laboratories. History taking should include a comprehensive account of the circumstances leading up to the suspect toxicosis, detailed daily records of production and the timing of appearance of clinical signs, any treatments of the birds or their environment, changes in husbandry, feed delivery dates and an estimate of when new feed was first eaten. Diagnosis of toxicoses in mammals is aided by meticulous clinical examinations of individual sick animals, but the breadth and depth of such investigations are impractical or unreliable in poultry. In poultry, toxicoses are approached mainly as a flock problem and a thorough necropsy of several birds, with subsequent rapid histopathological examinations, may be most helpful. Field visits are essential, not just by the attending veterinarian but in more difficult cases also by toxicologists, specialist epidemiologists, poultry pathologists and nutritionists.

Differentiation of toxicoses from infectious or production diseases is often difficult but the classical presentation, typical of some toxicoses, of peracute or acute onset with high morbidity in a short period of time is easy to detect in the large numbers of birds in commercial flocks. If there is an apparent association between the manifestation of production loss and/or clinical signs and ingestion of a new batch of feed, then it is often judicious to immediately change the feed, even before receiving results from the laboratory. In all poultry units, farmers should be instructed to always save 1 kg samples from each shipment of feed given, until after the flock has been processed. This will allow the laboratory the possibility of detecting toxicants producing subacute or chronic manifestations some time after the contaminated batch of feed has been totally consumed.

Laboratory analysis for toxicants is essential for a definitive diagnosis. It is, in broilers in particular, often more urgent than in mammals raised for meat production because of the short production cycle. This necessitates reporting of results within a few days. One should always be aware of the limitations of analytical laboratories, which examine about 1–25 g of feed for each potential toxicant. This may or may not be representative of the several tons of feed received, because insufficient mixing, which often occurs at the feedmill, results in different aliquots containing widely differing levels of constituents. To minimize this possibility, about 5 kg of feed should be sent to the laboratory. If possible this should comprise about 10 subsamples from differing areas (see Taking a feed sample in Ch. 2). It should also be appreciated that no laboratory can determine if a feed is 'toxic'. Neither can any one laboratory determine all causes of toxicoses, and analyses for specific substances must be directed to specialist laboratories that perform those analyses. Many veterinary laboratories have a resident toxicologist who may be able to direct the analyses to a more likely chemical cause. An often quoted empirical diagnostic option is to feed suspect feeds to healthy birds in an effort to recreate the toxicosis, but this is unreliable and usually ineffective, since many toxicoses have a low morbidity and the feed sample may not be representative of the feed that the sick birds actually ate. Experimentally, toxicosis is difficult to recreate in small numbers of birds when mild changes (in bodyweight or feed conversion, for instance) can only be detected in large numbers of birds.

As modern poultry husbandry regimens become more widespread and accepted globally, 'backyard' production becomes less common on a total production basis. This chapter will therefore refer only to commercial production, for which the sole feed source is a balanced feed supplied by feedmills. However, backyard poultry production does continue, and the raising of chickens under such uncontrolled conditions is even encouraged in less developed countries, where families still depend on such husbandry for a reliable source of protein; specific backyard production problems are discussed in a specific smallholder website. The commoner feed-related sources of toxicoses include coccidiostats (especially ionophores), mycotoxins, sodium, calcium, tannic acid and some drugs. Drinking water may be important if used as a means of therapy, and various drugs, quaternary ammonium disinfectants and copper sulphate are potential toxicants. Toxicants in the air include ammonia and some sprayed insecticides, and, much less commonly, carbon monoxide. Litter (bedding) may uncommonly contain toxic fungicides and, if suspect, the source and any treatment of the litter should be thoroughly investigated. Injected drugs rarely cause toxicosis, except for those interacting with ionophore coccidiostats.

Many toxicoses are related to feedmill practices. These may be the use of poor-quality feed constituents, insufficient mixing of mixed feed ingredients, inappropriate constituents or quantities added or incorrect delivery/destination of the feed. Feedmills may inadvertently acquire feed constituents of poor quality or contaminated with mycotoxins. Excessive amounts of correct feed constituents may be added. Insufficient mixing of the feed may result in stratification, with part of the feed containing too much, causing an overdosage, and part of it containing an underdosage; in this manner ionophores, sodium or calcium may be the causes of a dietary imbalance responsible for illness due to too much or to too little, especially in a large batch of feed. Compounding incorrect constituents is not common, but these may be those destined for another species or from other chemicals used or stored in the feedmill. Much more common is supplying feed made for one species, type or age to another species, type or age that is more sensitive toxicologically to a specific additive – for example providing growing turkeys with a broiler diet containing narasin or salinomycin.

Mistakes with premix formulation (mainly ionophores, vitamins, minerals) may be made by feedmill suppliers and are not common, but if they occur, mass toxicoses (or deficiencies) will occur. Mistakes made by farmers involve drinking water additives, or incorrect husbandry leading to excessive ammonia or carbon monoxide production. Negligence or ignorance may be due to insufficient avoidance of known, potential problems such as ionophore interactions with some therapeutic agents administered simultaneously. This may often be beyond the control or knowledge of the farmer and more in the realm of veterinary supervision. Malicious toxicoses are rare but, if toxicants such as cholinesterase-inhibiting insecticides, for example, are added to the water supply, the resulting toxicosis may be very serious.

FEED- OR WATER-RELATED TOXICOSES

Mycotoxins

Grains comprise the main bulk of poultry feed, and mycotoxin contamination of grains is probably one of the most common and certainly most under-reported causes of toxicoses in poultry. Mycotoxins, discussed in more detail in Chapter 38, are ubiquitous natural contaminants of grains and are being increasingly regarded as natural environmental contaminants rather than appearing in animal feeds sporadically and uncommonly at potentially toxic levels. If no or few feed analyses are made, the incidence of mycotoxicosis may appear to be zero, and those conducting surveys and more exhaustive analyses find, not coincidentally, more evidence of toxicoses. The type of toxin and degree of contamination depends on the grain and its moisture content, the genotype of the toxigenic fungus that might infest the grain and, of most importance, environmental conditions during growth, harvest, transport and storage. The origin of the grains in the feed is therefore of the utmost importance in risk assessment.

Field cases of mycotoxicoses in poultry are uncommonly reported in the literature, in part because of a dichotomy of data reported between levels needed to invoke toxicosis derived from experiments and those actually found in field manifestations. For example, the most common of the more toxic mycotoxins in feeds is aflatoxin B1, usually comprising about 80% of total aflatoxins, and, whereas aflatoxins are known to have a minimum toxic level (MTL) in the feed of more than 2 ppm, in the field very low contamination levels of about 50 ppb have caused nonspecific manifestations of reduced production and at even lower levels probable immunosuppression, although this is practically impossible to prove in a field setting. Low-level feed contamination may also be manifested as low absorption of nutrients, leading to the appearance of undigested feed particles in the faeces, and anaemia. The higher feed levels that produce typical hepatotoxicity and increased capillary fragility and haemorrhage are rarely encountered in most countries but may be common in less developed countries. Wild cranes and ducks have been poisoned after ingesting grains and peanuts contaminated with aflatoxins.

Ochratoxin is found mainly in some European climes and lesions associated with ochratoxin toxicosis may be more evident at necropsy, with accompanying nephrotoxicity (mainly proximal tubule necrosis) demonstrated by histopathology; co-contaminants have caused mainly hepato-toxicity. Levels above about 300 ppb of ochratoxin should be avoided.

Toxins produced by *Fusarium* spp. are numerous. The fusariotoxin trichothecenes, typified by T-2 toxin and diacetoxyscirpenol (DAS), often induce easily identified manifestations of charac-teristic lesions in the oropharynx and feed refusal, often with lymphocyte depletion in the bursa of Fabricius, spleen and thymus; when seen together, these findings serve as good grounds for a diagnosis. These trichothecene mycotoxicoses are probably quite common in countries with *Fusarium* grain contamination but are not often diagnosed, mainly because of nondetection of multifusariotoxin contamination of grains (this being the rule rather than the exception), an insufficient appreciation of additive or even synergistic toxic effects, poor sampling and the con-duction of insufficiently comprehensive analyses. These factors and the misleadingly high toxic feed levels reported in the literature derived from nonstressful laboratory trials using pure toxin deter diagnosticians from committing themselves to a firm diagnosis. Levels of T-2 and DAS as low as 150 ppb in the feed are probably toxic.

The common but only relatively recently discovered fusariotoxin fumonisin apparently has low toxicity in poultry. At 50 ppm in the feed, fumonisin was toxic to poults but not to broiler chicks fed to market age, whereas the MTL for most poultry is more than 100 ppm; lesions seen are mainly multifocal hepatic necrosis and hepatocellular and biliary hyperplasia. Moniliformin may be a co-contaminant with fumonisin and was found experimentally to reduce production in most domestic poultry species at more than 50 ppm, which would be an exceedingly rare finding in animal feeds; cardiotoxicity was the main lesion found. The fusariotoxin fusarochro-mane caused tibial dyschondroplasia in broilers.

Two fusariotoxins with only mild–moderate toxicity to poultry, zearalenone and deoxyniva-lenol (DON), have been used as indicators of the possible presence in grains of much more serious fusariotoxin co-contaminants. Zearalenone in the feed was associated with prolapse of the oviduct in laying hens. The MTL (reduced growth rate) of DON in broilers was estimated to be over 1000 ppb, although in one source it was given as about 250 ppb. It is interesting, and highly relevant to producers using grains from differing climates, that a risk assessment of mycotoxicosis in poultry in Europe (using their grains) regarded DON as being the only prob-lematic mycotoxin (especially in so-called '*Fusarium* years' when such toxins are found in high concentrations).

Poultry are less sensitive than mammals to ergot, with a MTL of more than 3000 ppm needed to reduce feed intake (an effect of the bitter taste of the constituent alkaloids) and growth; lay-ing hens tolerate twice this level.

Aflatoxin, ochratoxin and T-2 toxin have been found to be strongly immunosuppressive in poultry, affecting both humoral and cellular components and manifested as causing a higher disease susceptibility and poor vaccinal protection, with no suspicion in the field of a toxicosis (proven with aflatoxin and Newcastle disease or *Eimeria tenella* infection, and with ochratoxin with *Escherichia coli*). Only the combination of an inspired clinician and the analysis of stored feed samples from batches already consumed would bring about such a diagnosis, although such 'toxicoses' in poultry are probably not uncommon. Fumonisin has also recently been found to be immunosuppressive, although feed levels capable of such a clinical syndrome are unlikely to be found in countries with developed poultry industries feeding locally grown corn. The pathogenic fungus *Aspergillus fumigatus* has been shown to produce gliotoxin in infected turkey tissues, thus possibly adding to the damage caused by the pathological lesions; gliotoxin has immunosuppressive effects. DON is also immunosuppressive.

Despite the carcinogenicity of aflatoxin, ochratoxin and fumonisin in humans, the likelihood of harmful exposure by ingestion of poultry food products is slight from flocks properly monitored for manifestations of ill-health and production. The main risk is with aflatoxin and ochratoxin; fusariotoxin residues in poultry products are not regarded as a risk to human health.

Many feed additives are marketed as 'detoxifiers' or adsorbents, with the aim of neutralizing the effects of mycotoxins in feeds. While several of these preparations are efficacious against specific toxins, it is unlikely that any one product can ameliorate the deleterious effects of all the mycotoxins that can affect poultry. The prudent use of these additives would comprise an evaluation of the cost involved and the risk of feed contamination in the country involved, when only known and unavoidable contamination would best warrant use of these additives.

Other natural toxicants

Biogenic amines in spoiled animal byproduct feedstuffs were not found to be a potential problem in poultry. However gizzerosine, derived from histidine in overheated fish meal, causes the gizzard erosion syndrome 'vómito negro' in broilers aged about 3 weeks, manifested by mortality and dark gizzard and sometimes dark-coloured intestinal contents. Changing feed to ground corn for 2–3 days stops the effect of the toxicant.

Plant toxins contaminating feed from unselected strains of rapeseed contained large amounts of erucic acid in rapeseed oil, causing in the past reduced production, anaemia and cardiomyopathy in fowl, turkeys and ducks. Excess glucosinolates in rapeseed meal caused egg tainting or massive liver haemorrhage in hens and hepatopathy in turkeys. Modern rapeseed strains (e.g. canola) have neither contamination problem in the grains.

Gossypol (MTL 400 ppm in broilers) from cottonseed has an accumulative effect over weeks and induced most prominently congestive heart failure in one study and enlarged gall-bladders and biliary hyperplasia in another study. Another natural toxicosis is from excess (>0.5%) tannic acid in some sorghum strains that causes reduced production in fowl by simply reducing feed intake. Naturally occurring phytates may reduce calcium availability. Nitrite (MTL 200 ppm in fowl, 400 ppm in turkeys) is usually not found in grains. Nitrite toxicoses were reported from condensed water vapour containing nitrite formed from excessive ammonia in the air; dyspnoea and brown blood colour were seen.

Nutrient additives

As added vitamins and elements are usually formulated in premixes, separately or together, specific for each species and type of bird, mistakes involving one vitamin or most added elements are most unlikely. However toxicoses have been rarely caused by excess of vitamin A (signs, particularly in turkeys, of reduced production, severe conjunctivitis, osteoporosis, osteodystrophy) and vitamin D (osteodystrophy with signs of gait and varus/valgus abnormalities).

Feed-supplemented elements including iron (MTL, in broilers and hens 1000 ppm; signs of reduced production), zinc (MTL in broilers 2000 ppm, hens >2000 ppm; signs of reduced production, but 1000 ppm caused lymphoid cell degeneration in thymus), cobalt (MTL about 5 ppm; signs of reduced performance), manganese (MTL in broilers 2500 ppm; signs of anaemia), iodine (MTL in hens 600 ppm, in turkey hens about 350 ppm; signs of reduced production and hatchability), selenium (MTL in broilers >5 ppm, hens 3 ppm; signs of reduced production) and copper (MTL in broilers 600 ppm, turkeys 1000 ppm; signs of reduced production) could cause toxicosis. Selenium toxicity was greater with sodium selenite than with organic selenium, with the former at 10 ppm causing pale, enlarged livers showing oedema and necrosis.

More likely is toxicosis due to calcium, which is usually added separately by the feed mill, when toxicoses are most likely to be caused by misdelivery of layer feed (MTL 5%) to meat-type birds (MTL about 1.5%), or incomplete incorporation of particles into the feed and their subsequent preferential selection by birds; manifestations are secondary to nephrotoxicity.

Sodium toxicosis caused by excessive dietary salt is relatively common, as it is also added separately by the feed mill. Toxicosis is age dependent and is invariably seen only in immature birds – broiler chicks up to 3 weeks of age and in turkey poults up to 2 weeks of age (MTL about 2000 ppm sodium). The main clinical manifestations are polydipsia, diarrhoea, ascites, hydropericardium, dyspnoea, some sudden death, and sometimes central nervous system (CNS) signs (if water is restricted). In 30% of male chicks large, usually bilateral, cystic testes are seen. Sodium may also be a significant contaminant of the drinking water and, as twice as much water as feed is ingested on a weight basis, this may be enough to precipitate toxicosis in a marginally toxic feed. Excessive sodium is the main toxic inducer of the ascites (pulmonary hypertension) syndrome. An electrolyte imbalance of sodium, potassium and chloride may reduce broiler performance. Excess bicarbonate (MTL 6000 ppm) may increase water intake and urate deposition. It should also be noted that a very severe deficiency (e.g. of calcium or sodium in layers) may cause abrupt changes in production that more resemble an acute toxicosis.

Toxicoses from contaminating elements

Birds under modern conditions of husbandry are most unlikely to be exposed to toxic levels of inorganic salts of the heavy metals arsenic (MTL 100 ppm), cadmium (MTL 50 ppm, 10 ppm caused anaemia after chronic exposure), mercury (MTL 250 ppm) and lead (MTL 500 ppm in broilers, >25 ppm in hens, but only 1 ppm in laying quail) and therefore toxicoses are improbable. However, dietary imbalances caused 1 ppm of lead to be toxic in broilers. Chronic lead toxicoses in wild ducks and geese are commonly seen consequent to ingestion of lead gunshot in wetlands, with signs including marked weight loss and weakness, thus comprising by far the most common lethal toxicosis of wild birds, with millions of ducks dying each year. Cadmium may be found at high levels in some dicalcium phosphate sources added to feed. Cadmium fed at more than 1 ppm would not affect performance but could cause unacceptable tissue residues; cadmium may also cause cellular immunocompetency that was prevented with added zinc. Chronic hexavalent chromium exposure reduced cellular and humoral immunocompetency. Fluoride (MTL 500 ppm in broiler feed; signs of reduced production) may contaminate water in some parts of the world and also bonemeal or some rock phosphates added as a source of phosphorus.

Coccidiostats

Incorporation of coccidiostats into the feed of commercial poultry is very widespread and broilers may be fed coccidiostats continuously until a few days before, or up to, slaughter. Some of these compounds have low toxicity but others have a narrow therapeutic index, which, together with mistakes or insufficient mixing, and interactions with therapeutic agents, results in toxicoses being widespread.

Polyether ionophores

This group is probably the leading cause of toxicoses in poultry. Mechanisms of ionophore toxicosis in poultry are by a simple overdose, by interaction with chemotherapeutic agents or by administration to a wrong species or type or age of bird; all these are relatively commonly seen and have been very well documented. Interaction with certain therapeutic agents induces a typical ionophore toxicosis usually indistinguishable from excess dietary ionophores, even though normal levels are present in the feed. Therefore in typical clinical cases, examination for both ionophores and chemotherapeutic agents may have to be made. Diagnosis is best made by manifestations of clinical signs (initial feed refusal, lethargy, less weight gain, diarrhoea, paresis, paralysis, wing extension, legs stretched out caudally, dyspnoea). Whereas necropsy and histopathological manifestations of myonecrosis are inconsistent (sometimes found in skeletal or less often in heart muscle), elevated levels of the serum enzymes creatine kinase, aspartate transaminase and lactic dehydrogenase may be reliable effect biomarkers in recently recumbent birds. Male birds may be affected more than females – usually a function of their greater weight (especially in turkeys). Breeder chickens and turkeys may also show lowered egg production, less often reduced hatchability and uncommonly less fertility. Conclusive diagnosis of ionophore toxicosis is by feed analysis. There is no specific treatment for ionophore toxicoses.

Monensin is very much used in broilers, and turkeys (<10 weeks of age). Several times the normal feed level may produce a feed refusal that effectively precludes a serious toxicosis if it is monitored and corrected, whereas a mildly elevated level of 150–200 ppm may be readily eaten, inducing a toxicosis. The MTL is about 150 ppm in broilers, 200 ppm in hens and about 60 ppm in adult turkeys (poult MTL about 200 ppm). Clinical signs in fowl and turkeys typically include recumbency with one or both legs stretched out caudally. This is characteristic of ionophore toxicosis if seen simultaneously in many birds in a short period of time. Birds usually die of dehydration. Deleterious interactions were recorded with normal feed or drinking water or parenteral administration of enrofloxacin, tiamulin, chloramphenicol, sulfachlorpyrazine, sulfadimethoxine, sulfamethazine, oleandomycin and erythromycin. Monensin increased liver levels of lead and iron, and decreased selenium liver levels.

Lasalocid is the least toxic of the ionophores used in poultry but the few toxicoses seen are usually very similar to that of monensin. The MTL is about 200 ppm in broilers and turkeys. In addition, a unique neurotoxicological manifestation may be seen. This may be mild and observed in a very small proportion of a flock given even normal levels, when a 'walking on tiptoes' gait is seen, or it can be more severe, with sitting or shuffling on hocks and paralysis, with a much higher morbidity when chloramphenicol is administered simultaneously. Deleterious interactions were recorded with normal levels of sulfadimethoxine also.

Salinomycin has a particularly high toxicity to turkeys, in which the MTL is only about 15 ppm compared with about 90 ppm in broilers; guinea fowl are also very sensitive to this toxicosis. Vitamin E plus selenium, and zinc were suggested as antioxidants to counter the oxidative damage (manifested as anaemia) in such toxicoses in broilers. Deleterious interactions were recorded with normal levels of tiamulin, sulfachlorpyrazine, sulfadimethoxine, sulfaquinoxaline and erythromycin.

Narasin has been implicated in turkey toxicoses (MTL about 30 ppm), with dyspnoea and flaccid paralysis of wings and legs. Deleterious interactions were recorded in broilers with normal levels of tiamulin, sulfachlorpyrazine, sulfaquinoxaline and erythromycin.

Maduramicin is used in broilers and turkeys but has not been recorded as a cause of toxicoses in poultry. This is surprising, as one study showed that even the recommended level of 5 ppm for 3 weeks induced growth retardation, diarrhoea and depression, with a hypochromic anaemia (possibly due to lowered blood copper). Deleterious interactions were recorded experimentally between normal administered levels of maduramicin and tiamulin.

Residues of ionophore coccidiostats could reach human foods through overdosage, an undiagnosed toxicosis or noncompliance with withdrawal times, and so could theoretically pose a health risk to humans with existing cardiac disease.

Other coccidiostats

Many compounds are used before and after an ionophore in shuttle programmes to reduce the likelihood of ionophore resistance. An overdose of amprolium (MTL about 800 ppm in broilers, 1000 ppm in hens) may lead to signs of thiamine deficiency, with CNS signs and weak chicks at hatch. Nicarbazin is not used in broilers reared at high ambient temperatures because of its hyperthermic effect at normal feed levels (not so when combined with narasin); the MTL is about 200 ppm, with signs related to less feed intake. In hens, even less than the normal levels given to broilers caused reduced egg lay and size, eggshell thinning, depigmentation of brown shells, egg-yolk mottling and poor hatchability due to early embryonic mortality. In males 200 ppm retarded development of testes, with poor sperm quality. In halofuginone toxicity (MTL 6 ppm in broilers and hens) most signs were secondary to less feed intake. In arprinocid toxicity (MTL about 90 ppm in broilers) less feed intake and vent pecking were seen. With dinitolmide toxicosis (MTL about 250 ppm in broilers) specific signs are CNS-derived, including torticollis or extended neck and staggering; pigeons were found to be very sensitive.

Antibiotics

Antibiotics such as chlortetracycline and neomycin that have been added to poultry feed, or oxytetracycline, doxycycline, norfloxacin, enrofloxacin, flumequine, ampicillin, colistin, spectinomycin, neomycin, lincomycin, tylosin and spiramycin that may be administered in the drinking water, have low toxicity by this route and toxicosis is unlikely. Parenteral administration with oxytetracycline, norfloxacin, danofloxacin, penicillin G, amoxicillin, streptomycin, gentamicin and kanamycin should also have a low risk of toxicosis if used correctly; parenteral polymyxin B may produce renal and CNS toxicity.

Sulphonamides

Sulphonamides are potentially more hazardous than most other therapeutic agents against infectious diseases because of their low therapeutic indices, and overdosage may occur most often when medicating water in hot weather, when water consumption rises considerably. Sulfadimidine, sulfachloropyrazine, sulfachloropyridazine, sulfadimethoxine, sulfadiazine, sulfamethoxazole and sulfaquinoxaline are usually given in the water, and some infrequently in the feed. Toxicosis is due to induced vitamin K deficiency with severe anaemia, widespread haemorrhages, jaundice and pale bone marrow being typical findings.

Nitrofurans

Members of this group have been banned from use in food-producing animals in many countries because of public health concerns, so toxicity is now very unlikely to be encountered. Furazolidone in the feed to turkeys (MTL 250 ppm) caused a severe round heart syndrome, and ascites and cardiomyopathy in fowl and ducks. In broilers (MTL about 300 ppm) there may be acute signs of CNS manifestations and less weight gain and smaller combs. In breeder fowl and turkeys (MTL 110 ppm), flocks showed reversible signs of smaller testes, poor sperm production and quality, less hatchability, and in layers (MTL 220 ppm) reduced lay. Immature ducks may also show grossly cystic testes with tubular dilatation. Nitrofurazone in broiler feed (MTL 500 ppm), and even at normal levels in broiler feed given to ducklings, gave CNS manifestations of hyperexcitability.

Growth-promoting additives

The recent European Union ban on the use of such antimicrobial growth-promoting feed additives for fear of resistance to human antibiotics may bring about similar restrictions elsewhere. Virginiamycin, bacitracin, oleandomycin and bambermycin are antibiotics that have been used as feed additives to promote growth and have extremely low toxicity in poultry. Organoarsenicals such as 3-nitro-4-hydroxy-phenylarsonic acid (MTL about 200 ppm in broilers, 50 ppm in turkeys) and 4-nitrophenylarsonic acid may cause acute or chronic toxicoses with mainly CNS signs such as ataxia, neck extension, paresis, paralysis, hock-sitting, curled toes, and also diarrhoea, sometimes haemorrhagic in nature. Copper sulphate may be added to broiler and layer feed or drinking water to improve production and excess induces poor growth and a few erosive oropharyngeal lesions; layers exhibit reduced lay.

Other drugs

Piperazine, phenothiazine, mebendazole, flubendazole and ivermectin anthelmintics have low toxicities in poultry and toxicoses are unlikely. Levamisole has low toxicity in fowl but geese are more sensitive to this drug. The antiprotozoan dimetridazole (MTL in turkeys about 1500 ppm) caused CNS signs, also seen in ducks and geese with drinking water medicated at the correct level for turkeys.

Other contaminants

In the period 1960–1980, ascites found in broilers was invariably of a toxic origin, but the chick oedema and toxic fat syndromes then caused by polychlorinated biphenyls (PCBs) and their contaminants are now unrecorded and broiler ascites seen now is invariably a common manifestation of the ascites syndrome, an undesirable byproduct of intensive phenotypic broiler selection. However recent mass contamination of poultry products in Europe from feed contaminated with PCB-related dioxins and dibenzofurans from the illegal incorporation of non-natural oils into fats has brought about renewed thinking on ways to avoid such incidents, largely based on improved quality control of all feed ingredients.

Quaternary ammonium disinfectants may be added to drinking water to reduce microorganism contamination but dosing in excess, particularly for several days, causes erosive lesions in the oropharynx very similar in nature to those caused by some trichothecene mycotoxins; however, the lesions with the disinfectants are much more widespread than the smaller, localized lesions found with T-2 and DAS.

PESTICIDE TOXICOSES

Insecticides

Under normal conditions of poultry husbandry, birds may be exposed to insecticides by spraying of the building or spot treatment of litter against flies or beetles, or against ectoparasite infestations. Insecticides approved for these uses and applied correctly will not be deleterious, whereas incorrect usage has caused toxicoses.

Chlorinated hydrocarbon insecticides (OCls) such as DDT, aldrin, dieldrin, chlordane, heptachlor, heptachlor epoxide and methoxychlor have largely been banned or phased out because of prolonged persistence in animals and in the environment, high toxicity and potential carcinogenicity in humans. Some OCls are still used for termite control in building foundations. Apart from universal, very low, residue level contamination of the feed, there is a negligible risk of exposure or toxicosis due to OCls in commercial poultry. Lindane and especially endosulphan are still intensively used in many countries; lindane was found to be immunosuppressive (cellular and humoral components) in chicks at a level of 25 ppm. Signs of OCl toxicoses are manifestations of CNS involvement, mainly tremor and convulsive muscle movements.

Organophosphorus (OP) insecticides used in ectoparasite control have chiefly been malathion, tetrachlorvinfos and coumaphos. They are cholinesterase-inhibiting in their mode of action, are characterized by moderate to high toxicity, low persistence and rapid action and have efficacious treatments. Some OP compounds, such as diazinon, fenthion and parathion, are particularly toxic to birds and have caused wild bird mortality. Signs of OP toxicosis are profuse ropy salivation, locomotor and respiratory muscular weakness, dyspnoea and paralysis. High morbidity and mortality may be seen within minutes or at most several hours of exposure, and within 24 h birds usually recover or die. Some compounds are well absorbed through the skin after aerial spraying and drift to poultry flocks. Diagnosis is by determination of a reduction in plasma (or brain) acetylcholinesterase levels, with residue analysis of feed/water/bedding/skin or crop/gizzard content. Treatment is with atropine sulphate at a dosage of 50 mg/kg bodyweight intramuscularly (a dose much higher than in mammals) with or without oximes (pralidoxime chloride, 2-PAM, at 50–100 mg/kg bodyweight intramuscularly). Adult hens are the animal model for testing OP compounds for delayed neurotoxicity, an axonal degeneration associated with inhibition of neurotoxic esterase in the CNS.

Carbamate anticholinesterase insecticides, such as carbaryl, have very low toxicity (MTL 3000 ppm) and are used on birds against ectoparasites, whereas other carbamates such as carbofuran, methomyl, bendiocarb and aldicarb are highly toxic but practically should not get to poultry, although methomyl-containing fly baits may be used on farms. Signs are similar to the OP but are even more rapid, with tremor and convulsions being much more marked. Diagnosis is as for OP, but blood or brain acetylcholinesterase levels may regenerate rapidly and give false-negative results. Treatment is best performed with atropine sulphate as for OPs. Organophosphorus and carbamate insecticides are a major cause of toxicoses in wild birds but atropine and oximes have been extremely efficacious treatments.

Pyrethroid insecticides such as permethrin, cypermethrin and deltamethrin have low toxicity and are being continuously improved to be used at lower concentrations. These pyrethroids and others are used in bird ectoparasite and farm pest insect control but only very rarely cause (nonfatal) toxicoses; characteristic signs are hyperactivity, tremor and salivation. Deltamethrin at 100 ppm in broiler feed reduced weight gain, as a result of overproduction of free radicals.

Rodenticides

Rodents may be severe pests in poultry buildings and so toxic baits may be used and could be eaten by poultry. Most rodenticides are acute in action.

First-generation anticoagulants such as warfarin, chlorphacinone, diphacinone and coumatetralyl are characterized by moderate toxicity with repeated, continuous ingestion over several days needed to cause toxicosis, with subacute onset of a haemorrhagic syndrome. Second-generation anticoagulants such as brodifacoum, bromadiolone, difenacoum, difethialone and flocoumafen are by far the most commonly used rodenticides worldwide. They are highly toxic and, despite the low levels used in the baits, kill rodents (and some nontarget animals) after only one ingestion. Livers of domestic poultry inadvertently exposed sublethally to such rodenticides could be deleterious to human health. Liver residues in exposed animals persist for months and these rodenticides, particularly brodifacoum, are a major cause of raptor and owl mortality in wild bird populations.

Other rodenticides are used less commonly and are of less toxicological importance to poultry. Sodium fluoroacetate is considerably less toxic to birds than to mammals; sudden death is the main finding in birds. Zinc phosphide causes liver necrosis and respiratory distress. Strychnine is used in some countries and is somewhat less toxic to birds than mammals – tonic convulsions and hyperaesthesia are the main manifestations. Cholecalciferol (vitamin D equivalent) is highly toxic to mammals, but ducks, for example, were found to be highly resistant.

Other pesticides

Despite a multitude of herbicides and their very wide use, modern compounds have low toxicity to animals and are used at low application rates, essentially precluding toxicoses. Commercial poultry invariably are not exposed to herbicides, whereas the husbandry of some yarded birds could result in exposure to herbicides. Paraquat is the most toxic herbicide in mammals but was not found to cause toxicosis in turkeys even when used at higher than recommended levels.

Very many fungicides are much used, but the more selective compounds used now present a very low risk to farm animals that are exposed only to grains in feedstuffs. Copper oxychloride has been used as a grain fungicide but only on grains destined for planting; the compound was shown experimentally to cause atrophy of fowl testes. Organomercury fungicides used on (seed) grains caused severe CNS manifestations but these dangerous compounds (for human health too) have been universally banned from such use. Thiram caused depressed growth with tibial dyschondroplasia in broilers and soft eggshells in hens. Pentachlorophenol could be a contaminant of wood shavings used as litter, mainly causing reduced body weight, diarrhoea, egg or meat taints, or lowered hatchability. The molluscide metaldehyde used in a vegetable bait caused CNS signs in fowl, ducks and geese.

TOXICOSES FROM THE AIR OR LITTER

Ammonia is produced in wet litter and toxicoses may be common, subtle and much underdiagnosed. Levels in the air as low as 25 ppm in broilers and turkeys worsen feed conversion, cause eye and lung lesions and increase condemnations; 50 ppm is toxic in hens. The human nose can detect less than 10 ppm, making it the most practical sensor for adverse levels. Toxicosis due to carbon monoxide from poorly maintained gas heaters is possible; 400 ppm is the toxic level, causing head shaking, ataxia and dyspnoea, with bright red blood. Carbon dioxide toxicosis is extremely unlikely, with 12 000 ppm being the toxic level. Formaldehyde overuse in the hatchery caused gasping and eye lesions in newly hatched chicks; in poults high mortality and mouth lesions were seen. Phenolic disinfectants may be used on floors, could contaminate bedding and have mainly deleterious respiratory effects with coughing, dyspnoea and rales. Litter may be contaminated with fungicides, or other compounds such as ferrous sulphate, added to reduce ammonia production; improper mixing may result in ingestion of this chemical and signs of ulcerative ventriculitis and hepatopathy. A unique case of very high acute mortality was recorded in brooding chicks due to the use of new polytetrafluoroethylene (PTFE (Teflon®))-coated heat lamps. The sublimated PTFE after the initial heating of the coating was pneumotoxic, with dyspnoea, pulmonary congestion and oedema being found. Such toxicoses are not uncommon in pet birds after the first use or overheating of PTFE-coated kitchen utensils.

FURTHER READING

Adams H R 2001 Veterinary pharmacology and therapeutics, 8th edn. Iowa State University Press, Ames

Anon 1999 Biotoxins. In: Field manual on wildlife diseases, general field procedures and diseases of birds. USGS, Washington DC. Available on line at: www.nwhc.usgs.gov/publications/field_manual/index.jsp

Anon 1999 Chemical toxins. In: Field manual on wildlife diseases, general field procedures and diseases of birds. USGS, Washington DC. Available on line at: www.nwhc.usgs.gov/publications/field_manual/index.jsp

Anon 2003 Mycotoxins: risks in plant, animal and human systems. Task Force Report number 131. CAST, Ames

Anon 2006 Network for smallholder poultry development. Available on line at: www.poultry.kvl.dk/

Bedford M 2000 Removal of antibiotic growth promoters from poultry diets: implications and strategies to minimize subsequent problems. Worlds Poult Sci J 56: 347–365

Bishop Y 2005 Veterinary formulary, 6th edn. Pharmaceutica Press, London

Brown T P, Julian R J 2003 Other toxins and poisons. In: Saif Y M (ed) Diseases of poultry, 11th edn. Iowa State University Press, Ames, p 1133–1159

Danicke S 2002 Prevention and control of mycotoxins in the poultry production chain: a European view. Worlds Poult Sci J 58: 451–467

Dowling L 1992 Ionophore toxicity in chickens: a review of pathology and diagnosis. Avian Pathol 21: 355–368

Hamilton P B 1982 Mycotoxins and farm animals. Refuah Vet 39: 17–45

Hoerr F J 2003 Mycotoxicoses. In: Saif Y M (ed) Diseases of poultry, 11th edn. Iowa State University Press, Ames, p 1103–1132

Kan CA 2002 Prevention and control of contaminants of industrial processes and pesticides in the poultry production chain. Worlds Poult Sci J 58: 159–167

Keshavarz K 1982 Anticoccidial drugs: growth and performance depressing effects in young chickens. Poult Sci 61: 699–705

Plumlee K H 2004 Clinical veterinary toxicology. Mosby, St Louis

Shlosberg A 2001 Natural mycotoxicoses in fowl induced by diacetoxyscirpenol and T-2 toxin – a diagnostic enigma. In: De Koe W J Samson R A (eds) Mycotoxins and phycotoxins in perspective at the turn of the millennium. De Koe, Wageningen

Shlosberg A, Bellaiche M, Hanji V et al 1997 New treatment regimens in organophosphate (diazinon) and carbamate (methomyl) insecticide-induced toxicoses in fowl. Vet Hum Toxicol 39: 347–350

Viera S L 2003 Nutritional implications of mould development in feedstuffs and alternatives to reduce the mycotoxin problem in poultry feeds. Worlds Poult Sci J 59: 111–122

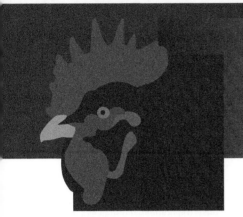

CHAPTER 45

Tom Pennycott

Diseases of game birds

An estimated 30–35 million game birds are reared and released each year in the UK for sporting purposes, made up of approximately 25 million pheasants (*Phasianus colchicus*), 5–10 million red-legged or French partridge (*Alectoris rufa*) and 1 million grey or English partridge (*Perdix perdix*) (figures provided by the Game Conservancy Trust and the British Association for Shooting and Conservation, January 2006). There are many different management systems used to produce the hatching eggs, to artificially incubate the eggs, to rear the progeny to a stage at which they can be released into a semi-wild environment, and to manage the birds following their release. Further details of such systems can be found in the standard game-bird-rearing guides listed below. Recent years have seen increasing numbers of pheasants and partridges being imported to the UK, mostly as hatching eggs and day-old chicks from France, but also older birds.

Several factors combine to make reared game birds susceptible to many different infectious and noninfectious diseases. The birds are often managed in large groups and at high stocking densities, and frequently in accommodation that has been used for other batches of game birds in the same year or in previous years. The birds are neither truly wild nor fully domesticated but are expected to adapt to both situations, and birds that have been released into a semi-wild environment may be caught up again and used for breeding purposes. Problems of egg hygiene, contact with wild birds, limitations on medication and fewer trained gamekeepers rearing increasing numbers of birds add to the difficulties.

Pheasants make up the bulk of the game birds reared and released, and most of the conditions described below will relate to this species. Where appropriate, additional reference will be made to red-legged or grey partridges. Some of the conditions also occur in chickens and turkeys, and fuller discussion of such diseases will be found elsewhere in this book.

The diseases considered below are divided into those affecting birds in the first 3 weeks of life, those affecting older birds in the rearing pens and after release, and those affecting adult birds, although some conditions can affect several age groups.

DISEASES AFFECTING GAME BIRDS IN THE FIRST 3 WEEKS OF LIFE

Young game birds are reared under conditions not unlike those of commercially reared chickens and turkeys. Group size varies from under 100 birds to several thousand, with heat most often provided by gas-fired heaters or 'electric hens' (heated elements under which the birds congregate to keep warm). Birds receive commercial crumbed or pelleted diets, with particle size increasing and protein content reducing as the birds grow older. Water may be delivered in manually filled or automatic drinkers, and there is increasing interest in the use of nipple drinkers. Bedding is usually in the form of wood shavings, sometimes preceded by corrugated paper, but other materials such as pea gravel and cardboard squares may be used. Birds often have access to grass runs within the first 3 weeks of life, weather permitting. Alternatively, young partridges may be allowed access to elevated runs with wire floors. As in chickens and turkeys, young pheasants and partridges can die from yolk sac infections, as starve-outs or nonstarters, from aspergillosis, from environmental factors such as overheating, chilling and carbon monoxide poisoning, and from colisepticaemia. These conditions are discussed elsewhere. Other important conditions of young game birds in this period are *Rotavirus* infection and salmonellosis. It may be worthwhile agreeing target mortality figures with the gamekeeper, for example 4% mortality in the first 2 weeks of life, with veterinary help sought if the target figure is likely to be exceeded.

ROTAVIRUS INFECTION

Rotavirus infection is seen most often in pheasants and partridges between the ages of 4 and 14 days but can be seen later in the rearing period. Birds become dull, huddle together and stop feeding. Others are found dead or comatose and, as the disease progresses, signs of diarrhoea may be seen. Most deaths occur in the first 2 weeks of life but some of the survivors may appear stunted, especially if *Salmonella* spp. are also present. Additional problems include vent pecking and susceptibility to chilling. Overall mortality can approach 70%, but more often is in the range 10–30%.

Post-mortem examination usually reveals watery intestinal contents and caeca that are distended by frothy yellow fluid (Fig. 45.1). Pasting of the vent with dried faeces may result in impaction of the rectum. The birds are often small for their age with evidence that they have started to feed but stopped again, and there may be signs of a secondary bacterial infection such as pericarditis, perihepatitis, hepatomegaly or splenomegaly.

Game birds may be affected by group A and non-group-A (atypical) rotaviruses. Both can be detected in caecal contents by electron microscopy or polyacrylamide gel electrophoresis (PAGE), but kit tests that employ a latex agglutination test or enzyme-linked immunosorbent assay (ELISA) for group A *Rotavirus* will not detect the atypical rotaviruses.

The epidemiology of rotavirus infection still remains unclear but the organism appears to be widespread. It is suggested that adult pheasants may carry this virus and shed it in the faeces. Faecal contamination of the shell of their eggs can then occur, providing the route of entry of virus into the incubators and subsequently into the chicks that hatch. Lateral spread to other chicks can then occur in the hatcher, during transport or in the brooder huts. If two consecutive batches of birds are reared in the same brooder accommodation, even if the unit is cleansed

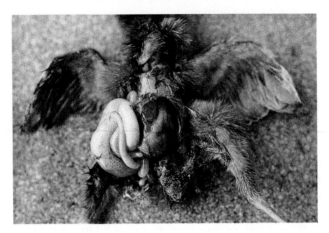

Fig. 45.1 Pheasant chick with *Rotavirus* infection. Caeca distended with frothy fluid.

and disinfected between batches, an overwhelming challenge to the second batch of chicks may occur, resulting in clinical disease. Birds being reared in large multiage houses are also susceptible to *Rotavirus* for the same reasons.

Although there is no specific treatment, electrolytes in the drinking water may be beneficial, and antimicrobial therapy in the drinking water may reduce losses from secondary bacterial infections – mortality is highest in the presence of concurrent salmonellosis or colibacillosis, as is stunting of survivors. The use of probiotics after the antimicrobials may be helpful. Measures must also be taken to prevent the spread of disease to other susceptible batches of young chicks.

Control measures are aimed at breaking the cycle of infection from adults to chicks and preventing a build up of virus numbers in the birds' rearing accommodation. Eggs must be collected frequently and carefully sanitized or disinfected as quickly as possible, and subsequent hygiene of the egg store, setters and hatchers must be of a high standard. Ideally chicks should be reared in accommodation that has not previously been used in the current season for rearing game birds and not in the same air space as older chicks. If this is not possible, the accommodation should be thoroughly cleansed and disinfected before the new birds go in. Currently there is no commercially available vaccine against *Rotavirus* infection in game birds.

SALMONELLOSIS

The number of reported outbreaks of salmonellosis in game birds rose between 1993 and 1997 but has steadily fallen again since then. Serotypes such as *Salmonella* Binza and *Salmonella* Orion are probably only significant as secondary infections, for example following a primary rotavirus infection. Other serotypes such as *Salmonella* Typhimurium and *Salmonella* Enteritidis are of primary importance and can result in high mortality, especially in the first 2–3 weeks of life, with post-mortem lesions including pericarditis, perihepatitis and caseous caecal cores.

Also of concern is disease in young pheasants caused by *Salmonella* Pullorum, in which mortality can reach 50% in the first 2–3 weeks of life, with stunting in some of the survivors. Post-mortem lesions include infected yolk sacs, pale nodules in the wall of the caeca and rectum, caseous caecal cores and white or fawn-coloured nodules in the lungs. Fine foci of liver necrosis are seen less frequently, as is pericarditis and perihepatitis. Following the trend seen with other serotypes of *Salmonella*, the number of incidents of *S.* Pullorum in game birds has fallen substantially since

1997, but that does not preclude the possibility of transfer of infection from pheasants to poultry in the future.

S. Typhimurium, *S.* Enteritidis and *S.* Pullorum can spread vertically from one generation to the next, either in or on the unhatched egg. Egg hygiene measures will reduce the risk of egg transmission but will be unsuccessful if true transovarian infection is occurring rather than external contamination of the eggshell. During an outbreak, losses may be reduced by the use of an appropriate antibacterial in the drinking water. Hygiene measures should also be enforced to reduce spread to other birds, especially if another batch of younger chicks is on site or due to be delivered. The reasons for the decline in salmonellosis in game birds are unclear but possibly reflect improved hygiene at breeding sites and hatcheries, aided by a reduction in the numbers of smaller sites producing hatching eggs and day-old chicks.

DISEASES AFFECTING OLDER GAME BIRDS IN REARING PENS AND AFTER RELEASE

As the birds in the rearing pens grow older, they spend more time in outdoor runs (where they are exposed to fluctuating weather conditions), supplementary heat is gradually removed and there may be further dietary changes. To reduce the risks of cannibalism the birds may be beak trimmed, or alternatively a plastic 'bit' may be placed between the upper and lower beaks, clipped into the nostrils. Further changes take place when the birds are transferred to release pens, temporary holding pens that help the birds to acclimatize to a semi-wild existence. These management procedures can be stressful and deaths may occur after bitting, in birds that fail to adjust to conditions in the release pens, and in birds that have become chilled or smothered. These management-related deaths can form a substantial part of 'normal mortality' – in a study of mortality on one game bird rearing site where mortality from 1 day to 6 weeks old was an acceptable 6.5%, over half of the 1273 deaths were due to suspected or confirmed chilling, smothering or postbitting stress (Fig. 45.2). Birds in this age group can be affected by mycoplasmosis, helminthiasis and marble spleen disease, conditions that also affect adults. Protozoal diseases such as spironucleosis (hexamitosis) and coccidiosis are important in this age group, and to a lesser extent bacterial diseases. Disease caused by the protozoan *Histomonas meleagridis* (histomoniasis or blackhead) is occasionally seen in pheasants and partridges, and infection with the yeast *Candida albicans* is not uncommon in partridges – these diseases are described more fully elsewhere. Target mortality for the period from 1 day old to release should be around 10%, although many gamekeepers achieve better figures than this. Mortality figures after release are difficult to establish because the carcasses are not readily found.

DISEASES ASSOCIATED WITH THE PROTOZOA *SPIRONUCLEUS (HEXAMITA)*, *TRICHOMONAS* AND *BLASTOCYSTIS*

Disease caused by *Spironucleus (Hexamita) meleagridis*, a small, leaf-shaped motile protozoon found in the small intestine, is very common in the summer months. Large numbers of organisms cause weight loss (sometimes leading to emaciation), frothy yellow diarrhoea, dehydration and eventually death. At post-mortem examination the intestinal contents are found to be very watery, with small boluses of semi-solid material, and the caecal contents are frequently frothy and yellow. Spironucleosis (hexamitiasis) can be seen in pheasants and partridges during the

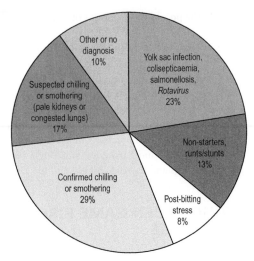

Fig. 45.2 Causes of death of 1273 pheasant chicks from 1 day to 6 weeks old.

rearing and releasing stages, and also in adult partridges. Other protozoa such as the motile *Trichomonas phasiani* and the nonmotile *Blastocystis* species may also be found in large numbers in the caeca of game birds with clinical signs and post-mortem features similar to spironucleosis. However these organisms can also be found in healthy birds and their presence in large numbers may be indicative of an imbalance of the normal caecal flora caused by other factors.

Trichomonas and *Spironucleus* are motile protozoa that are difficult to detect microscopically unless they are actively moving. Material for examination should therefore be as fresh as possible, and live birds showing signs typical of the flock problem should be submitted for euthanasia and full examination. Fresh material is less critical for the detection of the nonmotile *Blastocystis*.

Historically the control of motile protozoal infections of game birds relied on the inclusion of dimetridazole in the feed during the rearing period and for the first few weeks after release. Outbreaks of clinical disease were treated with the same drug in the drinking water. However dimetridazole is no longer authorized for use in turkeys and game birds in the UK. As an alternative, tetracycline antibiotics administered in the feed or drinking water may be used as part of the treatment and control measures, sometimes in conjunction with electrolytes. It is unclear if any response is due to the effect of the tetracyclines on the protozoa or on bacteria that have over-proliferated in the digestive tract.

When spironucleosis (hexamitiasis) was first described in turkey poults in 1955, a resistant non-motile cyst was described as part of the life cycle of the organism. The existence of such a cyst was disputed for many years, but recent work (Wood & Smith 2004) conclusively showed that clusters of cysts could be found in thick clots of intestinal mucus. Extrapolating from work carried out in turkeys many years ago, such cysts can remain infective at room temperature for a week and for up to 6 weeks at 4°C. Similarly, previous work showed that 30% of infected turkeys that survived became carriers, and the same may be true for infected game birds. Mucus-containing infective cysts could contaminate naturally occurring sources of drinking water and could adhere to boots, equipment, feeders, drinkers, etc., enhancing the spread of the organism. If the shells of eggs laid by carrier hen pheasants became contaminated by intestinal mucus, chicks hatching from the eggs could perhaps become infected, helping to explain the unexpected appearance of disease in the rearing pens. The findings of Wood & Smith reinforce the importance of improved hygiene, reduced stocking density and increased biosecurity in the control of spironucleosis.

COCCIDIOSIS

The most pathogenic coccidia of game birds are *Eimeria colchici* and *Eimeria legionensis*, which inhabit the caeca of pheasants and partridges, respectively. *Eimeria duodenalis* and *Eimeria phasiani* are found in the duodenum and small intestine of pheasants but are less pathogenic than those found in the caeca. An unidentified species of coccidium found in the duodenum and upper intestine of partridges has also been associated with significant mortality.

Coccidiosis has been diagnosed in birds as young as 1 week of age that had been placed in a heavily contaminated environment. More commonly, disease is seen in the rearing fields around 3–5 weeks of age, and in older birds after transfer to the release pens. Clinical signs may be relatively mild, with depression, reduced appetite and ruffled feathers. Diarrhoea may be present but rarely with any blood. If the challenge dose is high, the birds may lose weight, become dehydrated and die. In the case of partridges, coccidiosis can result in apparent sudden deaths. Post-mortem lesions include off-white cheesy cores in the caeca, or frothy caecal contents similar to those found in birds with spironucleosis. The intestinal contents may be fluid, and undigested food may be found in the small intestine and caeca.

Control depends on keeping the coccidial challenge as low as possible, by attention to hygiene (especially of the feeders and drinkers and the areas around them), avoiding the reuse or overstocking of pens, and incorporating anticoccidial drugs such as clopidol and lasalocid into the feed, often from 1 day old until after transfer to the release pens. However, if there is a heavy challenge the medication in the feed may not be sufficient to prevent disease and medication of the drinking water with an appropriate anticoccidial drug will be required. At the time of writing there are no products licensed to treat coccidiosis in game birds. Unlicensed products that have been used include amprolium, sulphonamides and toltrazuril.

STAPHYLOCOCCUS AUREUS, PASTEURELLA MULTOCIDA, ERYSIPELOTHRIX RHUSIOPATHIAE, YERSINIA PSEUDOTUBERCULOSIS

Staphylococcus aureus is typically associated with a unilateral or bilateral tenosynovitis in pheasants 7–10 days after transfer to release pens. Affected birds become lame, with distension of the hock joints and extensor tendons above the hock joints with purulent material. The bacteria may gain entry through minor wounds acquired when the birds are being caught in the rearing pens, during transport or in the first few days after transfer to the release pens. A concurrent reovirus infection has also been described.

Outbreaks of mortality due to *Pasteurella multocida* and *Erysipelothrix rhusiopathiae* occur in well-grown pheasants after release or less commonly in partridges or adult pheasants. Signs of septicaemia are found at post-mortem examination, and in birds with pasteurellosis the lungs are often congested or consolidated, resulting in confusion with marble spleen disease (see below). Haemorrhages on the muscles of the legs and breast are seen in some birds with erysipelas, and occasionally a hock joint arthritis.

Yersinia pseudotuberculosis usually causes problems in red-legged partridges, either well-grown released birds or adults. Sudden death of birds in good condition is often seen but wasting, diarrhoea and death may also occur. Post-mortem lesions of septicaemia are seen in birds dying suddenly, and in the more chronic form pale necrotic foci are frequently found in the liver, spleen and intestine.

More details of these bacterial conditions can be found elsewhere. Affected flocks can be treated in the drinking water with an appropriate antibacterial, although this can present practical problems if there are other sources of drinking water available to the birds. Strict adherence to withdrawal times must be observed. Lame or emaciated birds should be culled.

NEWCASTLE DISEASE AND PHEASANT ATAXIA

Newcastle disease in poultry is discussed elsewhere. Pheasants are also susceptible to Newcastle disease, with small outbreaks in England in May 1996 and July 2005. Affected birds show depression, diarrhoea and central nervous signs. A sharp drop in egg production may be seen in adult birds. Depending on the degree of risk, vaccination of game birds against Newcastle disease may be required.

A condition that must be differentiated from the nervous form of Newcastle disease has been described, referred to here as pheasant ataxia. Pheasants aged 8 weeks and above are most commonly affected, although the disease has also been seen in adults. Small numbers of birds (less than 2% of the flock) show nervous signs such as loss of balance, torticollis and lateral recumbency. Initially, affected birds remain bright despite the nervous signs, but loss of weight and death eventually results from the birds' inability to feed properly. No significant gross post-mortem lesions are present but perivascular cuffing of the blood vessels of the brain with mononuclear inflammatory cells, often with focal gliosis and malacia, is usually noted on histopathology. An avian reticuloendotheliosis virus may be involved.

DISEASES AFFECTING ADULT GAME BIRDS IN THEIR BREEDING ACCOMMODATION

Breeding pheasants are usually kept on grass in groups varying from one cock plus six hens to large flocks of several-hundred birds. Red-legged partridges are often kept in breeding pairs on grass or in wire-floored raised pens, or in flocks of up to 50 birds on grass. Grey partridges must be kept in pairs, either on wire or on grass. Most breeding pheasants are around 1 year old, but partridges may be kept for several breeding seasons. For many years it was standard practice to form breeding flocks in the spring months by catching pheasants that had been released in the summer/autumn and had survived the shooting season. However, there is now a trend to overwinter potential breeding pheasants in enclosed pens or buildings. As in chickens, turkeys and ducks, reproductive tract problems such as prolapse or impaction of the oviduct and egg peritonitis are common, as are deaths from traumatic injuries, and together may be responsible for about one half of all deaths in the breeding accommodation. Avian tuberculosis can be a problem in older game birds or those kept in grass breeding pens that have been in use for many years, and an ulcerative enteritis associated with *Clostridium colinum* occurs in adult red-legged partridges – these conditions are described elsewhere. Other important diseases seen in adults are infectious sinusitis, *Pheasant coronavirus*-associated nephritis, marble spleen disease and helminthiasis, and in recent years lymphomatous tumours of adult pheasants have been seen. A mortality figure of 5% is usually considered acceptable for the 5 months in which adult pheasants are kept in their breeding pens.

INFECTIOUS SINUSITIS

A condition of pheasants and partridges in which there is swelling around one or both eyes, referred to as infectious sinusitis, has been recognized since the mid-1950s. Infectious sinusitis has been associated with several different species of mycoplasma (of which *Mycoplasma gallisepticum* is probably the most important) but is probably of multifactorial aetiology. On some sites disease may be precipitated by exposure to viruses such as *Avian pneumovirus* and *Avian coronavirus*.

Clinical disease is seen most often in adults but has also been seen in younger birds. There is unilateral or bilateral swelling of the infraorbital sinus between the eye and nostril, resulting in shaking of the head, an oculonasal discharge, respiratory noises and dyspnoea. A purulent conjunctivitis and keratitis may develop, with loss of feathers around the eyes. In severe cases purulent material fills the nasal passages and reaches the mouth through the palatine slit, and affected birds may die or require culling because of their inability to feed. In laying birds there is often a concurrent drop in egg numbers and the production of pale-shelled eggs.

Mildly affected released birds can recover but may become carriers of *M. gallisepticum*. When these birds are caught up for breeding at the end of the winter, stress may cause the birds to re-excrete the organisms in large numbers, with spread to other birds in the group. The close contact between birds at this stage enables rapid spread of infectious agents within the group. In common with mycoplasmosis in other avian species, egg transmission also occurs.

Control measures include prophylactic treatment for *M. gallisepticum* at times of stress, hygiene of feeders and drinkers, culling when necessary, and ideally obtaining stock from mycoplasma-free sources. Several different therapeutic agents have been used to control or treat *M. gallisepticum*, such as tylosin, tiamulin, enrofloxacin and a combination of lincomycin and spectinomycin. These products may be administered at strategic times, such as at catching up, the onset of lay or transfer to release pens if there have been earlier problems. None of these products is licensed for use in game birds. Off-licence vaccination of future breeding flocks against *Avian pneumovirus* has also been used on some sites, although the efficacy is unclear. Releasing pheasants in the summer/autumn and catching them for breeding purposes in the spring increases the likelihood of diseases such as infectious sinusitis occurring in the laying pens. However recent years have seen an increase in the number of breeding sites maintaining closed flocks of future breeding pheasants over the winter months rather than releasing/catching birds, and this practice may result in a reduction in sinusitis and other infectious diseases.

PHEASANT CORONAVIRUS-ASSOCIATED NEPHRITIS

Gross enlargement and pallor of the kidneys, impaction of one or both ureters with urate casts and the deposition of urates on the surface of the liver and heart can be found in adult pheasants dying in their laying accommodation. Affected birds, both males and females, are often found dead in good body condition but may be seen alive, showing nonspecific signs of ill health and sometimes staining of the vent with white urates. Reduced egg numbers, quality and hatchability are a feature on some estates, and early in an outbreak egg peritonitis may be the predominant post-mortem feature. This condition, usually referred to as *Pheasant coronavirus*-associated nephritis or pheasant urolithiasis, was first recorded in Hampshire in 1983 but has since spread to many other areas of the UK. It is essentially a disease of adults but a similar condition has also been seen in pheasants aged 8 weeks. Mortality rates approaching 50% have been described. Significant mortality may be seen on the same site in subsequent years, but on some sites the condition becomes part of normal mortality.

Histologically there is dilation of the kidney tubules, with flattening of the tubular epithelium and distension of the collecting ducts with casts made up of necrotic cells and granulocytes. These changes may be severe, with areas of tubular necrosis and mineralization. An interstitial infiltration of mononuclear inflammatory cells occurs in many cases. A virus designated 750/83 has been isolated from the tissues of pheasants with such kidney lesions and has the appearance of a coronavirus on electron microscopy. This virus is different from the strains of *Coronavirus* recovered from poultry with infectious bronchitis, including the *Infectious bronchitis virus* strains M41, 793/B, D274 and D1466, and has been termed *Pheasant coronavirus*. However, attempts to isolate virus from kidney or caecal tonsil are often unsuccessful and the diagnosis is usually made on the basis of the history and post-mortem findings.

Although recognized for several years, the epidemiology is still largely conjecture. It is possible that the initial kidney damage occurs earlier in life, with kidney failure precipitated later by factors such as chilling, water deprivation, the stress of birds moving into breeding pens and the requirement to mobilize calcium for egg production. Equally uncertain is the approach to the treatment and control of this disease. The injection of inactivated vaccines against the M41 strain of infectious bronchitis of poultry has been used on some estates for control purposes but the results are equivocal. During an outbreak of disease measures should be taken to prevent dehydration in the birds, such as the provision of extra drinkers or drinkers that are easier to use. Electrolyte solutions in the drinking water may help but there is no evidence that the use of antibacterials against secondary bacteria reduces mortality.

MARBLE SPLEEN DISEASE

Marble spleen disease is another viral condition of pheasants resulting in sudden death. It is caused by a type II *Avian adenovirus* related to the virus causing haemorrhagic enteritis of turkeys and was first diagnosed in the UK in 1972. Although initially described in poults from 3 months of age, disease is most often seen in adult pheasants in the breeding pens, causing a flurry of sudden deaths.

Post-mortem examination demonstrates a bird that has died in good body condition, with food in the digestive tract and with heavily congested and oedematous lungs. Dark serosanguinous fluid may also be found in the rib spaces and trachea. The spleen of affected birds is usually enlarged and with confluent grey foci, giving a 'marbled' appearance, but some birds die with a grossly normal spleen. Histological lesions in the spleen include depletion and necrosis of lymphoid follicles, eosinophilic hyaline deposits in the sinusoids, reticuloendothelial cell hyperplasia and degeneration, and the formation of large, pale, faintly basophilic inclusion bodies in the nuclei of reticuloendothelial cells. Diagnosis can be confirmed by histopathology or by demonstrating viral antigen in the spleen using a gel diffusion test.

Marble spleen disease virus appears to be widespread in some populations of pheasants. Stress factors such as those encountered in the breeding pens may precipitate viral shedding, resulting in disease in birds that have not yet met the virus. This is especially likely to occur if the breeding flock is made up of birds from several different sources. The number of birds affected can be very small or may exceed 50%, presumably depending on the immune status of the birds. There is no specific treatment for marble spleen disease and there is no vaccine licensed for use in pheasants in the UK. Control must therefore depend on keeping stress factors that could precipitate disease to a minimum.

PARASITIC WORMS

The commonest parasitic worms found in pheasants and partridges are *Syngamus trachea* (the gapeworm), *Heterakis gallinarum* (the caecal worm) and hairworms of the subfamily Capillariinae. More information about the life cycles of these nematodes can be found in Chapter 39. Adult pheasants caught up for breeding often carry these parasites and, although usually wormed at this stage, they frequently become re-infected with *Syngamus* and *Heterakis*. Worms are also found in younger birds, especially from August onwards, and gapeworms in particular can sometimes cause problems in the rearing pens.

The gapeworm *S. trachea* is probably the most important parasitic worm of pheasants and partridges. Adult worms live in the trachea, resulting in coughing, sneezing, head shaking, neck stretching and gaping. There may be loss of weight, reduced egg production and sometimes death, especially in partridges. *H. gallinarum* lives in the caecum of game birds and usually causes few problems. However it transmits the protozoan organism *Histomonas meleagridis*, the cause of blackhead or histomoniasis, and work by the Game Conservancy Trust has also suggested that heavy burdens of *H. gallinarum* may affect breeding performance and body weight, especially if the birds are on a poor plane of nutrition. The closely related *Heterakis isolonche* creates more damage than *H. gallinarum* because it burrows deeply into the wall of the caeca of pheasants, creating large nodules that can result in emaciation, diarrhoea and even death.

Hairworms can be found in game birds, especially red-legged partridges. Hairworms that invade the upper digestive tract can cause progressive weakness, anaemia, weight loss and sometimes death. Regurgitation or difficulty in swallowing may be seen, and post-mortem examination may reveal roughened thickening of the upper digestive tract, with severely affected areas becoming easily detached. Hairworms that burrow into the intestinal wall result in weight loss, diarrhoea (sometimes with blood) and eventually death, and at post-mortem examination the wall of the intestine is thickened and the intestinal contents watery.

Flocks with helminthiasis should be treated with a licensed wormer in the feed or drinking water. Measures should be taken to prevent a build-up of helminth eggs or larvae in the environment of the birds by rotating pens on a regular basis, avoiding high stocking densities and ensuring good hygiene of feeders and drinkers. Potentially infected birds should receive a suitable anthelmintic before or on transfer to new accommodation, such as when adult pheasants have been caught up from the semi-wild and are being transferred to laying pens. Periodic medication when birds are on infected land will also help to reduce environmental contamination. Wild birds such as rooks and other members of the crow family should be discouraged from entering pens because these wild birds can carry large numbers of gapeworms.

LYMPHOMATOUS TUMOURS

Lymphomatous tumours of domestic fowl and turkeys are described elsewhere, and may be caused by Marek's disease virus, avian leukosis virus, reticuloendotheliosis virus and lymphoproliferative disease virus. Similar lymphomatous tumours have also been found in adult pheasants. Post-mortem lesions include enlargement of the liver, often with pale foci, enlargement of the spleen and thymus glands, focal or diffuse thickening of the mucosa of the proventriculus and nodular lesions in the duodenum, caecum, pancreas and kidney. Cutaneous and oropharyngeal lymphomas are also seen (Fig. 45.3), in which nodular swellings occur in the skin around the eyes and external ear openings, and large pale nodular swellings may be seen on the hard palate. In some birds the scaled areas of the legs are affected, resulting in diffuse swelling, crustiness of

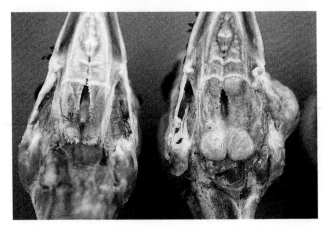

Fig. 45.3 Adult pheasant with cutaneous and oropharyngeal lymphomas on right; normal bird on left.

the skin and displacement of the scales. Histologically the tumours are composed of a pleomorphic mixture of lymphoblasts and lymphocytes, with some macrophages and reticulum cells. The cause of these tumours has yet to be determined, although *Reticuloendotheliosis virus* has been demonstrated in some of the tumours.

REFERENCE

Wood A M, Smith H V 2004 Spironucleosis (hexamitiasis, hexamitosis) in the ring-necked pheasant (*Phasianus colchicus*): detection of cysts and description of *Spironucleus meleagridis* in stained smears. Avian Dis 48: 138–143

FURTHER READING

Beer J V 1988 Diseases of gamebirds and wildfowl. Game Conservancy Booklet No 6. Game Conservancy, Fordingbridge, Hampshire

Game Conservancy 1983 Pheasant rearing and releasing. Game Conservancy Booklet No 8. Game Conservancy, Fordingbridge

Game Conservancy 1993 Egg production and incubation. Game Conservancy Booklet No 5. Game Conservancy, Fordingbridge

Lister SA 1989 Diseases of gamebirds. In Pract 11: 170–174

Pennycott T W 2000 Causes of mortality and culling in adult pheasants. Vet Rec 146: 273–278

Wise D R 1993 Pheasant health and welfare. Piggott, Cambridge

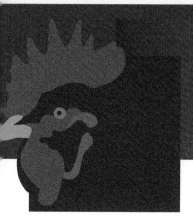

APPENDIX

1

Frank T. W. Jordan and
Paul F. McMullin

SOME USEFUL DATA

Contents

Some factors affecting optimal production

Housing and environment

Feed and water

Eggs

Blood volume – normal values

Heart rate

Blood collection from chickens

Respiration – chicken

Fumigation with formaldehyde gas

Some conversion factors

References

Further reading

SOME FACTORS AFFECTING OPTIMAL PRODUCTION

Genetic constitution

Growth
Food conversion
Egg production and quality
Conformation
Fertility, hatchability
Disease – resistance/susceptibility: gene abnormality
Behaviour

Environment – physical and chemical

Management – intensive, semi-intensive or free range, cage: size and structure, perchery, aviary
Housing: site, design, height and width, insulation
Cleanliness, cleanability and hygiene at turn-around
Ventilation, lighting duration, intensity and colour
Temperature, humidity
Litter: composition and condition, fresh/stale
Ammonia, carbon monoxide, carbon dioxide, hydrogen sulphide, dust
Equipment: feeders, drinkers, nests
Vermin, wild birds, animal pets, insects and human visitors
Panic; noise, particularly if discontinuous, predators
Single or multiple age groups in same area; movement of stock

Environment – social

Poultry population: total, density per pen/cage, sex ratios

Nutrition/feed

Deficiencies, excesses or imbalances
Water supply, physical and microbiological quality, ease of access by stock (drinker type, flow rate)
Food contaminants
Medication: antimicrobial substances, growth promoters, probiotics
Poisons/toxins

Disease (aetiologies/influencing factors)

External living agents – bacteria, mycoplasmas, chlamydia, viruses, fungi, protozoa, helminths, arthropods: live vaccines
External non-living agents – trauma, toxins and poisons, allergens
Unknown influencing factors – stressors, point of lay, movement of stock
See also genetic factors

HOUSING AND ENVIRONMENT

Area requirements for poultry (stocking densities)

These have been introduced for the welfare of stock and include cage, deep litter and free-range management. Particular attention has been given to laying cages and legislation has been introduced in the EU and certain individual countries stipulating minimum areas and other requirements for stock kept in this way. Further welfare legislation will be introduced in the future and the areas given below serve only as an illustration of current legislation and codes of practice.

Recommended stocking densities for poultry

POULTRY TYPE	SYSTEM TYPE	STOCKING DENSITY		REFERENCE
Chickens, rearing for laying	Cages	1 kg live weight/250 cm² (max. 2 kg)		
	Deep litter	17 kg/m²		
Adult laying birds	Conventional cages (EU ban expected from 2012 and no new cages introduced since 2003)	At least 550 cm² of cage area per hen		The Welfare of Farmed Animals (England) (Amendment) Regulations 2002
	Enriched cages	750 cm² to include at least 600 cm² useable area		
	Noncage (barn)	9 birds per m² (from 1 January 2007)*		
	Free range†	Within building as for barn above		EC Egg Marketing Regulations
		Outdoors 2500 birds/ha		
	Deep litter‡	17 kg/m² (max. 7 birds/m²)		EC Egg Marketing Regulations
	Straw yards‡	No information available		
	Perchery	No information available		
Broilers		Maximum recommended 34 kg/m² (1.8–3.0 kg)		Code of Recommendations (possible proposed Directive will alter this)
Broiler breeders		Maximum of 25 kg/m²		Code of Recommendations
Turkeys, rearing	Tier brooders	515 cm²/kg (19.4 kg/m²)		Codes of Recommendations for the Welfare of Turkeys
	Hay boxes or verandahs	300 cm²/kg (33.3 kg/m²)		
	Pole barns	410 cm²/kg (24.4 kg/m²)		
Turkeys, breeding	Hens	515 cm²/kg (19.4 kg/m²)		
	On range	17 m² per bird (590 birds/ha)		
	Males kept for AI	1 bird/m²		
Ducks, rearing	Age (days)	Perforated floors (birds/m²)	Solid floors (birds/m²)	Codes of Recommendations for the Welfare of Ducks
	1–10	50	36	
	10–21	25	14	

POULTRY TYPE	SYSTEM TYPE	STOCKING DENSITY		REFERENCE
	21–56	8	7	
	21–56 on grass	2500 ducklings/ hectare or maximum of 5000/hectare in well-grassed runs		
Ducks, breeding		5	3	
Ducks, breeding (on grass)		4000/ha		

* There is a derogation for establishments that were in operation prior to the Welfare of Farmed Animals (England) (Amendment) Regulations 2002 coming into force: they are permitted to maintain a higher stocking density of up to 12 hens/m².

† Organic is treated the same as free range for welfare requirements but is differentiated by marketing requirements.

‡ Systems referred to as Deep Litter and Straw Yards are no longer recognized systems for laying hens.

N.B. The 2002 Welfare Directive also stipulates minimum requirements for feeders, drinkers, nest box space, flooring and litter, which must be complied with.

Nest boxes – chickens

The Welfare of Farmed Animals (England) (Amendment) Regulations 2002 state that there shall be 'at least one nest for every seven hens. If group nests are used, there must be at least 1 m² of nest space for a maximum of 120 hens.'

No requirements have been set for the size of turkey, duck and goose nest boxes.

Transport

Stocking density of transport crates for chickens: up to 57 kg/m²; floor space per bird 296–488 cm²; height of cage 22 cm (1.8 kg) to 25.5 cm (>1.8 kg).

Temperatures

Brooding and rearing (for chickens and turkeys)

The aim should be to provide the birds with temperatures which they find most comfortable for themselves – a 'self comfort zone'.

For the commencement of brooding the brooder temperature is at about 30–35°C, the centre of the brooder 38–40°C and the house temperature about 24°C; however, with whole-house brooding do not exceed 31°C.

For pullets reduce temperature gradually to 18°C (i.e. by about 3°C per week).

For broilers reduce temperatures gradually to 21°C by 3 weeks of age.

The laying fowl

The optimal temperature range is 21–24°C. Below this, egg production is reduced by half an egg per hen-housed per year for each 0.5°C decrease. Above this range the number, size and quality of the eggs will be reduced.

The critical (lethal) environmental temperature is that which causes the rectal temperature of the bird to approach 45°C.

Humidity

The optimum relative humidity for poultry houses is 40–60% with a maximum of 75% for chicks during the first 2 or 3 days after hatch.

Ventilation and some environmental gases

The required ventilation will depend on the environmental temperature and humidity, type of housing and stocking density. It may be calculated on food consumed, which itself is associated with the metabolic rate. Minimum to maximum requirements are 3–25 m^3/s · tonne food consumed per day. It may also be accepted as 6–11 m^3/h · kg body weight for light breeds in cages to heavy breeds on litter in exceptionally warm conditions. Aerial contaminants should be kept at levels which comply with COSHH regulations which are averaged over an 8-h period. The maximum levels are as follows:

Ammonia	25 ppm
Carbon monoxide	50 ppm
Carbon dioxide	5000 ppm
Hydrogen sulphide	10 ppm
Inhalable dust	10 mg/m^3

Environmental ammonia – its effect on people and chickens

AMMONIA (PPM)	HUMANS	CHICKENS			
		Fall in egg production	Weight loss	Respiratory lesions	Ocular lesions
20	Smell perceptible			Slight +	
25–30			Slight +	Slight +	
50–60	Increasing smell		+	+	+
100	Eye and	+	++	+	+
200	Nose irritation	++	+++	++	++

The preferable level of ammonia is a maximum of 15 ppm and oxygen at a minimum of 18%.

Light and lighting – chickens

The control of lighting can only be efficiently practised under systems where there is complete exclusion of natural light. Lighting requirements are influenced by the age and type of bird and commonly practised programmes are as follows:

For broilers

First 5–14 days on 24 h light (10–20 lux) to encourage feeding. Then 23 h light (1–2 lux) and 1 h dark (0.2 lux) each day. Alternatively, an intermittent programme may be practised of 3 h light (10–20 lux) and 1 h dark (0.2 lux).

For layers

Day-old–1 week	22 h light (5 lux) per day
2–18 weeks	Gradually reduced to 8 h or 6 h light (5–10 lux) per day
19–22 weeks	Increase by 45–60 min/week (10–25 lux)
23 weeks–end of lay	Increase by 20–30 min/week (10–25 lux) to maximum of 15–18 h continuous light per day

When natural and artificial light are involved, approximations to the above can be made.

For turkeys

Recommendations by British United Turkeys are:
First 36h, 3h light followed by 3h dark and then it is important that the birds have at least 8h continuous darkness per day for optimal development of 'healthy' legs.

Manure – droppings

Droppings from the digestive tract are a mixture of faeces and urine mixed in the cloaca.
A laying hen produces about 100–150g of droppings per day.

Analysis (%) of manure from various species				
SPECIES	**MOISTURE**	**NITROGEN**	**P_2O_5**	**K_2O**
Chicken, battery	70–80	1.5	1.1	0.6
Broiler, litter	28	2.4	2.2	1.4
Duck, straw litter	32–60	0.8–3.2	1.4–2.3	0.6–2.2
Geese, fresh	75	0.6	0.6	0.8

Source: MAFF 1980.

Heat output per hen

A hen weighing 2 kg produces 26.4 kJ/h (6.3 kcal/h).

FEED AND WATER

Feed intake

Feed intake is influenced by the ingredients, presentation (pellets, crumbs, mash, grain and free range material), taste and nutritive value, the breed, age and sex of the stock, environmental factors, housing (intensive, semi-intensive, range), disease and whether management practices deliberately restrict feed intake. The following figures are therefore only a guide to food requirements with age. For optimal feed intake for production and breeding stock, the advice of the breeders should be sought with reference to the feed available and the gradual advance in the production of stock that grow faster and mature earlier.

AGE (WEEKS)	CHICKENS (G/BIRD PER WEEK) LAYERS	BROILERS MALE	FEMALE	TURKEYS (KG/BIRD PER WEEK) MEDIUM MALE	FEMALE	LARGE MALE	FEMALE
1	84	115	95	0.14	0.13	0.16	0.15
2	125	210	205	0.29	0.26	0.34	0.30
3	160	340	320	0.49	0.43	0.57	0.49
4	195	480	420	0.72	0.62	0.85	0.71
5	230	630	510	0.98	0.83	1.16	0.95
6	265	740	590	1.27	1.06	1.51	1.23
7	300	830	655	1.58	1.30	1.86	1.52
8	335	905	720	1.88	1.52	2.19	1.79
9	365	965	785	2.12	1.69	2.46	1.99
10	390	995	850	2.37	1.86	2.74	2.20
11	420	1010	910	2.59	2.01	2.99	2.39
12	450	1025	970	2.78	2.15	3.22	2.57
13	470			2.94	2.27	3.43	2.73
14	490			3.11	2.38	3.63	2.88
15	520			3.28	2.46	3.84	3.01
16	525			3.47	2.52	4.07	3.13
17	565			3.60	2.51	4.23	3.18
18	574			3.79	2.52	4.45	3.28
19				3.99	2.51	4.68	3.37
20				4.19	2.49	4.92	3.47
21				4.33	5.07		
22				4.54	5.32		
23				4.73	5.55		
24	Up to 900			4.73	5.78		

Calculating food consumption

$$\frac{\text{Total food consumed (kg)}}{\text{Average no. of birds}} \times \frac{1000\ (g)}{\text{No. of days}} = \text{g/bird per day.}$$

Rate of passage of food in the chicken

The passage of food along the digestive tract is influenced by the environment, the temperature, the age of the bird and the physical and chemical state of the diet. A feed of mash passes from the beak to the vent in 4h in growers, 8h in layers and 12h in the broody hen. Hard grains will remain in the tract for longer periods.

Feed space requirements

Troughs/chain feeders

Chickens

1 day–4 weeks	2.5 cm/bird
4–8 weeks	5.5 cm/bird (7.5 for broilers)
8–12 weeks	7.5 cm/bird (9.0 for broilers)
12–18 weeks	10.0 cm/bird
Adult	10.0 cm/bird

Turkeys (chain feeders are not used for turkeys)

1 day–16 weeks	2.5 cm/bird for both males and females
Over 16 weeks	2.5 cm/bird for females
	5.0 cm/bird for males

Ducks

1 day–8 weeks	5.0 cm/bird
Over 8 weeks	6.0 cm/bird

When troughs are used, the total length may be divided by 2 provided that the birds can use both sides.

Pans/tubular feeders of 300–400 mm diameter

Chickens

1–4 weeks	One per 35 birds
4–10 weeks	One per 25 birds
10–20 weeks	One per 20 birds

Water

Drinking water of adequate quality and amount should be provided with easy access for birds at all times.

Drinker space requirements for chickens

Trough/bell

1–12 weeks	12–20 mm per bird
12–25 weeks	25 mm per bird (one bell drinker per 80 birds)

Nipple drinkers

1 per 8–12 birds
2 per cage

Water consumption

The following is only a guide since the strain, age and gender of the bird and environmental temperature, humidity, feed and type of drinker can influence requirements and the advice of the breeders can be helpful.

AGE (WEEKS)	CONSUMPTION (L/100 BIRDS PER DAY)	
Chicken		
1	2–3	
2	4–6	
3	6–9	
4	9–10	
5	10–11	
6	13	
7	15	
8	17	
9	19	
10	20	
Adult hens	Up to 27.5 mL/bird per day, depending on lay	
Turkeys		
1	4–5	Water to food is in the ratio of 2:1 by weight early
2	7–8	in life and later in the ratio of 1.7:1
3	9–10	
4–7	14–32	
8–13	35–57	
14–19	58–70	

It is important that birds do not have to walk more than 3 m to any drinking point. Water consumption is often presented as volume of water per mass of feed.

EGGS

Passage of egg from ovulation to oviposition in the chicken is about 22–25 h.

Calculating production

Hen-housed production (%)

$$\frac{\text{Total eggs laid to date}}{\text{No. of hens when housed} \times \text{No. days from first egg}} \times 100.$$

Hen-month production (%)

$$\frac{\text{Total eggs laid in one month}}{\text{Average no. of hens for month} \times \text{No. days in month}} \times 100.$$

Hen-day production (%)

$$\frac{\text{Total eggs laid in one day}}{\text{No. hens alive on that day}} \times 100.$$

Egg mass

$$\text{Egg mass} = \frac{\text{Average egg weight} * \times \text{hen-day production}\%}{100}$$

* This is determined by weighing about 150 eggs of the day, none of which is double-yolked.

Egg weight/size

Chickens*

XL	Very large	$\geqslant 73\,g$
L	Large	$63\text{–}73\,g$
M	Medium	$53\text{–}63\,g$
S	Small	$<53\,g$

Turkeys

| Medium-sized birds | 122 eggs per 24 weeks of lay |
| Large birds | 107 eggs per 24 weeks of lay |

Egg size varies from 70 g (early lay) to 90+ g.
* Eggs graded to European Community Egg Marketing Standards.

Hatching eggs and incubation

Storage

After 7 days' storage it is essential to minimize water and carbon dioxide loss by storing in plastic bags in an atmosphere of nitrogen.

PREINCUBATION STORAGE (DAYS)	TEMPERATURE (°C)	RELATIVE HUMIDITY (%)
1–3	20	75
4–7	13–16	75
8–14	11–12	75

Periods of incubation

SPECIES	TOTAL PERIOD (DAYS)	TRANSFER FROM SETTER TO HATCHER (DAYS)
Chicken	21	18–19
Turkey	28	25
Duck (except Muscovy)	28	24
Muscovy duck	35–37	31
Goose, small breeds	30	26
Goose, large breeds	33–35	28
Japanese quail	16–17	14
Bobwhite quail	23–24	21
Partridge	23–25	21
Pheasant	23–24	21
Guinea fowl	28	24

Incubation temperatures and humidity

Still air incubators
Set at 38.4°C to ensure correct conditions within the eggs; relative humidity 60%.

Forced air incubators
Setter: for the first 18 days, 37.5–37.8°C; relative humidity 60%.
Hatcher: 18–21 days, 36.9–37.5°C; relative humidity 60%.
Ventilation rate: 6 L/egg per hour; oxygen should not be less than 17.5% and carbon dioxide not more than 0.4%. It is essential to turn eggs (preferably about seven times a day) during the first 18 days of incubation to prevent adhesion of the embryo to membranes.

After a journey, eggs should be allowed to 'settle' for 24 h before setting and it is important to avoid jarring eggs, particularly during the first 2 h of incubation, when the vitelline blood vessels are forming.

Microorganisms that may be present in the chicken egg

Microorganisms may be found in the chicken egg as a result of infection of the developing ovum, infection of the oviduct and/or contamination through the shell of the egg, before or after laying, with infected droppings, debris or by other means such as injection, washing or immersion in contaminated antimicrobials.

Infection from droppings, through the shell, may occur as the egg passes through the cloaca at oviposition or contamination of the shell after the egg has been laid. Infection of eggs may also result from environmental contamination following lay when eggs are subjected to unhygienic conditions. (This will include 'spoilage bacteria' and bacterial pathogens of the chicken.)

The following is a list of the more common organisms that may be found in the chicken egg, including chicken pathogens that may be transmitted through eggs. They are classified as viruses, bacteria, mycoplasmas, chlamydia and fungi. Spoilage bacteria, which are environmental contaminants, are also mentioned.

Organisms that are only rarely found in eggs are indicated as such and those for which only circumstantial evidence is suggestive of egg transmission are described as doubtful.

Viruses

Retroviridae	*Oncovirinae* – the leukosis/sarcoma group of avian type C oncoviruses
	Reticuloendotheliosis viruses of the REV group
	Other neoplastic viruses (rarely)
Picornaviridae	Avian enteroviruses – *Infectious avian encephalomyelitis virus*
Reoviridae	Avian reoviruses
	Avian rotaviruses (doubtful)
Adenoviridae	Avian group I adenoviruses
	Avian group II adenoviruses, *Splenomegaly virus* (marble spleen disease)
	Egg drop syndrome virus
Orthomyxoviridae	Avian influenza virus
Caliciviridae	*Avian hepevirus* (BLS/HSS) (doubtful)
Circoviridae	*Chicken anaemia virus* (doubtful)

Bacteria

Salmonellas	A very large number of serovars
Escherichia coli	A number of strains (although the strains infecting chickens relatively rarely affect mammals, including humans)
Staphylococci	Several species
Streptococci	Several species
Mycobacterium avium	Avian tuberculosis (rarely)
Campylobacter species	(Rarely – possibly through shell damage)
Ornithobacterium rhinotracheale	Many strains

Mycoplasma gallisepticum, Mycoplasma meleagridis, Mycoplasma iowae and *Mycoplasma synoviae.*

Chlamydia psittaci.

Fungi

Aspergillus fumigatus. Other *Aspergillus* species may also be egg-transmitted.

Spoilage organisms

These include a wide variety of Gram-negative and Gram-positive organisms, most of which are contaminating commensals. Examples of spoilage organisms that have been isolated from chicken and turkey eggs and associated with spoilage are *Proteus* spp., coliform bacteria, *Pseudomonas* group, *Klebsiella* spp., *Enterobacter* spp. and Gram-positive cocci.

BLOOD VOLUME – NORMAL VALUES

Chickens

Breed: White Leghorn (inbred strain) (Medway & Kare 1959)

AGE (WEEKS)	MEAN BODY WEIGHT (G)	MEAN BLOOD VOLUME (ML) (AS PERCENTAGE OF BODY WEIGHT)
1	62	12.0
2	115	10.4
3	163	9.7
4	250	8.7
6	399	8.3
8	572	8.4
16	1310	7.6
32	1789	6.5

Turkeys

Breed: White Holland, age 1 year (McCartney 1952)

Mean body weight	$5692 \pm 61.5\,g$
Mean blood volume	$410.2 \pm 10.0\,mL$
Mean corpuscular volume	$35.9 \pm 2.89\,g/L$

HEART RATE

SPECIES	RATE (BEATS/MIN)
Goose	200
Turkey	200–280
Fowl	350–470
Quail	500–600

BLOOD COLLECTION FROM CHICKENS

SITE	AGE	NEEDLE GAUGE (MM)	NEEDLE LENGTH (MM)	VOLUME THAT MIGHT BE TAKEN (ML)
Heart	Adult	17/22	50	At least 20
	3 weeks	22	19	5
	Day-old	22	19	0.5–1
Wing or right	Adult	21/20	37.5	At least 5
jugular vein	3 weeks	23	37.5	1–2

RESPIRATION – CHICKEN

Respiratory frequency	Male	12–21 breaths per minute
	Female	20–37 breaths per minute
Panting threshold	Ambient temperature	27–29°C
	Body temperature	41.9–42.0°C

FUMIGATION WITH FORMALDEHYDE GAS (MAFF 1977)

Fumigation cabinets or incubators containing eggs before commencement of incubation:
45 mL formalin (40%) + 30 g potassium permanganate/m^3.

Buildings up to 330 m^3 capacity:
20 mL formalin (40%) + 14 g potassium permanganate/m^3

or

paraformaldehyde granules (vaporized by heat) 360 g/100 m^3

or

aerosol generation using 275–500 mL formalin (40%) with an equal volume of water per 100 m^3.

For buildings over 330 m^3 use half above amounts.

Safety notes when using formalin + potassium permanganate fumigant

- Operator should wear rubber gloves when handling formalin.
- Formaldehyde gas must not be used where chlorine-containing chemicals (hypochlorites) are present.
- The reaction produces heat. Take steps to avoid risk of fire. Use metal containers.
- Not more than 1 L of formalin should be used per container. Containers should be at least 2 L capacity to avoid reactants boiling over the side of the vessel.
- Site containers along the length of the building with the required amount of potassium permanganate in each. Place formalin nearby.
- Operator should add formalin to the permanganate in the container furthest from the exit door.
- Operator should be kept under observation while mixing the reactants. The operator should wear a canister-type respirator.
- Fix a notice to the door of the poultry house indicating that fumigation is being carried out.
- Ventilate well following fumigation and before allowing staff to work in the building.

SOME CONVERSION FACTORS

CONVERT	TO	MULTIPLY BY
Length		
inch	millimetre (mm)	25.40
millimetre (mm)	inch	0.0394
centimetre (cm)	inch	0.394
inch	centimetre (cm)	2.54
foot (ft)	metre (m)	0.3048
metre (m)	foot (ft)	3.2808

CONVERT	TO	MULTIPLY BY
Area		
sq. ft	m^2	0.0929
m^2	sq ft	10.764
Volume		
cu. ft	m^3	0.0283
m^3	cu. ft	35.31
gallon (imperial)	litre (L)	4.54
litre (L)	gallon	0.22
gallon (US)	gallon (imperial)	0.83
gallon (imperial)	gallon (US)	1.22
Velocity		
ft/min	m/s	0.0051
cu. ft/min	m^3/h	1.699
Light		
lux	foot candle	0.0929
foot candle	lux	10.76
Weight (mass)		
gram (g)	ounce (oz)	0.035
ounce (oz)	gram (g)	28.35
kilogram (kg)	pounds (lb)	2.205
pound (lb)	kilogram	0.454
Energy		
watts	BTU/h	3.4121
BTU h^{-1}	kcal/h	0.2520
Temperature		
°C	°F	multiply by 9/5 and add 32
°F	°C	deduct 32 and multiply by 5/9

Equivalents

1 Therm = 100 MJ
1 BTU = 252 cal = 0.3 W/h
1 kW = 3413 BTU

REFERENCES

McCartney M G 1952 Total blood and plasma volume in turkey hens. Poult Sci 31: 184–185

MAFF 1977 Incubation and hatchery practice, Bulletin 148. HMSO, London

MAFF 1980 Ducks and geese, reference book 70. HMSO, London

Medway W, Kare M R 1959 Blood and plasma volume, haematocrit, blood specific gravity and serum protein electrophoresis of the chicken. Poult Sci 38: 624–631

FURTHER READING

Akester A R 1971 The heart. In: Bell D J, Freeman B M (eds) Physiology and biochemistry of the domestic fowl, vol 2. Academic Press, London, p 745–781

Anon 1987 Guidelines for the care of laboratory animals and their use for scientific purposes: 1 housing and care. Royal Society and Universities Federation for Animal Welfare, London

Code of Accepted Farming Practice for the Welfare of Poultry. State of Victoria, Department of Natural Resources and Environment, PO Box 500, East Melbourne, VIC 3002, Australia

Department for Environment, Food and Rural Affairs 2002 Code of recommendations for the welfare of livestock – laying hens. DEFRA, London

Department for Environment, Food and Rural Affairs 2002 Code of recommendations for the welfare of livestock – meat chickens and breeding chickens. DEFRA, London

Ewbank R, Kim-Madslien F, Hart C B (eds) 1999 Management and welfare of farm animals. 4th edn. Universities Federation for Animal Welfare, Wheathampstead

Farm Animal Welfare Council 1991 Report on the welfare of laying hens in colony systems. PB 0734. MAFF, Surbiton

Farm Animal Welfare Council 1992 Report on the welfare of broiler chickens. PB0910. MAFF, Surbiton

Farm Animal Welfare Council 1995 Report on the welfare of turkeys. PB2033. MAFF, Surbition

Farm Animal Welfare Council 1997 Report on the welfare of laying hens. PB3221. MAFF, Surbiton

Farm Animal Welfare Council 1998 Report on the welfare of broiler breeders. PB3907. MAFF, Surbition

Freeman B M 1971 Biochemical and physiological data. In: Bell D J, Freeman B M (eds) Physiology and biochemistry of the domestic fowl, vol 5 appendix. Academic Press, London

HMSO 1987 Animals prevention of cruelty: the Welfare of Battery Hens Regulations. HMSO, London

Kouwenhoven B 1993 Environment, husbandry, genetic and nutritional interactions in infectious diseases in poultry. In: Proceedings of the Xth World Veterinary Poultry Association Congress, Sydney, p 113–126

Ministry of Agriculture, Fisheries and Food 1987 Codes of recommendations for the welfare of livestock – ducks. MAFF, London

Ministry of Agriculture, Fisheries and Food 1987 Codes of recommendations for the welfare of livestock – turkeys. MAFF, London

Ministry of Agriculture, Fisheries and Food 1988 Codes of recommendations for the welfare of livestock – domestic fowls. Leaflet 703. MAFF, London

Stationery Office 2002 The Welfare of Farmed Animals (England) (Amendment) Regulations. Stationery Office, London

DEFRA websites relating to the welfare of:
Laying chickens: http://www.defra.gov.uk/animalh/welfare/farmed/layers/index.htm
Meat chickens: http://www.defra.gov.uk/animalh/welfare/farmed/meatchks/index.htm

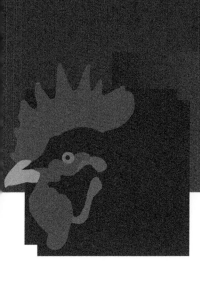

INDEX

Note: Page numbers in *italics* refer to tables and figures.

A

Abscess, subdermal, 194
Accredited Hatcheries Scheme, 129
Accredited Poultry Breeding Stations Scheme, 129
Acetyl CoA carboxylase, 526
Acetylisovaleryltylosin, *87*
Actinobacillus salpingitidis, 148
Adenoviruses, 367–81
    classification of, 367, *368*
    in eggs, 582
    preferred testing method, *43*
    unclassified, 381
Aeromonas formicans, 243
Aeromonas hydrophila, 243
Aerosol vaccination, 69–70, *70, 73, 78*
Aflatoxicosis, 435–6, 550, 551, 552
Africa
    meat consumption, 4
    meat production, *3,* 3–4
Agar gel immunodiffusion (AGID) test
    big liver and spleen (BLS) disease, 412–13
    infectious laryngotracheitis, 270
    Marek's disease virus, 264
    parvoviruses, 408
Agar gel precipitation test (AGP)
    infectious bronchitis (IB), 347
    Ornithobacterium rhinotracheale, 165
Aggressive pecking, 97–8
Air quality, 537

Air toxicoses, 558
Air sacculitis, 57, 143
Aldehydes, 60, 64
α-tocopherol, 517
Alpha toxin, 203
Alphaherpesvirinae, 267, 272
Alpharetrovirus, 277
Alphavirus, 416, 416–17
Alternative management systems, 512–13
Amidostomum anseris, 462, *462*
Aminocyclitol, *86*
Aminoglycosides, *86*
Ammonia, 508, 575, *575*
    toxicosis, 558
Ammonia blindness, 541
Amoebotaenia cuneata, 464
Amoxicillin, *86*
Amplified fragment length polymorphism (AFLP), 150
Amprolium toxicosis, 555
Amyloidosis, 486
Analgesics, 88
Anatid herpesvirus 1, 272
Aneurin, 519
Angara disease, 373
Angular (valgus/varus) deformities, 480–1
Animal By-Products Order 1999, 123
Animal Health and Welfare (AHAW) panel, 101
Anti-inflammatories, 88
Antibacterials *see* Antimicrobials
Antibiotics *see* Antimicrobials
Antibody testing *see* Serology/serotyping
Anticoccidial agents, *455,* 455–6

Antimicrobials, 88–9
    adverse reactions to, 85
    assessment of in clinical settings, 90–1
    Bordetella avium, 179
    botulism, 211
    Campylobacter, 182
    Chlamydophila, 241
    Clostridium perfringens, 205, 206
    colisepticaemia, 139
    coryza, 158
    enterococci, 199
    erysipelas, 218
    fowl cholera, 152–3
    Gallibacterium, 162
    multiple therapy, 92
    Mycoplasma gallisepticum, 227
    Ornithobacterium rhinotracheale, 169
    pharmacodynamic properties of specific,
        86–7
    pharmacological considerations relevant to,
        89–90
    responsible and prudent use of, 91–2
    Riemerella, 174
    Salmonella, 116
        S. Arizonae, 136
        S. Gallinarum, 132
        S. Pullorum, 129
    Staphylococcus, 195
    streptococci, 199
    toxicants, 555
    yersiniosis, 145
Antinutritional factors, feed, 511
Antioxidant deficiencies, 484
Antiparasitics, 88
Antiseptics, 88
Antiviral products, 88
Aortic rupture, 546
API-20NE identification strip, 165
Apramycin, *86*
Arboviruses, 415–24, *416*
Argas persicus, 460, 466
Arizonosis *see Salmonella* Arizonae
Arsenic, 553
Arthritis
    Escherichia coli, 143
    reoviral, *384,* 384–5
    Staphylococcus, 193
    viral, 66, 373

Arthropod-borne viruses, 415–24, *416*
Articular osteochondritis, 483
Artificial insemination, 36
Ascaridia, 22, 461, 462, *462, 463*
Ascites, 541, 545
Ascorbic acid *see* Vitamin C
Ash, 489
Asia
    egg production, 10–11
    meat consumption, 4
    meat production, *3,* 3–4
    meat trade, 5, 8
    vaccination programme for broiler breeders,
        77
Aspergillosis, 428–31
Aspergillus
    A. flavus, 428, 435
    A. fumigatus, 57, 428, 551
    A. glaucus, 428
    A. niger, 428
    A. parasiticus, 435
    A. terreus, 428
Asphyxiation, 539
Assured British Chicken scheme, 95
Astroviridae, 392, 392–7
Atadenovirus, 367, 368, 378–81
Ataxia, pheasant, 566
Avastrovirus, 392
Aviadenovirus, 367, 368, 369, 370
    in domestic fowl, 370–4
    of other birds, 374–5
Avian adenovirus splenomegaly (AAS), 377
Avian bordetellosis, 176–80
Avian chlamydophilosis, 235–42
    clinical signs, 238–9
    control, 241
    diagnosis, 239–41
    in eggs, 582
    epidemiology, *236,* 236–8, *237*
    legislation, 242
    pathogenesis, 238
    public health issues, 242
Avian encephalomyelitis (AE), 350–4
    control, 353–4
    diagnosis, 351–3
    epidemiology, 350–1
    preferred testing method, *43*
    vaccination, 47, 66, 75, *76, 77, 78*

Avian enterovirus-like viruses, 357
Avian hepatitis E virus (HEV), 411
Avian herpesvirus, *43*, 258–75
Avian influenza virus (AIV), 317–32, *320*
    clinical signs, 324
    control, 328–31
    diagnosis, 324–7
    effect on meat consumption, 4
    epidemiology, 317–23
    isolation, 42
    lesions, 324–5
    preferred testing method, *43*
    vaccination, 67, *77*
    wild birds, 59
    zoonosis, *331*, 331–2
Avian intestinal spirochaetosis (AIS), 243–6, 460
    control, 246
    diagnosis, 246
    epidemiology, 244–5
    lesions, 246
    pathogenesis, 245
    public health considerations, 246
    signs, 245–6
Avian leukosis/sarcoma group viruses (ALSV), *43*,
  276, 277–88
    control, 287–8
    diagnosis, 284–7
    epidemiology, 277–81
    exogenous and endogenous, 278–80, 287–8
    genetic resistance, 281
    neoplastic transformation of the cell, 278
    pathogenesis, 281–4, *282*, *284*
    public health issues, 288
    signs and lesions, 284–5, *286*
    virus subgroups, 278, *279*
Avian nephritis virus (ANV), 395–7
Avian paramyxovirus type 2 (APMV-2), 305–7
Avian paramyxovirus type 3 (APMV-3), 79, 307–8
Avian paramyxoviruses, 79, 294–316, *295*
Avian pneumovirus (APV) *see* Pneumovirinae
Avian rhinotracheitis (ART), 31–2
    see also Turkey rhinotracheitis (TRT)
Avian sarcoma virus (ASV) *see* Avian leukosis/
  sarcoma group viruses (ALSV)
Avian tuberculosis, 250–4
    control, 253–4
    diagnosis, 252–3
    epidemiology, 250–1
    lesions, 252
    public health considerations, 254
    signs, 252
Avibacterium, 146–8
    A. avium, *147*
    A. gallinarum, *147*, 159
    A. (Haemophilus) paragallinarum, *43*, *147*,
      148 (*see also* Coryza)
    A. (Pasteurella) avium, 148
    A. (Pasteurella) gallinarum, 148
    A. (Pasteurella) volantium, 148
    A. volantium, *147*
Avibirnavirus, 359
Avipoxvirus, 333
Avulavirus, 294

B

Bacteria
    in eggs, 582
    hatchery, 38
    resistance of, 91–2
Bacterial diseases, 110–256, *474*
    see also specific disease
Bactericidal drugs, 89, 90
    see also Antimicrobials
Bacterin, 174–5
Bacteriology, 21
Bacteriophages
    colisepticaemia, 140
    Salmonella, 123
Bacteristatic compounds, 89, 90
    see also Antimicrobials
Beak
    necrosis, 539
    trimming, 97, 540
Beetles, biosecurity, 58–9
Bell type drinkers, 25, 578
    colisepticaemia, 139
    vaccination administration, 69
Beta lactam, *86*
Bias, 501–3
Bicarbonate, toxicosis, 553
Big liver and spleen (BLS) disease, 410, 411–13
Bioavailability, systemic, 89
Biofilms in drinking water, 58
Biogenic amines, 552

Biosecurity, 48–65
    components of programmes, 52–9
    concepts of, 49–50
    management practices, 49, *49*
    Marek's disease virus (MDV), 266
    need for, 50–1
    Newcastle disease, 304
    operational, 53, 55–9
        equipment, 56–7
        feed, 57
        insects and beetles, 58–9
        litter, 57
        people, 55
        poultry, 56
        site decontamination, 59
        vehicles, 56
        vermin, 58
        water, 57–8
        wild birds, 59
    physical, 52, 53–4
    procedural, 52, 53
    salmonellosis, 118–19
    veterinary health and welfare planning, 51
    see also specific issue e.g. Hygiene
Biotin, 37, 513, *514,* 524–7
    average retention after feed processing, *511*
    deficiency, *525,* 525–7
Birnaviridae, 359–66
Blackhead, 458–9
Blastocystis, 563–5
Blindness from ammonia, 541
Blood sampling procedure, 18–19
Blood spirochaetes, 460
Blood volume, 582–3
Bone
    ash, 489
    calcium, 489
    deformities, 470, 472, *473,* 475, *476*
    disorders, 198, 470–1
    fractures, 483, 543
    fractures in hens, 98
    growth, 471, *471*
    infectious disorders, 477–80
    mineral content, 477
    phosphorus, 489
Bone marrow lymphoma, *474*
Bordetella avium, 176–80
Bordetellosis, avian, 176–80

Borrelia anserina, 460
Botulism, 208–11
    clinical signs, 210
    control, 211
    diagnosis, 210–11
    epidemiology, 208–9
    pathogenesis, 210
    public health considerations, 211
Brachial (wing) vein, blood sampling, 19
Brachyspira, 243–6
Brazil, meat trade, 6, 7–8
Breakfast therapy, 89
Breast burn, 96
Breeding birds
    broilers *see* Broiler breeders
    history establishment for investigation, 16
    house hygiene, 63–4
    layers *see* Layer breeders
    production figures for, 15, *15*
Breeding companies, 12
Bristol Gait Score, 96
Bristol Welfare Assurance Programme, 95
Broiler breeders
    Campylobacter, 182
    disease due to poor management, 542–5
    hatching failures, *33*
    investigation of disease in, 28–31
    lameness, 478–9
    production figures for, 15, *15*
    stocking density, *573*
    vaccination programmes, 74–6, *76,*
       77, 78
Broilers
    antibodies in, 23
    breeding companies, 12
    Campylobacter, 182
    coccidiosis, 448–51, 453–6
    disease due to poor management, 540–2
    feed intake, 576–7
    history establishment for investigation, 16
    hyperthermia, 537
    investigation of disease, 22–6
    lameness in, 96–7
    leg weakness in, 470
    legislation specific to, 103–5
    lighting, 575
    meat production, 4–5
    serological testing difficulty, 23, 40

skeletal disorders, infectious, 477–80
skeletal disorders, noninfectious, 480–4
stocking density, 103–5, *573*
vaccination programmes, 72–4, *74*
world trade, 6–10
Bronchitis *see* Infectious bronchitis (IB)
Brooder pneumonia, 428–31
Bunyaviridae, 416, 423–4
Bursa of Fabricus, 361–4
Bursal disease *see* Infectious bursal disease (IBD)

C

Cadmium toxicosis, 553
Cage layer fatigue, 484–6, *485,* 530
Cages, laying hens, 102
Calcium, 529–31
  bone, 489
  deficiency, 481
  malabsorption, 470
  osteopenia, 484, 485–6
  toxicosis, 553
Calcium tetany, 544
Caliciviridae, 410–14, *411,* 582
Campylobacter, 181–8
  C. coli, 181, 182
  C. fetus, 181
  C. jejuni, 181, 182, 183, *184,* 186, 187
  C. lari, 181, 182
  control, 186, *186*
  darkling beetles, 59
  diagnosis, 185
  epidemiology, 182–4
  legal requirements, 188
  preferred testing method, *43*
  public health considerations, 186–8
Canarypox virus (CNPV), 334
Candida albicans, 432–4
Candidiasis, 432–4
Cannibalism, 97–8, 545, 563
Capillaria, 21–2, 461, *462, 463,* 569
  C. obsignata, 461
Capsular polysaccharide (CP), 192
Carbamate anticholinesterase insecticides
  toxicosis, 557
Carbohydrate, 533
Carbon dioxide, 558, 575

Carbon monoxide, 575
  toxicosis, 558
Cardiac puncture, blood sampling, 19
Case–control studies, 500
Causal hypotheses, 499–500
Ceftiofur, *86*
Cellulitis, 542
  clostridial, 211–13
  Escherichia coli, 142–3
  Streptococcus, 197
Cestodes, 464, *464*
Chaetomium trilaterale, 439
Chalazae problems, *30*
Chelopistes meleagridis, 465
Cherry hip, 142
Chick antidermatitis factor (niacin), *511, 514,*
  523
Chicken anaemia virus (CAV), *43,* 398–401, *399*
Chicken astrovirus, 397
Chicken infectious anaemia (CIA), 66, 75, *76, 78*
Chicken(s)
  blood collection from, 583
  blood volume, 582–3
  coccidiosis in, 448–51, 453–6
  eastern equine encephalitis (EEE), 419
  egg weight/size, 580
  feed intake, 576–7
  heat output, 576
  Pneumovirinae diagnosis, 314
  respiration, 583
  stocking density, *573*
  see also Broiler breeders; Broilers; Layer
    breeders; Layers
Chicks
  Campylobacter, 183
  hatcher fluff examination, 38
China
  egg production, 10–11
  meat consumption, 4
  meat trade, 5, 6, 8–9
Chlamydiosis *see* Avian chlamydophilosis
Chlamydophila, 235–42, *236, 237*
Chlamydophilosis *see* Avian chlamydophilosis
Chloride, 25
Chlorinated hydrocarbon insecticides (OCIs)
  toxicosis, 556–7
Chlortetracycline, *87*
Choanotaenia infundibulum, 464

Cholangiohepatitis, 200–6

Cholecalciferol, 515

Cholera, fowl *see* Fowl cholera

Choline, *511,* 513, 528–9

Chondrodystrophy, *473,* 482, 523

Chondronecrosis, bacterial, 193, *194*

Circoviridae, 398–404, *403,* 582

Citrinin, 439

Citrobacter, 110

Claviceps, 440

Cleaning, 59

    see also Disinfection

Clostridium, 200–14

    C. botulinum, 200, 208–11

    C. colinum, 200, 205, 206–8

    C. novyi, 212

    C. septicum, 200, 212

Clostridium perfringens, 200–6

    clinical signs, 203

    control, 205–6

    diagnosis, 204–5

    disease, 202–4

    epidemiology, 201–2

    gangrenous dermatitis, 212

    lesions, 203–4

    pathogenesis, 202–3

    public health considerations, 206

Clubbed down, 521, *521*

Cnemidocoptes, 465–6

Cobalamin, *511*

Cobalt, 552

Coccidiosis, 21, 444–56

    chicken, 448–51, 453–6

    clinical signs and diagnosis, 453

    control, 453–6

    diagnosis, *446*

    duck, 452

    epidemiology, 447–8

    game bird, 452–3

    in game birds, 565

    geese, 452

    immunology, 447

    life cycle/biology, 444–6, *445*

    oocyst counts, *448*

    pigeon, 453

    turkey, 451, *452,* 456, *456*

    vaccination, 67, *74,* 75, *75, 76, 77*

Coccidiostats, 553–5

Cohort studies, 500, *501*

Colibacillosis

    respiratory, 90

    vaccination, 66–7

    see also Escherichia coli

Coligranuloma, 142

Colisepticaemia, 137–40

    clinical signs, 138–9

    control, 139–40

    diagnosis, 139

    epidemiology, 137–8

    lesions, 139

    pathogenesis, 138

Colistin, *87*

Collagen adherence protein (CNA), 192

Commission Directive 2002/4/EC, 102

Competitive exclusion (CE)

    Campylobacter, 186

    Salmonella, 121–2

Complement fixation tests (CFT), 241

Concept 2000 vehicle, 99, *99*

Confounding, 502–3

Contact dermatitis, 96

Conversion factors, 584–5

Copper, 552

Copper oxychloride toxicosis, 558

Coronaviridae, 340–9

Coronavirus-associated nephritis, pheasant, 567–8

Coryza, 155–9

    clinical signs, 157

    control, 158–9

    diagnosis, 158

    epidemiology, 155–7

    lesions, 157–8

    pathogenesis, 157

    turkey *see* Turkey coryza

    vaccination, 66, *77*

Council Directives

    98/58/EC, 101, 102

    1999/74/EC, 101, 102

    91/628/EEC, 101, 102–3

    93/119/EEC, 101, 103

Council of Europe Convention for the Protection of Animals Kept for Farming Purposes, 101

Crazy chick disease, 198, *198,* 518, *518*

Crimean–Congo haemorrhagic fever virus (CCHFV), 423–4

Critical control points (CCPs), 49, *49,* 53
    see also Hazard analysis and critical control
        point (HACCP) principles
Crop mycosis, 432–4
Cross-sectional studies, 500
Cryptosporidiosis, 21, *457,* 457–8
Cuclotogaster heterographus, 465
Culicoides midges, 460
Culls, hatchery, 35
Curled toe paralysis, 521, 522, *522*
Cyathostoma bronchialis, 461
Cytodites nudis, 466

D

Dactylariosis, 431–2
Danofloxacin, *86*
Davainea proglottina, 464
Deep pectoral myopathy, 483–4
Definitions, 493–5
Degenerative joint disease, 483
Dehydration, 538
Deoxynivalenol (DON), 438, 551
Department of Environment, Food and Rural
    Affairs (DEFRA) disinfectant approval system,
    61
Dermanyssus gallinae, 465, *465*
Dermatitis
    contact, 96
    foot-pad, 483
    gangrenous, 194, 211–13
    necrotic *see* Cellulitis
Derzsy's disease, 405
Diacetoxyscirpenol (DAS), 438
Diagnosis
    bias in, 502
    pitfalls of, 495–9
    signs and lesions, 352
Diagnostic sensitivity (D-SN), 41
Diagnostic specificity (D-SP), 41
Diaphysis, 471
Dietary electrolyte balance (DEB), 482
Differentiation of infected from vaccinated animals
    (DIVA), 330
Difloxacin, *86*
Dinitolmide toxicosis, 555
Directigen® Flu A kit, 327

Disinfectants, 88
    application of, 61–2
    selection of, 60–1
Disinfection
    improving biosecurity, 50
    procedures, 60–3
    salmonellosis control, 121
    terminal, of poultry houses, 62–3
Disk diffusion test, 91
DNA fingerprinting
    avian chlamydophilosis, 240
    Mycoplasma gallisepticum, 222
    Mycoplasma meleagridis, 232
    Mycoplasma synoviae, 230
    Riemerella, 172–3
Dosing machines, 69
Doxycycline, *87*
Drag swabs, 114
Drinkers/drinking water, 54
    biofilms, 58
    biosecurity, 57–8
    dehydration, 538
    disease transmission through, 83
    medication through, 83–4, 85
    placement of, 25
    sanitization, 62
    space requirements, 578
    vaccination administration, 68–9, *69*
Droppings, 24, 576, *576*
Drug(s)
    adverse reactions and side effects, 85
    classes used in poultry, 88–9
    coccidiosis control, *455,* 455–6
    effect on fertility, 36
    regulations, 92
    sensitivity surveys, 90
    toxicants, 556
    withdrawal for human consumption, 92
    see also specific drug
Duck enteritis herpesvirus (DEHV), 272
Duck plague, 272
Duck viral enteritis (DVE), 79, 272–5
    clinical signs, 273
    control, 274–5
    diagnosis, 273–4
    epidemiology, 272–3
    lesions, 274
Duck virus hepatitis (DVH), 79, 354–6, *355*

Duck virus hepatitis (DVH) type II, 394–5
Duck(s)
circoviruses, 401–4
coccidiosis in, 452
eastern equine encephalitis (EEE), 419
gas killing of, 100
meat production, 4
stocking density, *573–4*
vaccination programme, 79, *80*
world trade, 6
Dust, 508, 575
Dyschondroplasia, 20, *473, 474*, 475–6, 517
tibial, 470, 481–2
Dyspnoea, 268–9

E

Eastern equine encephalitis (EEE), 418–20
Echidnophaga gallinacea, 466
Echinostoma revolutum, 464
Ectoparasites, 465–6
Egg drop syndrome (EDS), 378–81, *379*
preferred testing method, *43*
vaccination, 66, *77*
Egg(s), 579–82
abnormalities, *29–30*
consumption, 11
contaminated, 36
cracked, 36
dipping, 90–1
hatch debris examination, 34–6
hatching and incubation, 580–1
hatching failures, *33*
hygiene and hatching care, 63–4, 120
infertile, 35–6
microorganisms present in, 581–2
peritonitis, 140–1
production, 10–11, *11*, 15, *15*, 579–80
production problems, 26–8, 373, 544–5
quality in infectious bronchitis, 343–5, *344*
quality problems, 28, *29–30*
Salmonella, 111, 136
trade, 12
viruses in, 581–2
weight/size, 580
see also Shell
Eijkman test, 137

Eimeria, 444
characteristics of various, *449–50*
diagnosis, *446*
E. acervulina, 205, 447, 448, *450, 451*
E. adenoides, 451, *452*
E. anseris, 452
E. brunetti, 205, *449*, 451
E. colchici, 452, 453, 565
E. columbanum, 453
E. dispersa, 452
E. duodenalis, 452, 565
E. gallopavonis, 451, *452*
E. grenieri, 453
E. hagani, 448
E. labbeana, 453
E. legionensis, 453, 565
E. maxima, 447, 448, *450*, 451, *451*
E. meleagridis, 451, *452*
E. meleagrimitis, 451, *452*
E. mitis, 448–51, *450*
E. mivati, 448
E. necatrix, 449, 451
E. nocens, 452
E. numidae, 453
E. phasiani, 452, 565
E. praecox, 448–51, *450*
E. tenella, 445, 446, 447, *449*, 451
E. truncata, 452
E. tsunodai, 453
in game birds, 565
life cycle /biology, 444–6, *445*
see also Coccidiosis
Electron microscopy, 389, *390*
Elementary bodies (EBs), 236, 238
Emaciation, 538
Embryonic mortality, 34–6
Encephalomalacia, 198, *198*, 518, *518*
Encephalomyelitis *see* Avian encephalomyelitis (AE)
End-of-lay hens, welfare issues, 99
Endemic disease, 493
Endocarditis
Enterococcus, 198
Staphylococcus, 194
Streptococcus, 198
Endochondral ossification, 471
Enriched cages, 102
Enrofloxacin, *87*
Enteric disease, *44, 51*

Enteritis
  duck viral, 79
  goslings, 381
  haemorrhagic, 67
  mild, 470
  necrotic, 200–6
  rotaviral, 388
  turkey haemorrhagic, 367, *369, 375,* 376–7
  ulcerative, 206–8
Enterobacteriaceae, 110–45
Enterococci, 196–9
  control, 199
  diagnosis, 198–9
  disease, 197–8
  E. durans, 196, 198
  E. faecalis, 196, 198
  E. faecium, 198
  E. hirae, 196, 198, *198*
  epidemiology, 196–7
Enterovirus-like viruses, 357
Environment
  control of, 25
  effect on hatchability, 36
  for egg production, 28
  factors affecting optimal production, 572
  gaseous, 36, 575
  improving biosecurity, 50
  requirements, 573–6
  respiratory disease complex, 508
Enzyme-linked immunosorbent assay (ELISA), 41
  avian encephalomyelitis, 353
  avian influenza, 327
  big liver and spleen disease, 412
  Bordetella avium, 179
  Chicken anaemia virus, 401
  Chlamydophila, 241
  Crimean–Congo haemorrhagic fever virus, 424
  hepatitis-splenomegaly syndrome, 414
  infectious bronchitis, 347
  infectious laryngotracheitis, 270, 271
  Mycoplasma gallisepticum, 225
  Mycoplasma meleagridis, 232
  Mycoplasma synoviae, 230
  mycotoxicoses, 440–1
  Ornithobacterium rhinotracheale, 165, 169
  Pneumovirinae, 315
  Riemerella, 174
  rotaviruses, 390

Salmonella Arizonae, 136
Salmonella Pullorum, 128
  salmonellosis, 115–16
Enzymes, 512
Epidemic disease, 493
Epidemic tremor *see* Avian encephalomyelitis (AE)
Epidemiology of poultry disease, 492–503
  definitions, 493–5
  diagnostic pitfalls, 495–9
  formulating a causal hypothesis, 499–500
  observational studies types, 500–1
  study pitfalls, 501–3
  see also specific disease
Epiphyseal osteochondrosis, 483
Epiphysis, 471
12,13-epoxytrichothecenes T-2, 438
Equipment
  biosecurity, 56–7
  damage caused by, 540
Ergocalciferol, 515
Ergotism, 440
Erratic ovulation and deformed egg syndrome
  (EODES), 544
Erysipelas, 79, 215–19
  clinical signs, 217
  control, 218
  diagnosis, 217–18
  epidemiology, 215–16
  lesions, 217
  pathogenesis, 216–17
  public health considerations, 219
  vaccination, 66
Erysipeloid, 219
Erysipelothrix rhusiopathiae (insidiosa), 66, 215–19,
  565–6
Erythroblastosis, 283, *286*
Erythroid leukosis, 283, *286*
Erythromycin, *87*
Escherichia, 110
Escherichia coli, 137–43
  cellulitis, 142–3
  coligranuloma, 142
  colisepticaemia, 137–40
  egg peritonitis, 140–1
  in eggs, 140–1, 582
  peritonitis, 140–1, 544
  preferred testing method, *43*
  swollen head syndrome, 142

Escherichia coli (*contd*)
    vaccination, 66–7
    yolk sac infection, 141–2
Europe
    egg production, 11
    meat consumption, 4
    meat production, *3,* 3–4
    meat trade, 5, 10
European Commission (EC), 101
European Food Safety Authority (EFSA), 101
European Parliament's Intergroup on Animal
    Welfare and Conservation, 101
European Union legislation, 101–5
Euthanasia, 18
    see also Killing
Exudative diathesis, 518
Eye drops vaccine, 71

F

Faeces, 24, 576, *576*
Fat, 26
Fat-soluble vitamins, 88
Fattening birds *see* Broilers
Fatty acids, 35
Fatty liver and kidney syndrome (FLKS), 526
Fatty liver haemorrhagic syndrome (FLHS), 533–4,
    545–6
Fatty liver syndrome, 533–4
Favus, 434–5
Feather pecking, 97–8
Feed
    additive regulations, 92, 205
    analysis of broilers, 23–4
    antinutritional factors, 511
    biosecurity, 57
    consumption calculation, 577
    disease transmission through, 83
    factors affecting optimal production, 572
    intake, 576–7
    medication through, 83–4
    physical form, 511
    rate of passage of, 577
    Salmonella contamination, 119–20
    sampling, 46
    space requirements, 577–8
    taking a sample of, 24

    toxicants in, 548, 549–50, 550–6
    vaccine administration, 72
    see also Nutrition
Female infertility, 35
Femoral head necrosis, *474, 475, 476,* 477–8
Femur fractures in broiler breeders, 543
Field investigation *see* Investigation
Flagellates, 21
Flaviviridae, 416, 417–18, 421
Flavobacteriaceae, 146–8
Fleas, 466
Flies, 28, 59
Flock testing, pullorum disease, 128–9
Flumequine, *87*
Fluorescence in situ hybridization (FISH), 162
Fluoride, 553
Fluoroquinolones, *86–7*
Fogging, 63
Folacin *see* Folic acid
Folate inhibitors, *87*
Folic acid, 37, *511, 514,* 527–8
Foot-pad dermatitis, 96, 483
Formaldehyde, 60
    egg fumigation, 64
    housing/equipment fumigation, 584
    toxicosis, 558
Fowl cholera, 149–54
    clinical signs, 151
    control, 152–3
    diagnosis, 152
    epidemiology, 149–51
    lesions, 151–2
    pathogenesis, 151
    vaccination, 66, 79
Fowl coryza *see* Coryza
Fowl plague, 317
Fowl pox virus (FPV), 333–9
    clinical signs, 336
    control, 338–9
    diagnosis, 336–8
    epidemiology, 333–5
    recombinant vaccines, 81
    vaccination, 66, *77,* 79
Fowl typhoid *see Salmonella* Gallinarum
Free-range flocks, 32, 512–13
Freedom Foods Scheme, RSPCA, 95
Fumigation, 63, 584
Fumonisin, 551, 552

Fungal diseases, 428–41
Fungi in eggs, 582
Fungicides toxicosis, 558
Furazolidone, 132
Fusarium, 438, 440, 551
Fusarochromanone (TDP-1), 440, 551

G

Gallibacterium, 146–8, 160–2
    clinical signs and lesions, 161
    control, 162
    diagnosis, 162
    epidemiology, 160–1
    G. anatis, 147, 148
Gallid herpesvirus 1, 267
Gallid herpesvirus 2, 259
Gallid herpesvirus 3, 259
Game birds
    breeding accommodation, 566–9
    causes of death in pheasant chicks, *564*
    coccidiosis in, 452–3, 565
    diseases of, 560–70
    Erysipelothrix rhusiopathiae (insidiosa), 565–6
    infectious sinusitis, 567
    lymphomatous tumours, 569–70, *570*
    marble spleen disease, 568
    Newcastle disease virus (NDV;APMV-1), 566
    parasites, 569
    Pasteurella multocida, 565–6
    Pheasant coronavirus-associated nephritis, 567–8
    protozoal diseases, 563–5
    rotaviruses, 561–2, *562*
    salmonellosis, 562–3
    Staphylococcus aureus, 565–6
    vaccination programme, 79
    worms, 569
    Yersinia pseudotuberculosis, 565–6
Gammaherpesvirinae, 259
Gammaretrovirus, 289
Gangrenous dermatitis, 194, 211–13
Gapes, 461, *461*
Gaseous environment, 36, 575
Gastrocnemius tendons, 478–9, 482
Geese
    circoviruses, 401–4

coccidiosis in, 452
    meat production, 4
    respiratory disease in, 381
Gel diffusion precipitin tests, 149
Genetics
    avian leukosis/sarcoma group viruses (ALSV), 281, 288
    coccidiosis control, 454
    factors affecting fertility, 36
    factors affecting optimal production, 572
    improving biosecurity, 49
    Marek's disease virus (MDV), 266
    resistance to *Salmonella* Gallinarum, 133
Gentamicin, *86*
Gizzerosine, 552
Gliotoxin, 551
Global meat trends, 2–3, *3*
Glucose, 533
Glucosinolates, 552
Glutaraldehydes, 60
Glutathione peroxidase (GSH-Px), 533
Goniocotes gallinae, 465
Goose parvovirus (GPV), 405–9
Gorging, 542
Gossypol, 552
Grains, 550
Granuloma, 194
Grille damage, 540
Growth-promoting additives toxicosis, 556
Guillain–Barré syndrome, 187
Gumboro disease, 58–9

H

Haemagglutination inhibition test
    infectious bronchitis (IB), 347
    Mycoplasma gallisepticum, 225
    Newcastle disease virus (NDV; APMV-1), 302
Haemagglutinin, 317, 326, 330
Haemophilus paragallinarum, 66
Haemorrhage, 20
Haemorrhagic enteritis, 67
Hairworms, 569
Halofuginone toxicosis, 555
Handling of poultry, 98–9
Hardware disease, 540

Hatchery
    cleaning and disinfection, 64–5
    design, 38
    hatch debris examination, 34–6
    history establishment for investigation, 17
    hygiene, 38, 63–5
    investigation of disease, 32–8
    management, 64
    salmonellosis control, 120–1
    site security, 64
Hazard analysis and critical control point
    (HACCP) principles, 49, *49*, 51–2, 53, 95–6,
    117
Health plans, 51–2
    see also Medication
Heart rate, 583
Heat output, hens, 576
Heating of houses, 25
Helminth parasites, 460–1, *462, 463,* 464
Henipavirus, 294
Hepatic lipidosis, 546
Hepatitis
    duck viral, 79, 354–6, *355,* 394–5
    turkey viral, 357–8
Hepatitis E, 411
Hepatitis-splenomegaly syndrome (HSS), 410,
    413–14
Hepatovirus, 350
Hepeviruses, 410–14
Herbicides toxicosis, 558
Herpesviridae, 43, 258–75
Herpesvirus of turkeys (HTV), 74, 81
Heterakis, 22, 461, *462, 463*
    H. gallinarum, 458, 462, 569
    H. isolonche, 462
Highlands J virus, 416–17
Highly pathogenic avian influenza (HPAI), 318,
    320, 321
        Asian H5N1 virus, 322–3
        clinical signs, 324
        lesions, 324
        vaccination, 329–30
Hip joints, 472–4, *475, 476*
Histology, 22
Histomonas meleagridis, 458
Histomoniasis, 458–9
Histopathology, 42
    Clostridium perfringens, 204

Hjärre's disease, 142
Hock-burn, 26, 96
Hock joints, 472, 478–9
Hong Kong meat trade, 6
Host defence mechanisms, 89
Housing/houses
    design, 54
    heating of, 25
    requirements, 573–6
    see also Environment
Humans
    factors affecting egg fertility, 35
    factors affecting egg production, 28
    hatchery hygiene, 38
    operational biosecurity, 55
Humidity, 508, 537, 538, 574
Husbandry
    alternative management systems, 512–13
    as a cause of disease, 536–47
        in broiler breeders, 542–5
        in broilers, 540–2
        in layers, 545–6
        in turkeys, 546
    effect on medication outcomes, 82–4
    improving biosecurity, 50
Hydrogen sulphide, 575
Hydropericardium, 373, 541
Hydroxy T-2 (HT-2), 438
Hygiene
    coccidiosis control, 454
    hatchery, 38
    Newcastle disease, 304
Hymenolepis
    H. cantaniana, 464
    H. carioca, 464
Hyperthermia, 537–8
Hypoglycaemia, 526
Hypothermia, 538

I

Iceberg effect, 83, *83*
Iltovirus, 267
Immunity and nutrition, 534
Immunofluorescence, reovirus, 385, *386*
Immunosuppressive agents, 508
Importation of Processed Animal Protein Order
    (1981), 120

In ovo
    drug administration, 90–1
    vaccines, 72
Incidence of disease, 493
Inclusion body hepatitis, *370, 372*–3
Incubation of eggs, 580–1
Indian meat trade, 9–10
Infection
    routes of, 83
    source of, 46
    welfare issues, 94–5
    see also specific infection
Infectious bronchitis (IB), 312, 340–9, *341*
    clinical signs, 342–5, *343*
    control, 347–8
    deep pectoral myopathy, 484
    diagnosis, 342–7
    epidemiology, 341–2
    lesions, 345
    preferred testing method, *44*
    vaccination, 66, 73, 74, *74, 76, 77, 78*
Infectious bursal disease (IBD), 20, *359,*
    359–66
    clinical signs, 362, *362*
    control, 365–6
    diagnosis, 362–5, *364*
    epidemiology, 360–1
    lesions, 362–3, *363*
    pathogenesis, 361–2
    preferred testing method, *44*
    vaccination, 66, 73, *74,* 75, *76, 77, 78*
Infectious coryza *see* Coryza
Infectious laryngotracheitis (ILT), 267–71
    clinical signs, 268–9
    control, 271
    diagnosis, 268–71
    epidemiology, 267–8
    lesions, 269–70
    preferred testing method, *44*
    vaccination, 66, *77*
Infectious runting, 503–6
Infectious stunting syndrome (ISS), 503–6
Infectious synovitis, 228
Infertility
    female, 35
    male, 35
Inflammatory process *see* Cellulitis
Influenza *see Avian influenza virus* (AIV)

Influenzavirus A, 317
Inhalation euthanasia, 18
Injected vaccines, 71, *71, 72*
Injection euthanasia, 18
Insecticide toxicoses, 556–7
Insects
    biosecurity, 58–9
    disinfection, 62, 63
Interaction
    epidemiology, 503
    nutrient, 513
Intestinal flora, 85, 121–2
Intestinal nematodes, 461–2
Intestinal spirochaetosis *see* Avian intestinal
    spirochaetosis (AIS)
Intranasal vaccines, 71
Intravenous blood sampling, 19
Intravenous pathogenicity index (IVPI),
    325–6
Investigation
    carrying out a field, 14–38
    categories of, 14–15
    defining the problem, 15–16
    establishing the history, 16–17
    laboratory tests *see* Laboratory tests
    process of, 13
Iodine, 552
Iodophors, 60, 61
Ionophores
    anticoccidials, 455
    toxicity, 484, 553–4
Iron, 552
Israel turkey meningoencephalitis, 417–18

J

Japanese meat trade, 6
Joint disease
    degenerative, 483
    Enterococcus, 198
Jugular vein, blood sampling, 19

K

Kauffmann–White scheme, 110–11
Killed vaccines, 67

Killing
    compulsory for notifiable disease, 100–1
    legislation, 103
    for post-mortem, 17–18
Kinky back, *473*
Klebsiella, 110
Kume serotyping scheme, 156

L

Laboratory tests, 39–47
    management of results, 47
    preferred tests for specific infections, *43–5*
    for toxicants, 549
    see also specific test
Lameness, 96–7, 470, *473–4*
Laminiosioptes cysticola, 466
Laryngotracheitis *see* Infectious laryngotracheitis
    (ILT)
Lasalocid toxicosis, 554
Latency to Lie (LTL) test, 96
Layer breeders, vaccination programmes, 74–6
Layers
    bone fractures in, 98
    disease due to poor management, 545–6
    end-of-lay welfare issues, 99
    EU legislation specific to, 102
    fatty liver syndrome, 533–4
    feather pecking, 97–8
    feed intake, 576–7
    history establishment for investigation, 17
    investigation of disease, 26–8
    lighting, 575–6
    production figures for, 15, *15*
    production problems, 26–8
    skeletal disorders, 484–6
    stocking density, *573*
    vaccination programmes, 76–7
LAYWEL, 102
Lead toxicosis, 553
Legislation
    Campylobacter, 188
    Chlamydophila, 242
    European Union, 101–5
    Newcastle disease virus (NDV; APMV-1), 302
    salmonellosis control, 123
    welfare, 94–106

Legs
    splayed, 539
    weakness, 470
Lentogenic Newcastle disease vaccines, 303
Leucocytozoonosis, 460
Leukosis *see* Avian leukosis/sarcoma group viruses
    (ALSV); Lymphoid leukosis
Lice, 28, 465
Light/lighting, 575–6
    effect on egg production, 27
    reducing to control cannibalism, 97
    tenosynovitis, 543
Limberneck, 208–11
Lincomycin, *87*
Lincosamides, *87*
Linoleic acid, 35
Lipeurus caponis, 465
Lipid hydroperoxides, 533
Liponyssus sylviarum, 465
Lipopolysaccharide (LPS) antigen, 115
Listeriosis, 247–9
Litter
    biosecurity, 57
    normal, 24
    problems of wet, 24–6
    salmonellosis contamination, 119
    toxicoses, 558
Live vaccines, 67
Liver disease, 200–6
Location
    of hatchery, 64
    of poultry farms, 53–4
Low pathogenic avian influenza (LPAI), 318, 321,
    322, 329–30, 507
Lymphoid leukosis, 263, 282, *282, 286*
Lymphoid neoplasia, chronic, 290
Lymphomas
    bone marrow, *474*
    Marek's disease, 261–2
Lymphomatous tumours in game birds, 569–70, *570*
Lymphoproliferative disease virus of turkeys
    (LPDV), 276, 291–2

M

Macrolides, *87*
Maduramicin toxicosis, 554

Magnesium, 25
Malabsorption, 470, 503–6
Male infertility, 35
Malignant oedema, 211–13
Mamastrovirus, 392
Management *see* Husbandry
Manganese, 37, 482, 532, 552
Manure, 576, *576*
Marble spleen disease, 377, 568
Mardivirus, 259
Marek's disease virus (MDV), 258–66, *473*
    cell-associated vaccine, 68
    clinical signs, *260,* 260–1
    control, 265–6
    darkling beetles, 59
    diagnosis, 260–4, *263*
    epidemiology, 259–60
    isolation, 42
    lesions, 261–2, *262, 263*
    pathogenesis, 263, *264*
    preferred testing method, *44*
    vaccination, 66, 74, *74, 76, 77, 78*
    zoonotic potential, 266
Maternal immunity
    infectious bursal disease (IBD), 360, 365–6
    Newcastle disease, 303
Mating damage, 540
MDCC-MSB1 cells, 400–1
Measuring and monitoring farm animal welfare, 95
Meat
    consumption, 4–5
    global trends, 2–3, *3*
    production, *3,* 3–4, *7*
    world trade, *5,* 5–10, *7*
Medication
    approaches to under field conditions, 84–5
    factors affecting the outcome of, 82–4
    improving biosecurity, 50
    individual, 82
    planning programmes, 51–2
    see also Drug(s); Vaccination/vaccines
Medicines *see* Drug(s)
Medullary bone, 485
Megabacteria, 249
Menadione *see* Vitamin K
Meningoencephalitis, Israel turkey, 417–18
Menocanthus stramineus, 465
Mercury toxicosis, 553

Mesogenic Newcastle disease vaccines, 303
Metaldehyde, 558
Metaphylaxis, 84–5
Metapneumovirus, 309
Meticillin-resistant *Staphylococcus aureus* (MRSA),
    195
Mexican meat trade, 6, 7
Mice, 28
    biosecurity, 58
    salmonellosis contamination, 119
Microbial surface components recognizing adhesive
    matrix molecules (MSCRAMMs), 192
Microbiological testing, 47
Microsporum gypseum, 434
MIDI system, 178
Minerals, feed levels, 25
    see also specific mineral
Minimal inhibitory concentration (MIC), 89, 91
Misting, 63
Mites, 28, *465,* 465–6
Molecular detection methods
    Avian influenza virus, 326–7
    Newcastle disease virus (NDV; APMV-1), 300–1
    poxviruses, 337
Mollicutes, 220
Molluscides toxicosis, 558
Monensin toxicosis, 554
Moniliformin, 440, 551
Monitoring disease, 51–2
Monoclonal antibodies, poxviruses, 337
Moore's swabs, 114
Moraxellosis, 250
Morbidity, broiler investigations involving, 22–3
Morbillivirus, 294
Mortality
    broiler investigations involving, 22–3
    embryonic, 34–6
Moths, 28
Multicentric histiocytosis, 283
Multifactorial conditions, 503
Multivitamins, 88
Muscle lesions, 472
Muscovy duck parvovirus (MDPV), 405–9
Muscular dystrophy, nutritional, 518–19
Musculoskeletal disease, 470–89
    glossary, 486–8
    post-mortem examination, 472–7
Mushy chick disease, 141–2

Mycobacterium avium, 250–4
    control, 253–4
    diagnosis, 252–3
    epidemiology, 250–1
    lesions, 252
    signs, 252
Mycoplasma, 220–33, *221*
    egg dipping, 90
    in eggs, 582
    infectious bone disorders, 479–80
    infectious sinusitis, 567
    M. iowae, 44, 220, 232–3
    M. meleagridis, 220, 230–2
    respiratory disease complex, 507
    serology testing, 41
    vaccination, 66
Mycoplasma gallisepticum, 220, 221–8
    clinical signs, 224
    control, 226–8, *227*
    diagnosis, 225–6
    epidemiology, 222–3
    infectious sinusitis, 567
    lesions, 224–5
    pathogenesis, 223–4
    preferred testing method, *44*
    vaccination, 66, *77*
Mycoplasma synoviae, 220, 228–30, 479
    preferred testing method, *44*
    vaccination, 66
Mycotoxins, 435–41, 550–2
    control, 441
    deep pectoral myopathy, 484
    diagnosis, 440–1
    feed sampling, 46
Myeloblastosis, 283, *286*
Myelocytomatosis, 283, *286*
Myeloid leukosis, 283, *286*

N

Narasin toxicosis, 554
Neck dislocation, 17–18
Necrotic dermatitis *see* Cellulitis
Necrotic enteritis, 200–6
Negative contrast electron microscopy, 389, *390*
Nematodes
    intestinal, 461–2
    respiratory tract, 461, *461*

Neomycin, *86*
Nephritis
    avian *see Avian nephritis virus* (ANV)
    Pheasant coronavirus-associated, 567–8
Nerves, peripheral, 261–2, *262*
Nest boxes, 63–4, 574
Neuraminidase, 330
Newcastle disease virus (NDV; APMV-1), 294, 295, 296–305
    aerosol vaccination, 69
    clinical signs and lesions, 298
    control, 302–4
    diagnosis, 298–302
    epidemiology, 296–7
    in game birds, 566
    isolation, 42
    preferred testing method, *44*
    vaccination, 66, 73, 74, *74, 76, 77, 78,* 79
    wild birds, 59
    zoonosis, 304–5
Niacin, *511, 514,* 523
Nicarbazin toxicosis, 555
Nicotinamide, 523
Nicotinic acid, 523
Nipple drinkers, 25, 58, 538, 578
Nitrite, 552
Nitrofurans toxicosis, 555
Noncage systems, 102
Notifiable diseases/notification, 13
    avian influenza, 318–19
    compulsory slaughter for, 100–1
    fowl cholera, 153
Nucleic acid, 46
Nutrients
    additives, toxication, 552–3
    deficiencies, 512
    see also specific nutrient
Nutrition
    disorders, 510–34
    effect on fertility, 35
    for egg production, 27
    factors affecting optimal production, 572
    and hatchability, 36
    in relation to immune status and disease, 534
    and wet litter, 25–6
Nutritional deficiency lesions, 37

O

Obesity, 539
Observational studies, 500–1, *501*
Occurrence of disease, 493
Oceania
    meat consumption, 4
    meat production, *3, 3–4*
Ochratoxicosis, 437–8
Ochratoxin, 551, 552
Odds ratio, 501
Oedema, malignant, 211–13
Omphalitis, 141–2
Oocysts, 21, 445–6, 447, *448, 451*
Oosporein, 439–40
Oral lesions, 539
Orbivirus, 382
Organomercury fungicides toxicosis, 558
Organophosphorus (OP) insecticides toxicosis, 557
Ornithobacterium, 146–8
Ornithobacterium rhinotracheale, 147, 148, 164–71, *168*
    clinical signs, 166–8
    control, 169–70
    diagnosis, 168–9
    epidemiology, 164–6
    lesions, 168
    number of isolates, 166, *167*
    vaccination, 67
Ornithosis *see* Avian chlamydophilosis
Orthomyxoviridae, 317–32, 582
Orthoreovirus, 382
Ossification, 471
Osteoarthritis, 483
Osteochondrosis, 483
Osteodystrophy, *474*
Osteomalacia, *473,* 485, 516
Osteomyelitis, *474, 475*
    spinal, 478
    Staphylococcus, 193, *194*
Osteopenia, 484–6, *485,* 530
Osteopetrosis, 284, *284,* 486
Osteoporosis, 98, *473,* 485, *485,* 516, 530–1
Oxolinic acid, *87*
Oxytetracycline, *87*

P

Page serotyping scheme, 156
Pale bird syndrome, 503–6
Pandemic disease, 493
Panophthalmitis, 143
Pantothenate, *511*
Pantothenic acid, *514,* 524
Para-aminobenzoic acid (PABA), 527
Paraformaldehyde prills, 120
Paramyxoviridae, 79, 294–316, *295*
Paramyxovirinae, 294–309
Parasites
    biosecurity, 58–9
    effect on egg production, 28
    free-range flocks, 32
    game birds, 569
Parasitic diseases, 444–67
Parasitology, 21–2
Paratyphoid *see* Salmonellosis (paratyphoid)
Partridges, 560
    see also Game birds
Parvoviridae, 405–9
    clinical signs and lesions, 407
    control, 408–9
    diagnosis, 407–8
    epidemiology, 405–6
Passive haemagglutination test, 149
Pasteurella, 146–8
Pasteurella multocida, 148
    differential diagnosis, *147*
    in game birds, 565–6
    preferred testing method, *44*
    vaccination, 66
    see also Fowl cholera
Pasteurellaceae, 146–63, 162–3
Pecking, feather, 97–8
Penicillin V, *86*
Penicillium citrinum, 439
Pentachlorophenol toxicosis, 558
People *see* Humans
Performance, investigation of suboptimal in broilers, 23–4
Peritonitis, 140–1, 544–5, 546
Pesticide toxicoses, 556–8
Pests, 28
Pharmacodynamics, 89

Pharmacokinetics, 89
Pheasant ataxia, 566
Pheasant coronavirus-associated nephritis, 567–8
Pheasants, 560
    causes of death in chicks, *564*
    marble spleen disease, 377
    rotaviral enteritis, 388
    see also Game birds
Phenolics, 60, 61
    toxicosis, 558
Phenotypic switching, 224
Phosphorus, 35, 37, 470, 481, 489, 529–31
Phylogenetic studies
    Newcastle disease virus (NDV;APMV-1), 301
    parvoviruses, 408
Phytase, 529
Phytates, 552
Picornaviridae, 350–8, 582
Pigeon paramyxoviruses type 1 (PPMV-1), 297
Pigeon pox, 335
Pigeonpox virus vaccine, 338
Pigeon(s)
    circoviruses, 401–4
    coccidiosis in, 453
Plant toxins, 552
Plasma sampling, 18
Pneumonia
    brooder, 57, 428–31
    Staphylococcus, 194
Pneumovirinae, 309–16
    control, 315–16
    diagnosis, 313–15
    epidemiology, *310*, 310–12
    pathogenesis, 312–13
    preferred testing method, *43*
    signs and lesions, 313–14
    zoonotic implications, 316
Pododermatitis, 483
Poisoning *see* Toxicants
Polychlorinated biphenyls (PCBs) toxicosis, 556
Polyether ionophores, 553–4
Polymerase chain reaction (PCR), 22, *44, 46*
    avian chlamydophilosis, 240
    Avibacterium paragallinarum, 158
    big liver and spleen (BLS) disease, 412
    Chlamydophila, 241
    Erysipelothrix, 218
    fowl cholera, 149, 150, 152

    Gallibacterium, 162
    infectious laryngotracheitis, 270
    Marek's disease virus, 264
    Mycoplasma gallisepticum, 226
    Mycoplasma meleagridis, 232
    Mycoplasma synoviae, 230
    Ornithobacterium rhinotracheale, 165, 169
    parvoviruses, 408
    poxviruses, 337–8
    see also Real time RT-PCR (rRT-PCR)
Polymyxin B, *87*
Polypeptide, *87*
Polytetrafluoroethylene (PTFE) toxicosis, 558
Polyvalent vaccines, 265
Porcine circovirus type 1 (PCV1), 401–2, *403*
Post-mortem examination
    killing birds for, 17–18
    musculoskeletal disease, 472–7
    procedure, 18, 19–21
Postantibiotic effect (PAE), 89
Potassium, 25
Poult enteritis and mortality syndrome (PEMS),
    385, 393–4, 506–7
Poultry
    harvesting machines, 98
    incoming, 56
    industry, 2–13
Poultry Breeding Flocks and Hatcheries (Registra-
    tion and Testing) Order 1989, 123
Poultry Health Scheme, 129–30
Poultry Stock Improvement Plan, 129
Poxviridae, 333–9
    clinical signs, 336
    control, 338–9
    diagnosis, 336–8
    epidemiology, 333–5
    preferred testing method, *45*
Prevalence of disease, 493, *497*
Processed Animal Protein Order 1989, 123
Production
    factors affecting optimal, 572
    world meat, 2–3, *3*
    world poultry meat, *3*, 3–4
Proportioners, 69
Prosthogonimus macrorchis, *464*
Protein, 25–6
Proteus, 110
Protozoa, 21, 563–5

Proventriculitis, transmissable, 381
Provitamin A, 513
Pseudomoniasis, 254–6
Pseudotuberculosis, 143–5
Psittacosis *see* Avian chlamydophilosis
Public health issues
    avian leukosis/sarcoma group viruses (ALSV), 288
    avian tuberculosis, 254
    botulism, 211
    Brachyspira, 246
    Campylobacter, 187–8
    Chlamydophila, 242
    Clostridium perfringens, 206
    erysipelas, 219
    listeriosis, 249
    reticuloendotheliosis, 291
Pullorum disease *see Salmonella* Pullorum
Pulsed field gel electrophoresis (PFGE), 150
Pyrethroid insecticides toxicosis, 557
Pyridoxine, *511, 514,* 522–3

Q

Quaternary ammonium compounds (QACs), 60, 61
    toxicosis, 556
Quinolones, *87*

R

Rachitic deformities, 515
Raillietina, 464
Rapid plate agglutination test
    Riemerella, 174
    Salmonella Arizonae, 136
    Salmonella Pullorum, 128–9
Rapid serum agglutination (RSA) test
    Mycoplasma gallisepticum, 225
    Mycoplasma meleagridis, 232
    Mycoplasma synoviae, 230
    Ornithobacterium rhinotracheale, 169
Rapid slide agglutination test, 137
Rats, 28
    biosecurity, 58
    salmonellosis contamination, 119

Real time RT-PCR (rRT-PCR), 301, 327
Rearing management, 27
Recombinant vaccines, 80–1
    avian influenza, 330
    Fowl pox virus, 339
    Marek's disease virus (MDV), 265–6
Red mites, 28, 58–9
Reoviruses, 382–7, 382–91, *383*
    clinical signs, *384,* 384–5
    control, 386
    diagnosis, *384,* 384–6
    in eggs, 582
    epidemiology, 382–4
    in leg disorders, 479
    preferred testing method, *45*
    vaccination, 66, 75, *76, 77, 78*
Respiration, 583
Respiratory disease
    aviadenoviruses, 373
    in geese, 381
    organisms, 51
Respiratory disease complex, 507–9
Respiratory tract nematodes, 461, *461*
Respirovirus, 294
Restriction endonuclease analysis (REA)
    fowl cholera, 150
    infectious bronchitis (IB), 346–7
Restriction enzyme fragment polymorphism (RFLP) profiling, 337–8
Reticular bodies (RBs), 236
Reticuloendotheliosis viruses (REV), 276, 288–91
    fowl pox vaccines, 339
    preferred testing method, *45*
Reticulum cell neoplasia, acute, 289–90
Retinol, 513
Retroviridae, 276–92, 581
Reverse-transcription polymerase chain reaction (RT-PCR)
    astroviruses, 394
    avian influenza, 326–7
    hepatitis-splenomegaly syndrome (HSS), 414
    infectious bronchitis (IB), 346–7
    real time *see* Real time RT-PCR (rRT-PCR)
Rhinotracheitis, avian (ART), 31–2
    see also Turkey rhinotracheitis (TRT)

Riboflavin *see* Vitamin B₂

Ribotyping, 150

Rickets, *473*, 475–6, *477*, 481, *516*

Riemerella, 146–8, 172–5

    clinical signs, 173–4

    control, 174–5

    diagnosis, 174

    epidemiology, 172–3

    lesions, 174

    pathogenesis, 173

    R. anatipestifer, 147

Ring tests, 46

Ringworm, 434–5

Risk factor, 495

Rispens, 74

RNA, *Rotavirus* detection, 389, *390*

Rodenticides toxicosis, 557–8

Rodents *see* Mice; Rats

Rotational (torsional) bone deformities, 480–1

Rotaviruses, 387–91, *390*

    clinical signs, 388–9

    control, 390–1

    diagnosis, 388–90

    epidemiology, 387–8

    in game birds, 561–2, *562*

    lesions, 389

    preferred testing method, *45*

RSPCA Freedom Foods Scheme, 95

Rubulavirus, 294

Runting and stunting syndrome, 503–6

Russian Federation meat trade, 5–6

S

Salinomycin toxicosis, 554

Salmonella

    classification, 110

    darkling beetles, 59

    in eggs, 582

    feed sampling, 46

    identification, 114–15

    isolation of, 114

    preferred testing method, *45*

    rats and mice, 58

    S. Agona, 111

    S. bongori, 110

S. enterica, 110, 112

S. Hadar, 111

Salmonella Arizonae, 110, 133–7

    clinical signs, 135

    control, 136–7

    diagnosis, 135–6

    epidemiology, 134

    lesions, 135

Salmonella Enteritidis, 111

    in game birds, 563

    serology, 115

    vaccination, 66, 75, 122

Salmonella Gallinarum, 130–3

    clinical signs, 131

    control, 132–3

    diagnosis, 132

    epidemiology, 130–1

    lesions, 131–2

    serology, 115

    vaccination, 66, 110, 122

Salmonella Pullorum, 110, 126–30

    clinical signs, 127

    control, 129–30

    diagnosis, 127–9

    epidemiology, 126

    in game birds, 563

    lesions, 127, *128*

    serology, 115

Salmonella Typhimurium, 110, 111

    in game birds, 563

    serology, 115

    vaccination, 66, 75, 122

Salmonellosis (paratyphoid), 111–24

    clinical signs, 113

    control, 116–23

    cycle of infection, *118*

    diagnosis, 113–16

    epidemiology, 112

    in game birds, 562–3

    lesions, 113

    pathogenesis, 112–13

    vaccination, 66, *76*

Salpingitis, 546

Salpingoperitonitis, 546

Sample sizes, 497–8, *499*

Sarcoma *see* avian leukosis/sarcoma group viruses (ALSV)

Saudi Arabia meat trade, 6

Schizonts, 21
Scientific Committee on Animal Health and
  Welfare (SCAHAW), 101
Scoliosis, *473*
Security, hatchery site, 64
Selenium, 533, 552
Sensitivity of tests, *496*, 496–7, 498
Septicaemia
    erysipelas, 219
    Staphylococcus, 193
    Streptococcus, 197
Serology/serotyping, 18–19, 39–42
    astroviruses, 397
    aviadenoviruses, 374
    avian encephalomyelitis, 353
    avian influenza, 327
    avian leukosis/sarcoma group viruses, 287
    Avian paramyxovirus type 3, 306, 308
    Avibacterium paragallinarum, 158
    big liver and spleen disease, 412–13
    Bordetella avium, 179
    botulism, 210–11
    Campylobacter, 185, 187
    Chicken anaemia virus, 401
    Chlamydophila, 241
    coryza, 156
    difficulty in broilers, 23
    eastern equine encephalitis, 419–20
    egg drop syndrome, 380
    factors influencing the approach to, *40*
    fowl cholera, 152
    Gallibacterium, 162
    hepatitis-splenomegaly syndrome, 414
    infectious bronchitis, 347
    infectious bursal disease, 364–5
    infectious laryngotracheitis, 270–1
    Marek's disease virus, 264
    Mycoplasma meleagridis, 232
    Mycoplasma synoviae, 230
    Newcastle disease virus, 301–2
    Ornithobacterium rhinotracheale, 165,
      169
    parvoviruses, 408
    Pneumovirinae, 315
    poxviruses, 337
    reoviruses, 386
    reticuloendotheliosis, 290
    rotaviruses, 390

Salmonella, 115–16
Salmonella Arizonae, 136
Salmonella Gallinarum, 133
Salmonella Pullorum, 127–9
    to support diagnosis, 39–41
    test interpretation, 41–2
Serum agglutination test (SAT), 115
Shell
    calcium and phosphorus, 530–1
    quality problems, *29*
Shigella, 110
Short-chain fatty acids (SCFA), 122
Siadenovirus, 367, *368*, 375–9
Sinusitis, infectious, 567
Site decontamination, 59
    see also Disinfection
Slaughter *see* Killing
Smothering, 539
Sodium, 25
    toxicosis, 553
Sodium chloride, 531–2
South America
    meat consumption, 4
    meat production, *3*, 3–4
    meat trade, 5
    vaccination programme for broiler breeders,
      78
Southern blotting, 337
Soya, 26
Specificity of tests, *496*, 496–7, 498
Spectinomycin, *86*
Spiking, 223
Spiking mortality of broilers, 541–2
Spinal osteomyelitis, 478
Spinal pathology, 472, *475*
Spindle-cell proliferative disease, 283
Spiramycin, *87*
Spirochaetosis *see* Avian intestinal spirochaetosis
    (AIS); Blood spirochaetes
Spironucleus meleagridis, 459, 563–5
Splayed legs, 539
Splenomegaly, 377
Spondylolisthesis, *473*
Spondylopathies, *473*, 480
Sporadic disease, 493
Sporulation, *Eimeria*, 446
Spray vaccines, 69–70, *70*, *73*, *78*
Stachybotrys, 438

Staphylococci, 191–5, *194*
    clinical signs and lesions, 193–4
    control, 195
    diagnosis, 195
    diseases, 192–4
    in eggs, 582
    epidemiology, 191–2
    femoral head necrosis, 478
    pathogenesis, 192–3
    preferred testing method, *45*
    S. hyicus, 193
Staphylococcus aureus, 191–2, 193, 194
    in game birds, 565–6
    gangrenous dermatitis, 212
Starve out, 539
Statistical association, 494–5
Stifle joints, 472
Stocking densities, 103–5, *573*, 573–4, *573–4*
Straw for bedding, 57
Streptobacillosis, 256
Streptococci, 196–9
    control, 199
    diagnosis, 198–9
    disease, 197–8
    in eggs, 582
    epidemiology, 196–7
    S. bovis, 196, 197
    S. gallinaceus, 196, 198
    S. gallolyticus, 196, 197
    S. zooepidemicus, 196, 198
Streptomycin, *86*
Stunning, 103
    see also Killing
Subdermal abscess, 194
Sudden death syndrome
    of broiler breeders, 543
    of broilers, 541
Sugar, 26
Sulphonamides, *87*
    toxicosis, 555
Supplementation, nutritional, 510–11
Swollen head syndrome, 142
Syngamus trachea, 461, *461, 462,* 569
Synovitis, *474*
    Escherichia coli, 143
    infectious, 228
Systemic bioavailability, 89

T

Tannic acid, 552
Temperature, 537–8, 574
    disinfectant activity, 60–1
    effect on fertility, 36
Tendons
    infectious disorders, 477–80
    lesions, 472
    rupture in reoviral arthritis, 384, *384*
Tenosynovitis, 384–5, *474*
    from feed distribution problems, 542–3
    induced by rearing at low light intensity, 543
    Staphylococcus, 193
    viral, 373
Terrestrial Animal Health Code 2005, 318–19
Tests
    general discussion, *496*, 496–7, *497, 499*
    sensitivity/specificity, *496*, 496–7, 498
Tetany, calcium, 544
Tetracycline, *87*
Thailand meat trade, 5, 9
Thiamine, *511, 514,* 519–20
Thiram toxicosis, 558
Thrush, 432–4
Tiamulin, *87*
Tibial dyschondroplasia, 470, 481–2
Ticks, 466
Tilmicosin, *87*
Tocopherol, 517
Toe trimming, 540
Togaviridae, 416, 416–17
Torsional (rotational) deformities, 480–1
Toxicants, 548–58
    from the air or litter, 558
    antimicrobials, 555
    coccidiostats, 553–5
    in feed, 548, 549–50, 550–6
    growth-promoting additives, 556
    heavy metals, 553
    nitrofurans, 555
    nutrient additives, 552–3
    pesticide, 556–8
    sulphonamides, 555
    in water, 550–6
Trace elements, toxicants, 552–3

Tracheal organ cultures (TOC)
    infectious bronchitis (IB), 346
    Pneumovirinae, 314–15
Tracheitis, 143
Transport of poultry
    handling and, 98–9, *99, 100*
    legislation, 102–3
    stocking density, 574
Trematodes, 464, *464*
Tremor, epidemic *see* Avian encephalomyelitis (AE)
Trichomonas, 459
    in game birds, 563–5
    T. gallinae, 459
Trichophyton
    T. megninii, 434–5
    T. simii, 434
Trichostrongylus tenius, 462, *462*
Trichothecene mycotoxicosis, 438–9
Trickle infection, 447
Trimethoprim, *87*
Tube agglutination test
    colisepticaemia, 137
    Pasteurella multocida, 149
    Salmonella Arizonae, 136
Tuberculin test, 253
Tuberculosis, avian *see* Avian tuberculosis
Turkey coryza, 176–80
    clinical signs, 178
    diagnosis, 178–9
    epidemiology, 176–7
    lesions, 178
    pathogenesis, 177
Turkey haemorrhagic enteritis (THE), 367, *369,* 375, 376–7
Turkey meningoencephalitis virus, 417–18
Turkey rhinotracheitis (TRT), 66, *74,* 309
    vaccination, *76, 78, 79*
Turkey viral hepatitis, 357–8
Turkey(s)
    astrovirus, *392, 393*–4
    blood volume, 583
    coccidiosis in, 451, *452,* 456, *456*
    disease due to poor management, 546
    eastern equine encephalitis (EEE), 419
    egg weight/size, 580
    Europe trade, 10
    feed intake, 576–7
    hatching failures, *33*

herpesvirus of, 74, 81
investigation of disease, 31–2
lighting, 576
lymphoproliferative disease virus of, 276, 291–2
meat consumption, 5
meat production, 4
Mexico trade, 7
Pneumovirinae diagnosis, 313–14
production figures for, 15, *15*
Salmonella Arizonae, 134, 136
stocking density, *573*
vaccination programmes, 78–9, 79, *80*
Tylosin, *87*
Tyzzeria perniciosa, 452

U

Ulcerative enteritis, 206–8
Un-enriched cage systems, 102
United Kingdom
    vaccination programme for broiler breeders, *76*
    vaccination programme for broilers, *74*
United States of America
    egg production, 10
    meat consumption, 4
    meat production, *3, 3*–4
    meat trade, 5, *6*–7
Usutu virus (USUV), 421

V

Vaccination/vaccines, 66–81
    avian encephalomyelitis, 47, 353–4
    Avian influenza virus, 329–31
    Bordetella avium, 179
    broiler breeders, 30
    coccidiosis control, 454–5
    colisepticaemia, 139–40
    consideration factors, 67
    coryza, 159
    duck viral enteritis, 274–5
    duck virus hepatitis, 356
    effect on serology, 40–1
    erysipelas, 218

Vaccination/vaccines (*contd*)
    fowl cholera, 153
    Gallibacterium, 162
    improving biosecurity, 50
    infectious bronchitis, 348
    infectious bursal disease, 365–6
    infectious laryngotracheitis, 271
    killed, 67, 71
    live, 67, 68
    Marek's disease virus, 265–6
    methods of administration, 68–72, *70, 71,*
        72, 73
    Mycoplasma gallisepticum, 227–8
    Newcastle disease virus, 302–4
    Ornithobacterium rhinotracheale, 169–70
    parvoviruses, 408–9
    poxviruses, 338
    programme types, 72–80, *74, 75*
    recombinant, 80–1
    reoviruses, 386
    Salmonella Arizonae, 136
    Salmonella Gallinarum, 132–3
    salmonellosis, 122
    types of, 67
Valgus/varus (angular) deformities, 480–1
Vehicles, biosecurity, 55, 56
Venezuelan equine encephalitis (VEE),
    420–1
Vent pecking, 97
Ventilation, 25, 537–8, 575
    broilers, 540–1
    hatchery, 64
Venugopal nair *see Marek's disease virus*
    (MDV)
Vermin, 28, 119
    biosecurity, 58
    disinfection, 62, 63
    see also specific pest
Vertically transmitted infections, 51
Veterinarians role, 12–13
Veterinary health planning, 51–2
Veterinary Medicines Regulations 2005, 92
Viral diseases, 258–424
    see also specific disease
Virus neutralization (VN) test
    avian encephalomyelitis (AE), 353
    infectious bronchitis (IB), 347
Visitors, site, 55

Vitamin A, 513–15, *514*
    average retention after feed processing, *511*
    deficiency, 514, *515*
    excess, 515
    toxicants, 552
Vitamin B_1, *511, 514,* 519–20
Vitamin B_2, 37, *514,* 520–2
    average retention after feed processing, *511*
    deficiency, *473,* 520–2, *521, 522*
Vitamin B_3, *511, 514,* 523
Vitamin B_5, *514,* 524
Vitamin B_6, *511, 514,* 522–3
Vitamin B_{12}, 37, *514,* 528
Vitamin C, 529
    average retention after feed processing, *511*
    deficiency, *474*
Vitamin D, *514,* 515–17
    deficiency, 481, 515–16, *516*
    excess, 516
    toxicants, 552
Vitamin D_3, *511*
Vitamin E, *514,* 517–19
    average retention after feed processing,
        511
    deficiency, 37, 517–19, *518*
Vitamin H *see* Biotin
Vitamin K, *511, 514,* 519
Vitamins
    average retention after feed processing, *511*
    B complex, 513
    fat-soluble, 88, 513
    general information about, *514*
    toxicants, 552
    water-soluble, 88
    see also specific vitamin
Vómito negro, 552

W

Waste disposal, 54, 64
Water, 578
    biofilms, 58
    consumption, 25, 84, 85, 578–9
    for egg production, 27–8
    hardness effect on disinfectants, 61
    salmonellosis contamination, 119
    toxicants, 550–6

volumes of vaccine-containing, *69*
    see also Drinkers/drinking water
Water sensitive paper (WSP), 69, *70*
Water-soluble vitamins, 88
Waterways, dangers of, 54
Welfare
    assessment of, 95–6
    legislation, 94–106
    planning, 51–2
Welfare Assessment System, 95
Welfare Assurance Schemes, 94
Welfare of Farmed Animals (England) Regulations
    2000, 101
Welfare Quality scheme, 95
West Nile virus, 421–3
Western equine encephalitis (WEE), 420
Wet litter problems, 24–6
White comb, 434–5
Whole-blood, stained antigen agglutination test,
    253
Whole blood test (WBT)
    Salmonella Pullorum, 128–9
    salmonellosis, 115
Wild birds
    biosecurity, 59
    Salmonella contamination, 119
Wildlife hosts, free-range flocks, 32
Wing flapping, damage from, 483–4
Wing web vaccination, 72
Wood shavings for bedding, 57

World scene, 2
Worms, 21–2, 569
    see also specific worm

Y

Yersinia pseudotuberculosis, 143–5, 565–6
Yersiniosis, 110, 143–5
Yolk
    antibody testing, 42
    quality problems, *29–30*
    sac infection, 141–2
Yucaipa-like viruses, 305–7

Z

Zearalenone, 438, 551
Zinc, 35, 37, 532–3, 552
Zoonoses
    antibiotic resistance of, 91
    avian influenza, *331,* 331–2
    fowl cholera, 153
    free-range flocks, 32
    Marek's disease virus (MDV), 266
    Newcastle disease virus (NDV; APMV-1),
        304–5
Zoonoses Order 1989, 123

Printed and bound by CPI Group (UK) Ltd, Croydon, CR0 4YY

08/05/2025

01864673-0001